Anthropology and Public Health

Anthropology and Public Health

Bridging Differences in Culture and Society

Second Edition

Robert A. Hahn, PhD, MPH
Coordinating Scientist, Violence Prevention Review
  and Excess Alcohol Consumption Review
Guide to Community Preventive Services
Division of Health Communication and Marketing
National Center for Health Marketing
Coordinating Center for Health Information and Service
  Centers for Disease Control and Prevention

Marcia C. Inhorn, PhD, MPH
William K. Lanman Jr. Professor of Anthropology
  and International Affairs
Department of Anthropology
The Whitney and Betty
  Macmillan Center for International and Area Studies
Council in Middle East Studies
Yale University

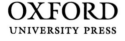

OXFORD
UNIVERSITY PRESS

2009

OXFORD
UNIVERSITY PRESS

Oxford University Press, Inc., publishes works that further
Oxford University's objective of excellence
in research, scholarship, and education.

Oxford New York
Auckland Cape Town Dar es Salaam Hong Kong Karachi
Kuala Lumpur Madrid Melbourne Mexico City Nairobi
New Delhi Shanghai Taipei Toronto

With offices in
Argentina Austria Brazil Chile Czech Republic France Greece
Guatemala Hungary Italy Japan Poland Portugal Singapore
South Korea Switzerland Thailand Turkey Ukraine Vietnam

Copyright © 2009 by Oxford University Press, Inc.

Published by Oxford University Press, Inc.
198 Madison Avenue, New York, New York 10016

www.oup.com

Oxford is a registered trademark of Oxford University Press

Library of Congress Cataloging-in-Publication Data
Anthropology and public health : bridging differences in culture and
society / [edited by] Robert A. Hahn, Marcia C. Inhorn.—2nd ed.
p. ; cm.
Rev. ed. of: Anthropology in public health. 1999.
Includes bibliographical references.
ISBN 978-0-19-537464-3 (cloth : alk. paper)
1. Public health—Anthropological aspects. I. Hahn, Robert A., 1945-
II. Inhorn, Marcia Claire, 1957- III. Anthropology in public health.
[DNLM: 1. Anthropology, Cultural. 2. Public Health Practice.
3. Community Health Planning. 4. Developing Countries. 5. Health
Services, Indigenous. WA 30 A628 2008]
RA418.A655 2008
362.1–dc22
2008006682

Foreword

When, almost 40 years ago, as a young physician with 14 months of field experience in Taiwan under my belt, I began studying anthropology at Harvard, medical anthropology was just about as marginal in anthropology as it was in public health and medicine. At that time there were a few dozen medical anthropologists and most were highly applied: like laboratory technicians, they were field assistants who did all the practical things needed for public health experts to conduct research and service projects in Asian, African, and Latin American countries, or among indigenous American Indian and enclave ethnic groups. A number of thoughtful public health leaders knew from experience that anthropologists could help them better understand and change what was then typically viewed as the resistance or ignorance of local populations to enlightened public health practices. Benjamin Paul's influential volume— *Health, Culture and Community*—represents a more sophisticated example of how anthropologists and public health practitioners thought of the utility of anthropology in organizing and carrying out more effective preventive and treatment interventions in low-resource societies.

My generation of medical anthropologists, even the ones who were most involved with public health projects, bridled at what we regarded as an excessively narrow and overly utilitarian understanding of what anthropology was about and what it could do for the nation's and the world's health. We did not see anthropology as the handmaiden of biomedicine and public health, and so our cohort led the way in the building of a new medical anthropology, a field rich in theory, in finely grained ethnographies, and one in which anthropologists were increasingly becoming principal investigators on research grants, many of which stepped outside established biomedical and public health approaches to reframe the object of enquiry so that social, political and moral processes became legitimate causal and outcome subjects. We also conceived of anthropology as advocacy and as policy.

The time was right. The theoretical interests of medical anthropologists—cultural meanings of the body, social suffering, lived experience in local worlds, globalization, political economy of health, and so on—not only moved toward the center of anthropology as a whole but also became one of the sources of new critical approaches to international health. A younger generation of medical anthropologists, including MD–PhD and PhD–MPH researchers, who followed after us broke out of the anthropological mode of the solo researcher and created interdisciplinary teams that they themselves directed. This cohort also emphasized social justice, structural violence, health disparities, and implementation research. The new global era of central concern with AIDS, other emergent infectious diseases, disability rights, tobacco-related diseases, epidemic diabetes, trauma from political and social violence, substance abuse, suicide, and dementia was the time for medical anthropology. And the book you hold in your hands is an outstanding illustration of what anthropology in public health is now about and where medical anthropology approaches to global health are headed. In fact, it is even more than this because global public health itself is undergoing a sea change. And the anthropologists whose work is represented in this book are part of a remarkable interdisciplinary cohort of social scientists of many types, epidemiologists, biostatisticians, public health practitioners, maternal–child health experts, mental health experts, health services researchers, and policy experts who are remaking public health in our times. This new public health is more critical of political and economic realities; more likely to combine health policy and social policy; more centered in local worlds and more collaborative with local professionals; more focused on explicitly ethical issues with more powerful analytic approaches; more willing to engage qualitative data and the humanities; and simultaneously more theoretically interested and more involved with implementation of programs and outcome evaluations.

Across campuses in the United States, there is a new social movement of undergraduates, graduate students, and professional school students who see global health as a way of changing the world. They see global health as infused with prosocial values, poised to apply high technology interventions even among the poorest, ready to address poverty and inequality via practicable strategies, and concerned with quality as much as efficiency of services. This new generation of students will find this book's structure appealing, for it makes clear not only how anthropological understanding of public health problems and anthropological design of public health interventions advance the agendas of global and domestic health, but also how anthropological evaluations of public health practices and anthropological critiques and reformulations of public health policies can have local effects that remake people's lives as well as their worlds.

Anthropology and Public Health does not just project anthropology into the health arena, it also projects public health into anthropology. The upshot is important, because we see in rich detail how anthropologists actually incorporate quantitative methods into ethnographic research; how ethnographers work in interdisciplinary teams; how biosocial framing of public health interventions enrich and expand what anthropology is as a practice; and, not the least, why anthropology can be a crucial bridge between social theory and practical policy work. Doubtless, the anthropology of the future will be increasingly defined by this platform.

In the course of my career for four decades as a medical anthropologist, I have often been asked by professionals and laypersons to explain what anthropology actually does in the real world and why it should be supported. This book provides detailed examples of answers to both questions. It is in these concrete case illustrations that we see both the extraordinary possibilities and perhaps also the limits of anthropologically informed public health practices. Because it is not only anthropology and public health that will remake health and social welfare but also political science, ethics, social medicine, sociology, social policy, and the humanities. Moreover, as anthropology is drawn into public policy and public health institutions, it will inevitably also contribute to unintended consequences of social action, bureaucratic rationalization, and institutional resistance. Here, perhaps more than other fields, anthropology—the "uncomfortable science" as Raymond Firth once called it—has a built-in advantage, also illustrated in the chapters that follow. Cultural analysis, based in hands-on fieldwork, routinely opens a space for critical self-reflection on one's own projects that is often a crucial counterpoise to the hyping of solution—frameworks and the blinkered commitment to institutional practices that turn out to be inappropriate, weak, or even at times dangerous.

Looking backward over the past four decades, it is impressive to see how far anthropological approaches to public health have come, and not just on the well-traveled road of infectious disease research and programs but also for noncommunicable diseases, mental illness, substance abuse, the female reproductive life-cycle, and health systems. And yet, when compared to the stark reality of serious threats to public health and public health systems in low-resource countries and among low-resource communities in rich countries, the prospect is more daunting. The way we need to evaluate anthropology in public health goes beyond how far it has come, and must ask the perturbing question: what has it in fact accomplished with respect to improved health and health systems, and reduced dangers? As this strong collection shows, the answer to this question is still in the making. For what we read in these pages is either new research to build programs, early programs, or longer-term assessments that are not yet completed. Hence this is exactly the moment to examine what is now underway. One of the most attractive features of this book is that the editors have asked the authors to lay out in more detail than we usually find in textbooks the specific methods of their research projects and programs, so that the reader can come to a sense of where this field is going. That is no small achievement.

I will myself use this book to teach medical anthropology, social medicine, and global health. And I believe many others will do the same.

Arthur Kleinman
Harvard University

Contents

ix

Part IV. Anthropological Critiques of Public Health Policy

Contributors

Antoine A. Abu-Musa is associate professor of obstetrics and gynecology in the Reproductive Endocrinology and Infertility Unit at American University of Beirut Medical Center. He is interested in both male and female infertility and the use of assisted reproductive technologies to overcome these problems. He is currently focusing on how war affects reproduction and infertility.

Aimee Afable-Munsuz is a research specialist in the Department of Clinical Pharmacy, University of California, San Francisco. Her research focuses on understanding the social mechanisms that mediate racial/ethnic disparities in health, cultural differences in childbearing and how they mediate disparities in unintended pregnancy; cultural variation in sense of personal control and its influences on preventive behavior; and more recently, how immigrant's social context might explain acculturation's influence on health.

Alexis Avery is a maternal and child health epidemiologist for the state of New Mexico. She earned her MPH from Tulane University in 1999 and is currently completing her doctoral degree in public health, also at Tulane.

Johnny Awwad is associate professor of obstetrics and gynecology in the Reproductive Endocrinology and Infertility Unit at American University of

Beirut Medical Center. He is interested in both male and female infertility and the use of assisted reproductive technologies to overcome these problems.

Nicole S. Berry is an assistant professor in the Faculty of Health Sciences at Simon Fraser University in Vancouver, British Columbia. She graduated from the University of Michigan's program in anthropology. Her articles have appeared in *Social Science and Medicine* and *Medical Anthropology*, among others.

João Biehl is associate professor of anthropology at Princeton University. He earned a doctorate in anthropology from the University of California at Berkeley and a doctorate in religion from the Graduate Theological Union. He is the author of *Will to Live: AIDS Therapies and the Politics of Survival* (2007) and *Vita: Life in a Zone of Social Abandonment* (2005). He is the co-editor of *Subjectivity: Ethnographic Investigations* (2007).

Astrid Blystad is educated as a nurse and anthropologist. She is associate professor in the Department of Public Health and Primary Health Care at the University of Bergen and at the Centre for International Health, Norway. Her research interests include religion and reproduction, gender and health, violence, health systems, and international health policy with a geographical emphasis on East Africa.

Jeannine Coreil is professor of community and family health in the College of Public Health at University of South Florida. A medical anthropologist with more than 30 years of experience working on public health issues in Haiti, her research has included studies of child health, maternal mortality, HIV/AIDS, and tropical diseases. For more than a decade she has collaborated with Gladys Mayard on community health projects in Léogane, Haiti.

Elaine M. Drew joined the Center for Alaska Native Health Research (CANHR) at the University of Alaska Fairbanks in 2004 after completing her PhD in anthropology at the University of Kentucky. Her dissertation research led to an in-depth ethnographic examination of the cultural politics surrounding women's experiences with hysterectomy in rural Central Appalachia. Now holding a joint appointment in CANHR and the Department of Psychology, Dr. Drew teaches courses in medical anthropology and social science research methods while building a research program on health disparities among Alaska Natives.

Michael H. Fakih is associate professor in the Department of Obstetrics and Gynecology at the Michigan State University College of Human Medicine. He is the clinical director of IVF Michigan, FIRST IVF (Beirut, Lebanon), and two IVF centers in the Arab Gulf. He is interested in both male and female infertility and the use of assisted reproductive and donor technologies to over-come these problems.

George M. Foster was professor emeritus in the Department of Anthropology, University of California, Berkeley. His research interests included peasant society, applied anthropology, international health, ethnomedicine, and culture change. In addition to long-term research in Mexico and Spain, he served as consultant with USAID, WHO, and other organizations in Asia, Africa, and Latin America. Prof. Foster died in 2006.

Namino Glantz, as an engaged medical anthropologist, aims to render insight from health research visible to local populations and to catalyze community problem-solving initiatives. To learn more about her work in Mexico and the United States, visit www.HealthandCulture.org.

Ellen Gruenbaum, professor and head, Department of Anthropology, Purdue University, has studied female genital cutting practices in Sudan and Sierra Leone and has been a research consultant for UNICEF and CARE. She is the author of *The Female Circumcision Controversy: An Anthropological Perspective* (2001) and numerous articles.

Robert A. Hahn has served as an epidemiologist at the U.S. Centers for Disease Control and Prevention in Atlanta since 1986. He has conducted anthropological and public health research in Peru, Mexico, Brazil, the United States, Niger, and the Cameroon, and published studies on a variety of topics. He is the author of *Sickness and Healing; An Anthropological Perspective* (1995). Dr. Hahn is currently coordinating scientist of systematic reviews on excess alcohol consumption and violence prevention for the CDC Guide to Community Preventive Services.

Najwa Hammoud is the nurse manager of the Assisted Reproductive Technology Unit at American University of Beirut Medical Center. She is interested in both male and female infertility and the use of assisted reproductive technologies to overcome these problems.

Antoine B. Hannoun is associate professor of obstetrics and gynecology in the Reproductive Endocrinology and Infertility Unit at American University of Beirut Medical Center. He is interested in both male and female infertility and fertility preservation through assisted reproductive technologies.

Ann D. Herring is professor of anthropology at McMaster University, Hamilton, Canada. Her research centers on the anthropology of infectious disease. She has a special interest in emerging infections and the social circumstances that permit them to flourish, aboriginal health in Canada, and nineteenth and twentieth century epidemics (particularly influenza and tuberculosis).

Marcia C. Inhorn is William K. Lanman Jr. Professor of Anthropology and International Affairs at Yale University. A medical anthropologist specializing in gender and health issues, she has studied infertility, assisted reproductive technologies, and reproductive tourism in several Middle Eastern countries and among Arab-Americans in Michigan. She has published 9 books on these subjects, including 3 ethnographies about infertility and in vitro fertilization in Egypt and 6 edited volumes on reproductive health, global health, and infectious disease.

Craig R. Janes is professor and associate dean of education programs in the Faculty of Health Sciences at Simon Fraser University in Burnaby, British Columbia, Canada. He is continuing his work in Mongolia, and has just completed a project that examines the impact of environmental degradation wrought by climate change, mining, and political economic reform on Mongolia's rural herders. He is also the team leader for the Canadian Coalition on Global Health Research's project to support development of the Mongolian national health research system.

Vinay R. Kamat is assistant professor in the Department of Anthropology at the University of British Columbia. A medical anthropologist with specialization in international health, he has conducted fieldwork in India and Tanzania. Dr. Kamat is currently conducting a 3-year study on how and why some of the radical shifts in malaria control strategies have occurred in sub-Saharan Africa in the last few years, and what these changes mean for those who are most severely affected by malaria.

Cary S. Kart is senior researcher at Scripps Gerontology Center at Miami University (Ohio) and research professor of sociology, Department of Sociology and Anthropology (Ret.), University of Toledo (Ohio). His research broadly focuses on the experience of aging and managing chronic conditions, including diabetes.

Carl Kendall is professor of medical anthropology and international health in the Department of International Health and Development, and Director of the Center for Global Health Equity, Tulane University School of Public Health and Tropical Medicine, New Orleans, Louisiana. His career has focused on improving public health practice. His research focuses on applications of anthropology to public health, including health seeking behavior, health disparities, and program monitoring and evaluation. He has worked in more than 40 countries.

Loulou Kobeissi is assistant research professor, Center for Research on Population and Health, in the Epidemiology and Population Health Department of the Faculty of Health Sciences, American University of Beirut. Her research interests include reproductive health, especially male infertility and breast cancer.

Joan D. Koss-Chioino is professor emerita in anthropology at Arizona State University, currently research professor at George Washington University and adjunct professor in the Department of Psychiatry and Neurology, Tulane Medical Center. Her current research interests include cultural psychology, cultural psychiatry, medical anthropology, religion and spirituality, and art and ritual. She has carried out research in Puerto Rico, Mexico, New Mexico and Bali, Indonesia, as well as among Puerto Ricans, Mexican Americans, Mexican immigrant families and adolescents, and African Americans in clinical settings in the United States. She has published 5 books on these subjects.

Da'ad Lakkis is an obstetrician–gynecologist in practice at FIRST IVF (Beirut, Lebanon). She is interested in both male and female infertility and the use of assisted reproductive technologies to overcome these problems.

Tom Leatherman is professor and chair of the Anthropology Department at the University of South Carolina, Columbia. His research in Peru, Mexico, and the United States addresses the impacts of poverty and inequality on human biology and health and the nutritional consequences of dietary globalization.

Stacy Lockerbie is a PhD candidate at McMaster University, Hamilton, Ontario, Canada. She has a special interest in East and South East Asia. While her previous research centered on diet and well-being in Vietnam, her current research looks at transnational adoption from China.

Gladys Mayard was trained in ethnology and development sciences at the University of Haiti. She has directed numerous public health research and intervention projects, and serves as a consultant to international development organizations. She is the founder and director of the Centre de Recherche et de Service Socio-Humanitaire in Port-au-Prince, Haiti.

Abdelwahed Mekki-Berrada is assistant professor in the Department of Anthropology at the University of Laval, Quebec City, Canada. He has conducted research on traditional providers in Morocco and India, migrant adaptation in Montreal, and sexual risk in Mumbai.

Greg Mirhej, a member of the research team at the Center for Community Research at the Hispanic Health Council, served as project coordinator for the Drug Monitoring Study in Hartford, CT.

Karen Marie Moland is educated as a nurse and political scientist. She is research fellow at Centre for International Health, University of Bergen and associate professor at Bergen University College, Norway. Her research interests include gender and reproductive health, birth and breastfeeding, health systems, health policy and HIV/AIDS. Her research is based in Kenya, Ethiopia and Tanzania.

Zaher Nassar is an obstetrician–gynecologist in practice at FIRST IVF (Beirut, Lebanon) and IVF Michigan. He is interested in both male and female infertility and the use of assisted reproductive technologies to overcome these problems. He is currently conducting studies of donor ova and assisted hatching.

Bonnie K. Nastasi is a school psychologist and associate director of the Walden Center for Research, Walden University, Minneapolis. She has conducted research and intervention on sexual risk among youth and adults in Sri Lanka, India, and the United States.

Mark Nichter is Regents Professor of anthropology at the University of Arizona where he coordinates the graduate medical anthropology training program. He specializes in the anthropology of health and development, global health, political ecology, and medical anthropology. He has conducted significant ethnographic fieldwork in South and Southeast Asia as well as in the United States and has been a social science advisor for the International Network of Clinical Epidemiology.

Mimi Nichter is associate professor of anthropology at the University of Arizona where she holds joint appointments in the College of Public Health and the Department of Family Studies and Human Development. For the past 15 years, she has been actively involved in tobacco-related research both in the United States and the developing world. Dr. Nichter was a faculty scholar with the Tobacco Etiology Research Network (TERN) of the Robert Wood Johnson Foundation. Presently, she is the head of the Alcohol, Tobacco, and Drug Study Group for the American Anthropological Association.

Siwi Padmawti is a medical anthropologist and member of the Indonesia Quit Tobacco International Group. After completing her graduate education at Ateneo de Manila University in the Philippines, she has worked as a health social science researcher at Gadjah Mada University where she presently serves as Vice Director, Center for Bioethics and Medical Humanity in the Faculty of Medicine. She is also head of the training and research division for INCLEN (International Clinical Epidemiology Training Unit).

Mark B. Padilla is assistant professor in the Department of Health Behavior and Health Education and adjunct assistant professor in the Department of Anthropology at the University of Michigan. He is a medical anthropologist with cross-training in public health, and has worked since 1999 in HIV/ AIDS research and interventions in several countries in Latin America and the Caribbean. His books include *Caribbean Pleasure Industry: Tourism, Sexuality and AIDS in the Dominican Republic* (2007) and a co-edited volume on *Love and Globalization: Transformations of Intimacy in the Contemporary World* (2007).

Adriana Petryna is associate professor of anthropology at the University of Pennsylvania. Her research addresses the social dimensions of scientific knowledge in contexts of crisis and in U.S.-based pharmaceutical research. She is the author of *Life Exposed: Biological Citizens after Chernobyl* (2002) and the co-editor of *Global Pharmaceuticals: Ethics, Markets, Practices* (2006). Her forthcoming book, *When Experiments Travel*, explores patient protection in the context of globalizing clinical trials.

Elisha P. Renne is associate professor in the Department of Anthropology and the Center for Afroamerican and African Studies at the University of Michigan. Her research focuses on reproductive health; the anthropology of development; gender relations; and religion and textiles, specifically in Nigeria. Her books include *Population and Progress in a Yoruba Town* (2003) and the co-edited volume *Regulating Menstruation: Beliefs, Practices, Interpretations* (2001).

Niranjan Saggurti is a demographer and program associate at the Population Council, New Delhi. He has conducted research and interventions on sexual risk in Mumbai and among migrants in South India.

Hassan Saleheen is a member of the research team at the Center for Community Research at the Hispanic Health Council, where he served as data analyst for the Drug Monitoring Study in Hartford, CT.

Claudia Santelices is an ethnographer and project coordinator at the Center for Health, Research and Intervention, University of Connecticut. Having conducted ethnographic research in Chile with domestic workers, in rural Connecticut with farm workers, and in Hartford, CT with street drug users, pregnant teenagers, and other vulnerable populations, Dr. Santelices was the coordinator of the ethnographic data collection for the Drug Monitoring Study in Hartford.

John Santelli is professor and chair of the Heilbrunn Department of Population and Family Health at the School of Public Health at Columbia University and a senior fellow at the Guttmacher Institute, following a career at the Centers for Disease Control. He is trained in adolescent medicine and has conducted research on sexual and reproductive health, HIV/STD risk behaviors, and programs to prevent STD/HIV/unintended pregnancy among adolescents and women. He has been a national leader in insuring that adolescents are appropriately included in health research.

Stephen L. Schensul is professor of community medicine and health care and director of the Center for International Community Health Studies at the

University of Connecticut School of Medicine. He has conducted anthropological research on sexual risk since 1991 in Mauritius, Sri Lanka, India, and in the United States.

Norine Schmidt is currently program manager for the Infectious Disease Section of the Department of Epidemiology at Tulane University School of Public Health and Tropical Medicine in New Orleans.

Nancy E. Schoenberg is Marion Pearsall Professor of behavioral science at the University of Kentucky's College of Medicine. Her research examines the cultural context of aging and the intersection between chronic health conditions and health inequities, with an emphasis on applying anthropological and other social science principles to address social problems. Her current research includes several projects for the NIH/National Cancer Institute on cancer in Appalachia related to screening, control, and prevention of cancer involving faith communities, provider practices, and research networks.

Merrill Singer is senior research scientist at the Center for Health, Intervention, and Prevention and the Center for Health Communication and Marketing at the University of Connecticut. Formerly the director of research at the Hispanic Health Council in Hartford, he has been involved in community-based AIDS research and prevention since 1988 and drug research since 1979.

Sandy Smith-Nonini is a research assistant professor of anthropology at the University of North Carolina, Chapel Hill. She is the author of *Healing the Body Politic: El Salvador's Struggle for Health Rights—From Civil War to Neoliberal Peace* (2008).

Ilene Speizer is a research associate professor in the Department of Maternal and Child Health at the University of North Carolina at Chapel Hill. She is also a faculty fellow of the Carolina Population Center. Her primary research interests focus on adolescent reproductive health; intimate partner violence; and HIV prevention. She has undertaken research in the United States, sub-Saharan Africa, Latin America, and the Caribbean.

Eric A. Stein is assistant professor of anthropology at Evergreen State College. He earned his PhD in anthropology and history at the University of Michigan in 2005. His work draws on ethnography, archives, and memory to understand rural experiences of public health in Indonesia since the late Dutch colonial period, with an emphasis on issues of gender and power. He is concerned more broadly with understanding technology, sanitation, reproduction, and inequality in Southeast Asia.

Eleanor Palo Stoller, research professor at Wake Forrest University, has also held faculty positions at State University of New York, University of Florida, and Case Western Reserve University where she was the Selah Chamberlain Professor of Sociology. She is interested in the ways in which older people and their families manage frailty and disease in late life. She is the co-editor of *Worlds of Difference: Inequality and the Aging Experience* (2000).

R. Brooke Thomas is professor emeritus of anthropology at the University of Massachusetts, Amherst. Since the 1960s, he has conducted research on bio-cultural adaptations of the high Andean Quechua and on the impact of mass tourism on the lowland Maya of the Yucatan Peninsula, Mexico.

C.U. Thresia is a senior research fellow at the Achutha Menon Centre in Kerala, India, and is a member of the Quit Tobacco International Group. She is a cultural anthropologist, who received her PhD at Jawaharlal Nehru University, Centre of Social Medicine and Community Medicine, in New Delhi, India. Her research has focused on women's work, gender relations, and rural development in Kerala.

David Van Sickle is a Robert Wood Johnson Foundation Health and Society Scholar at the University of Wisconsin—Madison. Previously, he worked as an epidemic intelligence service officer at the U.S. Centers for Disease Control and Prevention. He received his PhD in medical anthropology from the University of Arizona in 2004, focusing his research on chronic disease in India.

Ravi K. Verma is a psychologist and director of the Asia Regional Office of the International Center for Research on Women in New Delhi. He has conducted research and intervention on sexual risk in India since 1995 among adults, youth, men who have sex with men (MSM), and migrants in rural and urban areas throughout India.

Introduction

ROBERT A. HAHN AND MARCIA C. INHORN

This book is about anthropological contributions to public health at the dawn of the new millennium.[1] At the beginning of the twenty-first century, there is cause for great hope *and* great concern in the world of public health. On the positive side, advances in global health have occurred at a rate that is unprecedented in human history. In both the developed and the developing worlds, longevity has increased markedly, owing largely to basic research and application of discoveries and inventions in biomedicine and public health.[2] Causative agents of major infectious disease have been discovered, and antibiotics have prevented the deaths of millions. Simple therapies for diarrhea have significantly reduced morbidity and mortality in the developing world, especially among children. Immunization can now prevent infection, morbidity, and death from many diseases that were previously mass killers. Indeed, the global eradication of smallpox by campaigns of vaccination based on public health surveillance may be counted as one of the major global achievements of the twentieth century. In the twenty-first century, new public health philanthropists, such as the Bill and Melinda Gates Foundation, have channeled their resources and energies into the development of new vaccines and other low-cost, appropriate health technologies for the developing world.

Beyond infectious diseases, principal causes of major chronic diseases, such as lung cancer and heart disease, have been identified. The use of screening

1

technologies can prevent death from cervical, breast, and colorectal cancers. Injuries (both intentional and unintentional) are now seen as matters of public health, and their prominent modifiable risk factors are recognized. Although the demonstrated capacity to control chronic diseases and injuries has been less dramatic, modification of the physical and social environment has been shown to reduce exposure to prominent risk factors for many of these conditions. Overall, biomedicine and public health have made major contributions to human health during the twentieth century (Centers for Disease Control and Prevention [CDC] 1999).

Yet, the challenges to global public health in the twenty-first century are still formidable. Since the year 2000, a number of major natural disasters, including the South and Southeast Asian tsunamis, devastating earthquakes in Pakistan and China, Hurricane Katrina in the southern United States, major famines in parts of East and West Africa, and recent cyclones in Bangladesh and Burma (Myanmar) have tested public health infrastructures, both locally and globally, in terms of their ability to deliver timely relief. Reemerging infectious diseases continue to take millions of lives each year. Africa and Asia have also suffered from virulent viral epidemics of ebola, SARS, and avian flu—generating concern about the resurgence of a deadly global flu pandemic. In particular, the emergence and resurgence of three "global killers"—HIV/AIDS, malaria, and tuberculosis—can perhaps be counted as *the* most pressing challenge to global health in this new millennium. The HIV/AIDS pandemic has taken more than 20 million lives, has left more than 12 million AIDS orphans and many child-headed households, and threatens to take the lives of the more than 30 million people now living with the virus as well as the lives of millions more who will become infected, including in the populous nations of China, India, and Russia.

Chronic "lifestyle" diseases, now epidemic in the United States, are spreading to the rest of the world as a result of changing diet and lifestyle—including the so-called "McDonaldization" effect of globalization and the spread of Western fast food to developing countries. In addition, more than half of the world's men smoke, leading to epidemics of tobacco-related diseases and death, including in family members who suffer the effects of secondhand smoke and the diversion of family resources into tobacco consumption. Tobacco-related diseases are increasingly a global problem of women, and girls and women have been the targets of commercial tobacco campaigns (World Health Organization 2001).

Although major improvements in child health have been achieved during the twentieth century, children in many parts of the world are still at risk of low birth weight, childhood malnutrition, and death from a variety of infectious diseases, including malaria, a major killer of children. Mothers—who are "counted upon" within public health initiatives to save the lives of their children—may themselves be dying from HIV/AIDS and childbirth-related maternal mortality, the latter of which has been singularly recalcitrant to so-called "Safe Motherhood" initiatives around the world. In fact, so many women and children who are living in poverty continue to die from preventable conditions that two of the eight Millennium Development Goals (MDGs) developed by the United Nations as a global blueprint for action by the year 2015 focus on reducing child mortality and improving maternal health.

The first priority of the UN MDG initiative is to halve the rate of extreme global poverty by the year 2015—an indication of the extent and severity of poverty in many parts of the world and in almost every continent. That some continents, including Latin America, Africa, and parts of Asia, are more severely affected by poverty than others bespeaks the major global inequalities and health disparities between rich and poor nations. Such disparities have been exacerbated through structural adjustment programs (SAPs) and neoliberal economic policies that reinforce the dependence of needy "recipient" nations on wealthy "donor" nations through donor–recipient models of economic aid, including in health development.

As a result of these various factors, wide gaps separate public health capacities to advance global health and the actual fulfillment of these capacities in countries around the world. Available public health knowledge and resources potentially allow far more control of human suffering than has been achieved at this point in the twenty-first century. An index of this gulf is the difference in longevity between Japan, with the highest life expectancy, and Sierra Leone, with the lowest. The Japanese can expect to live more than twice as long as the Sierra Leonese do (men 78 and 37 years, respectively; women 85 and 40 years, respectively) (WHO 2000). However, if *healthy* life expectancy at birth is measured, then the Japanese can be expected to live *three times* as long in good health as do Sierra Leone the Sierra Leonese. Because of HIV/AIDS-related morbidity, men and women from can be expected to live healthy for only 27 years and 30 years, respectively. Because of HIV/AIDS, the overall life expectancy in sub-Saharan Africa has dropped precipitously in the new millennium, with AIDS now being the leading cause of death and far outstripping other life-threatening diseases, such as malaria, tuberculosis, diarrheal disease, and pneumonia. The 155-fold difference between health care expenditures in the high-income economies of the developed world and the low-income economies (World Bank 2007) undoubtedly contributes in part to the disparities in longevity, by affecting efforts to both prevent and treat disease, including through provision of antiretroviral (ARV) therapies to prolong life expectancy in AIDS patients. In short, when considered on a global scale, health care expenditure may be inversely proportional to need.

Obstacles to Achieving Global Health in the New Millennium

It can be argued that there are four major obstacles to closing the gaps in morbidity and mortality worldwide. First is the ongoing *deliberate production of illness, suffering, and death* by human acts such as warfare, genocide, homicide, torture, and persecution. In 2000, the World Health Organization estimated that 269,000 people died and 8.44 million disability-adjusted life years (DALYS)[3] were lost to death and disabilities in 1999 as the direct and immediate effects of all the wars, both civil and international, being fought in that year (Ghobarah, Huth, and Russett 2004). Since 2000, the United States has launched major war efforts in Afghanistan and Iraq, adding to the list of 30 current conflicts being fought around the world in the year 2008. In 2006, there were approximately 20 million people "of concern" to UNHCR (United Nations High Commission on Refugees), the UN refugee agency worldwide (UNHCR 2008). The exodus of more than 2 million Iraqis, mostly to the neighboring countries of Syria and Jordan, has reversed 5-year declines in the global refugee population, bringing the global total to nearly 10 million people.

A second obstacle to solving public health problems is *inequitable allocation of resources, including misallocation and inefficient allocation,* both within and between nations of the world. Discrimination and unequal access to resources based on gender, race/ethnicity, age, religion, socioeconomic status, and region are well recognized (Doyal 1995). Lack of access to resources based on such discrimination can have substantial detrimental effects on health, leading to so-called "health disparities" between populations living within a given society. In addition, ethnocentrism and nationalism, as well as racism, sexism, ageism, and other forms of prejudice, have been, and continue to be, underlying factors in the unequal distribution of resources among and within nations. The beliefs that one's own culture and society are the only true and worthy ones and that other societies are fundamentally less deserving of the fruits of prosperity and good health underlie global inequalities in health. Such inequalities are a manifestation of so-called "structural violence," or the violence of poverty, social and political marginalization, and other forms of structured inequalities that affect people's lives, health, and overall well-being (Farmer 2003, 2004).

A third and related obstacle is *lack of commitment of needed resources—* including health care services, technologies, pharmaceuticals, and personnel— to suffering populations. Public health rests on a moral assumption that response to the perceived suffering of others is a worthy action, deserving commitment of resources and effort. Implementation requires the agreement, if not the active participation, of national governments in efforts to improve public health within a country's borders. Some public health initiatives fail because of lack of national and/or international commitment to projects designed to address the perspectives and concerns of the populations in need. The concept of "political will" has been invoked to describe the issue of political commitment to public health efforts. Indeed, public health is a very political field of action, involving complex forms of collaboration among governments, international agencies, ministries, and various nongovernmental organizations, including faith-based organizations, the latter of which are increasingly involved in the delivery of public health services around the world.

A fourth obstacle is the *inadequate translation of public health knowledge into effective action*, largely because of social and cultural boundaries. Such boundaries may separate those who have specific preventive and curative capacities and resources from those who may need them. The failure of some public health programs to study and take into account the culture and society of the community toward which the program is being directed has sometimes led to only partial success or even demise of the program. Indeed, for public health programs to be maximally effective, social and cultural differences must be bridged, and communities receiving public health programs must "buy into" program efforts. The participatory research approaches developed in public health are a promising move toward cross-cultural bridge building (Cargo and Mercer 2008). But the failure of some public health agencies to reflect on their own cultural assumptions or to base programs on misleading concepts and erroneous theories and information remains a serious challenge to global health in the new millennium.

Anthropology and Public Health: Four Approaches

This anthology is devoted primarily to the fourth obstacle—the need for nuanced social and cultural assessment in overcoming public health problems. We argue that the lack of routine and systematic use of anthropological theory and methods has been detrimental to the field of public health. Public health needs anthropology to be maximally effective. Yet, anthropologists have not been consistently collaborative, nor have they made their perspectives understandable for the cultures of others—for example, the public health community.

The authors in this anthology are motivated by their desire to explore interdisciplinary intersections between anthropology and public health and to translate their research in ways that are useful and meaningful for public health audiences. Most of the authors in this book are trained in the subfield of medical anthropology, and many have received additional training in public health. As a result, they are heavily invested in the study and solution of public health problems in both the developed and developing worlds. The chapters in this anthology illustrate the salience of anthropological theory and methods for the public health community through 24 case studies of a diverse range of public health topics in a variety of global sites. The anthology is divided into four sections, based on four different approaches taken by anthropologists to the study of public health issues.

The first section of the anthology, "Anthropological Understandings of Public Health Problems," examines the ways in which anthropologists attempt to understand public health problems within a larger social, cultural, historical, and political–economic context, yet stopping short of developing public health education or promotion programs. Such contextualized studies of public health problems are imperative, not only to understand what local communities think and believe about the causes of their health problems, but also to understand how they grapple with them. In this respect, the importance of indigenous (i.e., local) health culture, including people's own understandings of and solutions to local health problems, is emphasized in the chapters in this section. Anthropologists studying indigenous perspectives on public health problems can provide rich data on knowledge, attitudes, and practices surrounding health; social organization and norms that affect care-giving; and the "local moral worlds," including local religious norms, that surround therapeutic decision making and the acceptance (or rejection) of public health innovations (Kleinman 1996).

The second section of the anthology, "Anthropological Design of Public Health Interventions," introduces the principles, methods, and approaches of so-called "applied" medical anthropology in public health settings. The chapters in this section highlight the work of anthropologists who attempt to develop effective public health education and intervention programs. The expertise offered by anthropologists in public health interventions often focuses on so-called "formative research," or the conceptualization stage of an intervention, in which knowledge of and from the local community is imperative. However, as shown in several of the chapters, anthropologists are now also taking leading roles in multiple facets of public health intervention projects. These roles include design, management, and evaluation of the intervention, including follow-up on intervention outcomes many years after the project. The long-term engagement of anthropologists facilitates local participation and uptake and increases sustainability.

The third section of the anthology, "Anthropological Evaluations of Public Health Initiatives," emphasizes the importance of evaluation—of local, small-scale intervention projects, as well as of major, internationally funded public health initiatives being carried out around the world. The anthropologists in this section of the book critically analyze notions of health "development," often pointing to the difficulties of developing effective, long-term, public health interventions for many of the most serious global health problems. This is especially true when local-level realities are ignored in public health initiatives emanating "top down" from international agencies. The importance of local change initiatives, coming from *within* affected communities, will be apparent in this section of the book.

Finally, the fourth section of the anthology, "Anthropological Critiques of Public Health Policy," challenges many of the major policy initiatives being invoked in global public health in the twenty-first century. The theory of neoliberalism, which focuses on privatization of public health and biomedical services around the globe, is critically assessed, as are the public health bureaucracies from which such policies emanate. In addition, many public health policies have emerged in reaction to perceived imminent public health threats. In states of emergency, policies of questionable nature are sometimes enacted, with detrimental outcomes for local populations. Examining macrolevel public health policies with a critical eye is therefore an essential endeavor. Such critiques can determine where mistakes have been made and can suggest what lessons might be relevant for future policy makers. Anthropologists are trained in critical theory; thus, as a group, they excel in this critical evaluative role. However, it is important to note that anthropology also excels in auto-critique; anthropologists pride themselves on "reflexivity" (self-reflection) about their research motives, their relationship to those studied, the power differentials between researcher and subject, and what might be described as "best practices" in research methodology, or how different methods are needed for different research problems. The field is also characterized by a strong ethical orientation, with "do no harm" to research subjects as the first principle.

Given the focus of this book on the "value added" by anthropology to public health, the remainder of this introduction briefly

- describes the underlying principles of anthropology, indicating their application to public health;
- gives an overview of anthropological methods; and
- proposes directions for the future of anthropology in public health.

Principles of Anthropology

Anthropology is a discipline that examines diverse aspects of human social life, its processes and causes, the interrelations of its elements, and its relations with phenomena studied by other disciplines, for example, human biology, ecology, economics, politics, and religion. The annual meetings of the American Anthropological Association, undoubtedly the largest regular gatherings of anthropologists in the world, indicate the field's rich variety as its practitioners examine facets of social life taken for granted by most.

Anthropology is commonly divided into four major subfields: *archaeology* examines the physical remains of societies—most often societies of the past— to reconstruct as much of their social and cultural life as possible; *physical anthropology* focuses on human biology and its relation to society, culture, and history; *linguistic anthropology* examines various facets of human language and its relationship to social and cultural life; and *social and cultural anthropology* examines the organization of societies and their cultural systems, that is, their beliefs, values, norms, and patterns of behavior. Although the division into four subfields reflects differences in interests, theories, and methods, these also may be shared among the subfields.

Medical anthropology, which focuses on the interrelationships of society, culture, and biology on the one hand and sickness and healing on the other, might be considered a component of social and cultural anthropology, incorporating the other fields as well; or it might be regarded as a fifth subfield. With nearly 1,300 members of the Society for Medical Anthropology (SMA) of the American Anthropological Association, medical anthropology is the anthropological field most central to public health. In the remainder of this introduction, medical anthropology is the subfield to which we refer when we use the term *anthropology*.

Like scholars in other disciplines, anthropologists have diverse views and approaches to their discipline. Nevertheless, there are perspectives shared by most anthropologists. The following discussion summarizes four basic anthropological premises and their corollaries, indicating their application in public health. The chapters in this book illustrate these assumptions.

Premise One: Cultural Relativism

Undoubtedly, the most basic premise of anthropology is *cultural relativism*, the assumption that "cultures" (the systems of beliefs, values, and norms of behavior found in all societies) are more or less coherent, systematic, and rational within their own context. Beliefs about health and sickness, and their causes and treatment, commonly referred to as *ethnomedicines*, are elements of these cultural systems. Politics, the economy, and religion are also cultural elements; in many technologically less developed societies, there is considerable overlap of ethnomedicines and other cultural elements. Cultural relativism is essentially the opposite of ethnocentrism, cited earlier as a source of failure to address major global health problems. Although there are limits to the anthropological acceptance of cultural relativism (e.g., few if any anthropologists would find slavery or the culture of Nazi Germany in the 1930s and 1940s to be legitimate), most anthropologists subscribe to some version of cultural relativism and value the integrity and worthiness of all human societies.

A question of relativism critical to the role of anthropology when working with public health is whether the predominant medical system of Western civilization, *biomedicine*, is superior entirely, in general, or in specific aspects—to the *ethnomedicines*, or indigenous health systems of non-Western societies (Hahn 1995). An operating principle of public health is that biomedicine and public health have at least some superior knowledge or technique that justifies addressing the health problems of others.

Several corollaries follow from the premise of cultural relativism. First, *societies and cultures are best understood as whole systems, that is, "holistically."* If the elements of a cultural system do not "make sense" on their own, then the way in which cultural elements fit together is critical for understanding the individual elements. Anthropology traditionally addressed this corollary of relativism by means of holistic studies of communities, referred to as *ethnographies*. These are studies that examine not simply a focal topic, but the interrelationships of physical environment, principal activities, economics, and social organization, including kinship and marriage, politics, science, and religion. In contemporary anthropology, holistic studies are exceptional, perhaps in response to the limitations of funding. Yet even focused, topical studies, which are now the rule, frequently provide contextual information, as shown in the chapters in this anthology.

Second, *Western civilization is also a culture, or rather a combination of many cultures.* Similarly, the discipline of anthropology, largely an intellectual product of the Western world, is itself a culture with many subcultures. A consequence of this corollary is that anthropologists have their own distinct worldviews; they have theories about the way the world is, along with their own, possibly distinctive, values and behavioral norms.

For public health, an implication of the culture of anthropology is that, to communicate with practitioners of other disciplines or even within their own society, anthropologists need to translate their concepts and methodologies into the concepts and languages of other disciplines and practices, for example, public health and policymaking. Although this corollary—the need to translate across cultural boundaries—seems basic to the discipline of anthropology, many anthropologists appear to ignore it in dealing with the nonanthropological world. Many anthropologists direct their discourse only to fellow anthropologists. Some anthropologists may resist translation because they regard the application of anthropology to the solution of real world problems as tainting the discipline with politics and values (as if their own studies were apolitical and value free). Anthropologists who do not acknowledge their own culture or who disdain application of their knowledge may fail to communicate their perspective, its methods, and usefulness across disciplinary boundaries adequately.

Third, *local populations, not the outsiders, are the experts on their own sociocultural environment.* If appropriately enlisted, community members can become the teachers of local perspectives, values, and social life. Anthropologists are schooled to be the students of others. They often acknowledge that, in many instances, they do not even know what knowledge is relevant in new cultural settings. When they do develop questionnaires, they do so on the basis of their understanding of the local culture and society, often based on months, if not years, of immersive fieldwork. The humble assumption that expertise resides in others—and particularly local community members—is common in anthropology, but rare in other academic disciplines. It is integral also to participatory research approaches now recommended by the Institute of Medicine, among others (Cargo and Mercer 2008).

Fourth, a corollary especially important to programs of public health is that those who seriously interact with foreign cultures have a moral obligation to take those cultures seriously, including their social organizations and values. Anthropologists have noted that public health programs in the past were often based on the assumption that the communities for which programs were planned were "empty vessels," lacking the relevant knowledge of how to improve some facet of their lives; it was assumed that the problem would be solved by introducing the Western "expert's" knowledge and techniques. Anthropologists reject this assumption.

Taking the culture and society of others seriously involves two related steps. First is coming to know the social organization and values of the other culture. The methods outlined below and exemplified in the chapters of this book indicate how such knowledge is achieved. This knowledge may make public health and other interventions more effective and efficient by being responsive to the local settings and enhancing local participation. But there is a second step, which some regard as essential, in taking the local social setting seriously and in using knowledge of this setting to develop local interventions. This is a *moral* step of respecting, attending to, and addressing local perceptions, interests, and ways of life. At the least, it requires listening and sympathetic understanding; at the most, it requires helping to serve local interests.

The challenge of taking others seriously may be couched as a question: "Are we providing a benefit that the recipient does not recognize or value as a 'benefit'?" Members of the recipient society may reject our offering because they do not understand it—at least in the same way that we do—or because they understand it but give this potential benefit a relatively low priority. We might then be motivated to act paternalistically—a morally hazardous course, particularly when dealing with communities that include adults. In the design or implementation of public health programs, local concerns are often not a critical consideration, but should be. The anthropological approach provides moral grounds for routinely making local concerns a primary criterion in public health decision making.

The 1998 Code of Ethics of the American Anthropological Association recognizes the many individuals and communities involved in research, including the anthropologist, his or her students and institution, the broader society, those who participate in an anthropologist's study, and the institutions and agencies that fund anthropological research (American Anthropological Association 1998).[4] First and foremost, the code emphasizes obligations to the populations studied:

> A. Responsibility to people and animals with whom anthropological researchers work and whose lives and cultures they study.
>> 1. Anthropological researchers have primary ethical obligations to the people, species, and materials they study and to the people with whom they work. These obligations can supersede the goal of seeking new knowledge, and can lead to decisions not to undertake or to discontinue a research project when the primary obligation conflicts with other responsibilities, such as those owed to sponsors or clients. These ethical obligations include:
>> - To avoid harm or wrong; understanding that the development of knowledge can lead to change which may be positive or negative for the people or animals worked with or studied
>> - To respect the well-being of humans and nonhumans
>> - To consult actively with the affected individuals with the goal of establishing a working relationship that can be beneficial to all parties involved (American Anthropological Association 1998)

Premise Two: Theoretical Foundations of Knowledge and Practice

A second anthropological premise is that anthropological *knowledge and practice are founded in theory,* that is, one's beliefs and actions are based on underlying beliefs about how the world works. The anthropological approach to knowledge, however, is more inductive than many disciplines in that anthropologists are especially open to having their theories shaped by their experience in the field. Thus, theoretical formulations in anthropology are often fully formulated after field-based research has been undertaken. The "grounded" nature of anthropological theory allows for a process of theoretical revision over time on the basis of new knowledge and observations gained "on the ground" within a research setting.

Because anthropological knowledge production emerges through a process of inductive theory building, many anthropologists eschew deductive approaches based on the testing of predetermined hypotheses. Hypothesis-testing approaches to research are less common in anthropology than in other social sciences and in public health. Although public health funding agencies may require hypothesis-testing approaches, major anthropological funders—including the Wenner-Gren Foundation for Anthropological Research, the National Science Foundation's Cultural Anthropology program, the Social

Science Research Council, and the Fulbright and Fulbright-Hays programs—
generally do not. Rather, research objectives and goals in anthropological
research are enumerated in relation to theory and methodology, but without
the requirement of a hypothesis-testing research design. In addition, conceptual models, which often "stand in" for theory in public health research, are
rarely part of the ethnographic approach favored within anthropology.

This is not to say that anthropology is theoretically underdeveloped. On the
contrary, anthropology is a very rich theoretical field, deriving inspiration from
such major social theorists as Max Weber, Sigmund Freud, Karl Marx, Pierre
Bourdieu, Michel Foucault, Antonio Gramsci, Paolo Freire, Anthony Giddens,
Immanuel Kant, Michel de Certeau, and many others. Contemporary theory
in anthropology is characterized by rich and productive ferment, with some
anthropologists favoring materialist perspectives, whereas others emphasize the
symbolic and interpretive (Dirks, Eley, and Ortner 1994). In an insightful review
of the late twentieth century development of anthropological theory, anthropologist Sherry Ortner wrote: "We are no longer sure of how the sides are to be drawn
up, and of where we would place ourselves if we could identify the sides" (Ortner
1994:372). In recent years—reflecting an intellectual movement in the social
sciences and humanities known as *postmodernism* or *poststructuralism*—anthropologists have recognized that cultures and societies are not always single, unified
systems. Rather, human social life is often fragmented and fractured along lines
of class, race, gender, and so on. Such fragmentation speaks to the social distribution of power within a society, and the crucial importance of understanding a
society's history. Together with historians, anthropologists are attending to these
relations of power, as noted by anthropologist Nicholas Dirks:

> Culture as emergent from relations of power and domination, culture as a form of
> power and domination, culture as a medium in which power is both constituted
> and resisted; it is around this set of issues that certain anthropologists and certain
> historians ... are beginning to work out an exciting body of thought (Dirks et al.
> 1994:6).

Relations of power and domination within societies suggest the need to attend
to the historical context of health programs, as well as to the political environment in which such programs are embedded. The importance of history and
politics cannot be overstated. They are crucial determinants of the success
of some public health programs, and the failure of others, as will be shown
by several authors in this book. Indeed, many anthropologists employ critical theoretical perspectives to understand how power differentials, including
those between donor and recipient in public health programs, may stymie public health efforts. Such anthropological critiques are generally keenly attentive
to history and politics on both the micro and macrolevels of analysis.

Anthropologists have proposed a wide range of theories to examine human sickness and health in different social and cultural settings. The range of theoretical positions is suggested by the following rough categorization (Hahn 1995):

- *Ecological/evolutionary theory* claims that the physical environment and human adaptations to it are the principal determinants of sickness and healing. Physical anthropologists employing a so-called *biocultural* approach to public health problems emphasize the interaction between human biology, ecology, and culture.
- *Cultural theory* posits that cultural systems of beliefs, values, and norms are the basic determinants of sickness and healing. So-called *phenomenological* or *interpretivist* approaches to public health problems emphasize local narratives of suffering and an analytical deciphering of cultural symbols and world view.
- *Political–economic theory* proposes that economic organization and relationships of power are the principal forces determining human sickness and health. So-called *critical medical anthropologists* who adopt a political–economic, or *materialist*, perspective tend to emphasize the tensions between *structure and agency*, or how economic factors may constrain health-promoting human action.

These theories have substantially different consequences for public health, in terms of whether biological, cultural, or economic determinants of health are emphasized in any given study. Yet, these theoretical orientations are not exclusive of one another; many anthropologists combine them productively.

It is important that public health practitioners recognize that knowledge and practice are founded in theory and that they need to be aware of their own theories. Awareness of underlying theory and theoretical assumptions allows deliberate assessment of the extent to which a theory's elements are reasonable and compatible with observations. If observations are incompatible with theory, then a theoretical approach may need further assessment and revision. Whereas there is a rich and ever-expanding literature on theory in anthropology, the theoretical literature in some key public health fields, such as epidemiology, is comparably sparse. (Theory is substantially richer in public health fields such as behavioral sciences, communication, and health education.) Many public health research projects lack explicit theoretical models in favor of methodological rigor. Although methods are important, they are insufficient to answer public health research questions if they are not used to explore, validate, or build theoretical understanding. In this regard, public health could benefit from greater theoretical cross-fertilization with anthropology, including anthropology's tendency toward critical (self-) reflection.

Anthropological theory may be useful in public health in at least two ways. First, theories may help explain particular circumstances, for example, the history and genesis of health problems within a particular community for which a program is being planned. Second, the varying anthropological theories of health determinants described above may expand upon the models of behavior and behavior change utilized in many public health intervention studies. Anthropologists are keenly attuned to the complexity of human behavior and belief; much health behavior does not fit neatly into conceptual models, suggesting that these models be expanded.

Premise Three: Research as a Sociocultural Process

A third basic premise of anthropology is that *research and intervention are sociocultural processes*. Research about (and by) human beings involves social relationships. In anthropology, and in many other disciplines as well, this relationship is frequently "cross-cultural." Within one's own sociocultural setting, it may be reasonable to assume that people share some of one's values, concepts, and behavioral norms; this assumption cannot reasonably be made when crossing sociocultural boundaries. For example, one cannot assume that information about a different setting will be provided just for the asking or absorbed when given. There are societal rules for interaction, including the proper way to ask questions; rules may differ for political and religious leaders, men and women, and children and elders; and such rules must be recognized to gather information effectively. Moreover, to interpret responses, it is important to know how one is regarded by the community being studied. For example, in communities where investigators are believed to represent "the government," information may be withheld or distorted so as to maximize the benefits (or minimize the losses) of a potential governmental response.

Similarly, *intervention, including public health action, is fundamentally a process of social and cultural exchange*. Again, there are at least two sociocultural systems involved, those of the "donor" and the "recipient." As in cross-cultural research, there are rules for behavior that must be recognized to effectively implement an intervention. Here, too, it is important to know how one is regarded by the community examined to know how to interpret community members' responses to an intervention. To this end, anthropologists commonly engage in a process of *reflexivity*, in which they carefully examine and attempt to articulate how their relationships with community members, including mutual perceptions about each other, may affect the research process and the information generated. Indeed, many anthropologists would argue that one of the key tools in anthropological research is the anthropologist himself/ herself. How well he or she is accepted by the community being studied will have major implications for the outcomes of research.

Another corollary given credence by many anthropologists is the *national and global context of local society and culture.* Anthropologists recognize that, although individual cultures are more or less internally coherent systems, they are also part of nations which are, in turn, connected with other nations of the world. Thus, local cultures are not autonomous systems; they are deeply connected to and influenced by international circumstances and events. Recent attention by anthropologists to processes of *globalization* indicates that the global context must be taken into account. Societies may once have lived in relative isolation, little affected by the activities of other societies. However, in the new millennium, such isolation is rare, if it still exists. Anthropologists studying the *glocal,* or the reception of things "global" on the "local" level, suggest that processes of globalization are uneven, with some societies achieving the fruits of globalization more than others. Furthermore, local societies may accommodate, refashion, or resist global forces; the local reception of the global is never guaranteed. The importance of globalization for public health cannot be underestimated: Local acceptance of global health programs—which are often designed in "headquarters" in the West—rests on the ability of public health professionals to "tailor," "hybridize," or "indigenize" top-down, "one-size-fits-all" interventions to the local level. This involves taking into account not only the society for which the intervention is intended, but also its social, economic, and political environment. Local programs may succeed or fail depending on the way in which these global public health initiatives are culturally tailored to the local level.

Premise Four: Human "Nature" is Also Cultural and Social

A fourth premise shared by most anthropologists is that human "nature" is not only natural (i.e., a matter of the "basic" sciences of physics, chemistry, and biology), but also cultural and social. Interdisciplinary connectedness has two basic facets, one substantive and the other methodological.

The subject matters of anthropology and other disciplines, including psychology, political science, and history, as well as biology and the physical sciences, are fundamentally connected. Many anthropologists assume, for example, that human culture and social organization are substantially affected by human biology and the physical environment, as shown by the contrast between arctic and desert cultures. Similarly, human biology is affected by human culture and social life, as suggested by studies of migrants whose health status often tends to change when they leave their country of origin to live in a new country. The integrated sociocultural and biological aspect of human nature is critical for public health, insofar as populations for whom programs are designed cannot be assumed to be biologically identical to the populations of the program designers. Population differences can lead to the success of a program in one setting and failure in another. The understanding of socio-cultural and biological effects on public health problems may be essential in addressing those problems. Thus, in addition to social and cultural anthropology, physical anthropology, with its attention to the biocultural basis of human health and well-being, may also be important in public health.

A second connection is methodological: If the subject matters of different disciplines are interconnected, then *the methodologies* of *those disciplines are also mutually relevant.* Anthropologists, for example, may need to be aware of the methodologies of fields closely linked with their particular study foci. In addition, different disciplines have developed methodologies that may be useful to the practices of other disciplines, independent of disciplinary subject matter; for example, anthropologists sometimes use techniques derived from biostatistics and epidemiology (Chapter 6; Hahn 1995; Inhorn 1995; Trostle 2005; Trostle and Sommerfeld 1996).

Anthropological Methods in Public Health

Foundations

Given its basic objectives and premises, anthropology's methodological challenge is to develop a theoretical and disciplinary framework through which the differing cultural frameworks and details of other societies can be understood. At least initially, the anthropologist has no choice but to use his or her own framework to know the culture of others. To this end, anthropological methods are designed to be flexible and to allow comprehension of other ways of seeing and organizing reality.

Many aspects of human social life, such as beliefs and values, are subjective and resist quantitative measurement. Such subjective phenomena may, nevertheless, be determinants of behavior and are thus critical to assess. Subjectivity of a research topic does not imply subjectivity of the research method used to assess the topic. Subjective characteristics may be measured by the qualitative approaches developed by anthropologists and others (Bernard 2005); once measured, individuals and communities may be systematically compared.

Within anthropology, there are two distinct views regarding quantification in anthropological research. This "qualitative–quantitative" division is associated with underlying differences in views of the discipline, its methods, and its results. Most anthropologists regard qualitative information, which examines the concepts, values, and meanings of sociocultural life, as the essence and foundation of anthropological knowledge. From this perspective, causation among social and cultural elements may not be an appropriate goal of anthropological inquiry; other forms of explanation, such as creating a coherent description or "making sense" of information, may be the primary goal. However, a vocal minority of anthropologists view quantitative information and statistical analysis as the basic sources of anthropological knowledge. From this perspective, causal or other quantified analysis is a central task, although "making sense" of information may also be a goal of quantitative analysis.

Increasingly, some anthropologists are taking the middle ground in this qualitative–quantitative division, using both approaches in a complementary manner, each indicating support for the other. Medical anthropologists, including contributors to this book, often adopt a *mixed-methods* approach, in which methodological *triangulation*, or multiple methods to determine the validity of research findings, is employed (Bernard 2005). It has been argued that, although there are differences in practice between quantitatively and qualitatively oriented disciplines—for example, between epidemiology and anthropology—there is no radical difference in underlying principles; indeed, both approaches implicitly use each other and may be enhanced by explicit combination and collaboration (Chapter 6; Hahn 1995; Inhorn 1995).

As in many disciplines, anthropological research usually has several phases. The anthropologist generally begins by posing a research question; reviewing prior approaches, theories, and results; and specifying research design. Next, a study is conducted and the findings analyzed; and finally a book, series of articles, or report is prepared. The anthropological research process gives primary importance to the societies being studied and their cultural perspectives. And, depending on the setting, anthropologists may encourage participation of the study population in the research process, in phases ranging from community participation in the formulation of the initial research question through review of the results and final report. Indeed, the participatory research approaches used in public health have roots in anthropology (Cargo and Mercer 2008).

Formulating a Research Question

Anthropological research commonly has many sources, including the personal interests of the researcher and colleagues; the perceived magnitude of the problem to be studied; the state of theory, method, and findings in the discipline; sources of support; and research opportunities. The anthropologist must select a focus, however general, and develop a coherent proposal balancing these realities. Much of the research being done in medical anthropology emphasizes public health problems of social significance, for which practical solutions may eventually be achieved.

Because the culture an anthropologist studies generally differs greatly from the anthropologist's own culture, it may be difficult to specify in advance the exact information sought in research. Respondents may think of the research topic in a manner entirely different from that of the researcher, a difference critical to the anthropologist's process of understanding. Thus, the phases of research do not always follow the same course. Newly discovered topics may be critical to the researcher's original interests and alternative methods of information collection or analysis may be indicated. Nevertheless, it is incumbent on the researcher to specify clearly at the start what he or she intends to do, why, to what end, and how. It is also an intellectual prerequisite that the researcher demonstrates how the proposed study responds to the theory, methods, and prior findings on the chosen topic.

Anthropology applied to public health problems may also differ in several ways from the approaches of other anthropological subdisciplines. Because it is directed toward solution of a problem, the questions it seeks to answer will generally have practical import, such as why some intervention did not work, or how new knowledge of a public health problem can suggest a way to overcome it. Research of social significance, with potential benefits to the society being studied, is prioritized in the anthropology of public health. Increasingly, anthropological funding agencies, particularly the National Science Foundation, are attentive to the social significance of anthropological research. On the basis of such policy-relevant research, the anthropologist may go on to develop a public health intervention and evaluate its outcome. Anthropologists participating in these initiatives may produce action-oriented reports of findings (and theory and methods) that may include recommendations to policy makers, public health practitioners, or the communities studied.

As suggested above, anthropological research, like all other research, needs to be funded. Traditionally, support was needed for prolonged field research in remote locales. Although such long-term, immersive anthropological research continues today, many anthropological research projects are more focused, are carried out over shorter periods, and may involve research teams, including teams in which local research assistants are trained to carry out anthropological methods of data collection. As noted earlier, a variety of funding agencies, including those that foster research in the non-Western world, support anthropological research projects. It is critical that researchers attend to funding sources, while also being aware of and nurturing institutional connections, particularly with host countries and study communities. The American Anthropological Association's Code of Ethics regards informed consent of the study community and its members as a prerequisite for anthropological research. Ethical issues should always be paramount in research design, and increasingly, funding agencies require ethical disclosure on the part of all grantees.

Fieldwork: Collecting and Analyzing
Anthropological Information

In anthropology, the research setting is typically referred to as *the field*. *Doing fieldwork* or *ethnography* is a rite of passage in anthropological training and an ongoing activity in the careers of many anthropologists. Basically, fieldwork means living or working for an extended period (often a year or more) at the site of one's research—an obvious precondition of participant observation, described subsequently. It also means a commitment to serious foreign language training, both before and during fieldwork. Anthropologists try to achieve fluency in one or more field languages, so that they can communicate effectively with those among whom they are living. Anthropologists refer to community members who provide them with information as *informants*. For anthropologists, the term does not carry the connotation of espionage associated with "informer"; moreover, it avoids the connotation of domination associated with anthropology's own history of research in colonial settings and with the term research "subject" used by other behavioral disciplines.

Anthropologists generally carry out their fieldwork alone, without a team of colleagues or research assistants. This "solo" model of research, sometimes called the *lone stranger* model, is valued and supported within the discipline of anthropology, including by anthropological funding agencies (Agar 1980). Increasingly, anthropologists are recognizing the value of taking others with them to the field, including spouses and children, students, and fellow researchers. Although group research is not the norm in anthropology, anthropologists are increasingly working in collaborative, cross-disciplinary teams, as shown in several chapters in this book.

Because fieldwork often fully and sometimes abruptly engages the anthropologist in a setting very different from his or her own home setting, it is commonly an intense and personal experience. It is often wonderful, but it sometimes results in *culture shock*, that is, a personal disturbance fostered by abrupt immersion in a new cultural setting where one may not understand the language, expectations, and one's standing, and where one's own sense of cultural and social order is not shared. Although many anthropologists experience such strains, most gradually transform their uncertainty into understanding.

Anthropologists recognize the need to establish *rapport* with the community in which they conduct their study, and particularly with the community informants. Rapport is a relationship of mutual trust. Building rapport is a critical step in research, because information given by informants may be substantially affected by their relationship with the researcher and by their understanding of what the researcher is doing. From an anthropological perspective, it involves the interaction of two social and cultural systems. Once rapport is established, the likelihood that informants will behave abnormally—out of character—in front of the newcomer diminishes. But rapport is not simply of methodological interest, as a tool for gathering information; it is of ethical importance as well in affirming the observer's obligations to the people studied.

A renowned principle of anthropological research is *participant observation*. Participant observation is not so much a specific method as an approach to the collection of information by means of the presence and participation of the researcher in the social life of the study setting. The participant observer makes anthropological observations while participating; participation is a means of observation. Anthropologists rarely attempt to *go native*, fully adopting local customs and beliefs: most retain some distance while participating. The observer's participation may diminish the effects his or her presence might otherwise have on "normal" events.

Anthropologists traditionally assess basic background information about the research setting. They make maps of the community, collect information on its physical environment, including the "man-made" environment, and approximate population size and demographic characteristics, sometimes through community censuses. Much of this information can be collected by use of unobtrusive measures, which do not involve the observer's presence in, and thus potential alteration of, the local setting (Scrimshaw and Hurtado 1987). Such information not only gives a sense of what the place is like but is also often critical to the substance of the project.

Beyond background information, basic anthropological information collected in the field may be roughly categorized into two types: *cognitive*, that is, mental or ideational (including local concepts, beliefs, attitudes, and values); and *behavioral*, that is, describing what people actually do and how they interact. Anthropologists have developed substantial expertise for eliciting local concepts of how things (e.g., types of diseases) are classified and defined (Bernard, 2005). They regard the understanding of concepts as a guide to local views of the world. Anthropologists have also developed techniques for assessing how concepts are woven into belief systems (e.g., about the etiology and treatment of diseases). And they have methods for the assessment of attitudes and values, that is, ideas about what is good and bad, right and wrong, beautiful and ugly. Values are important because they are associated with local priorities—for example, whether treatment of one person or one condition is regarded as more or less important than the treatment of another person or another condition.

Interviews are the principal sources of cognitive information collected by anthropologists in the field; anthropologists value the importance of *discourse*, or "talk," whether it is in naturally occurring conversations or through interviews guided by the anthropologist. Anthropological interviews, like interviews in other disciplines, are commonly described in terms of their degree of *structure*, that is, the extent to which they are intended to control interviewer–informant dialogue (Agar 1980; Bernard 2005; Fetterman 1998; Spradley 1979). Informal interviews are barely interviews at all; the researcher participates in normal conversation and records comments of interest to the research topic. Informal interviews are a side benefit of participant observation.

In formal interviews—classified as unstructured, semi-structured, or structured—interviewee and interviewer both know there is a specific goal: the interviewer's collection of certain information. Degrees of structure are the extent to which the interviewer is supposed to follow a fixed sequence of questions and the interviewee is supposed to choose from a fixed set of response options. In *unstructured interviews*, although the interviewer may have a chosen topic, he or she learns both by attempting to move the discussion to flesh out the topic and by allowing informants to explain their points of view on topics of interest and to lead in directions yet unknown to the anthropologist. Except for specific purposes, anthropologists carefully avoid *leading questions*, because rather than eliciting a response that reflects the respondents' own beliefs about the question, these might yield an answer that is thought to be expected by the questioner. Unstructured interviews are characterized by many *open-ended questions*, some of which may be included in a simple *interview guide* developed beforehand by the anthropologist, but others of which may arise during the course of the interview itself.

Bernard (2005) provides a list of *probes* useful in unstructured interviews to elicit different kinds of responses by informants. For example, the *echo probe* responds to an informant's statement with a brief summary of the statement; the *silent probe* waits silently for the informant to continue speaking; and the leading, or *baiting probe* (Agar 1980) suggests to the informant knowledge on the part of the interviewer, to encourage the informant to reveal information that might otherwise be secret. Since the rules of talk vary with the setting, the usefulness of probes depends on the cultural circumstances. For example, cultures differ in the time allowed between turns of speech, so that what the interviewer regards as a silent probe may be a normal wait in some settings, and thus not a probe at all.

A particularly useful probe for anthropology in public health is the question, "What happens when someone has such-and-such a disease?" The question may be about a current episode of the disease or a past one. When directed toward a specific informant's experience with a disease, it may lead to a rich and complex *illness narrative*, in which the informant reveals his or her *explanatory model* (EM) of the disease, and how he or she went about seeking treatment (Kleinman 1989). Illness narratives allow assessment of local theories of disease origin, perceived importance and implications, consultation and diagnosis, home and healer treatment, and follow-up; they may be complemented by observation of disease-related actions, such as when an anthropologist accompanies an informant on a trip to a healer. Illness narratives is an important part of the anthropological toolkit in public health. Many of the chapters in this book will provide case studies in which portions of illness narratives are presented.

Along with unstructured illness narratives, *semi-structured interviews* are among the most common forms of interviews used in the anthropology of public health problems. The anthropologist generally prepares an interview schedule containing a list of questions he or she wants addressed. The semi-structured interview schedule contains both close-ended and open-ended questions, which will be asked of multiple informants. Semi-structured interviews are particularly useful when there are time constraints on the interview, when there may not be subsequent opportunities for interviews, and when teams of interviewers must collect comparable information (Bernard 2005). Semi-structured interviews are particularly useful for determining *patterns* of knowledge and belief because the same questions are asked of multiple informants.

Finally, in *structured interviews*, the interviewer has a fixed set of questions or a questionnaire. Several structured interview techniques have been developed by anthropologists working within the subfield of *cognitive anthropology* to assess local concepts, beliefs, and values (Bernard 2005). These techniques include *free listing*, in which the informant is asked to list all items in a given category, such as skin diseases; *ranking*, in which the informant is asked to rank items by specified criteria, such as most severe or most common; *triad tests*, in which the informant is asked to indicate which two of three items are most similar and which are most different; and *pile sorts*, in which the informant is asked to put like items together in piles. These techniques allow analysis of how informants divide up their universe and what dimensions connect and distinguish the elements.

Anthropologists also use *questionnaires*, which are generally developed only after months of prior fieldwork and built on established knowledge of local concepts and beliefs. Although widely used in other behavioral disciplines, questionnaires raise special issues in anthropology, largely because of differences in culture and society between questioner and respondent. Not only literacy, but also, for example, rules of speech, privacy, and secrecy may affect the design, administration, and usefulness of questionnaires. Questionnaires presume that the researcher knows what to ask and how; thus, anthropologists tend to use them only in later stages of a study.

Each form of interviewing has its particular use: unstructured interviews are an excellent means of exploring new topics, exploring topics in greater depth, and in designing more structured interviews. Anthropologists use unstructured interviews in a variety of ways, for example, to develop genealogies, to elicit life histories from elders in a community, and to collect myths, fables, and other stories that a community deems important. Semi-structured interviews allow more directed exploration and facilitate systematic coverage of a topic and are thus particularly useful in more focused research on particular public health problems. Structured interviews are best suited for examining the range and distribution of specific beliefs in populations (Bernard 2005).

In recent years, anthropologists have also used *focus groups* as an interview technique (Krueger 1994). In focus groups, individuals from a community are selected by chosen criteria and interviewed together by a trained interviewer. The interviewer guides the discussion with a semi-structured list of questions and analyzes the results to assess group attitudes and practices on a given topic. Although focus group methodology suffers the anthropological handicap of occurring out of normal social context, it is useful for rapidly assessing a community's ideas about a topic, and for generating discussion about issues of potential concern to the community. Focus group questions must lend themselves to the group setting; interpretation of responses must reflect the group process involved in their creation.

Because language is a principal instrument of their research, particularly in interviews, anthropologists give great importance to the *local language* in conducting field research. Ideally, the researcher uses the local language. In practice, though, even if language instruction is available, it is often difficult, if not impossible, to learn the local language in advance, and it may require years to learn a language in the field. Anthropologists, therefore, sometimes use *interpreters*, when available. The use of interpreters, however, hinders a basic anthropological task—the recognition and comprehension of conceptual differences in culture, commonly represented in language. For this reason, anthropologists make every effort to learn the local language and to be careful about *translation*; for example, when they translate questionnaires or educational materials into a local language, they may *back translate*, that is, check the accuracy of the translation by translating the material back to the researcher's language.

Furthermore, many anthropologists attempt to *tape-record* interviews as much as possible, for the purposes of detailed transcription, translation, and analysis later. Although tape-recording allows for greater accuracy and precision, it may also arouse fear and suspicion among informants, especially if the information being collected is of a sensitive nature. For this reason, anthropologists typically ask informants whether they can tape-record interviews; tape-recording should never be done covertly, and the tape-recorder should never be used without an informant's explicit permission. When tape-recorders are not being used, the anthropologist generally takes handwritten notes during the interview or, increasingly, enters these notes directly into a laptop computer.

In addition to asking questions about the cognitive world of the local population, anthropologists also gather information through systematic *observation* of local behaviors and social interactions. The behaviors observed are not simply physical movements, but also actions that are intentional and meaningful to the actor, including "verbal behaviors" (speech). *Behavioral observations* form part of the background description of an anthropological report, allowing characterization of the basic activities of the population, such as work, rituals, and recreation. Systematic observation of behavior requires selection of settings and persons to be observed, as well as definition and classification of behaviors of interest. For purposes of public health, background information may indicate sources of exposure to various pathogenic agents, substances, or events.

Beyond background characteristics, anthropologists may also observe health-related behavior, such as how people recognize and respond to health conditions, consult and make decisions with family members and others regarding home treatment, and resort to healers of different sorts. By assessing behaviors in households and other social units, anthropologists can estimate the distribution of these behaviors in the population. On the basis of information collected in this systematic way, the researcher should be able to describe community response to health conditions of interest. The application of anthropological methods in settings such as clinics, hospitals, and health bureaucracies allows the analysis of treatments, healer–patient interactions, and the control of health resources.

The analysis of *social organization* is a common anthropological practice that involves both cognitive and behavioral information. Social organization is the framework in which the society operates; its components include institutions and other organizational structures as well as behavioral roles. Social organization is a broad notion that interrelates societal groups and membership, societal and community factions, and leadership and decision making, as well as marriage and postmarital residence, kinship, and inheritance. Law and its sanctions, as well as politics and economics, may be regarded as elements of social organization. Cognitive information indicates the rules and rationale of social organization, whereas behavioral information indicates what people actually do (including violation of organizational rules and consequent sanctions). Social organization may be important in public health for many reasons, including societal allocation of work and other activities (some of which may, in turn, be associated with harmful exposures), allocation of treatment resources and control of access, certification of healers and healing institutions, and provision of public education, health-related information, and programs.

The systematic recording of observations in the field is a critical step in anthropological research. This may be especially true with an open-ended research agenda, in which observations that do not make sense to the observer initially may become comprehensible later. Bernard (2005) provides a useful classification of types of information recorded in the field, including logs of intended and actual daily activities, a personal diary, and methodological and descriptive field notes of observations and analyses. Taking *field notes* is an important part of anthropological field research. Anthropologists typically carry a notebook with them at all times, to make *field jottings* of their observations and conversations. At the end of the day, these field jottings are transformed into more fully descriptive field notes at the computer. Computer software developed for anthropology allows for the analysis of such notes (Bernard 2005).

Traditionally, anthropological research required at least a year and sometimes more than 2 years of field study, followed by a thorough analysis and written account. Anthropology is often criticized by action-oriented professions as too time- and resource-consuming in producing results. Partly in response to such concerns, anthropologists have formulated a variety of quicker and more focused approaches to the collection of information. *Rapid Assessment Procedures (RAPs)* have been developed to survey the research setting and address particular health issues in 1 or 2 months, using a systematic set of questions and methods. First developed to understand issues of nutrition and primary care, RAP is applicable and has been used in the assessment of a broad array of issues (Scrimshaw and Gleason 1992). Scrimshaw and Hurtado (1987) provide guides for the rapid and systematic elicitation of health-related information at the community, household, and biomedical resource (i.e., clinicians and pharmacy) levels. These guides can be tailored to particular studies and particular settings; they are not rigid protocols. Both RAP and a similar approach, the *Focused Ethnographic Study (FES)*, directed toward the understanding of specific disease conditions and programs, have been used by applied medical anthropologists since the 1990s (Pelto and Pelto 1997). Although more time generally allows for the gathering of more and better information, the results of rapid, focused approaches may be more likely to meet the urgent needs of public health programs and personnel.

Computers have offered enormous benefits to qualitative as well as quantitative analysis in anthropology. Computers allow the filing, analysis, and transmission of vast amounts of information (Bernard 2005; Weitzman and Miles 1995). Without the assistance of computers, data analysis would (and formerly did) require enormous amounts of time and resources. But there are also hazards in the use of computers in anthropological (and other) research. Perhaps the greatest hazard is the distance that computers readily allow between the researcher and the information stored and manipulated, easily producing so-called results that do not accord with what the researcher has observed. Researchers may simply enter the information they have collected, decide on a coding strategy to sort the information, and establish an analytic approach to assess relationships in the sorted information. With a few computer keystrokes, an "analysis" is produced. What is missing is the intense scrutiny, pondering, review, and revision that are traditional in anthropology and that give the anthropologist a familiarity with what he or she has observed. Anthropologists must recognize the need to remain close to their information in the course of computer analysis and to use computers as tools to assist data collection and analysis guided by careful thought and experience.

Ethnographic and Other Reports

The format of anthropological reports often differs from that of other disciplines. Anthropology is a book-oriented field. The books that anthropologists produce are called *ethnographies*, a term that refers to both the process and product of fieldwork. Thousands, if not hundreds of thousands, of ethnographies have been written by anthropologists over the past century. These rich descriptions of cultures provide a veritable wealth of information, including about matters of health, sickness, and healing around the globe. Several of the contributors to this book have published such ethnographies.

Ethnographies are often lengthy, generally around 200 pages or more. Thus, they require time and effort to read and absorb. Furthermore, ethnographies may be written in a way that appeals to other anthropologists (e.g., full of jargon and esoteric language, abstract theoretical or methodological discussions, and factual details not clearly relevant to application). Although these characteristics may be efficient, if not necessary, for communication within the discipline of anthropology, they are inappropriate and ineffective in communication with non-anthropologists. In short, ethnographies may not be read outside of anthropology—an obvious obstacle to their effective use.

Increasingly, anthropologists studying public health issues are writing for broader audiences and publishing in peer-reviewed journals that are widely read within public health circles (e.g., *Social Science and Medicine*). Generally, these anthropological publications include descriptions of research objectives, methods used, results or findings obtained, and their implications. The contents, language, and accessibility of such publications are critical determinants of their use and application. Often, such anthropological publications also include recommendations for action or policy.

Integrating Anthropology and Public Health

The objectives of this anthology are to provide examples for public health of how anthropology is useful—even necessary—in public health. Given this conviction, we propose six courses of action to increase the integration of anthropology and public health.

Translating Anthropology into Public Health

Anthropologists are accustomed to communication within their own discipline. As in many other disciplines, much of what is produced is not readily comprehensible to those in other fields, and it is sometimes not clear to anthropologists in other schools or subfields. A major effort in the preparation of this book was the translation of anthropological studies into a language accessible to public health audiences. What would be useful, particularly for anthropologists who apply their scholarship to the solution of social problems, is the development and use of curricula to teach anthropologists how to communicate beyond the discipline. Such a curriculum should emphasize the following:

- Common language and concepts and the avoidance of jargon
- Clear description of methods
- Theoretical exposition focused on solution of the problem at hand
- Ethnographic detail focused on the problem
- Reports organized to clearly indicate the utility of the information provided, theories and methods used, findings, and implications
- Practical conclusions that address solutions to the problem, or that indicate that the problem should not be addressed or that the proposed project will be ineffective or should be revised or abandoned

Integrating Medical Anthropology into Schools of Public Health

Medical anthropology is a discipline of fundamental importance to public health, and as such should be routinely taught in schools of public health. Many schools of public health across the globe have begun to hire faculty with doctoral degrees in medical anthropology and to add medical anthropology courses to their curricula. Many medical anthropology faculty members around the world, including several contributors to this book, are jointly appointed between departments of anthropology and schools of public health. Indeed, one medical anthropologist has already served as the dean of a school of public health, whereas another is a provost. This trend toward integration of medical anthropology into schools of public health is heartening. The first edition of this book has been used in schools of public health around the world, and we imagine that the revised edition will be similarly well received. We hope that it might serve as an introduction to anthropology for public health students, faculty, practitioners, administrators, and policy makers, who will come to see why ethnographic research is invaluable to the understanding of and response to public health problems.

Training Anthropologists in Public Health

Just as public health has much to learn from anthropology, medical anthropology has much to learn from public health, particularly in the areas of epidemiology and biostatistics. Research design tends to be much more rigorous in public health studies than in anthropological ones; anthropologists could learn to strengthen their own research designs and to move beyond single case studies by receiving public health training. Increasingly, doctoral students of medical anthropology are receiving dual degrees in public health. Masters of public health (MPH) degrees in epidemiology and international health have been most popular to date. Receiving such training has made more and more anthropologists aware of the merits of public health approaches, and how anthropology can learn from public health, as well as vice versa. As noted earlier, several of the contributors to this book have received such dual training. Some anthropologists have even gone on to establish their own public health organizations, such as Partners in Health (PIH) (Chapter 21).

Establishing Links among Anthropological and Public Health Organizations

Establishing connections between anthropological and public health professional organizations would help facilitate interaction and integration of the fields. Closer working relations of, for example, the American Anthropological Association (AAA) and its Society for Medical Anthropology (SMA), with the World Health Organization (WHO), the US Centers for Disease Control and Prevention (CDC), the National Institutes of Health (NIH), and the many privately funded public health organizations that work around the world (e.g., the Ford Foundation, the Bill and Melinda Gates Foundation), would facilitate the exchange of relevant perspectives, information, and personnel. Increasingly, anthropologists present their work at the meetings of the American Public Health Association (APHA) and the Global Health Council (GHC). The GHC's official journal, *Global Public Health*, is edited by a medical anthropologist and includes several other anthropologists on its editorial board. Such professional linkages are vital in terms of integrating the two fields.

Employing Anthropologists in Public Health Organizations

Many anthropologists are not employed in academia. Rather, they are *practicing* or *applied medical anthropologists*, who bring their anthropological expertise to nonacademic work settings. In this regard, practicing anthropologists have been consulted and employed by public health agencies for decades. At the CDC, for example, there are more than 40 PhD anthropologists at work on diverse public health matters. Several anthropologists work at the NIH, and many others receive NIH funding for field research projects. Anthropologists also hold program officer positions in many of the major global health organizations, such as WHO, the Ford Foundation, the Population Council, and so on. Self-employed anthropological consultants are paid by agencies to provide expertise on a variety of public health initiatives, especially around HIV/AIDS. Public health agencies need to continue employing practicing medical anthropologists in the new millennium and to see the "value added" by anthropological expertise. Similarly, practicing medical anthropologists need to seek employment in the public health world, demonstrating why they can offer services that are novel and important in the solution of public health problems.

Working in Collaborative, Transdisciplinary Teams

In order for anthropologists to work in the world of public health, they need to embrace the concept of collaboration. As a discipline, anthropology has reveled in the solitary pursuit of knowledge, with lone ethnographers "going solo" into the field. However, public health projects usually rely on teamwork, with multiple investigators bringing their expertise to the solution of a common problem. Anthropologists who hope to work in public health need to value collaboration and the merits of multidisciplinarity. Increasingly, the term *transdisciplinarity* is being employed to emphasize the truly transactional and boundary-crossing nature of interdisciplinary collaborations that provide more than just the sum of their parts. Anthropology has much to offer to such transdisciplinary efforts to solve public health problems. Indeed, in the new millennium, medical anthropology may well make its most significant contributions "at the intersections" of other fields, including the field of global public health (Inhorn 2007). But to do so, anthropologists must be willing to move beyond the solo model of research, to turn intellectual curiosities outward beyond the field of anthropology, and to embrace the spirit of interdisciplinary dialogue and collaboration with openness and candor. Through such boundary crossings, anthropology can perhaps make its greatest contributions to the world in which we live.

This book represents one such attempt at boundary crossing. The book highlights four ways in which anthropology can contribute to public health: through anthropological understanding of public health problems, through anthropological design of public health interventions, through anthropological evaluation of public health initiatives, and through anthropological critiques of public health policies. A range of public health problems in a wide variety of geographic settings are highlighted to showcase the breadth and depth of anthropological contributions to the field of public health. HIV/AIDS receives special attention, given its pandemic status. However, many other issues of vital importance to public health in the twenty-first century are covered in this book. Ethnographic methods are spelled out in detail, and ethnographic findings are richly described. The stories of real lives found throughout most chapters, as well as the fieldwork photos, serve to humanize the accounts and to remind us of the unalleviated suffering caused by public health problems in many parts of the world. Alleviation of such suffering seems a worthy goal for the new millennium. In this respect, anthropology and public health are united by their common compassion.

Notes

1. The conclusions in this report are those of the authors and do not necessarily represent the views of the Centers for Disease Control and Prevention.

2. Biomedicine is distinguished from public health in its focus on pathology in individual patients and its orientation toward laboratory science and clinical practice (Hahn 1995). Public health focuses on the pathology and health of populations; it builds on biomedicine but examines a broader array of causes.

3. The DALY is a measure of disease burden that takes into account not only death from specific causes, but also the youthfulness of the decedent and the sickness, disability, and suffering associated with these causes.

4. The Code of Ethics is available on the Internet at www.aaanet.org/committees/ethics/ethcode.htm

References

Agar MH (1980) *The Professional Stranger. An Informal Introduction to Ethnography.* New York: Academic Press.

American Anthropological Association (1998) Code of Ethics of the American Anthropological Association, www.anthronet.org

Bernard HR (2005) *Research Methods in Anthropology. Qualitative and Quantitative Approaches*, 4th ed. Walnut Grove, CA: AltaMira.

Cargo M, Mercer S (2008) The value and challenges of participatory research: Strengthening its practice. *Annual Review of Public Health* 29:325–351.

Centers for Disease Control and Prevention (CDC) (1999) Ten Great Public Health Achievements—United States, 1900–1999. *MMWR* 48(12):241–243.

Dirks NB, Eley G, Ortner SB, eds. (1994) *Culture/Power/History. A Reader in Contemporary Social Theory.* Princeton, NJ: Princeton University Press.

Doyal L (1995) *What Makes Women Sick.* New Brunswick, NJ: Rutgers University Press.

Farmer P (2003) *Pathologies of Power: Health, Human Rights, and the New War on the Poor.* Berkeley, CA: University of California Press.

Farmer P (2004) Sidney W. Mintz Lecture for 2001: An anthropology of structural violence. *Current Anthropology* 45:305–325.

Fetterman DM (1998) *Ethnography. Step by Step*, 2nd ed. Thousand Oaks, CA: Sage Publications.

Ghobarah HA, Huth P, Russett B (2004) The post-war public health effects of civil conflict. *Social Science and Medicine* 59:869–884.

Hahn RA (1995) *Sickness and Healing. An Anthropological Perspective.* New Haven, CT: Yale University Press.

Inhorn MC (1995) Medical anthropology and epidemiology: Divergences or convergences? *Social Science and Medicine* 40:285–290.

Inhorn MC (2007) Medical anthropology at the intersections. *Medical Anthropology Quarterly* 21(3):249–255.

Kleinman (1989) *The Illness Narratives: Suffering, Healing, and the Human Condition.* New York: Basic Books.

Kleinman (1996) *Writing at the Margin: Discourse Between Anthropology and Medicine.* Berkeley, CA: University of California Press.

Krueger RA (1994) *Focus Groups: A Practical Guide for Applied Research.* Newbury Park, CA: Sage Publications.

Murray CJL, Kreuser J, Whang W (1994) Cost-effectiveness analysis and policy choices: investing in health systems. *Bulletin of the World Health Organization* 72:181–192.

Ortner SB (1994) "Theory in Anthropology Since the Sixties." In: *Culture/Power/History: A Reader in Contemporary Social Theory.* NB Dirks, G Eley, and SB Ortner, eds. Princeton, NJ: Princeton University Press, pp. 372–411. [Reprinted from *Comparative Studies in Society and History* (26):126–166.]

Pelto PJ, Pelto GH (1997) Studying knowledge, culture, and behavior in applied medical anthropology. *Medical Anthropology Quarterly* 11:147–163.

Scrimshaw NS, Gleason GR, eds. (1992) *RAP. Rapid Assessment Procedures: Qualitative Methodologies for Planning and Evaluation of Health Related Programmes.* Boston: International Nutrition Foundation for Developing Countries.

Scrimshaw SCM, Hurtado E (1987) *Rapid Assessment Procedures for Nutrition and Primary Health Care: Anthropological Approaches to Improving Programme Effectiveness.* Los Angeles: University of California, Latin American Center Publications.

Spradley JP (1979) *The Ethnographic Interview.* New York: Holt, Rinehart and Winston.

Trostle JA (2005) *Epidemiology and Culture.* Cambridge, UK: Cambridge University Press.

Trostle JA, Sommerfeld J (1996) Medical anthropology and epidemiology. *Annual Review of Anthropology* 25:253–274.

UNHCR (United Nations High Commission on Refugees) (2008) www.unhcr.org

Weitzman EA, Miles MB (1995) *Computer Programs for Qualitative Data Analysis.* Thousand Oaks, CA: Sage Publications.

World Bank (2007) http://econ.worldbank.org

World Health Organization (2000) www.who.int

World Health Organization (2001) *Women and the tobacco epidemic.* Canada: WHO.

Part I

ANTHROPOLOGICAL
UNDERSTANDINGS OF PUBLIC
HEALTH PROBLEMS

1

The Anthropology of Childhood Malaria in Tanzania

VINAY R. KAMAT

Introduction: Nature and Magnitude of Childhood Malaria

Malaria is an infectious disease transmitted by the bite of a female *Anopheles* mosquito, which acts as the vector for the disease.[1] Malaria affects some 300 to 500 million people worldwide. It is a leading cause of mortality and morbidity, with an estimated 1.5 to 2.7 million deaths per year. Ninety percent of these deaths occur in sub-Saharan Africa, mostly among children under the age of 5 (Kager 2002; Korenromp, Williams, Gouws, Dye, and Snow 2003; Nchinda 1998; Snow, Guerra, Noor, Myint, and Hay 2005; WHO 1994).[2] Fewer than 20% of these febrile episodes and deaths come to the attention of any formal health system, and the relatively few ill patients who have any contact with the health services represent the "ears of the hippopotamus" (see Breman 2001). In sub-Saharan Africa, malaria is responsible for approximately 40% of public health expenditure, 30% to 50% of inpatient admissions, and up to 50% of outpatient visits in places where malaria transmission is intense (Hay, Guerra, Tatem, Atkinson, and Snow 2005:81). In 2001, malaria was ranked the eighth highest contributor to the global Disability Adjusted Life Years (DALY) and second in Africa (Snow, Korenromp, and Gouws 2004; WHO 2002).

At present there is no effective vaccine to prevent malaria. However, relatively simple and effective preventive measures such as insecticide-treated nets (ITNs) and Intermittent Presumptive Treatment for pregnant women (IPTp) and treatments such as artemisinin-based combination therapy (ACT), derived from the herb *Artemisia annua*, do exist (see Barnes and Folb 2003; Bloland 2003; Bloland, Kachur, and Williams 2003; Kachur et al. 2004; Whitty 2004). Simply put, malaria is an avoidable infection and a curable disease, and the deaths it causes are preventable through simple, effective public health intervention strategies. Yet, the absolute numbers of malaria cases in sub-Saharan Africa are on the rise. More children die from malaria nowadays than they did 40 years ago (see Guerin et al. 2002:564; Malowany 2000; Snow, Trape, and Marsh 2001). Although the World Health Organization made a clear pledge in 1998 to halve deaths from malaria by 2010—a pledge that African heads of state endorsed at The African Summit on Roll Back Malaria held in Abuja, Nigeria in April 2000 it has yet to make much progress (see Alnwick 2000; Attaran 2004:932–993; Attaran and Barnes 2004; WHO 2000).

There are several reasons why malaria still persists as one of the "grand challenges" in global health. First, the majority of malarial infections in sub-Saharan Africa are caused by *Plasmodium falciparum*, which is the most virulent and therefore the deadliest of the four human malaria parasites. Second, the mosquito *Anopheles gambiae*, which is the main malaria vector, is widespread in Africa and is one of the most difficult vectors to control. Third, the increasing resistance of the malaria parasite to a range of antimalarials—especially chloroquine and sulfadoxine–pyrimethamine—has directly contributed to the rise in malaria-related mortality in sub-Saharan Africa (Plowe 2003; Snow, Craig, Deichmann, and Marsh 1999; Snow et al. 2001; White 2004). Finally, as with most vector-borne infectious disease, malaria is a disease of poverty and affects mostly the poor and marginalized people in poor countries (see Barat et al. 2004; Sachs and Melaney 2002; Worrall, Basu, and Hanson 2005).

There are numerous reasons why malaria-related deaths occur mostly among young children. First, malaria often occurs as an overwhelming acute infection in young children. In many cases, malaria manifests as seizure or coma (so-called "pure" cerebral malaria)[3] and may kill a child in as little time as 2 days (Greenwood et al. 1987; Maitland and Marsh 2004). Thus, mortality from severe malaria remains high among young children even when effective drugs are used in the best facilities. Patients and caretakers often arrive at health centers with their febrile children in an advanced state of disease that cannot be reversed by any form of antimalarial and/or ancillary therapies (Guerin et al. 2002:568). As Maitland and Marsh (2004:131) have recently documented in Kenya, most deaths in children admitted to hospital with severe malaria occur within the first 24 hours of admission. This implies that the majority of children die of the complications of severe malaria before they can benefit from the full effects of quinine—a powerful antimalarial that is generally administered intravenously. In other words, it is the delay in receiving adequate treatment that kills many people, especially children with malaria. With prompt diagnosis and medicinal treatment, most cases of malaria are entirely curable (Whitty et al. 2004). Second, repeated malaria infections contribute to the development of severe anemia compounding further the risk of death (Caulfield 2004; Crawley 2004; Premji et al. 1995). Third, low birth weight, frequently the consequence of malaria infection in pregnant women, is a major risk factor for newborn infants (see Anonymous—Africa Malaria Report 2003).

Faced with the enormous complexity of the problem of malaria in sub-Saharan Africa, there is a consensus among malaria researchers and health policy makers that prompt and effective treatment is probably one of the most cost-effective elements of malaria control (Guerin et al. 2002:567). Taking into consideration all these factors, the World Health Organization has reemphasized the importance of early diagnosis and effective biomedical treatment as one of the key factors in preventing high levels of malaria-related deaths in sub-Saharan Africa (WHO 2005).

The Anthropology of Childhood Malaria in Tanzania

This chapter provides an anthropological perspective on childhood malaria in Tanzania. It illustrates how examining the problem of childhood malaria from an ethnographic perspective can provide the contextual knowledge that traditional epidemiological research often fails to capture. The chapter focuses specifically on the question of why some mothers and caretakers delay in seeking early diagnosis and treatment at public health facilities for their young, febrile children. These understandings include insights into the local knowledge of malaria, including the perceived etiology, the language of illness/terminology used to describe "malaria" and also evidence-based policies aimed at reducing the burden of malaria.[4] It also offers a more detailed knowledge of cultural perceptions of malaria, which enables us to understand, among other things, the *logic* that underlies health and treatment-seeking behavior. As Helitzer-Allen, Kendall, and Wirima (1993:270–283) have noted:

> In order to assist the community in selecting and designing appropriate and potentially successful control programs, it is necessary to understand the context of the disease in the community. This context includes community characteristics, the community perception of the nature and etiology of the illness and its symptoms, and health seeking behavior for prevention and treatment, including the use of traditional and cosmopolitan medications....Programs which take local concerns into account are more likely to be successful (and sustainable) than those that adopt a simple strategy of providing information.

There are several methods or "tools" of data collection that one can employ to provide contextual insights into the nature of malaria in a given community. For example, one can draw up a taxonomy of illness terminology. Examining discourse also provides a conduit to understanding aspects of a community's health culture (Quinn 2005). As Hill (2005:159) points out, "discourse—the production of the talk and texts that are the vehicles of so much human interaction—is the most important place where culture is both enacted and produced in the moment of interaction." Further, documenting and analyzing stories told by mothers with young febrile children and eliciting illness narratives about children's sickness is important for designing and implementing successful community-based malaria control programs.

The chapter examines the complexities surrounding the process of treatment seeking for acute febrile illness among children under the age of 5 in a large periurban village on the outskirts of Dar es Salaam. The chapter draws on data from a larger ethnographic study of the impact of health sector privatization on health care seeking in post-socialist Tanzania (Kamat 2004). By drawing upon ethnographic examples, excerpts from illness narrative interviews, case materials and quantitative data, this chapter provides a more textured understanding of caretakers' treatment seeking for their young, febrile children. After discussing the research setting and methods, the chapter elaborates on the local cultural models of fever[5] and some of the reasons for treatment delays. The way mothers report symptoms to health care personnel in order to obtain the best available treatment for their sick children is highlighted. Excerpts from narrative interviews are presented to draw attention to the travails that mothers face in their efforts to deal with children's sickness and their search for therapy for febrile children. These contextualized stories and excerpts highlight how health care seeking surrounding childhood febrile illnesses is often affected by a multiplicity of factors—cultural meanings associated with certain illnesses, perceived severity and past experience with an illness, structural disadvantages affecting women's access to societal resources, unexpected circumstances, and the patterns of communication between patients/caretakers and health care providers in government health facilities.

Case studies are presented to illustrate the pragmatic considerations that inform mothers' negotiation of appropriate therapy for their febrile children in a medically pluralistic setting. The chapter concludes by calling attention to the role ethnographic research can play in highlighting the contextual factors and sociocultural dynamics at the household and clinical levels that influence patterns of treatment seeking and treatment negotiation for childhood malaria as a means to improve community-based health interventions to increase child survival.

Ecological Context of Malaria in Tanzania

More than a decade after its decision to liberalize the economy, Tanzania, with a population of 36 million, remains one of the world's poorest nations with a per capita GDP of $457 and a per capita income of $280 per year (Sanders 2001). This grim level of poverty coupled with an inadequate health infrastructure often translates into excessive childhood illnesses, especially malaria-related deaths. In Tanzania, morbidity and mortality rates, as well as rates of life-threatening infectious diseases, are exceedingly high (see Ministry of Health, United Republic of Tanzania 1997; Setel 1999). In 2002, for example, the infant mortality rate was 77.85 deaths per 1000 live births and the maternal mortality rate was 550 deaths per 100,000 live births. Each year, of the 100,000 to 125,000 people who die from the malaria and related complications, an estimated 70,000 to 80,000 are children under the age of 5. Malaria is the leading cause of deaths among hospitalized people, and it is also the main reason for admission of children younger than 5 years at medical facilities (MOH, Government of Tanzania 2003).

Dar es Salaam, the third fastest growing city in Africa, is Tanzania's commercial capital and the largest major urban center in the country. Its population is increasing at a rate of 4.39% each year. The current population is estimated at 3 million, and the metropolitan area population is expected to reach 5.12 million people by 2020. It hosts a major port on the Indian Ocean and comprises three independently governed municipalities—Kinondoni, Ilala, and Temeke. The Dar es Salaam region is characterized by a hot and humid tropical climate and two rainy seasons. Malaria is endemic and transmission occurs throughout the year. Malaria transmission is more intense in the periurban and rural areas of Dar es Salaam than it is in the urban areas. The deadly *Plasmodium falciparum* is the predominant malaria parasite, accounting for 90% of all cases. It is primarily transmitted by *Anopheles gambiae* and *Anopheles funestus*. The majority of people in Dar es Salaam perceive malaria (or *homa ya malaria*) as a very common illness (Stephens et al. 1995). Over the last 20 years or so, major public health interventions have been implemented in the Dar es Salaam region to control malaria. However, malaria remains the single most common clinical diagnosis at health facilities in the municipalities of this region (Kachur, Black, Abdulla, and Goodman 2006; Wang et al. 2006).

Reliable epidemiological data on morbidity and mortality due to malaria in Dar es Salaam are difficult to obtain. While some sources have estimated that as many as 1 million cases of malaria are reported at public health facilities in this region each year, others have argued that this could be an overestimation. There are important implications for the management of severe febrile illness, including the unnecessary treatment and consequent neglect of alternative diagnoses that could lead to avoidable morbidity and mortality (see de Castro et al. 2004; Wang et al. 2006; Whitty et al. 2004).[6] Notwithstanding the deliberations surrounding the exact number of malaria cases, the fact remains that more than two-thirds of malaria-attributable febrile illnesses are dealt with outside of the formal medical system. These cases are frequently unrecorded in the official vital statistics on morbidity and mortality due to malaria (see Williams and Jones 2004). Ethnographically grounded studies are often able to capture some of the "missing" cases of malaria as well as malaria-related childhood deaths that would otherwise go undocumented (see de Savigny et al. 2004; Setel, Whiting, Hemed, and Chandramohan 2006).

Fieldwork Setting and Methodology

Mbande,[7] the periurban village where I conducted 16 months of continuous fieldwork, has a population of about 5500 people and is located on the periphery of Chamazi Ward of Temeke District, Dar es Salaam. Mbande village came into being in 1974 during *Operation Vijijini*. As a state-designated registered *Ujamaa* (familyhood) village, Mbande's history is about three decades old. The people of this village share a common history with hundreds of other villages that were started during the *Operation* through the agglomeration of individual households into larger units. During the *Operation* people from all over Tanzania were moved, often under force, from their original settlements to start new villages or to merge with existing/neighboring larger villages. The villagization program involved the largest number of people in the history of African resettlements, relocating between 5 and 9 million rural Tanzanians (see Freyhold 1979).

Oral histories do not suggest that coercion and distress on a scale documented by researchers in the 1970s (Boesen, Madsen, and Moody 1977; Freyhold 1979; Hyden 1980; McHenry 1979) and further theorized by Scott (1999) in his book *Seeing Like a State* was part of people's resettlement and rehabilitation experience. This could be partly explained by the fact that between 1973 and 1974 there were fewer than 150 people living in and around what is now Mbande village. In fact, many still lived on their family farm (*shamba*) in the fertile valley nearby. One of the local leaders used his influence with the government bureaucrats and worked hard to unite the local people to avoid being amalgamated with one of the already existing larger villages. The district authorities yielded to the villagers' perseverance to subsist as a separate entity. Thus, the development of Mbande village began in earnest.

Clusters of houses in the village are locally referred to as the *sehemu ya Wamakonde* (the area of *Wamakonde*), the *Wamatumbi* area, the *Wamgindo* area, and so forth. These clusters of houses refer to areas where households from certain ethnic groups (*makabila*) settled down together in the village during the *Operation*. The completion of an all-weather road in 1996 marked the beginning of a new wave of migrants into the village, mostly from Northwestern Tanzania. The Sukuma and Nyamwezi youth quickly built a reputation for being extremely hard working and improved their economic situation in a very short period through the cultivation of okra and the selling of produce for a good price. The road facilitated the rapid transportation of people and goods between the village and the city. One of the important consequences of this ready accessibility to the village has been the increase in demand for land. Many people in Mbande are selling portions of their agricultural land to migrants from other parts of Tanzania—a trend that is intensified by the overall political and economic changes taking place in a country in an era of economic liberalization. The increased commoditization of village land witnessed in Mbande is similar to what scholars have reported from other places in Tanzania (see Askew 2006; Swantz 1995).

Of the 95% of the local residents who are Muslims, 40% identify themselves as Zaramo, the original inhabitants of Dar es Salaam (Swantz 1995; Tripp 1997). Subsistence-oriented farming is the economic base for the majority of the local people, while a small proportion of villagers engage in small business ventures such as the selling of *chapatis*, tea, fruits, fish, and vegetables in the marketplace. For most, cash income is scarce—the average per capita, per month cash income in the village is approximately TShillings 1475 (<$2).[8] The local health arena is pluralistic as villagers have access to "traditional" Swahili medicine as well as biomedicine and pharmaceuticals, provided that they can pay for therapy. Located 5 minutes away from the main marketplace is a municipal dispensary (*zahanati*) staffed by an experienced medical officer and three nurses, two of whom are Mother and Child Health specialists and an auxiliary trainee nurse. Although the practice of charging a fee is in place at the dispensary, patients, especially children, are rarely refused treatment even if they are unable to pay the required fees. In general, the dispensary is well equipped, but it does not have any field extension services. The health staffs are not trained in the Integrated Management of Childhood Illnesses (IMCI) (for details see Schellenberg et al. 2004).[9] Patients are occasionally referred to the Temeke district hospital, which is located some 20 km from the village. Each year, more than 1000 cases of fever, excluding those diagnosed with acute respiratory illness (ARI), are treated at the dispensary. Nearly all the cases are clinically diagnosed without the aid of a microscope. In most cases, mothers arrive at the dispensary 48 to 72 hours after they have first noticed that their child had a fever. Also within the village are three privately owned pharmacies. These are operated by unqualified pharmacists who sell a range of medicines across the counter, including antimalarials and antibiotics. There are four known "traditional healers" (*mganga*, plural *waganga*) who reside in the village. Only one of them, Mzee Tinyango, who is in his mid-80s, practices on a full-time basis from his home. On average, he attends to five to eight patients a week, many of whom come from distant places (see Kamat 2008a for details).

Methods

I conducted most of my ethnographic activities in Mbande, the main village, and eight surrounding hamlets. However, during the first few weeks of my research I also conducted fieldwork in three other villages—Charambe, Maji Matitu, and Chamazi—located along a 14-km all-weather road that connects Mbande with the large town Mbagala. I used a combination of ethnographic methods to gather data for this study—participant observation, key informant interviewing, oral life history interviews, illness narrative interviews, focus group discussions, a household census and a household socioeconomic and health survey. With the help of Mzee Ali, my research assistant who lived in Mbande, I elicited detailed oral life histories of 25 elderly people. This exercise enabled me to document the history and characteristics of the village within its larger regional, historical context. Further, with the help of a female research assistant, Mariam, I interviewed 45 mothers of young children who were diagnosed with severe malaria at the local dispensary. All of the interviews were conducted in Kiswahili. I also conducted a census in four sectors of the village, covering 354 households, and yielding a total population of 1513 inhabitants. A total of 116 of the households had at least one child of 5 years and younger. The heads of these 116 households were interviewed for the household socioeconomic and health survey, using a semi-structured interview schedule. I also participated in the everyday lives of the local people and built extensive contacts with them. I participated in various social and religious events, including a wedding ceremony and a *ngoma* dance, and was an observer at religious ceremonies. As a participant observer, I shared meals with the local people, listened to their stories, documented various ceremonies, and often sat down on a straw mattress for many hours with elderly people, catching up with local happenings and listening to their conversations.

This chapter draws mainly on direct participant observation data and illness narrative interviews with 45 mothers. Also briefly included are data from the household socioeconomic and health survey (n = 116). The 45 mothers were initially recruited at the local dispensary. To contextualize the interview data better, all in-depth interviews were conducted in the mothers' homes. At least half of them were interviewed twice to elicit additional details about their life histories. In-depth interviews, which lasted between 50 and 90 minutes, were audio-recorded, transcribed verbatim in Kiswahili by two research assistants, and later translated into English for analysis. The text data from the ethnographic interviews were processed using Microsoft Word® to do a line-by-line discourse analysis (see Hill 2005). Census and household survey data gathered as part of the larger study were processed using the software SPSS version 10.5 for Windows. Notes from my field diary were elaborated and incorporated into the analysis.

Cultural Models of Fever and Treatment Delays

Most malaria researchers and health policy makers agree on one thing about malaria in sub-Saharan Africa—that large numbers of children who are affected with malaria die each year because they do not get prompt medical attention. Therefore, the World Health Organization's primary strategy to reduce the high numbers of malaria-related mortalities especially in sub-Saharan Africa is to convince caretakers of young children with febrile illness to bring the child to a medical facility within 24 hours after first noticing any of the key symptoms of malaria—high fever, vomiting, malaise, and, occasionally, convulsions. One problem that stands out in this regard is that many caretakers do not recognize some of the key symptoms of malaria as indicative of malaria. Even when they do, in many cases, caretakers do not readily recognize the seriousness of these symptoms in their sick children. They treat these symptoms as indicative of an ordinary illness (*homa ya kawaida*) rather than of a life-threatening illness. In Mbande, for example, interviews with 45 mothers who had brought their febrile children to the local dispensary revealed that most of them had delayed bringing their children to the dispensary by at least 48 hours after the recognition of fever. Some mothers had waited for nearly a week before deciding to bring their feverish child to the dispensary. Mothers typically explained the delay by saying that they thought it was only "ordinary fever."

During follow-up interviews with these mothers in their homes a week or so after they had agreed to participate in this study, many mothers said that they were in fact very surprised when they found out that what they thought was ordinary fever had suddenly turned into a strong fever (*homa kali*) or malaria (*homa ya malaria*). They said this regardless of the fact that many of the mothers had dealt with several fever and malarial episodes on previous occasions either of the index child or their other children. In other words, past experience with a malaria episode did not necessarily lead mothers to initiate more prompt action during subsequent episodes. This has important implications not only for the kinds of assumptions on which malaria-related health education messages are based, but also for the quality of communication that takes places between providers of health care and parents/caretakers of febrile children. In a small number of cases, mothers explained that *homa kali* had dramatically turned into *degedege*, the indigenous name for a much feared life-threatening illness that in many cases people do not associate with malarial fever. From a biomedical perspective, however, the cultural representations of *degedege* resemble the characteristic features of cerebral malaria, which is a type or stage of malarial infection that kills a majority of young children (see Maitland and Marsh 2004; Winch et al. 1996).

Folk Etiology of Degedege

The Kiswahili word *degedege* literally translates into English as "bird bird." In coastal Tanzania, among the Zaramo people in particular, the illness is believed to be caused by a coastal spirit (*mdudu shetani*) that takes the form of a bird that casts its shadow on vulnerable children on moonlit nights. Children who come under the bird's shadow subsequently become seriously ill, develop convulsions, and in many cases succumb to the illness and die (see Kamat 2006; for variations in cultural explanations, see also Comoro, Nismba, Warsame, and Tomson 2003; Gessler et al. 1995; Hausmann-Muela, Ribera, Mushi, and Tanner 2002; Makemba et al. 1996; Tarimo, Lwihula, Minja, and Bygbjerg 2000; Winch et al. 1996; Winch 1999).

In the dominant local cultural model of fever, if *homa ya kawaida* is left untreated, it may lead to *homa kali*, which in turn, if untreated, may lead to *homa ya malaria*. Finally, if malarial fever is not successfully treated, it may lead to *degedege*—although some informants said that *degedege* is a distinct illness with an etiology that is not related to malaria (Figure 1.1). They believed that the illness is not an advanced stage of malarial infection but an illness that is caused by "spirits." While most mothers I interviewed shared the cultural understandings of the etiology of *degedege*, there was considerable variability and flexibility in how they interpreted the taxonomy of fevers and the trajectory of the illness or the "ultimate" cause of the illness.

Significantly, more than one-third of the mothers interviewed for this study had never witnessed a child suffering from *degedege*. Furthermore, only another one-third of the mothers reported that they had dealt with an episode of *degedege* in the past. Yet, more than two-thirds of the mothers were confident that if they were presented with a situation of fever-inducing

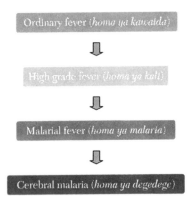

Figure 1.1. Illness taxonomy and the logic of illness transformation. Homa (fever) is a polysemic i.e., many–meaning term.

illnesses, they would certainly be able to distinguish *degedege* from other serious conditions. Despite this assuredness, many mothers who were interviewed had gained information about *degedege* in the form of "second-hand episodes" without having personally experienced the event, that is, by listening to stories about *degedege* episodes told by friends and neighbors (Price 1987). In other cases, while the illness label remained unchanged (e.g., *homa kali*), changes in perception of severity through visible symptoms or the failure of a home-based treatment greatly influenced the mothers' health care response.

Although the perceived severity of the symptoms was one of the key factors in the mother's decision to bring the child to the dispensary, an equally important factor that acted as a "prompt" for mothers to rush their child to the dispensary was the realization that "home treatment" had failed. Home treatment typically involved giving the child Panadol®, an antipyretic or a leftover dose of an antimalarial. Just as the way illness understandings may change through time, the subsequent treatment options that are pursued to treat the illness also change. Diagnoses and interpretations change in response to different outcomes of a range of attempts at treatment—either simultaneously or sequentially (see Amuyunzu-Nyamongo and Nyamongo 2006; Hausmann-Muela, Ribera, and Tanner 1998; Hunt, Jordan, and Irwin 1989; Nyamongo 2002).

In Mbande, people consider "bad luck" or "God's will" to render particular children to be more vulnerable than others to *degedege*. Thus, when asked why some children are more prone to contracting *degedege* than others, the majority of the people in the village responded that it was just "God's wish" or "God's work" (*kazi ya mungu*) and that it was not due to witchcraft (*uchawi*), sorcery (*kurogwa*), or someone's evil actions. This etiological belief significantly influences their acceptance of the fatal outcomes of the illness. Interviews with key informants and with local *waganga* who are known for their expertise in diagnosing and treating cases of *degedege* suggested that there is a general agreement that the illness is caused by a "spirit bird." However, a close analysis of audio-taped interviews with elderly people revealed that the information they provided varied greatly in terms of the details on the etiology, symptoms, susceptibility, treatment modality, and preventive measures for *degedege*. While elderly informants spoke with an element of confidence about the illness, younger informants, especially young mothers, spoke of *degedege* in terms of what they had gleaned by word of mouth. They stated that they had heard about *degedege* from others and knew that it was a dangerous illness that can strike any child without warning. In fact, they had not seen it or experienced it, but they knew definitively what it was, based on what they had learned from second-hand episodes.

Indigenous Therapy for Degedege. Elderly people in Mbande affirmed that the traditional therapy for *degedege* had significantly changed over the years. They attributed this change mainly to the greater presence of biomedicine in their lives, especially following the dramatic increase in the number of private health facilities in Dar es Salaam. Even so, several elders gave graphic accounts of the practice where, upon noticing the first signs of the illness (convulsions), a mother would rush the child to a latrine (*choo*). There, the child would be laid on a banana leaf and washed with the mother's urine. The smell of urine is believed to repel the spirit in possession of the child's body, at which point the child would likely stop convulsing. It is only after this stage that the child is taken to a *mganga* for treatment, who normally checks the patient carefully before prescribing medicinal bathing herbs. While some *waganga* simply use knowledge from previous experience in treating *degedege* patients, others resort to divination or *ramli* (Swahili from the Arabic Khatt-ar-raml), a system of divination by calculation and examination of Arabic books, which is widespread in East Africa (see Whyte 1997:64). The *mganga* may also use herbal medicines. Some medicinal leaves are rubbed on the patient's legs and often on the whole body, while some others are boiled and the decoction is given to the patient to drink. The patient usually rests for a few minutes and then passes urine or defecates. If the patient does either of these, it is concluded that the patient is on the way to recovery. If not, the patient is still in danger of dying.

Depending upon the patient's condition, the *mganga* may treat the patient for 3 to 4 days or until he/she has completely recovered. If a patient recovers, he/she is permitted to return home with her parents and no further treatment is recommended. The parents may then pay the *mganga* his fees or they will pay at a later date if the *mganga* is flexible. In case the parents are not satisfied with the treatment, they may decide to take the patient to another *mganga* in the hope that a different healer may offer more effective options. For example, they may go to a *mwalimu ya Quarani*, a traditional healer who uses *kombe*, a drinkable medicine. If all else fails, parents may even decide to take the child to a public or private hospital. If treatment at the hospital also fails, then the outcome is commonly described as "the patient's fate or predicament" (*bahati ya mtu*); there was little that anyone could have done to save the child from dying. Most people in Mbande said that they were unaware of any particular medicine or any specific procedure that could protect a child from getting *degedege*.

Importantly, however, in Mbande, people who believe that their child is suffering from traditional or Swahili illnesses such as *degedege* do not necessarily consult a *mganga* as a first resort, but instead may proactively seek help from a biomedical health facility (see also Comoro et al. 2003; de Savigny et al. 2004). Under particularly severe conditions, however, their efforts are constrained by the lack of easy and timely access to such facilities. As a consequence, many parents seek out *waganga* as an alternative to a biomedical facility because they are available for consultation at convenient hours, and because they provide treatment, consolation, and flexibility in the payment of fees. Many parents or caretakers of children who have developed high fevers do not simply follow a linear trajectory in their search for therapy based on some widely shared cultural model. Instead, despite the fact that cultural knowledge (including etiological beliefs) about *degedege* may be shared locally, there is a striking degree of variation in the therapeutic pathways that parents follow to deal with an *actual* episode of the illness (see Kamat 2008b for details).

Degedege and Injections: Objects of Ambivalence. In Mbande, injections are popular with mothers who bring their children into the dispensary for treatment. Most mothers were happy when the doctor or one of the nurses recommended an injection for their child, because in most cases the initial effect of the injection is indeed dramatic. During the entire course of my participant observation at the dispensary, not one mother or patient refused an injection. Thus, the decision whether to give an injection or not to a sick child was entirely up to the doctor or the nurse. Even if a mother told the nurse that she did not have the money to pay for the cost of the injection, it was at the nurse's discretion whether to go ahead and give the injection, or withhold it from the patient because of her inability to pay the nominal fees. However, what concerned most mothers were not prescriptions that entailed the injection, but a diagnosis that required the mother to return with her sick child to the dispensary for an additional four to five injections; this automatically escalated the cost of treatment, in addition to the trouble of having to travel to and from the dispensary. This factor had serious implications for treatment adherence and follow-up.

In examining people's beliefs about injections and treatment seeking for *degedege* in Kibaha district, Tarimo et al. (2000:182) found that "in a sample of 1492 mothers, 76.3% of the mothers held the belief that an injection in a child with high fever would either precipitate convulsions or cause death." Similarly, Makemba et al. (1996:312) have also reported that in their Bagamoyo study, parents were unanimous in their conviction that treating *degedege* with an injection results in the death of the child. In the present case, however, of the 45 mothers who were asked whether they would allow their child to be given an injection at the dispensary if their child was convulsing, the majority (58%) said that they would not object if the doctor or the nurse at the dispensary decided on an injection. However, 27% said that they would refuse. Interestingly, 15% said that they might refuse an injection at first, but would eventually accept if the doctor or the nurse insisted. As Hawa, a 21-year-old mother of three children, explained, "I believe that an injection will only aggravate my child's condition if he has *degedege*, but they [dispensary staff] are the experts [*watalam*]; they know what is best for my child. After all, what I want is that my child should get well."

Given the asymmetrical power relations between the dispensary staff and the patients, sentiments such as those expressed by Hawa shed important light on the context of social relations at the site of the dispensary. The question is whether or not mothers of young children are in a position to exercise agency in order to determine the course of treatment once the dispensary staff have made their authoritative decision. Of the 19 mothers in the study sample who said that they would initially refuse an injection for their child, two-thirds said that they had heard that if a child who has *degedege* is given an injection, the illness (fever) tends to worsen and the child eventually dies. The other 37% said that they would refuse the injection because they had heard from the elders in the family and the neighborhood that an injection is not an appropriate therapy for *degedege*, as it can bring bad luck and it can cause the child to die (*anapoteza maisha*). Two mothers were unsure of their response if they were faced with a situation where their child had *degedege* and the doctor or the nurse had decided on an injection. As Fatuma, a mother of two young children, explained:

> I will refuse the injection because neither I nor my children have experienced *degedege*. I have not seen any person having *degedege* either. So I don't even know what the symptoms of *degedege* are. I've only heard about it and they (the experts – *watalam*) say that an injection is not good for this illness; the child could die. There are others who say that an injection is good. I haven't asked anyone in particular why exactly a child who is suffering from *degedege* should not be given an injection. But still, I'm afraid because people say that an injection is not good for treatment of *degedege*. However, if the child dies, then it's God's plan because it's not possible to give birth to ten children and expect all of them to survive – some will die, and some will survive.

Notwithstanding the beliefs and convictions that mothers expressed with regard to the use of an injection in the treatment of *degedege*, I did not witness a single instance where a mother offered resistance to the nurse's decision to administer an injection to the sick child. Once inside the dispensary's arena, mothers had little choice but to defer to the staff the communicative privileges and the right to decide on the treatment modality by the dispensary staff. For the mothers to question the authority of the medical personnel, they needed a position from which they could negotiate the right to ask questions (see Ainsworth-Vaughn 1998; Mishler 1984, 1991, 1995; Wilce 1997).

Inevitability of Sickness Among Children

During the recruitment phase and initial conversations with mothers who were attending the local dispensary with their sick children, two things struck me the most. First, mothers commonly spoke of their children's illness as "routine" (*kawaida tu*). Illness is something they have come to live with as part of their everyday life and the praxis of raising children in a rapidly changing health and social environment. Second, nearly all the mothers I conversed with had come to the dispensary without the accompaniment of a family member or a member of their social network. Only occasionally were they accompanied by a friend or a neighbor who had also brought her child to the dispensary for diagnosis and treatment of an illness. Men were rarely seen at the dispensary with their sick children. Put simply, children's sickness is predominantly a woman's domain, and this has serious implications for how malaria control interventions are planned and implemented, whom they are directed at, and whether gender is given a prominent role while conceiving intervention programs (see Vlassoff and Manderson 1998; Tanner and Vlassoff 1998). The following story of Amina, whom I met the first time at the local dispensary, captures the essence of this phenomenon—the "ordinariness" of childhood febrile illnesses and the practice of mothers "going it alone" when it comes to taking care of their child's health and illness. This case sheds light on the importance of an anthropological understanding of the cultural, contextual factors that influence medical decision making with regard to childhood malaria and implications this has for understanding public health interventions aimed at child survival.

Amina's Story

Amina is a 30-year-old mother of five young children, two of whom are identical twins (*mapacha*). She lives in a hamlet located about 30 minutes walking distance from the market place in Mbande. Amina's husband is a subsistence farmer; he makes a living mainly by growing cassava and maize. In addition to working the land with her husband, Amina weaves mats (*mkeka*) and sells them for TShilling 6000 to 8000 ($6–8) a piece once every 2 months.[10] I first met Amina at the dispensary where I was observing and documenting doctor–patient interactions, and recruiting mothers for this study. That day, Amina was the first to arrive at the dispensary and the last one to leave. She had arrived at 8.00 a.m. in the morning with Msaikwa, her 1-year-old daughter (one of the twins), who had a fever of 40° C at the time when the nurse took her temperature. The nurse had promptly advised Amina to start sponging Msaikwa to bring down her body temperature. In the interim, the baby was given antipyretic syrup. By the time the baby's body temperature had come down to normal, and the nurse had decided to give the baby an antimalarial injection, Amina and Msaikwa had spent 6 hours at the dispensary. Amina was all too familiar with this routine, as she had come to the dispensary on several occasions for mother and child health (MCH) services and to get treatment for her other children. A week later, I visited Amina and her family at her home along with Mariam, my research assistant, for a pre-arranged interview.

With five children to look after, and hardly any cash income, Amina and her husband were leading an impoverished life. When asked how she managed her life with such a large family and such a meager income, she sighed:

> In this family, at any given time my children are sick; every day, every week, every month. One day this child has a fever, the next day that child has mouth sores, the third day this child is coughing, the fourth day that child has a stomach ache, and fifth day he has diarrhea, and on and on. That's how it has been for me. I'm really sick and tired of taking my sick children to the hospital all the time; I don't get to rest at all. I have several relatives in this area, but no one really helps me with taking care of my sick children. There is no help whatsoever. My husband is busy working the land, growing cassava; that's all we grow here; that's all we eat. We sell some cassava and get some money so that we can take our sick children to the hospital and pay for the treatment. I know it's normal for children to fall sick. I can't say that my children will not fall sick or should not become sick. They have to fall sick, and they have to get better. It would be inappropriate (*haramu*) to say that children shouldn't fall sick sometime or the other. After all, we are human beings; as God's children, we have to fall sick and get better.

As with many other families in Mbande and the surrounding hamlets, for Amina, sickness was a part of her everyday life. One way she coped with the perennial sickness in her family was to importune God to make sense of her suffering. These feelings echoed the sentiments of several other mothers interviewed during the course of my fieldwork. In addition to representations of her poverty, social relations are at the core of Amina's narrative as she repeatedly mentioned that although she has several relatives living nearby, she could not count on them for help: "There is no help whatsoever." This has important implications for our understanding of the social context and the social relations of health care seeking. While the popular impression about life in Tanzania is marked by sharing and cooperation among members of social networks, in reality, when it comes to dealing with children's sickness, the majority of the mothers interviewed for this study stated that they had absolutely no help whatsoever from members of their social network. One key informant summarized this by stating, "Everyone is preoccupied with his or her family problems, they struggle over scarce cash, and they do not have the economic or social resources, including time to spare for others."

"No Blood": Anemic Children and Local Perceptions of Vulnerability to Febrile Illness

As with Amina, other mothers who were asked why their children fell sick emphasized the "ordinariness" of child illness. They also repeatedly invoked God in their explanation by using the phrase, "It's God's wish." While several mothers attributed their child's sickness to "God's wish," that is, something that is beyond their immediate control, a few others gave a partial explanation saying that their children were predisposed to falling sick repeatedly because they did not have enough blood in their body. They spoke of "no blood" (*damu hana*, or *damu imepungua*) in the child's body by citing numbers—"only 40%" or "50%" or "0.5". These terms were influenced by English phrases they had learned from encounters with the staff at the local/private dispensary or government hospital that refer to the hemoglobin levels. Some mothers provided detailed explanations regarding their belief about "no blood" as a predisposing factor in their child's vulnerability to repeated episodes of fever, and the trouble they had to go through to try and "fix" the problem. The following excerpt from a narrative interview with one of the mothers with a very sick baby illustrates this point.

Zaituni's Story

Zaituni is a 40-year-old mother of nine children. She lives in a hamlet near Mbande with her husband and seven of her children. Two of her daughters are married and live elsewhere in Dar es Salaam. In explaining the condition of her youngest daughter Zainabu, who was 7 months of age at the time of this interview, Zaituni said:

> On the fourth or fifth day (after onset of fever), I took Zainabu to the dispensary. There they told me that Zainabu had malaria and that she had very little blood in her body. They gave me a referral slip (*cheti*) and told me to rush her to Temeke District Hospital. When I went to Temeke District Hospital, they referred me to Muhimbili National Hospital. At Muhimbili, Zainabu was admitted and treated for malaria. They checked her blood and found it was .3. They gave her some blood (i.e., blood transfusion), to increase her blood, and after three days, I returned to Mbande for follow-up. At the dispensary, they referred me again to Temeke Hospital and the people at Temeke Hospital referred me again to Muhimbili Hospital. So, Zainabu was once again admitted at Muhimbili Hospital for four days. Her blood level increased to 5.6, and her malaria was cleared. The doctor at Muhimbili gave Zainabu quinine injections and syrup. After she was discharged I brought her home and three weeks later, I went to the dispensary for follow-up. That day, Zainabu had high fever. At the dispensary, they found that Zainabu still had malaria (she had a fever of 40° C) and her blood level was .5. They told me to take Zainabu once again to Muhimbili Hospital. I went with Zainabu to Muhimbili; they examined her, gave her some medications and told me to return with her today.

In addition to Zainabu's mother, at least seven other mothers interviewed for this study had a similar story to tell. An analysis of their narratives suggests that there is little deviation in the sequence of events, especially with regard to the action of "shuttling" between the local dispensary, the district hospital, and the national hospital in search of blood and a cure for their young children's sickness. Significantly, when mothers were asked to talk about the most recent episode of their currently sick child, they would typically begin their illness narrative by going back several months and make a reference to their memory of the first time their child was sick—when he/she was taken to a health facility. Thus, for example, a mother would state: "Oh, my child has always been sick…since the time she was born," or, "My child has always been like this: fever, fever, fever." This observation reflects precisely what Hausmann-Muela et al. (2002) have also observed elsewhere in Tanzania: that "in the local notion, the personal history of ill health is not a series of independent illness episodes. Rather, illness is regarded as a continuous transformation from one condition to the next, whereby illness episodes are blurred."

Poor nutritional status thus contributed to a child's vulnerability to sickness. (see Kitua et al. 1997; Premji et al. 1995; Shiff et al. 1996). Repeated malarial and other parasitic infections made matters worse, as no amount of blood transfusions could address the "crux" of the problem—the economic and social vulnerability of poor people.

Sponging and Negotiating "Best" Treatment

During participant observation at the local dispensary, I found, that for the most part, the interactions between the dispensary staff and the mothers were routine. Occasionally, however, a nurse advised one of the mothers to begin sponging her feverish child so as to lower the child's body temperature. Typically, the mother would follow suit, sit on the floor, and start sponging her child with a wet cloth. This practice resulted in the lowering of the child's body temperature. However, the process was lengthy, and often took between 30 minutes and 4 hours. Most of the mothers who were recruited for this study had witnessed other mothers sponging their feverish child, or they had been advised to do so themselves during previous consultations at the dispensary. A little more than half (56%) the mothers had sponged their febrile child before bringing him/her to the dispensary. However, about 20% said that they were simply too scared to do anything by themselves. Their primary course of action was to bring their child to the dispensary to seek the doctor or the nurse's opinion. Thirteen percent of the mothers said that they had not resorted to sponging because they were not aware of this practice. Another 7% said that when they found that their child had high fever, their "mind stopped working" (akili yangu sio nzuri). Other mothers explained that when they had made the decision to bring their sick child to the dispensary, the child's body temperature was "still okay" and therefore they assumed it was only ordinary fever. However, upon arrival at the dispensary, the child's temperature alarmingly shot up. At this point, it was necessary for the mother to follow the nurse's advice to sponge the child. The question is, why do many mothers refrain from sponging their feverish child before bringing him/her to the dispensary?

Follow-up interviews with mothers and discussions with the dispensary staff revealed that many mothers do not sponge their child before bringing him/her to the dispensary because they do not want to "mask" the symptoms. Drawing upon their past experiences, many mothers believed that if they arrived at the dispensary with a child whose temperature had been lowered by sponging, the doctor and nurses would not take them seriously. They thus inferred that their child would not get the necessary level of attention and the right medicine. They also believed that the child would be given an antipyretic instead of an antimalarial injection. In essence, mothers were being "strategic" in the presentation of their child's illness in order to authenticate it, even if it meant that they were inadvertently putting the child at risk of developing more serious complications. They adopted this strategy so that the dispensary staff would take their child's illness seriously and provide the best treatment possible for their child. In this case, strategic symptom reporting did not denote "irrational" health behavior or lack of faith in biomedicine, but rather indicated a manipulation of the system toward "felt needs" (Nichter 1996:120–121; see also Nsimba et al. 2002:206–207).

The implications of this practice are immense because in contexts of limited, accessible health care options, mothers may put their children "at risk," albeit inadvertently, with the hope that the dispensary staff will take their child's illness more seriously. A proactive approach on part of health workers based on a demonstrated willingness and a responsibility to treat all febrile children seriously would be a first step in convincing mothers that they need not refrain from sponging their febrile children. This would perceivably lead to better treatment outcomes. As noted earlier, the dispensary staff had not received any IMCI training—training that would have prepared them to assume a proactive disposition toward their patients. Dissatisfaction with the quality of attention and medicine that mothers/caretakers receive for their sick children at the health center often leads them to seek alternative resources in order to meet their child's needs, as well as their own. This leads to further delays in seeking appropriate medical attention.

The Pragmatics of Negotiating Multiple Therapies: Fatuma's Story

The dynamics of medical decision making become all the more complex in places like Mbande, which are characterized by medical pluralism. For example, Fatuma is a 24-year-old single mother of two children. I met her the first time at the local dispensary. She had brought her 9-month-old daughter, Mariam, to deal with yet another fever episode. During our conversation, I expressed my concern regarding Mariam's health and asked why she was so "clingy" (*kamata kamata*) today. Fatuma responded, "No, she's fine; she's been very active. She laughs and plays like any other child, but for the last so many days, she's been sick. She's been having this fever. It's fever, fever, and fever [*homa, homa, homa tu*]. I'm really tired of having to deal with Mariam's fever episodes!" The dispensary medicines did not seem to be working at all. At the dispensary, Fatuma went through the routine of reporting Mariam's condition to the nurse in order to get the necessary medications, and to return home. Two days later while I was making some notes at the local *mganga* Mzee Tinyango's house, Fatuma and Mariam walked into the verandah. Mariam was flushed with fever, crying loudly and looking miserable. Fatuma looked exhausted, an indication that she had not slept the previous night. In all my previous conversations with Fatuma, she had never mentioned seeing Mzee Tinyango or any other *mganga* regarding matters of health or misfortune. Fatuma had given me the impression that despite the fact that she had never attended school, she preferred biomedicine, in that she had faith in modern pharmaceuticals and was unlikely to take resort to a "traditional healer." Thus, I was very surprised to see her in Tinyango's house with her daughter. "Mariam's not well so I've come to see the *mganga*," she told me.

It took me a while to compose myself after the surprise of seeing Fatuma with Mariam at Tinyango's *kilinge* (pl. *vilinge*) or consulting room. I felt Mariam's body temperature and noted that she had high fever. After about 15 minutes, Fatuma took Mariam to see Tinyango in his *kilinge*. I followed them inside and made notes on the dialogue that took place. Tinyango's treatment involved consoling Mariam and giving her a few drops of medicated honey (Figure 1.2). Importantly, Fatuma did not mention anything about Mariam's fever to Tinyango. Instead, she said that she had brought Mariam to him because she had been crying incessantly that night and had been waking up convulsing (*ana stuka*). After the therapy session was over, I asked Fatuma to explain to me again why she had come to Tinyango. She said, "I've already got medicines to deal with Mariam's fever. I came to Tinyango for some other illness—*shetani shetani*. Mariam has been waking up convulsing and crying continuously in the night. No, I did not come to Tinyango to get medicines for Mariam's fever." I also learned from Fatuma that 2 days earlier, when the dispensary was closed, she had gone to one of the local pharmacies in order to buy an antimalarial syrup. The pharmacist had sold her a bottle of amodioquin, an antimalarial, which she gave to Mariam, but to no avail. Mariam's fever had continued. Three days later, Fatuma showed up again with Mariam at the dispensary. A quick blood test revealed that Mariam's hemoglobin level had dropped to a dangerously low level. Again, Mariam received an antimalarial injection, and the nurse advised Fatuma to "do something" about Mariam's nutrition, and to return to the dispensary to complete the scheduled dosage of five injections within the

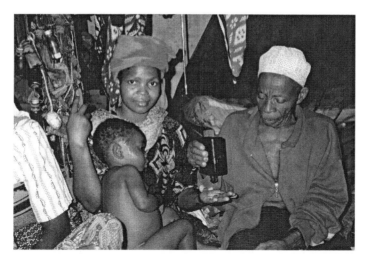

Figure 1.2. Fatuma's daughter being treated by a Zaramo healer. (Photo by Vinay R. Kamat).

week. While Fatuma adhered to the nurse's advice regarding the injections, as an impoverished single mother, she could do very little about improving her daughter's nutrition. A month after Mariam was treated at the local dispensary she was again diagnosed with severe malaria. The medical officer attributed the recrudescence of malaria to "treatment failure" and referred the patient to the district hospital. There she was hospitalized and given quinine intravenously, before being discharged 3 days later.

In search of appropriate therapy for her daughter, Fatuma had exhausted nearly all the local resources available to deal with fever-related illnesses. She had started by going to secular health facilities—the government dispensary and the private pharmacy, then to Mzee Tinyango, the local traditional healer, and then back to the dispensary again. In her pragmatic quest for therapy, Fatuma had routinely combined elements from diverse and even contradictory medical traditions (see Brodwin 1996:13). Fatuma thought that she was dealing with two different illnesses: Mariam's fever, which she knew would be best treated by modern pharmaceuticals and could be obtained either at one of the local pharmacies or the dispensary. Second, she was dealing with Mariam's convulsions, which she attributed to "spirits" (*mashaitani*) and therefore required the help of a *mganga*. However, from a biomedical standpoint, Mariam's different diagnoses are signs of the same illness (in this case, cerebral malaria) and require a single treatment modality. Fever with convulsions, in particular, has often been described as a separate illness requiring a different form of treatment (see Baume, Helitzer, and Kachua 2000; Makemba et al. 1996; Tarimo, Urassa, and Msamanga 1998).

Conclusion: Anthropology of Childhood Malaria and Implications for Public Health

Delay in seeking appropriate medical treatment is at the crux of the high malaria-related morbidity–mortality rates in Dar es Salaam. In this city, most children with a febrile illness are brought to a biomedical health facility at least 48 hours after the onset of fever. As the case studies have indicated, this delay is not primarily due to economic considerations alone, but a complexity of factors, including cultural factors that are amenable to ethnographic investigation. In the present case, what led most mothers to prolong their "wait and watch" period and to extend their practice of diagnosis by treatment was their belief that they were dealing with an ordinary fever, not a potentially life-threatening illness such as malaria. Additionally, when they did decide to take their sick children to the local dispensary, they practiced strategic symptom reporting, and this occasionally involved "inventing" and exaggerating symptoms to ensure quality diagnosis and treatment.

The point to bear in mind is that even if expensive but more efficacious antimalarials were made available in dispensaries such as the one described in this case study, in all probability many mothers would continue to delay in bringing their feverish children to a public health facility. Until the dispensary staffs are trained to proactively and effectively communicate the severity of the symptoms of malaria, mothers will continue to delay bringing their sick children to the local dispensary because they believe that they are dealing with an "ordinary" illness. Many poor patients in due course will turn to private pharmacies to purchase antimalarials that are less expensive, but of questionable efficacy (Goodman et al. 2004). This in turn leads to endless cycles of children developing high fevers and mothers becoming further frustrated with inefficacious treatment. The problem is also complicated by the fact that many private pharmacies in Tanzania are unlicensed and managed by unqualified or poorly trained pharmacists (Kachur et al. 2006). There is also the risk that patients will consume their medications in inappropriate dosages and thus compromise the clinical efficacy of the drugs. In short, carefully planned, anthropologically informed community-based health interventions that address differences in cultural, etiological, and nosological categories will go a long way in enabling the poor to mitigate their experience with high levels of malaria-related morbidities and mortalities.

Simply put, malaria must be dealt with as an economic and a social issue. Sociocultural factors are central in determining malaria risk, persistence, and popular treatment. Health planners must consider community beliefs and practices when developing and implementing health policies, as communities must be reasonably convinced of their value before they will embrace change. In public health programs, little attention is paid to social factors, such as gender, marginalization, and inequity. These factors constrain individual choices and the ability of an individual to exercise these choices in illness prevention and treatment (Manderson 1998; Sommerfeld 1998). At the community level, the most economically marginalized populations are at greatest risk from malaria because of limited resources, substandard education, and a lack of access to health care facilities (Durrheim and Williams 2005:178; Molyneux, Murira, Masha, and Snow 2002). Comprehending the vulnerability of the poor requires a careful consideration of the broader socioeconomic and political contexts in which health and disease are embedded. Ultimately, considering the social production of illness remains a key factor (see Baer 1996; Brown 1997; Brown, Inhorn, and Smith 1996; Farmer 1999, 2003; Inhorn and Brown 1997; Packard 1989).

Anthropological studies of malaria alone will not provide the best way forward in the global fight against malaria. Instead, these studies should be regarded as providing useful perspectives on how malaria as an illness is understood and dealt with in local communities. The utilization of anthropological methods in malaria control has the potential to act as a "corrective" in the overly technical and biomedically driven interventions that have come to dominate the global malaria control discourse and practice. The central role socioeconomic and cultural factors play in how illnesses are interpreted and dealt with in the household and health centers, and the context in which the majority of the illnesses are dealt with outside the formal health sector must be considered (Foster 1995). The potential for anthropological studies in malaria can best be harnessed in planning and implementing community-based health interventions, where knowledge of local terminology for febrile illnesses/taxonomies of fever and illness-related cultural beliefs and practices can go a long way in designing locally appropriate health interventions (Helitzer-Allen et al. 1993; Oberlander and Elverdan 2000; Winch et al. 1996). At a time when global discourses on malaria control are predominantly biomedically oriented and technical in nature, the goal of anthropology is to put "life" into the problem: to "bring the local to the attention of the global" (Janes 2004). In this lies the value of anthropology in malaria control.

Notes

1. There are about 400 species of *Anopheles*. However, only 60 of them transmit malaria under natural conditions, and 30 are of major importance. Of these, the *Anopheles gambiae* complex and *Anopheles funestus* are the most efficient vectors for *Plasmodium falciparum* transmission. The highest rates of sporozoite development are in *Anopheles gambiae*, the species that is widespread throughout sub-Saharan Africa (Breman 2001:4).

2. Malaria-related mortality is particularly difficult to measure because the symptoms of the disease are nonspecific and most deaths occur at home. Nonetheless, according to Hay et al. (2005), in the year 2000, there were 1,068,505 malaria deaths in Africa.

3. Cerebral malaria collectively involves the clinical manifestations of *Plasmodium falciparum* malaria that induce changes in mental status and coma. It is an acute, widespread disease of the brain, which is accompanied by fever. Clinical manifestations of cerebral malaria are numerous, but there are three primary symptoms common to both adults and children: (1) impaired consciousness with nonspecific fever; (2) generalized convulsions and neurological sequelae; and (3) coma that persists for 24 to 72 hours, with the patient initially in a semi-conscious state and then finally descending into a state of complete unconsciousness (see for details Maitland and Marsh 2004).

4. In the African context, there is a plethora of ethnographic studies that have documented how in many communities, the malaria–mosquito link as outlined in the biomedical model, is not readily appreciated by people who associate a range of etiologies with what is often biomedically diagnosed as malaria (see for example, Agyepong 1992; Gessler et al. 1995; Hausmann-Muela et al. 1998; Hausmann-Muela et al. 2002; Hausmann-Muela and Ribera 2003; Helitzer-Allen et al. 1993; Makemba et al. 1996; Mwenesi, Harman, and Snow 1995; Ramakrishna, Brieger, and Adeniyi 1988–89; Winch et al. 1996; 1999). However, these ethnographic insights are rarely incorporated into national malaria control programs (see Napolitano and Jones 2006; Williams and Jones 2004).

5. A cultural model is a cognitive schema that is intersubjectively shared by a social group. Such models typically consist of a small number of conceptual objects and their relations to each other (D'Andrade 1987:112).

6. There have been urgent calls to improve the problem of over-diagnosis/over-reporting of malaria cases. Hence improving diagnostic infrastructure is necessary, irrespective of which drugs are used, although with more expensive drugs, improved rational use of drugs increases their cost effectiveness. For example, a study conducted by Nsimba et al. (2002) in Kibaha district, 40 km northwest of Dar es Salaam, found that of the 461 children who were presumptively diagnosed with malaria, 449 were screened for malaria parasites. However, only 38% of these patients had malarial parasites in their blood. In Dar es Salaam, Wang et al. (2006) found that less than 5% of all fever-related consultations were likely to be due to malaria during the dry season of 2003 and this has important implications for fever case management. On the one hand, this leads to a substantial number of unnecessary treatments, a problem made much more serious with the introduction of the more expensive artemisinin-based combination therapy. On the other hand, overdiagnosed malaria patients may also distract from other causes of fever, some of which may be dangerous to the patient.

7. All names in this chapter are pseudonyms.

8. The per capita income was computed from a random sample survey of 116 households conducted as part of the larger ethnographic study.

9. Malaria as a febrile illness is included in the Integrated Management of Childhood Illness (IMCI) strategy, which aims to improve health systems, and to improve family and community practices regarding management of childhood illnesses (Gove 1997).

10. At the time of this study, a kg of regular store-bought rice was being sold at TShillings 650/kg.

References

Agyepong IA (1992) Malaria: Ethnomedical perceptions and practice in an Adangbe farming community and implications for control. *Social Science and Medicine* 35(2):131–137.

Ainsworth-Vaughn N (1998) *Claiming power in doctor–patient talk.* Oxford, UK: Oxford University Press.

Alnwick D (2000) Roll back malaria—what are the prospects? *Bulletin of the World Health Organization* 78(12):1377.

Amuyunzu-Nyamongo M, Nyamongo IK (2006) Health-seeking behaviour of mothers of under-five-year-old children in the slum communities of Nairobi, Kenya. *Anthropology and Medicine* 13(1):25–40.

Anonymous (2003) *The Africa malaria report 2003. The Burden of Malaria in Africa* 17–23.

Askew KM (2006) Sung and unsung: Musical reflections on Tanzanian postsocialisms. *Africa* 76(1):15–43.

Attaran A (2004) Where did it all go wrong? *Nature* 430:932–933.

Attaran A, Barnes KI, Curtis C, d'Alessandro U, Fanello CI, Galinski MR, et al. (2004) WHO, the Global Fund, and medical malpractice in malaria treatment. *The Lancet* 363 (January 17):237–240.

Baer H (1996) Toward a political ecology of health in medical anthropology. *Medical Anthropology Quarterly* 10(4):451–454.

Barat LM, Natasha P, Basu S, Worrall E, Hanson K, Mills A (2004) Do malaria control interventions reach the poor? A view through the equity lens. *American Journal of Tropical Medicine and Hygiene* 71(2):174–178.

Barnes K, Folb P (2003) The role of artemisinin-based combination therapy in malaria management. Global Health Council Technical Report—December 2003—Reducing Malaria's Burden. Washington, DC: Global Health Council, pp. 25–32.

Baume C, Helitzer D, Kachur PS (2000) Patterns of care for childhood malaria in Zambia. *Social Science and Medicine* 51:1491–1503.

Bloland PB (2003) A contrarian view of malaria therapy policy in Africa. *American Journal of Tropical Medicine and Hygiene* 68(2):125–126.

Bloland PB, Kachur SP, Williams HA (2003) Trends in antimalarial drug deployment in sub-Saharan Africa. *Journal of Experimental Biology* 206:3761–3769.

Boesen J, Madsen BS, Moody T, eds. (1977) *Ujamaa—Socialism from Above.* Uppsala, Sweden: Center for Development Research.

Breman JG (2001) The ears of the hippopotamus: Manifestations, determinants, and estimates of the malaria burden. *American Journal of Tropical Medicine and Hygiene* 64(1, 2):1–11.

Brodwin PE (1996) *Medicine and Morality in Haiti: The Contest for Healing Power.* Cambridge, UK: Cambridge University Press.

Brown PJ (1997) "Culture and the Global Resurgence of Malaria." In: *The Anthropology of Infectious Disease.* MC Inhorn, PJ Brown, eds. Amsterdam: Gordon and Breach Science Publishers, pp. 119–141.

Brown PJ, Inhorn MC, Smith DJ (1996) "Disease, Ecology, and Human Behavior." In: *Medical Anthropology: Contemporary Theory and Method (Revised Edition).* CF Sargent, TM Johnson, eds. Westport, CT: Praeger, pp. 183–218.

Caulfield LE, Richard SA, Black RE (2004) Undernutrition as an underlying cause of malaria morbidity and mortality in children less than five years old. *American Journal of Tropical Medicine and Hygiene* 71(2):55–63.

Comoro C, Nsimba SED, Warsame M, Tomson G (2003) Local understanding, perceptions and reported practices of mothers/guardians and health workers on childhood malaria in a Tanzanian district—implications for malaria control. *Acta Tropica* 87:305–313.

Crawley J (2004) Reducing the burden of anemia in infants and young children in malaria-endemic countries of Africa: From evidence to action. *American Journal of Tropical Medicine and Hygiene* 71(Suppl 2):25–34.

D'Andrade R (1987) "A Folk Model of the Mind." In: *Cultural Models in Language and Thought.* D Holland, N Quinn, eds. Cambridge, UK: Cambridge University Press, pp. 112–148.

de Castro CM, Yamagata Y, Mtasiwa D, Tanner M, Utzinger J, Keiser J, et al. (2004) Integrated urban malaria control: A case study in Dar es Salaam, Tanzania. *American Journal of Tropical Medicine and Hygiene* 71(Supplement 2):103–117.

de Savigny D, Mayombana C, Mwangeni E, Masanja H, Minhaj A, Mkilindi Y, et al. (2004) Care-seeking patterns for fatal malaria in Tanzania. *Malaria Journal* 3(27):1–15.

Durrheim DN, Williams HA (2005) Assuring effective malaria treatment in Africa: Drug efficacy is necessary but not sufficient. *Journal of Epidemiology and Community Health* 59:78–179.

Farmer P (1999) *Infections and Inequalities: The Modern Plagues.* Berkeley, CA: University of California Press.

Farmer P (2003) *Pathologies of Power: Health, Human Rights, and the New War on the Poor.* Berkeley, CA: University of California Press.

Foster SD (1995) Treatment of malaria outside the formal health services. *Journal of Tropical Medicine and Hygiene* 98:29–34.

Freyhold M von (1979) *Ujamaa Villages in Tanzania.* New York and London: Monthly Review Press.

Gessler MC, Msuya DE, Nkunya MHH, Schär A, Heinrich M, Tanner M. (1995). Traditional healers in Tanzania: The perception of malaria and its causes. *Journal of Ethnopharmacology* 48:119–130.

Global Health Council (2003) *Reducing Malaria's Burden: Evidence of Effectiveness for Decision Makers.* Washington, DC: Global Health Council.

Goodman C, Kachur PS, Abdulla S, Mwageni E, Nyoni J, Schellenberg JA, et al. (2004) Retail supply of malaria-related drugs in rural Tanzania: Risks and opportunities. *Tropical Medicine and International Health* 9(6):655–663.

Gove S (1997) Integrated management of childhood illness by out-patient health workers: technical basis and overview. *Bulletin of the World Health Organization* 75(Suppl):7–16.

Greenwood BM, Bradley AK, Greenwood AM, Byass P, Jammeh K, Marsh K, et al. (1987) Mortality and morbidity from malaria among children in a rural area of the Gambia, West Africa. *Transactions of the Royal Society of Tropical Medicine and Hygiene* 81:478–486.

Guerin PJ, Olliaro P, Nosten F, Druilhe P, Laxminarayan R, Binka F, et al. (2002) Malaria: Current status of control, diagnosis, treatment, and a proposed agenda for research and development. *The Lancet* 2(September):564–572.

Hausmann-Muela S, Ribera JM (2003) Recipe knowledge: A tool for understanding some apparently irrational behaviour. *Anthropology and Medicine* 10(1):87–103.

Hausmann-Muela S, Ribera JM, Tanner M (1998) Fake malaria and hidden parasites—the ambiguity of malaria. *Anthropology and Medicine* 5(1):43–61.

Hausmann-Muela S, Ribera JM, Mushi AK, Tanner M (2002) Medical syncretism with reference to malaria in a Tanzanian community. *Social Science and Medicine* 55:403–413.

Hay SI, Guerra CA, Tatem AJ, Atkinson PM, Snow RW (2005) Urbanization, malaria transmission and disease burden in Africa. *Microbiology* 3:81–90.

Helitzer-Allen DL, Kendall C, Wirima JJ (1993) The role of ethnographic research in malaria control: An example from Malawi. *Research in the Sociology of Health Care* 10:269–286.

Hill, J (2005) "Finding Culture in Narrative." In: *Finding Culture in Talk: A Collection of Methods*. N Quinn, ed. New York: Palgrave Macmillan, pp. 157–202.

Hunt LM, Jordan B, Irwin S (1989) Views of what's wrong: Diagnosis and patients' concepts of illness. *Social Science and Medicine* 28(9):945–956.

Hyden G (1980) *Beyond Ujamaa in Tanzania: Underdevelopment and an Uncaptured Peasantry*. Berkeley, CA: University of California Press.

Inhorn MC, Brown PJ, eds. (1997). *The Anthropology of Infectious Disease*. Amsterdam: Gordon and Breach Publishers.

Janes CR (2004) Going global in century XXI: Medical anthropology and the new primary health care. *Human Organization* 63(4):457–471.

Kachur PS, Black C, Abdulla S, Goodman C (2006) Putting the genie back into the bottle? Availability and presentation of oral artemisinin compounds at retail pharmacies in urban Dar es Salaam. *Malaria Journal* 5:25.

Kachur PS, Khatib RA, Kaizer E, Fox SS, Abdulla SM, Bloland PB (2004) Adherence to antimalarial combination therapy with sulfadoxine-pyrimethamine and artesunate in rural Tanzania. *American Journal of Tropical Medicine and Hygiene* 71(6):715–722.

Kager PA (2002) Malaria control: Constraints and opportunities. *Tropical Medicine and International Health* 7(12):1042–1046.

Kamat VR (2004) Negotiating Illness and Misfortune in Post-Socialist Tanzania: An Ethnographic Study in Temeke District, Dar es Salaam. PhD Dissertation. Atlanta, GA: Emory University.

Kamat VR (2006) I thought it was only ordinary fever! Cultural knowledge and the micropolitics of therapy seeking for childhood febrile illness in Tanzania. *Social Science and Medicine* 62(12):2945–2959.

Kamat VR. (2008a) Reconsidering the allure of the culturally distant in therapy seeking: A case study from coastal Tanzania. *Medical Anthropology* 27(2):1–30.

Kamat VR. (2008b) Dying under the bird's shadow: Representations of degedege and child survival among the Zaramo of Tanzania. *Medical Anthropology Quarterly* 22(1):67–93.

Kitua AY, Smith TA, Alonso PL, Urassa H, Masanja H, Kimario J, et al. (1997) The role of low-level plasmodium *falciparum parasitaemia* in anaemia among infants living in an area of intense and perennial transmission. *Tropical Medicine and International Health* 2(4):325–333.

Korenromp EL, Williams BG, Gouws E, Dye C, Snow RW (2003) Measurement of trends in childhood malaria mortality in Africa: An assessment of progress toward targets based on verbal autopsy. *The Lancet* 3:349–358.

Maitland K, Marsh K (2004) Pathophysiology of severe malaria in children. *Acta Tropica* 90:131–140.

Makemba AM, Winch PJ, Makame VM, Mehl GL, Premji Z, Minjas JN, et al. (1996) Treatment practices for *degedege*, a locally recognized febrile illness, and implications for strategies to decrease mortality from severe malaria in Bagamoyo District, Tanzania. *Tropical Medicine and International Health* 1(3):305–313.

Malowany M (2000) Unfinished agendas: Writing the history of medicine of sub-Saharan Africa. *African Affairs* 99:325–349.

Manderson L (1998) Applying medical anthropology in the control of infectious disease. *Tropical Medicine and International Health* 3(12):1020–1027.

McHenry D (1979) *Tanzania's Ujamaa Villages: The Implementation of a Rural Development Strategy.* Berkeley, CA: Institute of International Studies, University of California.

Ministry of Health, Government of Tanzania (2003) National Malaria Medium-Term Strategic Plan 2003–2007, pp. 1–66.

Ministry of Health, United Republic of Tanzania (1997) Policy Implications of Adult Morbidity and Mortality: End of Phase I Report. Dar es Salaam: Ministry of Health.

Mishler EG (1984) *The Discourse of Medicine: Dialectics of Medical Interviews.* Norword, NJ: Ablex Publishing.

Mishler EG (1991) Representing discourse: The rhetoric of transcription. *Journal of Narrative and Life History* 1(4):255–280.

Mishler EG (1995) Models of narrative analysis: A typology. *Journal of Narrative and Life History* 5(87):123.

MOH-AMMP (2002) http://research.ncl.ac.uk/ammp/

Molyneux CS, Murira G, Masha J, Snow RW (2002) Intra-household relations and treatment decision-making for childhood illness: A Kenyan case study. *Journal of Biosocial Science* 34:109–131.

Mwenesi Halima A, Harpman T, Snow RW (1995) Child malaria treatment practices among mothers in Kenya. *Social Science and Medicine* 40(9):1271–1277.

Nchinda TC (1998) Malaria: A reemerging disease in Africa. *Emerging Infectious Disease* 4:398–403.

Napolitano DA, Jones COH (2006) Who needs *pukka* anthropologists? A study of the perceptions of the use of anthropology in tropical public health research. *Tropical Medicine and International Health* 11(8):1264–1275.

Nichter M (2002) "The Social Relations of Therapy Management." In: *New Horizons in Medical Anthropology.* M Nichter, M Lock, eds. London and New York: Routledge, pp. 81–110.

Nichter M (1996) *Anthropology and International Health: Asian Case Studies.* Amsterdam: Gordon and Breach Publishers.

Nsimba SED, Massele, AY, Eriksen J, Gustafsson LL, Tomson G, Warasme M (2002) Case management of malaria in under-fives at primary health care facilities in a Tanzanian district. *Tropical Medicine and International Health* 7(3):201–209.

Nyamongo IK (2002) Health care switching behaviour of malaria patients in a Kenyan rural community. *Social Science and Medicine* 54:377–386.

Oberlander L, Elverdan B (2000) Malaria in the United Republic of Tanzania: Cultural considerations and health-seeking behaviour. *Bulletin of the World Health Organization* 78(11):1352–1357.

Packard RM (1989) *White Plague, Black Labor: Tuberculosis and the Political Economy of Health and Disease in South Africa.* Berkeley, CA: University of California Press.

Plowe CV (2003) Monitoring antimalarial drug resistance: Making the most of the tools at hand. *Journal of Experimental Biology* 206:3745–3752.

Premji Z, Hamisi Y, Schiff C, Minjas J, Lubega P, Makwaya C (1995) Anaemia and *Plasmodium falciparum* infections among young children in a holoendemic area, Bagamoyo, Tanzania. *Acta Tropica* 63:101–109.

Price L (1987) "Ecuadorian Illness Stories: Cultural Knowledge in Natural Discourse." In: *Cultural Models and Language and Thought*. D Holland, N Quinn, eds. Cambridge, UK: Cambridge University Press, pp. 313–342.

Quinn N (2005) "Introduction to Finding Culture in Talk: A Collection of Methods." In: *Finding Culture in Talk: A Collection of Methods*. N Quinn, ed. New York: Palgrave Macmillan, pp. 1–34.

Ramakrishna J, Brieger W, Adeniyi JD (1988–89) Treatment of malaria and febrile convulsions: An educational diagnosis of Yoruba beliefs. *International Quarterly of Community Health Education* 9:305–319.

Sachs A, Malaney P (2002) The economic and social burden of malaria. *Nature* 41:680–685.

Sanders T (2001) "Save our Skins: Structural Adjustment, Morality and the Occult in Tanzania." In: *Magical Interpretations, Material Realities: Modernity, Witchcraft and the Occult in Postcolonial Africa*. HL Moore, T Sanders, eds. London: Routledge, pp. 160–183.

Schellenberg AJ, Bryce J, de Savigny D, Lambrechts T, Mbuya C, Mgalula L, et al. (2004) The effect of integrated management of childhood illness on observed quality of care of under-fives in rural Tanzania. *Health Policy and Planning* 19(1):1–10.

Scott J (1999) *Seeing Like a State: How Certain Schemes to Improve the Human Condition Have Failed*. New Haven, CT: Yale University Press.

Setel PW (1999) *A Plague of Paradoxes: AIDS, Culture, and Demography in Northern Tanzania*. Chicago, IL: University of Chicago Press.

Setel PW, Whiting DR, Hemed Y, Chandramohan D (2006) Validity of verbal autopsy procedures for determining cause of death in Tanzania. *Tropical Medicine and International Health* 11(3):681–696.

Shiff C, Checkley W, Winch P, Premji Z, Minjas J, Lubega P (1996) Changes in weight gain and anaemia attributable to malaria in Tanzanian children living under holoendemic conditions. *Transactions of the Royal Society of Tropical Medicine and Hygiene* 90:262–265.

Snow RW, Trape J, Marsh K (2001) The past, present and future of childhood malaria mortality in Africa. *Trends in Parasitology* 17(12):593–597.

Snow RW, Guerra CA, Noor AM, Myint HY, Hay SI (2005) The global distribution of clinical episodes of Plasmodium falciparum malaria. *Nature* 434(7030):214–217.

Snow RW, Korenromp EL, Gouws E (2004) Pediatric mortality in Africa: Plasmodium falciparum malaria as a cause or risk? *American Journal of Tropical Medicine and Hygiene* 71(Supplement 2):16–24.

Snow RW, Craig M, Deichmann U, Marsh K (1999) Estimating mortality, morbidity and disability due to malaria among Africa's non-pregnant population. *Bulletin of the World Health Organization* 77:624–640.

Sommerfeld J (1998) Medical anthropology and infectious disease control (editorial). *Tropical Medicine and International Health* 3(12):993–995.

Stephens C, Masamu ET, Kiama MG, Keto AJ, Kinenekejo M, Ichimori K (1995) Knowledge of mosquitoes in relation to public and domestic control activities in the cities of Dar es Salaam and Tanga. *Bulletin of the World Health Organization* 73:97–104.

Swantz M (1995) *Blood, Milk and Death: Body Symbols and the Power of Regeneration among the Zaramo of Tanzania*. Westport, CT: Bergin and Garvey.

Tanner M, Vlassoff C (1998) Treatment-seeking behavior for malaria: A typology based on endemicity and gender. *Social Science and Medicine* 46(4–5):523–532.

Tarimo DS, Lwihula GK, Minja JN, Bygbjerg IC (2000) Mothers' perceptions and knowledge on childhood malaria in the holoendemic Kibaha district, Tanzania: Implications for malaria control and the IMCI strategy. *Tropical Medicine and International Health* 5(3):179–184.

Tarimo DS, Urassa DP, Msamanga GI (1998) Caretakers' perceptions of the clinical manifestations of childhood malaria in holoendemic rural communities in Tanzania. *East African Medical Journal* 75:93–96.

Tripp AM (1997) *Changing the Rules: The Politics of Liberalization and the Urban Informal Economy in Tanzania*. Berkeley, CA: University of California Press.

Vlassoff C, Manderson L (1998) Incorporating gender in the anthropology of infectious diseases. *Tropical Medicine and International Health* 3(12):1011–1019.

Wang S, Langeler C, Mtasiwa D, Mshana T, Manane Lusinge, Maro G, et al. (2006) Rapid urban malaria appraisal (RUMA) II: Epidemiology of urban malaria in Dar es Salaam (Tanzania). *Malaria Journal* 5(28):1–10.

White NJ (2004) Antimalarial drug resistance. *Journal of Clinical Investigation* 113(8):1084–1092.

Whitty CJM, Allan R, Wiseman V, Ochola S, Nakyanzi-Mugisha M, Vonhm B, et al. (2004). Averting a malaria disaster in Africa—where does the buck stop? *Bulletin of the World Health Organization* 82(5):381–384.

Whyte SR (1997) *Questioning Misfortune*. Cambridge, UK: Cambridge University Press.

Wilce JM (1997) Discourse, power, and the diagnosis of weakness: Encountering practitioners in Bangladesh. *Medical Anthropology Quarterly* 11(3):352–373.

Williams HA, Jones COH (2004) A critical review of behavioral issues related to malaria control in sub-Saharan Africa: What contributions have social scientists made? *Social Science and Medicine* 59:501–523.

Winch PJ (1999) "The Role of Anthropological Methods in a Community-Based Mosquito Net Intervention in Bagamoyo District, Tanzania." In: *Anthropology in Public Health: Bridging Differences in Culture and Society*. RA Hahn, ed. New York: Oxford University Press, pp. 44–62.

Winch PJ, Makemba AM, Kamazima SR, Lurie M, Lwihula GK, Premji Z (1996) Local terminology for febrile illnesses in Bagamoyo District, Tanzania and its impact on the design of a community-based malaria control programme. *Social Science and Medicine* 42(7):1057–1067.

World Health Organization (1994) World malaria situation 1992. *Weekly Epidemiological Record* 69:309–316.

World Health Organization (2000) The Abuja Declaration on Roll Back Malaria in Africa by the African Head of States and Governments. Abuja, Nigeria. Geneva: World Health Organization.

World Health Organization (2002) World Health Report. Reducing Risks, Promoting Healthy Life. Geneva: World Health Organization.

World Health Organization (2005) World Malaria Report 2005. Geneva: World Health Organization.

Worrall E, Basu S, Hanson K (2005) Is malaria a disease of poverty? A review of the literature. *Tropical Medicine and International Health* 10(10):1047–1059.

2

Diagnosis and Management of Asthma in the Medical Marketplace of India: Implications for Efforts to Improve Global Respiratory Health

DAVID VAN SICKLE

Introduction: Asthma as a Global Health Problem

Asthma, a chronic inflammatory disorder of the airways, is now one of the most common chronic diseases, affecting 300 million people worldwide (Global Initiative for Asthma 2004). Asthma emerged as a global public health problem in the second half of the twentieth century, when prevalence appeared to rise steadily in many countries, particularly among children, and most obviously in populations that had or were adopting a westernized lifestyle and becoming urbanized. This rise was accompanied by dramatic increases in the use of health-care services for asthma, in the sale of asthma treatments, and in deaths from asthma.

International epidemiological studies using standardized case definitions and methodologies have permitted comparisons of the patterns of disease prevalence and trends over time in different countries (Asher et al. 2006; Pearce et al. 2007). Overall, approximately 12% to 14% of children world-wide have symptoms suggestive of asthma (Pearce et al. 2007), but the prevalence varies widely across different populations (Asher et al. 2006; Global Initiative for Asthma 2006; Pearce et al. 2007). Recent evidence suggests that prevalence may have leveled off or even begun to decline in some western counties (Asher et al. 2006; Pearce et al. 2007). But in a number of low-income countries—which previously had lower rates of this disease—prevalence of asthma has continued to increase (Asher et al. 2006; Pearce et al. 2007).

Asthma is marked by variable and recurrent episodes of airflow obstruction and bronchial hyper-responsiveness that result in the characteristic symptoms of cough, wheeze, and difficulty breathing (National Asthma Education and Prevention Program 2007). Overall, the clinical manifestations, severity, progression, and response to treatment can vary among individuals and over an individual's lifetime. Its course, for example, may include remission or increasing severity, and may vary markedly in different age-groups. Although the etiology of asthma remains unclear, recent observations suggest that the origins of the disease often occur in childhood, when, for example, exposure to airborne allergens and viral respiratory infections may affect a developing immune system (National Asthma Education and Prevention Program 2007).

A number of common environmental exposures in low- and middle-income countries either increase the risk for the onset of asthma or cause exacerbations of existing disease. For example, exposure to outdoor air pollutants—the levels of which in Indian cities are among the highest in the world—is a major cause of asthma exacerbations and respiratory and all-cause mortality (Brunekreef and Holgate 2002; Global Initiative for Asthma 2004; National Asthma Education and Prevention Program 2007). Indoor air pollution—resulting from the widespread use of biomass fuels for cooking and heating, often in unventilated situations—and a high rate of tobacco smoking also represent major public health problems and important risk factors for respiratory disease, including asthma (Global Initiative for Asthma 2004; Smith 2000). In addition, high rates of occupational asthma (and other lung disease) occur in a range of common industries in these countries because of inadequate workplace protections (Bousquet, Dahl, and Khaltaev 2007; Ehrlich et al. 2005; Global Initiative for Asthma 2004; Jeebhay and Quirce 2007).

Major advances have been made in the management of asthma in recent years, but given the transient nature of its principal symptoms and the absence of a single objective diagnostic test, diagnosis of the disease remains a challenge (Global Initiative for Asthma 2006; National Asthma Education and Prevention Program 2007). Physicians often rely on a characteristic history of symptoms and the findings of a physical examination, although changes in lung function are used to corroborate the diagnosis whenever possible. The episodic treatment of symptoms with bronchodilators, which were the main line of defense in the past, has been largely supplanted by the development of anti-inflammatory medications, designed to prevent or minimize exacerbations of asthma by addressing the underlying pathology of asthma (Global Initiative for Asthma 2006). Although specific recommendations vary for different levels of severity, these medications have emerged as a mainstay of asthma therapy and a focus of clinical practice guidelines, and their prescription is a commonly used metric of the quality of care (Global Initiative for Asthma 2006). These therapies are largely effective in controlling symptoms and allow most people to achieve control of their disease and participate fully in the activities they choose.

Despite advances in the understanding of the pathogenesis of asthma and the development of more effective medications, morbidity and mortality from asthma have continued to increase. Worldwide, asthma accounts for 15 million, or approximately 1%, of the disability-adjusted life-years (DALYs) lost each year (Global Initiative for Asthma 2004)—a burden comparable to that of diabetes—and one in every 250 deaths is attributed to asthma (estimated at 255,000 in 2005); over 80% of these deaths occur in low- and middle-income countries (Global Initiative for Asthma 2004). The economic burden of asthma is considerable in terms of both direct medical expenditures (such as hospital admissions and medications) and indirect costs (such as absences from work and premature death).

These trends have prompted efforts to raise awareness of asthma among physicians and to provide recommendations for its diagnosis and management in clinical settings around the world (Ait-Khaled and Enarson 2005; Global Initiative for Asthma 2006). The development and dissemination of clinical practice guidelines, such as the Global Initiative for Asthma (Global Initiative for Asthma 2006), has been a primary strategy of the activities. These projects summarize the scientific evidence around diagnosis and treatment (among other topics) so that it can be transferred into local practices, with the aim of reducing asthma-related morbidity and mortality.

Global efforts to improve asthma care through guidelines have assumed that a primary determinant of the diagnosis and management of asthma is the level of knowledge of physicians. Evidence-based recommendations presented in an understandable and practical format were expected to improve and standardize the quality of asthma care. However, two decades and numerous updates later, asthma is still not well controlled among most populations, and many patients are not treated optimally (Global Initiative for Asthma 2006; Lalloo and McIvor 2006). Persistent questions remain about why, for example, many patients with symptoms of asthma do not receive a diagnosis of the disease, and why only a minority of patients receive appropriate medications (Global Initiative for Asthma 2006).

The failure of physicians to comprehensively implement asthma guidelines has brought the topic to the forefront of public health research (Ait-Khaled et al. 2006; Cabana et al. 1999, 2000; Cabana, Rand, Becher, and Rubin 2001; Chhabra 2005; Lalloo and McIvor 2006). Although acknowledging the particular problems posed by inadequate medical and limited financial resources in some areas, research has yet to consider other factors that determine how workable and relevant the recommendations of guidelines are in practice. Little attention has been given to the role that local level attributes and variables have on current patterns of practice or to how various incentives may drive the clinical practices of physicians to diverge from what they know.

This chapter uses ethnographic research among physicians in India to identify determinants of diagnosis and treatment of patients in real-world clinical settings, and to examine the factors limiting their implementation of asthma guidelines. I focus on the accuracy of diagnosis and labeling and the delivery of appropriate treatment, examine these in relationship to specific incentives and challenges that doctors face, and place the entire discussion within the context of a pluralistic health-care marketplace. By identifying some of the circumstances, incentives, expectations, and perceptions that influence clinical practices for asthma in India, I hope to provide potential alternative strategies and solutions for global efforts.

Fieldwork Setting and Methodology

This chapter is based on fieldwork conducted in 2001 and 2002, during which I interviewed 40 biomedical (or allopathic) practitioners, many on a number of occasions, and observed consultations with patients in a variety of clinics.[1]

The majority of the participants were located in Chennai—a city along the southeast coast of India—and in an outlying rural agricultural area, which included several villages and small towns. A small number of participants were located in other Indian cities, including Mumbai, New Delhi, and Trivandrum.

Chennai, formerly known as Madras, is the capital of the state of Tamil Nadu. With an estimated population of 7 to 8 million, Chennai is the fourth largest city in India and among the most densely populated cities in the world. It is a leading commercial and manufacturing center—marked by burgeoning electronics and information technology industries—with a diverse population that is much more literate and wealthy than the country as a whole. Yet the city struggles with water shortages, traffic congestion, and air pollution; approximately 20% of its population lives in slums. Similar contrasts characterize the health-care arena. Chennai is home to a number of technologically advanced, for-profit corporate hospitals. But the city is also the historic center of the traditional Tamil medical system known as Siddha, and has remained a setting of vigorous medical pluralism, with traditional Indian medicine (including Ayurveda and homeopathy) playing an important role in health and health care.[2]

Research Methodology

An initial purposive sample of practitioners was selected from the Chennai telephone directory for individual interviews. This group was chosen specifically to reflect a range of medical training and specialties, clinic types and sizes, and diverse geographical and socioeconomic neighborhoods in the city. In an outlying rural agricultural area comprised of several villages and small towns, I interviewed the majority of practitioners likely to treat asthma.

The sample of biomedical practitioners included physicians with a range of experience and training, from general practitioners to respiratory specialists. Seventy percent were men. On average, they reported 20 years in practice and the treatment of 50 patients per day. The individuals in this sample worked in a variety of, and often multiple, health-care settings, from simple private clinics and small hospitals (locally termed "nursing homes") to government health centers and large, modern, private hospitals. In this chapter, I limit materials and discussion to the private sector, where, as I will discuss, the overwhelming majority of health care for asthma is delivered (Das and Hammer 2007b).

Physicians who agreed to participate in individual interviews were met in their offices after consulting hours. They were free to respond in English or Tamil, the local Indian language (a native Tamil-speaking assistant was present at all times), but all physicians chose to speak English throughout the interview(s). Although equivalent terms for common asthma symptoms (including wheeze, cough, and dyspnea) exist in Tamil, English is the language of medical education in India, and practitioners use English throughout their training and in daily clinical practice. The interviews averaged 1 hour in length, and followed a semi-structured format with a prepared, ordered list of questions. Each interview was tape-recorded with the explicit permission of the practitioner and transcribed verbatim for analysis with qualitative software (TAMS Analyzer May Day Softworks, Akron, OH).

Some interviews were conducted using standardized audiovisual depictions of asthma to guide the discussion. This video questionnaire was developed for the International Study of Asthma and Allergies in Childhood (ISAAC), and has been used in many countries around the world to estimate prevalence of asthma among children (Asher et al. 1995, 2006; Pearce et al. 2007). My goal in using this video to lead interviews with physicians was to eliminate bias introduced by the term asthma, and to capture differences in how practitioners saw and treated a particular set of symptoms rather than only what they classified as asthma. Practitioners were not informed in advance either that the video was an instrument used in asthma epidemiology or that the purpose of the study involved asthma in any way. Complete details about the video methodology have been published elsewhere (Van Sickle 2005; Van Sickle and Singh 2008).

This chapter focuses on the results of interviews with biomedical physicians, which comprised one part of a larger ethnographic research project on the topic of asthma and allergy in India. A smaller sample of practitioners of traditional Indian medical systems (including homoeopathy, Ayurveda, and Siddha) was also interviewed, observed, and surveyed during this period. I also interviewed people with asthma and their families, and accompanied some of them to consultations at local clinics and hospitals in order to understand how asthma was perceived and managed, to describe patterns of health-care seeking and prescribed treatments, and to collect information on the frequency of symptoms and the costs of the disease. Another portion of the research was devoted to examining some of the forces driving public awareness and concern with asthma and allergy, including the frequency and content of coverage of the topic in the Indian print media, the role played by the spread of the English language, the marketing activities of the private Indian health-care industry, and the efforts of environmental organizations to use asthma to garner support for campaigns against air pollution. Finally, an emergent market of Indian asthmatics had understandably attracted the attention of the domestic pharmaceutical industry, one of the most vigorous sectors of the Indian economy. I conducted a series of interviews with executives and sales representatives of pharmaceutical companies to examine the way the industry had anticipated and reacted to the increasing prevalence of asthma through popular and professional education, and marketing and promotional efforts.

Diagnosis and Labeling

Although populations in India have previously reported some of the lowest prevalence of asthma in the world, recent reports suggest that prevalence of asthma, and of severe asthma, may be increasing, particularly among children and urban residents (Asher et al. 2006; Chakravarthy, Singh, Swaminathan, and Venkatesan 2002). Prevalence varies widely across age-groups and location, but current estimates suggest at least 5% of the Indian population, or approximately 55 million people, have symptoms of asthma (Asher et al. 2006). However, numerous studies have reported that only a fraction of persons with symptoms of asthma have a diagnosis (Khan, Roy, Christopher, and Cherian 2002; Shivbalan, Balasubramanian, and Anandnathan 2005). In one community study conducted in Mumbai, fewer than 10% of people with symptoms of asthma reported diagnosis by a physician (Chowgule et al. 1998). Despite this fact, there is very little information about how practitioners in India (or other developing countries) view the set of symptoms that characterize asthma, how they describe and label these presentations, or how these practices are influenced by local context and culture. In this section, I examine some reasons underlying when, why, and among whom the diagnosis of asthma is made.

Identifying Asthma—Differential Diagnosis in Indian Clinics

A primary goal of global asthma activities is to encourage practitioners to recognize and diagnose asthma; yet practitioners in India face a number of practical hurdles to doing so. Chief among them is a different overall burden of respiratory diseases, many of which have signs and symptoms that overlap with asthma, complicating the ability of providers to recognize certain typical manifestations of asthma.

Guidelines assume that physicians uniformly interpret and apply the diagnostic label of asthma (Ait-Khaled et al. 2006). But when practitioners in Chennai were shown the audiovisual questionnaire and asked to identify likely diagnosis for each scene, more than half of them attributed the presentations depicted in the video sequences to a variety of diseases other than asthma, including bronchitis, tuberculosis, acute respiratory infections and pneumonia, tropical pulmonary eosinophilia, and chronic obstructive pulmonary disease (Van Sickle 2005; Van Sickle and Singh 2008). In particular, practitioners found it difficult to distinguish presentations of asthma from those of infectious respiratory disease, which, as one specialist put it, "cloud the whole issue of respiratory symptoms in India." Not surprisingly, epidemiological studies conducted in India and other developing countries show that a significant percentage of children with asthma are diagnosed with recurrent pneumonia or tuberculosis (Ciftci, Gunes, Koksal, Ince, and Dogru 2003; Eigen, Laughlin, and Homrighausen 1982; Heffelfinger et al. 2002; Lodha, Puranik, Natchu, and Kabra 2002).

In India, acute respiratory infections account for 40% of all childhood illnesses and approximately 30% of deaths among children, and each year, 2.2 million new cases of tuberculosis are diagnosed across the country (Chadha 2005; Simoes et al. 2006). These patterns changed the symptoms that practitioners were attentive to and the way they interpreted a given presentation. Often, practitioners who viewed the ISAAC video did not report observing wheeze even when it was highlighted, and the majority of physicians attributed scenes featuring cough to something other than asthma (Van Sickle 2005; Van Sickle and Singh 2008). Many tied their interpretation to the local patterns of disease, emphasizing, for example, "In India, the first thing you should think of is tuberculosis." Some perceived conflict between guidelines for infectious respiratory disease and those for asthma. "WHO guidelines emphasize that any patient presenting with cough and wheeze of more than 2 weeks, here in this part of the world, should be suspected of having TB," one said. "But the most common cause of recurrent cough here is asthma, not tuberculosis."

The majority of physicians were overly influenced in their decision making by what was representative, or typically true, of their population, and attributed symptoms such as wheeze and cough to the wrong cause (Croskerry 2002, 2003). It is a common mistake, particularly when economic considerations limit the investigations that can be performed and the number of visits a person will make to a given provider. Although such errors could be minimized if physicians spent more time with patients (Croskerry 2002, 2003), time is short in clinics in India, where there are strong incentives to maximize the number of patients seen. The majority of consultations with general practitioners took 3 minutes—just enough time for 1 or 2 brief questions, a cursory examination, possibly an injection, and the writing of a prescription. A recent study of more than 4100 consultations reported similar results: an average visit to an MBBS doctor in the private sector took 4 minutes (Das and Hammer 2007b).

Physicians emphasized the need for symptom-based guidelines to help providers differentiate asthma from the other respiratory problems that are common in the population (Singh 2004). A number of them criticized the focus of existing guidelines on a single disease and emphasized the need for an approach best suited to a patient with a definitive diagnosis (Price and Thomas 2006). They urged that practical guides be developed to help providers diagnose asthma by providing structured, evidence-based rules for incorporating specific, readily available details from the patient history, such as the reported presence of nocturnal symptoms or a family history of allergy or asthma, together with the basic findings from examination. "Make it easier for clinicians to pick up asthma the moment they see it," one said. A recent World Health Organization initiative, the Practical Approach to Lung Health (PAL), has developed syndromic algorithms to guide primary health workers through patient assessment and referral for major respiratory diseases (ten Asbroek et al. 2005) and also suggests a way in which guidelines might evolve to remain both broadly applicable and connected to real-world clinical settings.

The Organization and Financing of Medical Care, and the Social Life of Asthma

Physicians in urban India diagnose and label asthma in the midst of a strikingly competitive private health-care marketplace. Indian cities, such as New Delhi, Mumbai, and Chennai, may have as many as 80 practitioners within 15 minutes' walking distance of every house (Das and Hammer 2007b). Since households in India overwhelmingly prefer to seek medical care in the private sector—it accounts for 82% of all visits nationwide (Mahal, Yazbek, Peters, and Ramana 2001)—many of these doctors are competing with each other for patients. Moreover, there are no substantial systems of medical insurance, so the bulk of health-care spending (82%, according to the World Health Organization) is private out-of-pocket payment made at the time of illness on a fee-for-service basis. Few organizational arrangements tie individuals to a particular physician or clinic; patients typically resort to numerous providers over time (or simultaneously), for different diseases, and often across medical systems, such as Ayurveda or homeopathy. In this environment, providers try to meet patient expectations about the type of care they will receive and to offer diagnoses and labels that are acceptable to them. The very real concern about losing patients to other providers leads physicians to limit the diagnosis and labeling of diseases with unpopular connotations, such as asthma.

Asthma has a variety of negative meanings among the Indian public and is widely considered a stigmatized disease (Aggarwal et al. 2006; Behera, Kaur, Gupta, and Verma 2006; Ghosh 2004; Gupta 1997; Khan et al. 2002; Kumar 1999); in some areas, sufferers are still forced to live separately from the community. Physicians ascribed the social significance to mistaken perceptions that it is a contagious (Shivbalan et al. 2005), debilitating, and untreatable chronic disease; many Indians also regard it as something that affects adults only (Shivbalan et al. 2005). As a result, physicians faced substantial resistance from patients and family members to a diagnosis of asthma, particularly in the case of children. "Patients don't like the word 'asthma.' They won't agree with the doctor. It's difficult to convince them that they have asthma." Other physicians felt compelled to help patients avoid the label. "I wouldn't like to brand a person as an asthmatic because that has a different connotation here. Even if they have severe wheezing, if I say 'asthma,' or ask them 'Any family history of asthma?' they will say, 'No, no. It's not asthma!' They wouldn't like to accept. They feel it is something that should not come to a person."

Practitioners looking to satisfy their patients and forge a stable relationship with them as customers are attracted to alternative, gentler diagnoses to help patients cope better with their ailments. These labels avoid stigma, play down the chronicity, and emphasize the potential for recovery, but they also contribute to the persistence of ambiguous and potentially harmful ideas about serious health problems (Nichter 1994). "Here we don't tell them it's asthma, due to the stigma attached. Instead we use all sorts of euphemisms, such as 'wheezy bronchitis' or simply 'wheezy child,' or if there is some allergy, we call it 'allergic bronchitis.'" Physicians underlined the potential for unpopular diagnostic labels to drive patients away, to the clinics of other practitioners. "If you tell them, 'Your child is suffering from asthma,' invariably they will shift to a different pediatrician who says, 'It is not asthma. It is only allergic bronchitis.' Or, 'wheezy bronchitis.' Or, 'This can be treated, it can be handled.'" The following excerpt from one interview summarizes the concerns about the power of the label:

> Suppose a child has a respiratory infection and wheeze. Parents don't want to hear that word "bronchial asthma." Even if one doctor tells them—they will take the treatment for respiratory infection and never come back to that doctor. They go to the next doctor … Wherever the parents are told that the child may be having asthma, they will try to avoid. They'll go to some other doctor, because every doctor, the first time he sees a patient, he won't tell it is asthma. Because the patient won't come back.
> *So what happens to those patients?*

> One doctor after the other. Very few people will tell them that it is asthma. They'll only say it is "allergic wheeze," or they will tell them it is "wheezy bronchitis," or they'll tell them "allergic bronchitis," but nobody uses this word "asthma."

A pediatrician at a large hospital noted that even patients who registered and attended the hospital's weekly "Asthma Clinic" resisted the label. "They come and get their routine drugs but even there nobody wants to be branded an asthmatic." Reacting to the unpopularity of the term asthma, another large hospital in Chennai renamed its pediatric asthma clinic the "Wheezy Child Clinic."

Practitioners sometimes misrepresented asthma or employed alternative labels to motivate patients to comply with treatment. As one told me, "We have to tell them, 'It is not a lifelong problem. Definitely you'll be getting cured if you take this medicine.' That way they are taking the medicines." Others used the social significance of disease labels to encourage patients to use inhaled medications, suggesting, "What I do is give them a hint. 'If you're careless, this allergic bronchitis can become asthma.' Then they're more likely to take the medicines carefully." As another explained, "In the first stage, I tell them that symptoms are like asthma or may take the form of asthma. I'm priming them that the patient has some problem, but not a 'big problem' like asthma. This motivates them to take their medication."

Some physicians temporarily offered patients a more neutral label, such as wheezing, and then, using allergy skin testing or another type of investigation, worked to identify something specific about the patient that could be incorporated into the diagnosis. In this way, persons with asthma received a diagnosis of "dust mite allergy." Other specialists described diagnosing closely allied conditions—such as allergic rhinitis or gastroesophageal reflux disease—which lacked the stigma of asthma but could be treated with relative sophistication. These physicians argued that these were reasonable substitutes shown to be linked to asthma, which allowed them to prescribe appropriate anti-inflammatory medications.

Commercial pressures in the marketplace have largely precluded the emergence of any system of patient referral. "Nobody wants to refer patients in private practice. The general practitioner doesn't want to let his patients go to the specialist," one told me. "Why should he refer? He would like to keep the patient with him. He gets his fees every week." Another said, "I know many people who say, 'You'd rather admit a few patients. You've got to keep a nursing home full. Because how are we going to keep running the nursing home?'" Because they feared losing the patient from their practice, general practitioners almost never referred to specialists. "At the end of the day," one physician explained, "I'm always concerned that the moment one of my patients goes into those types of clinics, I will lose track of them." General practitioners criticized specialists for devising ways to retain referred patients indefinitely. One said, "Such fellows can always find something someone is allergic to."

Patient resistance to the diagnosis of asthma limited the extent to which any physician could educate persons and family members about the disease (Singh 2004); few patients knew much about the disease or understood they suffered from asthma (Shivbalan et al. 2005). "It's medical apathy," one pediatric allergist told me. "Doctors are too afraid to give the diagnostic label asthma because they are able to perceive their distress when they are being told." Another said, doctors "have failed to educate the patients, and remove the stigma and fear that comes with asthma." He wanted patients to be made aware that "we have excellent medicines now which will give them a normal life," and believed that physicians had an obligation to take "a more positive attitude toward the label asthma" and to spend more time demystifying and destigmatizing asthma.

Popular awareness of asthma is increasing, prompted by accelerating coverage in the Indian media, the educational activities of environmental and physician organizations, and the promotion and marketing campaigns of pharmaceutical companies. Over time, these efforts may gradually dispel some of the negative connotations around asthma and encourage patients and clinicians to pursue appropriate diagnosis and management. Until then, guidelines will continue to face struggles in settings like India, where the social significance and meaning of asthma exert an influence on health-care seeking and medication taking, and there are incentives that encourage patients and providers to align around alternative disease labels.

Treatment

Despite its prevalence, there have been few systematic attempts to document how physicians in India manage asthma. A small study from one part of the country (Bedi 1994) and anecdotal reports (Ghosh 2004; Singh 2004) suggest that many practitioners in Indian communities do not manage the disease as recommended by international guidelines. By some estimates, fewer than 2% of persons with asthma in India use inhaled medication for asthma (Singh 2004). Lack of knowledge and awareness among physicians of the utility of inhaled and anti-inflammatory medications is not the only barrier to their use. Instead, a variety of social and medical calculations, as well as economic incentives, explain why many practitioners underused recommended asthma medications.

Symptomatic Treatment

Despite the emergence of inhaled therapies and anti-inflammatory medications designed to prevent asthma exacerbations, the majority of persons with asthma only received low-cost treatment to address symptoms as they occur. Very few general practitioners prescribed inhaled therapies (Bedi 1994; Gupta 1997). Instead, they relied on oral medications, including bronchodilators, methylxanthines, corticosteroids, antibiotics, antihistamines, and a variety of formulations that targeted cough and mucus production. Persons who presented with signs and symptoms of asthma (or during an exacerbation) often received (some of) these formulations as injections, a popular and preferred form of treatment in India (Lakshman and Nichter 2000). Although these strategies provide temporary relief from asthma and a variety of other respiratory problems, in the case of asthma they do little to prevent recurrence of symptoms or to slow the progression of the disease. Some have other potential downsides, such as the development of side effects resulting from the use of corticosteroids or the emergence of resistant strains of organisms from the inappropriate use of antibiotics.

The overwhelming tendency of general practitioners to address asthma through symptomatic treatment of exacerbations is the result of convergence between the preferences and expectations of patients and the motivation of physicians to demonstrate their skill and effectiveness as healers. Patients preferred symptomatic oral or injectable treatment for a variety of reasons including concern about inhaled medications. They also evaluated the skill and efficacy of a provider by assessing his or her ability to deliver prompt, symptomatic relief. As a result, providers felt compelled to deal conclusively with episodes using the most popular and accepted treatments, fearing that otherwise they would lose customers and income (Das and Hammer 2007a).

But many physicians had an additional incentive to treat the symptoms of asthma as they occurred. Although symptomatic treatment generally ended the exacerbation and generated revenue for the practitioner, it did little to prevent recurrence in cases of persistent disease. When, after some time, such patients experienced another exacerbation, they returned to the practitioner who effectively resolved the previous episode, seeking symptomatic relief and guaranteeing him or her additional revenue.

One of the obstacles to prescribing inhaled medications was the effectiveness with which they relieved symptoms in the short term, and, in the case of anti-inflammatories, their demonstrated long-term efficacy at preventing exacerbations. Physicians expressed concern that such treatments might mean the loss of a significant portion of their clinic revenue. Sales pitches for inhaled medications made by pharmaceutical representatives were interrupted by physicians who asked "How will I earn a living?" Some called the drugs "practice killers." Another pulmonologist summarized the situation:

> When it comes to asthma, most people get their asthma treatment from private practitioners. And when you see a private practitioner, one of the limiting things here is the private practitioner has to hang on to his patient. So he tends to give them something which gives them quick relief and also makes sure that the patient comes back to see him. Which means if you tell them straight away "You'll probably have it for the rest of your life," then it's good-bye to that patient. They wouldn't say that they have asthma. They might give this injection

that gives them a wonderful sense of relief within 24 hours and after a few days they get the same problem so they would come back to see the practitioner, and so then there's more fees. So, in fact, there may be a kind of disincentive to prevent patients from having any symptoms whatsoever for the rest of their lives, which will effectively be like shooting yourself in the foot, and preventing your income from improving. So, maybe I'm a little cynical here, but I think these are all the kinds of pressures that a private practitioner would have. He would have to make sure that the patient is not going to wander off to the next person down the road.

Inhaled and Anti-inflammatory Therapy

Many Indians had reservations about inhalers and declined to use them even when they had been recommended by their physician. Aside from concerns about cost, opposition arises from the popular belief that they are excessively powerful, and that an individual, particularly a child, might become addicted—"a life sentence." Others feared the drugs would turn them or their child into a lifelong asthmatic. In fact, the Indian public still widely considers inhalers drugs of last resort (Gupta 1997; Gupta, Sen Mazumdar, Gupta, and Sen Mazumdar 1998). Many believe that once they or their children begin to use them, no other medications will work in the future. Some considered the use of inhalers a sign of a desperate—or poorly qualified—practitioner, and stated that they would take their child to a "better doctor" if inhalers were prescribed.

Stigma surrounding asthma and the visibility of inhalers also played an important role in the lack of acceptance and use of inhaled medications. Because inhalers are emblematic of asthma, and cannot be readily used without drawing attention to the person, they are particularly unpopular among the poor (Lal, Kumar, and Malhotra 1994) and among women (Singh, Sinha, and Gupta 2002), perhaps because of the barrier the disease poses to the marriage prospects of young women.

In contrast to general practitioners, specialists defined their practice around the very medications shunned by the bulk of the population, and employed several strategies to encourage use of inhaled medications. Often, demonstrating the effectiveness of inhaled bronchodilators by giving them to symptomatic patients in the clinic was enough. "They realize that it can relieve the wheeze within 2 to 3 minutes and that it is much better than taking oral tablets," one told me. "So I try to convince them by showing them." Others tried to reassure patients about their safety, or emphasize the cost-effectiveness of the medications; some extended credit toward their purchase.

With the general public being reluctant to use inhaled medications that have a dramatic effect on symptoms, only specialist physicians ever tried to introduce the subtler, and more expensive, preventive anti-inflammatories. Recommended to be taken daily, regardless of whether the person has symptoms or not, they work by addressing the underlying pathology of the disease, eliminating most symptoms and exacerbations. But this leads many patients to wonder whether they need to continue taking them at all. Numerous studies have found that the majority of patients in India discontinue their use as soon as their symptoms have resolved (Gupta and Gupta 2001; Shivbalan et al. 2005).

Getting patients to try inhaled steroids required a variety of tactics. Specialists often asked patients initially to use them for 1 month, only to extend their treatment during follow-up appointments. Some never prescribed preventive therapy during the initial visit; only if patients returned with additional symptoms, and explicitly asked whether future attacks could be prevented, did they introduce daily medications. Specialists also often exaggerated the benefits of inhaled anti-inflammatory therapy. Patients were told that routine use of inhaled steroids would cure asthma, bring about "changes in your airways," or "make you immune to the effects of allergens," eliminating the need for future treatment. Other practitioners described the drugs as preventive medicine, able to lower the risk of asthma developing in patients at risk due to heredity or the change of seasons.

Many specialists criticized general practitioners for undermining confidence of their patients in the drugs and even intervening to stop inhaled therapy after it had been started. "Patients come back to us saying that inhaler treatment has been stopped by their primary care doctors," one allergist told me. "Grassroots doctors actually discourage inhalers!" Specialists routinely reinforced the need for inhaled therapy, trying to keep patients convinced of the need for and the safety of the medications. As one practitioner put it, "Even if we explain a hundred times, 'Inhaled steroids and inhaled drugs don't have any side effects,' they are not convinced. They still equate it to addiction."

Indian pharmaceutical companies have also tried to normalize use of inhalers and daily preventive therapy through public and professional education and awareness efforts. Their networks of sales representatives provide the companies with detailed information about the factors influencing the acceptance and use of their medications, allowing them to quickly respond and adapt their products to changing popular and professional mindsets (Kamat and Nichter 1998). This detailed information from the field guided a successful strategy of creating specific products to address the pressures and concerns of particular patients and physicians. For example, the companies marketed inhalers and nebulizers as providing lower dosages of medications to those concerned about the potential harmfulness of biomedical drugs, and emphasized less expensive dry-powder inhalers as an affordable alternative among those for whom cost was a barrier.

Affordability of Recommended Therapy

Guidelines take for granted that recommended drugs are available and affordable, an assumption that is not true in many parts of the world. In fact, in many countries, when they are available, essential asthma medicines and appropriate preventive asthma therapy remain unaffordable for the majority of the population (Ait-Khaled et al. 2000; Ait-Khaled, Enarson, and Bousquet 2001; Mendis et al. 2007; Watson and Lewis 1997). In one study of doctors in 24 developing countries, 83% reported that they would prescribe more inhaled corticosteroids if they were cheaper (Watson and Lewis 1997).

The preference of many physicians in India for treatments not recommended in asthma guidelines often represents a practical calculation of the affordability of medication for patients. Providers adjusted their practices to patient characteristics and routinely considered the socioeconomic status of patients when determining what medications to prescribe (see also Nichter 1989), taking into account whether the patient could afford to spend the money required to take the drugs as advised. "Although the cost of asthma medication is probably among the lowest in the world in India," one physician said, "even that is unaffordable to the majority of asthmatics." Physicians improvised with the options at hand, and attempted to make do with what the patient could afford. To see that physicians can meet these varied means, Indian pharmaceutical companies have developed and marketed class-specific products for patients at all levels of the socioeconomic continuum.

Some physicians criticized international guidelines for emphasizing the newest, most expensive formulations while overlooking issues about the affordability of asthma therapy in settings like India. "We need a common-sense approach to asthma that recognizes international criteria may not apply universally," one told me. "My view is we need studies of what is appropriate, acceptable, and possible, as well as what is optimum." In fact, by some estimates, only 10% of the Indian population can afford inhaled medications, and providing treatment currently recommended by international guidelines to every patient in India (assuming a 5% prevalence) would require 30% of the country's health-care budget (Singh 2004). There was widespread interest in a basic, affordable regimen of preventive therapy and "something like reasonable asthma care" for the general population of India. The search for low-cost treatment options led some physicians to suggest another look at managing asthma using old oral medications such as theophylline and corticosteroids. "We still don't know how bursts of oral steroids for exacerbations compare to inhaled steroids," one noted. "There is a great gap between optimum asthma care and what is available at present. And that might be one way of overcoming this."

Medical Pluralism

Efforts to raise the quality of care for asthma in countries such as India must also address the effects of a pluralistic health-care marketplace on clinical practice, health-care seeking, and the social meanings of medication and diagnostic labels. The increased popularity and visibility of traditional Indian medicine treatments for asthma sparked off contests over the public understanding and meaning of asthma, and the ability to define the appropriate treatment approach, as practitioners sought to portray asthma in ways that reinforced their specific position with respect to its management (Jackson 2001). Because these public debates contextualized and imbued asthma and its medications with social significance, they shaped the clinical practices of physicians and the health behaviors of patients and family.

Asthma is believed to have been well known in ancient India. Clear descriptions of its symptomatology and treatment appear in the ancient Ayurvedic text *Caraka Samhita*, where it is referred to as *tamaka swasa* (Chapter 6.3, Section 18), and (like other diseases) is thought to arise from an imbalance of the bodily humors, or *tridosha*. In particular, asthma is considered to be the result of excessive cooling of the body, which arouses the *kapha* humor, stimulating the production of phlegm and obstructing the airways (Nichter 1987; Obeyesekere 1976). Contemporary practitioners of traditional Indian medicine understand and explain asthma using a combination of these humoral theories and the hot–cold conceptual schema (Nichter 2003) linking health to the quality of the surrounding social and natural environment (Langford 1995, 2002).[3]

Practitioners of traditional Indian medicine used asthma to support radical critiques of orthodox biomedicine and its reliance on routine pharmaceutical therapy for chronic diseases. These practitioners promoted a return to traditional principles, lifestyles, and medical treatments as steps necessary to resolve the individual and social problems giving rise to asthma. They linked their approach to the popular interpretation of the disease as an outcome of the disordered westernization of Indian society, a more toxic environment, and an increasingly susceptible population. Many practitioners of traditional Indian medicine lured patients with advertisements and promises of a cure for asthma (Figure 2.1). Signs touting the ability of various medical systems or practitioners to cure the disease were visible throughout Indian cities, and editorials and articles making such claims appeared regularly in local newspapers and media outlets.

Practitioners of traditional medicine reinforced popular doubts about inhaled and anti-inflammatory treatments, characterizing them as icons of the false promises and quick, temporary fixes of biomedical pharmaceuticals. And they defined their approach in opposition to biomedical treatments, which, they warned, suppressed rather than cured symptoms, caused dangerous side effects, and created lifelong asthmatics. In addition, biomedicine was explained to hinder the effectiveness of Indian treatment, and traditional medicine practitioners encouraged patients taking biomedical treatment for asthma to give

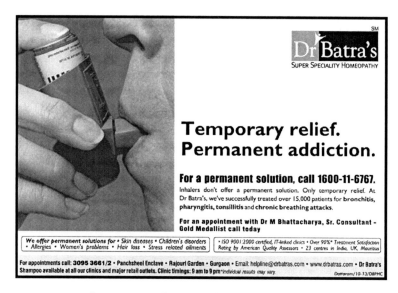

Figure 2.1. An advertisement for one of the largest chains of homeopathic clinics in India. (Photo by David Van Sickle)

up their medications as soon as possible, making this a prerequisite or explicit goal of successful therapy.

Biomedical practitioners believed that traditional practitioners undermined their ability to pursue accurate but unpopular diagnoses, to offer appropriate education about the disease, and to convince patients of the need for long-term therapy. As one said, "Quacks who are not physicians suddenly advertise, 'Complete cure for asthma!' The people rush." In the clinic, "They tell them that it is curable. It is the first thing they say. That they won't ever need to see a doctor for it again." Biomedical practitioners struggled to break a pattern of health seeking in which asthma patients attended their clinics during times of acute exacerbations but followed Indian medicine during intervening periods when they were free from symptoms. "They walk into an allopath when it is acute, but when it is not acute they experiment with all kinds of quackery, witchcraft and whatnot," one practitioner told me. Many biomedical clinicians tried to preempt use of Indian medicine by explaining to patients in consultations that alternative treatments would not resolve acute exacerbations. "When you get a sudden severe attack, Ayurveda and Siddha will not work," one said. "Then you will have to come back to an allopathic physician." He continued:

> What's the point when you have to run back to us when there is an emergency? Instead of spending 6 months or 10 months going for treatment and not really getting rid of it, let's follow the prescribed protocol of treatment. If it doesn't work for you then you go and try.

Biomedical physicians emphasized the problems posed by patients who simultaneously used treatments from multiple medical systems, many of whom concealed the use of alternative medicines from their physicians.

Specialists were particularly impatient with the fact that, having received only symptomatic treatments for asthma and allergy, many patients believed that they had tried everything biomedicine had to offer. "Nine out of 10 times they only receive oral bronchodilators. It never means a comprehensive plan with inhaled steroids." They blamed general practitioners for pushing the public toward alternative medicines and the treatments of traditional Indian medicine. "Our allopathic friends have failed miserably in educating the population about asthma and the treatment possibilities," one pediatric allergist said. "A lot of people have become resigned to the conclusion that allopathy is hopeless for long-term treatment of asthma, and that alternative medicines have a cure for asthma." Others emphasized the responsibility of general practitioners to improve their practices, noting, "the future of alternate medicine will be very bright if our fellow doctors continue to be in the dark as to the advances of asthma treatment in allopathy." In response, general practitioners argued that it was the chronic regimens of specialists that drove such patients to Indian medicines in search of a cure.

Others emphasized that biomedical practitioners would do well to study what drew patients to Indian medicine and forged confidence in their alternative treatments. One pulmonologist emphasized that their "holistic approach" of cultivated, lasting, and trusting relationships with their patients might explain the "totally different attitudes" of patients toward Indian medicine treatment and biomedicine. "The patient feels straightaway kind of indebted to this person who has spent so much time and energy understanding him as a person," he said. "After that, it doesn't matter what he says or what he does, he has full faith in him." He noted that such connections between patients and their Indian medicine practitioners explained why many of his patients made excuses for it when it failed, but "tied anything untoward onto allopathic practice." He said:

> You can tell them till the cows come home about the number of studies and the scientific approach to what we practice and how safe it is and how the safety is recorded and so on. It doesn't cut any ice there with them at all. Because they have this kind of emotional empathy for something which is traditional and which is holistic and which is supposedly harmless—which is untrue, incidentally.

As this pulmonologist saw it, biomedical physicians in India could learn a lot from Indian medicine, not the least of which was how "to make this allopathic system more acceptable—a friendlier system—so that patients like and accept it."

Biomedical physicians tried to undermine their patients' confidence in the safety and efficacy of the traditional treatments and the integrity of the practitioners, and rarely encouraged patients to continue using Indian medicines. In one consultation I observed, a biomedical practitioner seeing a young girl for wheezing asked about the use of Siddha medicine. "It is like this," he told the girl's father. "Say you have to get to Delhi. You can either fly to Delhi in an airplane, or you can go by foot. If you walk, you may arrive 2 or 3 months from now, or you may not arrive at all. If you fly you will be in Delhi in a matter of hours." Traditional Indian medicine practitioners don't deny that their cures will take longer, often months at a minimum. But they present this to patients as evidence that their treatments are, in fact, remedying the underlying problem giving rise to asthma. It is in part a strategy to reassure patients and families who might otherwise balk at the effort and expense of lengthy treatment.

A widespread discourse about the misuse of steroids and allegations of quackery underscores the competitive nature of medicine in India, and illustrates the struggle for popular authority and legitimacy in the pluralistic marketplace. Many physicians tried to foster the impression that legitimate medical practitioners in India were beleaguered by quacks and hucksters who deliberately misused corticosteroids, making it difficult to successfully treat a patient with asthma. "I don't advise steroids, but they are common here," one specialist told me, "especially among the general practitioners. There are a lot of quacks in this line. A lot of quacks. They immediately prescribe prednisolone, betamethasone, and dexamethasone." Quacks were said to be giving steroids "left and right" for any and all complaints—and asthma and allergy in particular—in order to demonstrate an immediate effect. "They want well-being. They want the patient to become alright soon," said one allergist. "And when they give steroids he will just immediately get up and improve." In fact, a number of specialists—blaming both general practitioners and practitioners of Indian medicine—indicated that they had difficulty gaining medical control of asthma because, as one put it, "Most patients are already so loaded with steroids that it is difficult to treat them."

In specialist clinics, warnings about the rampant prescription of steroids by general practitioners and their surreptitious use by practitioners of Indian medicine were a regular feature of consultations. General practitioners also cautioned their patients about the uncertainty and danger inherent in Indian medicines and the "burgeoning number of quacks and morally corrupt practitioners" willing to harm patients to build a reputation. "They will tell you it is herbal," one explained to a family, "but what they are actually doing is giving a high dose of steroid" to "work wonders" on asthma patients. "Naturally you're going to feel better, you're not going to get the wheeze or the allergy."

Specialists told me that patients often left their practice, or rejected preventive anti-inflammatory treatment, because the results were slow to materialize compared to what they had experienced with steroids. "Oral steroids are so effective at suppressing symptoms that patients think the doctor is really a magician," one told me. "Patients feel that your [inhaled] treatment is off, while this man has made the child active again, and there is no wheeze or anything." These practitioners attempted to stem increasing interest in Indian medicine by publicizing the "danger of Indian medicine treatment," and the "good drugs available in allopathy," in a variety of newspaper articles, editorials, and television interviews. But many found themselves on the defensive, as they struggled to differentiate inhaled steroids from the harmful steroids of quacks.

The Practical Management of Asthma in the Marketplace

This chapter suggests that the limited implementation of guideline recommendations among physicians in India is not entirely a result of providers not knowing what to do. Instead, when faced with persons with symptoms of asthma in their clinics, their behavior is often influenced by a variety of contextual factors and incentives; these rival medical knowledge as a determinant of the quality of diagnosis and treatment. By describing how the situation often rewards these practitioners for doing less or acting differently than they know they should, I have tried to illustrate how there are few mechanisms in the private sector, as it is currently organized, to drive physicians to implement the recommendations of guidelines (Bhat 1999).

In this setting, an abundant supply of physicians and the predominance of private payment, pressured physicians to forge a stable relationship with their patients, and often gave rise to important divergences between the knowledge of physicians and their clinical practices. Physicians tended to do what they were asked, or what patients expected and preferred, even when they knew that it was not always appropriate, optimal, or recommended. Other analyses have confirmed that the knowledge of practitioners is not the only determinant of the quality of care delivered. A detailed study of visits to practitioners in New Delhi concluded that households would be better off using less qualified private practitioners, who tended to do as much as they knew, rather than more qualified doctors in the public sector, whose effort was often minimal (Das and Hammer 2007b). In the United States, the supply of physicians and the capacity of health services have been shown to be an important determinant of the frequency of use of medical care (Center for the Evaluative Clinical Sciences 1998). Similarly, underuse of effective medications and services in the United States has been linked to discontinuity of care and a lack of mechanisms—for example, routine measurement and reporting of performance—to encourage and support compliance with treatment guidelines (McGlynn et al. 2003).

In Chennai, many patients and general practitioners emphasized symptomatic management of asthma exacerbations, and faced with a considerable variety of respiratory diseases with similar and overlapping presentations, physicians both mistakenly and deliberately applied alternative labels that patients found more acceptable. They had both financial and intellectual rationales for doing so. Office treatment of respiratory symptoms accounted for a significant portion of their income and represented an important source of care for patients who could not afford routine medications. In addition, many practitioners did not believe that much of what they saw was, in fact, asthma, and preferred to err on the side of treating potential respiratory infections or tuberculosis.

Biomedical specialists tried to raise awareness of asthma and the need for specialist attention, to remake the reputation of asthma medications, and to encourage patients to accept greater responsibility for the management of their disease. They attempted to overcome the stigma surrounding asthma and resistance to medications by changing the technological basis for the diagnosis, by educating patients and other practitioners, and by effectively preventing episodes through anti-inflammatory medications. Nevertheless, they treated only a small, often wealthy, fraction of the Indian population.

Clinical practices were also influenced by the behavior and rhetoric of other practitioners in the pluralistic marketplace. As the prevalence and awareness of asthma increased, different groups of practitioners attempted to identify and position themselves as the proper source of asthma care. Scientific and popular controversy about the origins of asthma—which tied the disease to collective anxieties about modernization and the social and environmental changes accompanying industrialization—presented practitioners of traditional systems of Indian medicine with the opportunity to reassert the cultural authenticity and relevance of their medical traditions to a modern world with new kinds of ailments (Ferzacca 2001). Competition among practitioners across medical systems turned on alternative conceptualizations of asthma and its appropriate therapy, as practitioners struggled to engage popular opinion about the causes of asthma and to package their approach in ways that appealed to their clients.

As these practitioners realized, the cultural explanations and social relations of a disease impact the selection of health-care providers and the decisions guiding treatment (Nichter 1994). Sometimes the diagnostic and treatment preferences of patients and their families are at odds with clinical guidelines (Mull 1999). In these situations, physicians often adjust their practices to meet the expectations of their clientele. This research suggests that changing popular ideas about the origins and meaning of asthma, as well as consumer perceptions of quality and appropriate asthma care, may be an important strategy to improve the timely diagnosis, appropriate treatment, and follow-up or referral of persons with asthma (Ait-Khaled et al. 2001; Das and Hammer 2007b).

Conclusion

The populations of India and other low- and lower middle-income countries will increasingly face a growing burden of chronic conditions—including asthma, cardiovascular disease (Reddy et al. 2006), chronic obstructive pulmonary disease (Barnes 2007; Global Initiative for Chronic Obstructive Lung Disease 2006), and diabetes (Yoon et al. 2006)—that require long-term medical management and routine pharmacotherapy (Nichter and Van Sickle 2002). Worldwide, the number of persons with asthma is predicted to rise by 100 million people (to 400 million) by 2025 (Global Initiative for Asthma 2004). Yet very little is known about how practicing clinicians in such settings have responded to the rising prevalence and growing public health importance of these diseases, or what role they expect to take in shaping management of these conditions over time. Whether clinical and public health strategies that have been successful elsewhere make sense and are desirable in these settings and under existing health-care arrangements requires further investigation.

For example, self-management of asthma—in which the patient assumes some responsibility for day-to-day treatment of their disease—has become a cornerstone of therapy in many industrialized countries. But the concept and tools of self-management will likely need to be rethought and adjusted to fit the particular medical circumstances and cultural settings of other populations. How can asthma management education be accomplished in India when many general practitioners barely communicate with patients at all during consultations and very few clinics have nurses or paramedical personnel? At the same time, the Indian health-care marketplace is changing rapidly, as evidenced by the recent launch of a network of private primary health-care centers, and the introduction of private health insurance. New strategies backed by anthropological research will be needed to align the care and treatment of chronic diseases under these arrangements with public health goals, and to ensure effective collaboration with health care delivered in the public sector (Sengupta and Nundy 2005).

Ethnographic fieldwork might identify promising, but entirely different, options for the organization and delivery of care for chronic diseases. For example, my interviews with persons with asthma revealed that many turned directly to pharmacists, rather than physicians, for advice and medication to treat their symptoms. As a result, I began to interview pharmacists and pharmacy attendants, and spent afternoons behind the counter, listening and watching sales take place. Later on, I conducted a simulated client study at pharmacies across Chennai to investigate the types of medications that pharmacy attendants recommend to customers seeking treatment for a standardized set of asthma symptoms, and to examine the quality of pharmacy services and the characteristics of consultations (Van Sickle 2006). The main lesson from that research is that a pharmacy attendant training program might go a long way toward improving the management of asthma in the community by helping staff to identify and refer persons with possible asthma, dispense appropriate advice and medications, and collaborate with other health professionals in the management of persons with known chronic respiratory disease. Given the importance of retail pharmacies in many low- and middle-income countries as a source of medication and advice for many health problems, their integration into global strategies to improve diagnosis and management of asthma (and other chronic diseases) should be considered.

Anthropological research on asthma and other chronic diseases in these settings might also provide insights into the quality or stability of measures of disease prevalence across populations. In this case, interviews with physicians revealed that their perceptions and interpretations of asthma symptoms could partly explain the low prevalence of diagnosed asthma reported by populations in India. The same physicians could, over time, become more aware of the symptoms of asthma and more likely assign the diagnosis of asthma to patients. As Dodge and Burrows (1980) suggested, "the epidemiology of asthma is a reflection of the diagnostic habits of physicians in the locale, as well as an indicator of the frequency of a specific syndrome." Ethnographic fieldwork can help identify which instruments and estimates of asthma prevalence best reflect the true burden of disease (Fuso et al. 2000).

Until pharmacological or public health measures become available to prevent or lower the prevalence of asthma, the priorities must be to limit exposures that cause asthma exacerbations, and to make the cost-effective approaches proven to reduce asthma-related morbidity and mortality available to as many people as possible. Nowhere will these strategies be more important than in developing countries such as India and China, where, because of the size of their populations and their unprecedented rates of economic development, urbanization, and associated lifestyle and environmental changes, the greatest burden of increasing asthma prevalence is likely to occur (Global Initiative for Asthma 2004).

This chapter has examined the multiple rationales behind the limited implementation of recommended clinical practices and treatments among a sample of physicians in India. It suggests that as long as more knowledge is not necessarily reflected in improvements in the practices of these physicians, attempts to raise the quality of asthma care built solely on increasing the knowledge of practitioners will have a fundamental, but limited role. Global efforts to ensure the delivery of quality asthma care should incorporate a situational and contextually informed understanding of the factors limiting asthma diagnosis and management. Multilevel work that takes into account the positions of multiple stakeholders, ranging from patients and their families to the practitioners and the pharmaceutical industry, will suggest additional potential strategies to align incentives around quality care and population health.

Acknowledgments

This research was generously supported by the U.S. National Science Foundation (BCS-0001494) and the Robert Wood Johnson Foundation Health and Society Scholars Program. I would also like to thank Manjula Datta, Mark Nichter, and Anne Wright.

Notes

1. This research was approved by the Institutional Review Board at the University of Arizona and by the Ministry of Human Resource Development, Government of India.

2. The label "Indian medicine" is routinely used in India to differentiate these types of practitioners, treatments, and products from those of allopathy or biomedicine. Although I use the term biomedicine throughout this chapter, for the most part physicians in India refer to the biomedical system as allopathy; I have retained that term in quotations.

3. Readers interested in reviews of traditional Indian medical systems should consult Langford (2002); Leslie (1976); Leslie and Young (1992); Nichter (1992); Obeyesekere (1992); Tabor (1981); Trawick (1987, 1992); and Zimmermann (1980, 1988).

References

Aggarwal AN, Chaudhry K, Chhabra SK, D'Souza GA, Gupta D, Jindal SK et al. (2006) Prevalence and risk factors for bronchial asthma in Indian adults: A multicentre study. *Indian Journal of Chest Diseases and Allied Sciences* 48:13–22.

Ait-Khaled N, Auregan G, Bencharif N, Camara LM, Dagli E, Djankine K et al. (2000) Affordability of inhaled corticosteroids as a potential barrier to treatment of asthma in some developing countries. *The International Journal of Tuberculosis and Lung Disease* 4:268–271.

Ait-Khaled N, Enarson D, Bousquet J (2001) Chronic respiratory diseases in developing countries: The burden and strategies for prevention and management. *Bulletin of the World Health Organization* 79:971–979.

Ait-Khaled N, Enarson D (2005) *Management of Asthma: A Guide to the Essentials of Good Clinical Practice*. Paris: International Union against Tuberculosis and Lung Disease.

Ait-Khaled N, Enarson DA, Bencharif N, Boulahdib F, Camara LM, Dagli E et al. (2006) Implementation of asthma guidelines in health centres of several developing countries. *The International Journal of Tuberculosis and Lung Disease* 10:104–109.

Asher MI, Keil U, Anderson HR, Beasley R, Crane J, Martinez F et al. (1995) International Study of Asthma and Allergies in Childhood (ISAAC): Rationale and methods. *European Respiratory Journal* 8:483–491.

Asher MI, Montefort S, Bjorksten B, Lai CK, Strachan DP, Weiland SK et al. (2006) Worldwide time trends in the prevalence of symptoms of asthma, allergic rhinoconjunctivitis, and eczema in childhood: ISAAC phases one and three repeat multi-country cross-sectional surveys. *Lancet* 368:733–743.

Barnes PJ (2007) Chronic obstructive pulmonary disease: A growing but neglected global epidemic. *PLoS Medicine* 4:e112.

Bedi RS (1994) Asthma management by private general practitioners of Punjab. *Indian Journal of Chest Diseases and Allied Sciences* 36:9–13.

Behera D, Kaur S, Gupta D, Verma SK (2006) Evaluation of self-care manual in bronchial asthma. *Indian Journal of Chest Diseases and Allied Sciences* 48:43–48.

Bhat R (1999) Characteristics of private medical practice in India: A provider perspective. *Health Policy Plan* 14:26–37.

Bousquet J, Dahl R, Khaltaev N (2007) Global alliance against chronic respiratory diseases. *European Respiratory Journal* 29:233–239.

Brunekreef B, Holgate ST (2002) Air pollution and health. *Lancet* 360:1233–1242.

Cabana MD, Rand CS, Powe NR, Wu AW, Wilson MH, Abboud PA et al. (1999) Why don't physicians follow clinical practice guidelines? A framework for improvement. *The Journal of American Medical Association* 282:1458–1465.

Cabana MD, Ebel BE, Cooper-Patrick L, Powe NR, Rubin HR, Rand CS (2000) Barriers pediatricians face when using asthma practice guidelines. *Archives of Pediatric and Adolescent Medicine* 154:685–693.

Cabana MD, Rand CS, Becher OJ, Rubin HR (2001) Reasons for pediatrician nonadherence to asthma guidelines. *Archives of Pediatric and Adolescent Medicine* 155:1057–1062.

Center for the Evaluative Clinical Sciences (1998) *The Dartmouth Atlas of Health Care*. Hanover, NH: Dartmouth Medical School.

Chadha VK (2005) Tuberculosis epidemiology in India: A review. *The International Journal of Tuberculosis and Lung Disease* 9:1072–1082.

Chakravarthy S, Singh RB, Swaminathan S, Venkatesan P (2002) Prevalence of asthma in urban and rural children in Tamil Nadu. *National Medical Journal of India* 15:260–263.

Chhabra SK (2005) Guidelines for management of asthma: The gaps between theory and practice. *Indian Journal of Chest Diseases and Allied Sciences* 47:77–80.

Chowgule RV, Shetye VM, Parmar JR, Bhosale AM, Khandagale MR, Phalnitkar SV et al. (1998) Prevalence of respiratory symptoms, bronchial hyperreactivity, and asthma in a megacity. Results of the European community respiratory health survey in Mumbai (Bombay). *American Journal of Respiratory and Critical Care Medicine* 158:547–554.

Ciftci E, Gunes M, Koksal Y, Ince E, Dogru U (2003) Underlying causes of recurrent pneumonia in Turkish children in a university hospital. *Journal of Tropical Pediatrics* 49:212–215.

Croskerry P (2002) Achieving quality in clinical decision making: Cognitive strategies and detection of bias. *Academic Emergency Medicine* 9:1184–1204.

Croskerry P (2003) The importance of cognitive errors in diagnosis and strategies to minimize them. *Academic Medicine* 78:775–780.

Das J, Hammer J (2007a) Location, location, location: Residence, wealth, and the quality of medical care in Delhi, India. *Health Affairs (Millwood)* 26:w338–w351.

Das J, Hammer J (2007b) Money for nothing: The dire straits of medical practice in Delhi, India. *Journal of Development Economics* 83:1–36.

Dodge RR, Burrows B (1980) The prevalence and incidence of asthma and asthma-like symptoms in a general population sample. *American Review of Respiratory Disease* 122:567–575.

Ehrlich RI, White N, Norman R, Laubscher R, Steyn K, Lombard C et al. (2005) Wheeze, asthma diagnosis and medication use: A national adult survey in a developing country. *Thorax* 60:895–901.

Eigen H, Laughlin JJ, Homrighausen J (1982) Recurrent pneumonia in children and its relationship to bronchial hyperreactivity. *Pediatrics* 70:698–704.

Ferzacca S (2001) *Healing the Modern in a Central Javanese City.* Durham, NC: Carolina Academic Press.

Fuso L, de Rosa M, Corbo GM, Valente S, Forastiere F, Agabiti N et al. (2000) Repeatability of the ISAAC video questionnaire and its accuracy against a clinical diagnosis of asthma. *Respiratory Medicine* 94:397–403.

Ghosh G (2004) Optimal care for asthmatic children—do we need special clinics? *Indian Pediatrics* 41:907–911.

Global Initiative for Asthma (2004) *Global Burden of Asthma.* Bethesda, MD: National Institutes of Health; National Heart, Lung, and Blood Institute.

Global Initiative for Asthma (2006) *Global Strategy for Asthma Management and Prevention.* Bethesda, MD: National Institutes of Health; National Heart, Lung, and Blood Institute.

Global Initiative for Chronic Obstructive Lung Disease (2006) *Global Strategy for Diagnosis, Management, and Prevention of COPD.* Bethesda, MD: National Institutes of Health; National Heart, Lung, and Blood Institute.

Gupta PP, Gupta KB (2001) Awareness about the disease in asthma patients receiving treatment from physicians at different levels. *Indian Journal of Chest Diseases and Allied Sciences* 43:91–95.

Gupta SK (1997) Approach to aerosol therapy in management of asthma at primary care level. *Journal of the Indian Medical Association* 95:595–596.

Gupta SK, Sen Mazumdar K, Gupta S, Sen Mazumdar A (1998) Patient education programme in bronchial asthma in India: Why, how, what and where to communicate? *Indian Journal of Chest Diseases and Allied Sciences* 40:117–124.

Heffelfinger JD, Davis TE, Gebrian B, Bordeau R, Schwartz B, Dowell SF (2002) Evaluation of children with recurrent pneumonia diagnosed by World Health Organization criteria. *The Pediatric Infectious Disease Journal* 21:108–112.

Jackson M (2001) Allergy: The making of a modern plague. *Clinical and Experimental Allergy* 31:1665–1671.

Jeebhay MF, Quirce S (2007) Occupational asthma in the developing and industrialised world: A review. *The International Journal of Tuberculosis and Lung Disease* 11:122–133.

Kamat VR, Nichter M (1998) Pharmacies, self-medication and pharmaceutical marketing in Bombay, India. *Social Science and Medicine* 47:779–794.

Khan S, Roy A, Christopher DJ, Cherian AM (2002) Prevalence of bronchial asthma among bank employees of Vellore using questionnaire-based data. *Journal of the Indian Medical Association* 100:643–644, 655.

Kumar L (1999) Consensus guidelines on management of childhood asthma in India. *Indian Pediatrics* 36:157–165.

Lakshman M, Nichter M (2000) Contamination of medicine injection paraphernalia used by registered medical practitioners in south India: An ethnographic study. *Social Science and Medicine* 51:11–28.

Lal A, Kumar L, Malhotra S (1994) Socio-economic burden of childhood asthma. *Indian Pediatrics* 31:425–432.

Lalloo UG, McIvor RA (2006) Management of chronic asthma in adults in diverse regions of the world. *The International Journal of Tuberculosis and Lung Disease* 10:474–483.

Langford J (1995) Ayurvedic interiors: Person, space and episteme in three medical practices. *Cultural Anthropology* 10:330–366.

Langford J (2002) *Fluent Bodies: Ayurvedic Remedies for Postcolonial Imbalance*. Durham, NC: Duke University Press.

Leslie CM, ed. (1976) *Asian Medical Systems: A Comparative Study*. Berkeley, CA: University of California Press.

Leslie C, Young A, eds. (1992) *Paths to Asian Medical Knowledge*. Berkeley, CA: University of California Press.

Lodha R, Puranik M, Natchu UC, Kabra SK (2002) Recurrent pneumonia in children: Clinical profile and underlying causes. *Acta Paediatrica* 91:1170–1173.

Mahal A, Yazbek A, Peters D, Ramana GNV (2001) *The Poor and Health Service Use in India*. Washington, DC: World Bank.

McGlynn EA, Asch SM, Adams J, Keesey J, Hicks J, DeCristofaro A et al. (2003) The quality of health care delivered to adults in the United States. *New England Journal of Medicine* 348:2635–2645.

Mendis S, Fukino K, Cameron A, Laing R, Filipe A, Jr, Khatib O et al. (2007) The availability and affordability of selected essential medicines for chronic diseases in six low- and middle-income countries. *Bulletin of the World Health Organization* 85:279–288.

Mull DS (1999) "Anthropological Perspective on Childhood Pneumonia in Pakistan." In: *Anthropology in Public Health: Bridging Differences in Culture and Society*. R Hahn, ed. New York: Oxford University Press, pp. 84–114.

National Asthma Education and Prevention Program (2007) *Expert Panel Report 3: Guidelines for the Diagnosis and Management of Asthma*. Bethesda, MD: US Department of Health and Human Services; National Institutes of Health; National Heart, Lung, and Blood Institute.

Nichter M (1987) Cultural dimensions of hot, cold and sema in Sinhalese health culture. *Social Science and Medicine* 25:377–387.

Nichter M (1989) "Paying for What Ails You: Sociocultural Issues Influencing the Ways and Means of Therapy Payment in South India." In: *Anthropology and International Health: South Asian Case Studies*. Dordrecht, Netherlands: Kluwer Academic Publishers, pp. 214–231.

Nichter M (1992) *Anthropological Approaches to the Study of Ethnomedicine*. Langhorne, PA: Gordon and Breach Science Publishers.

Nichter M (1994) Illness semantics and international health: The weak lungs/TB complex in the Philippines. *Social Science and Medicine* 38:649–663.

Nichter M (2003) "Hot/Cold." In: *South Asian Folklore: An Encyclopedia*. MA Mills, PJ Claus, S Diamond, eds. New York: Routledge, pp. 289–290.

Nichter M, Van Sickle D (2002) "The Challenges of India's Health and Health Care Transitions." In: *The Challenges of India's Health and Health Care Transitions*. A Ayres, P Oldenburg, eds. Armonk, NY: ME Sharpe for The Asia Society, pp. 159–196.

Obeyesekere G (1976) "The Impact of Ayurvedic Ideas on the Culture and the Individual in Sri Lanka." In: *Paths to Asian Medical Knowledge*. C Leslie, A Young, eds. Berkeley, CA: University of California Press, pp. 201–226.

Obeyesekere G (1992) "Science, Experimentation, and Clinical Practice in Ayurveda." In: *Paths to Asian Medical Knowledge*. C Leslie, A Young, eds. Berkeley, CA: University of California, pp. 160–176.

Pearce N, Ait-Khaled N, Beasley R, Mallol J, Keil U, Mitchell E et al. (2007) Worldwide trends in the prevalence of asthma symptoms: Phase III of the International Study of Asthma and Allergies in Childhood (ISAAC). *Thorax* 62:758–766.

Price D, Thomas M (2006) Breaking new ground: Challenging existing asthma guidelines. *BMC Pulmonary Medicine* 6(Suppl 1):S6.

Reddy KS, Prabhakaran D, Chaturvedi V, Jeemon P, Thankappan KR, Ramakrishnan L et al. (2006) Methods for establishing a surveillance system for cardiovascular diseases in Indian industrial populations. *Bulletin of the World Health Organization* 84:461–469.

Sengupta A, Nundy S (2005) The private health sector in India. *British Medical Journal* 331:1157–1158.

Shivbalan S, Balasubramanian S, Anandnathan K (2005) What do parents of asthmatic children know about asthma? An Indian perspective. *Indian Journal of Chest Diseases and Allied Sciences* 47:81–87.

Simoes EAF, Cherian TH, Chow J, Shahid-Salles S, Laxminarayan R, John TJ (2006) "Acute Respiratory Infections in Children." In: *Disease Control Priorities in Developing Countries*. DT Jamison, JG Breman, AR Measham, G Alleyne, M Claeson, DB Evans, P Jha, A Mills, P Musgrove, eds. New York: Oxford University Press and the World Bank, pp. 483–497.

Singh RB (2004) Asthma in India: Applying science to reality. *Clinical and Experimental Allergy* 34:686–688.

Singh V, Sinha HV, Gupta R (2002) Barriers in the management of asthma and attitudes towards complementary medicine. *Respiratory Medicine* 96:835–840.

Smith KR (2000) Inaugural article: National burden of disease in India from indoor air pollution. *Proceedings of the National Academy of Sciences USA* 97:13286–13293.

Tabor DC (1981) Ripe and unripe: Concepts of health and sickness in Ayurvedic medicine. *Social Science and Medicine* [B]15:439–455.

ten Asbroek AH, Delnoij DM, Niessen LW, Scherpbier RW, Shrestha N, Bam DS et al. (2005) Implementing global knowledge in local practice: A WHO lung health initiative in Nepal. *Health Policy Plan* 20:290–301.

Trawick M (1987) "Death and Nurturance in Indian Systems of Healing." In: *Paths to Asian Medical Knowledge*. C Leslie, A Young, eds. Berkeley, CA: University of California Press, pp. 129–159.

Trawick M (1992) "An Ayurvedic Theory of Cancer." In: *Anthropological Approaches to the Study of Ethnomedicine*. M Nichter, ed. Langhorne, PA: Gordon and Breach, pp. 207–222.

Van Sickle D (2005) Perceptions of asthma among physicians: An exploratory study with the ISAAC video. *European Respiratory Journal* 26:829–834.

Van Sickle D (2006) Management of asthma at private pharmacies in India. *The International Journal of Tuberculosis and Lung Disease* 10:1386–1392.

Van Sickle D, Singh RB (2008) A video-simulation study of the management of asthma exacerbations by physicians in India. *The Clinical Respiratory Journal* 2:98–105.

Watson JP, Lewis RA (1997) Is asthma treatment affordable in developing countries? *Thorax* 52:605–607.

Yoon KH, Lee JH, Kim JW, Cho JH, Choi YH, Ko SH et al. (2006) Epidemic obesity and type 2 diabetes in Asia. *Lancet* 368:1681–1688.

Zimmermann F (1980) Rtu-Satmya: The seasonal cycle and the principle of appropriateness. *Social Science and Medicine* 14B:99–106.

Zimmermann F (1988) The jungle and the aroma of meats: An ecological theme in Hindu medicine. *Social Science and Medicine* 27:197–215.

3

Situating Stress: Lessons from Lay Discourses on Diabetes

NANCY E. SCHOENBERG, ELAINE M. DREW,
ELEANOR PALO STOLLER, AND CARY S. KART

Introduction

Type 2 diabetes (previously known as non–insulin-dependent diabetes mellitus or adult-onset diabetes, and hereafter referred to as DM or diabetes) accounts for approximately 90% to 95% of the total diagnosed cases of diabetes in the United States and is a major cause of morbidity, disability, and mortality globally (National Institute of Diabetes and Digestive and Kidney Diseases [NIDDK] 2002). In the United States alone, DM directly affects approximately 17 million people, or 6.2% of the population, and is the leading cause of non-traumatic amputations, new cases of blindness in adults, and end-stage renal disease. Individuals with diabetes are also at greater risk for stroke, high blood pressure, central nervous system disease, periodontal disease, and depression. In 1999, approximately 450,000 deaths, or nearly one-fifth of all deaths in the United States, were attributed to diabetes (Centers for Disease Control and Prevention [CDC] 2002).

The heavy burden that diabetes places on health is likely to increase through the first half of the 21st century owing to the decreasing age of onset of DM, the escalating incidence of DM, and the increase of disproportionately affected groups in the United States. The number of new cases of diabetes has already reached approximately 800,000 annually, or 2200 each day, with a predicted

165% increase in the number of those with diagnosed diabetes by 2050 (Boyle et al. 2001).

Etiology of Diabetes and Risk Factors

The etiology of diabetes involves a complicated and interactive mixture of genetic, metabolic, behavioral, and ecological factors (NIDDK 2002). Epidemiologists have associated the risk of diabetes with older age, family history, lower socioeconomic status (SES), and specific ethnic groups (Harris 2001). In 2000, the age-adjusted prevalence of diabetes was 18.8% among Native Americans, 15.0% among non-Hispanic African Americans, 13.6% among Mexican Americans, and 7.4% among non-Hispanic Whites (NIDDK 2002).

Although there is clear evidence of dramatic global interpopulation differences in diabetes prevalence, it is difficult to disentangle the relative contribution of factors that increase the likelihood of diabetes (Harris 2001). Although the health disparities literature frequently focuses on race/ethnicity as a key predictor of suboptimal health, low SES and residence patterns similarly undermine health status; the precise mechanisms and processes engendering these risks are yet undetermined (Moss and Krieger 1995).

Stress and Diabetes

Stress constitutes another risk factor linked to economic marginalization and is implicated in the diabetes epidemic (NIDDK 2002). In the biomedical diabetes stress literature, researchers have examined both acute stressors (e.g., loss of a spouse) and chronic stressors (e.g., income insufficiency and subsequent physiological responses). Although some studies suggest that stress can directly affect blood glucose (BG) through the release of stress hormones or by disrupting self-care practices (Cox and Gonder-Frederick 1992; Peyrot, McMurry, and Kruger 1999), methodological shortcomings complicate arriving at definitive conclusions. For clinical practice, many medical texts discuss stress as playing a role in diabetes in a distinctly limited way—i.e., stress *may* elevate blood sugar and, thus, needs to be "managed" by the patient (Havel and Taborsky 2003). With some exceptions (Hinkle and Wolf 1952), attention to life history and circumstances has fallen outside the purview of biomedical research and practice, but has been a defining characteristic of anthropological inquiry into diabetes (Walrath 2003).

Anthropological Contributions to Stress Research

Recent findings from anthropologists and other social scientists on lay knowledge of diabetes, disease causation, and stressful life situations highlight the various and nuanced ways in which individuals from diverse backgrounds associate stress with diabetes. Oftentimes, anthropologists have grounded these discussions in explanatory models (EMs), a construct most commonly associated in anthropology with Arthur Kleinman et al. (1980; 1988), who maintains that all groups (patients, healers, etc.) have ideas about sickness and health that presumably affect their approaches to prevention and healing. EMs generally take the following five elements into consideration: (1) etiology (explanation for causes of the condition); (2) proximal (precipitating) factors and symptoms; (3) physiology; (4) course of the condition (e.g., timeline) and appropriate behavioral response; and (5) treatment. Medical anthropologists have argued that making these EMs explicit may optimize treatment approach and ultimately improve health.

For example, in a study conducted by Mercado-Martinez and Ramos-Herrera (2002), Mexicans and Mexican Americans provide diabetes EMs that implicate emotional stress or a stressful event as an etiological factor. Participants reported social, economic, or relational factors that produced strong emotions, either a "fright" (*susto*) or an event of serious anger or rage, which caused their diabetes. In addition, although most participants were cognizant of biomedical perspectives toward diabetes etiology (e.g., diet or exercise factors), they actively discounted biomedical claims of diabetes causality, particularly regarding heredity. Weller et al. (1999:724) described concordance with biomedical perspectives on diabetes among Latinos of varying national origins, but found that the "Mexican sample differed from the others by consistently identifying emotional causes of diabetes: fright (*susto*), anger, and strong emotions." Studies among Mexican Americans in the U.S. and aboriginal communities in Canada have also demonstrated how participants link changing life circumstances and increases in life stressors to diabetes onset, even when the acculturation of biomedical beliefs with traditional health beliefs results in a blending of the participants' overall explanation of diabetes (Garro 1995; Hunt, Valenzuela, and Pugh 1998; Poss and Jezewski 2002).

When researchers have compared patient and practitioner diabetes EMs, they have frequently found stress to occupy a central role in lay diabetes models, alongside the tendency of practitioners to either minimize or disregard the potential influences of stress (Cohen, Tripp-Reimer, Smith, Sorofman, and Lively 1994). Loewe and Freeman (2000) found important patient–provider differences in EMs of diabetes along many dimensions, including the role of stress in diabetes onset and management. They found that patients attributed diabetes onset to a particular trigger or precipitating event that tended to be complex, contextually situated, and consistent with existing social arrangements. The authors suggest that given the tendency of providers to discount claims about stress as either a trigger to diabetes onset or significant factor in glycemic control, it is not surprising that patients reiterate standard biomedical explanations in their etiological narratives, even as they later interject views about the role of a stressful event or emotion in the onset or exacerbation of BG levels. As Rock (2003) points out, the biomedical emphasis on the individual body, versus the social context and the life world of the sufferer, is related to the reliance of biomedicine on a precise scientific diagnostic definition of diabetes that differs from the experiences of sufferers and the more comprehensive definitions of the disease.

As Loewe and Freeman (2000:388) conclude, despite decades of research that documents the relationship between psychosocial stress and physiological responses, "clinical medicine remains highly reductionist and the vectors of disease point from soma to psyche, rarely in the other direction." Concomitantly, health-care providers and diabetes educators continue to underscore lifestyle changes, namely diet, exercise, and medication adherence to enhance glycemic control, and relegate stress to a regimen management issue. As a result, psychosocial factors linked to diabetes continue to be minimized in physician training and patient care, "depriving patients of a comprehensive approach to their problems" (Helz and Templeton 1990:1275). As Scheder (1988) has argued, a continued emphasis on individual health behaviors, although relevant to diabetes, obscures the importance of oppressive and stress-producing social and political-economic factors related to negative health outcomes.

In this chapter, we will expand the discussion of stress in the context of diabetes by demonstrating how a multiethnic sample of adults with diabetes implicated stress in the onset and management of the disease. We focus on how informants describe varying arenas in which stress intersects with diabetes, how they situate stress within their lives and the experience of the disease, and the implications of these findings for diabetes research and medical practice worldwide.

Research Methods

Study Participants

In-depth interviews were conducted with 20 respondents aged 50 years or older with DM from each of the following groups: African Americans, Mexican Americans, Great Lakes Indians, and rural Whites. Great Lakes Indians, all of whom lived off reservation in the Detroit metropolitan area, is an amalgamated term for the major tribal groups in the upper midwest including Pottawatomie, Ojibway, and Odawa (Chapleski, Lichtenberg, Dwyer, Youngblade, and Tsai 1997). Rural Whites from Appalachian Kentucky were included because of the high prevalence of DM and because they face many of the same risk factors for poor diabetes outcomes as other disproportionately affected ethnic groups, including compromised health access and low SES (CDC 2002).

Although determination of the sample size using theoretical saturation (the point at which no new themes or surprises emerge) is optimal, our sample size was preestablished and limited because of resource constraints and time-consuming open-ended protocols. While we included individuals from racial/ethnic groups most likely to be affected by DM, our findings cannot necessarily be considered representative of each group or used to provide a cross-cultural comparison. Table 3.1 highlights key characteristics of our sample.

Recruitment

Our study sites were located in Cleveland and Toledo, Ohio (for the African Americans and Mexican Americans, the latter of whom were both immigrants and native born); Detroit, Michigan (for the Great Lakes Indians); and a rural county in Appalachian Kentucky (for the rural whites). Since these four groups are most accessible in different areas of the country, we maintained four distinct research sites, with one coinvestigator at each site. The coinvestigators, a medical anthropologist (Schoenberg), two medical sociologists (Stoller & Cart), and a gerontologist (Chapleski), remained in close contact via telephone and face-to-face meetings to ensure consistency in project protocol and analysis. Aside from actually conducting the interviews, the investigators were responsible for all research components (i.e., research design, obtaining project funding, ensuring protection of human subjects, training, data transfer and management, analysis, and development of publications and presentations). All protocols were approved by the Institutional Review Board at each participating institution.

Participants were recruited either at senior centers (American Indians and Mexican Americans) or at local health clinics (rural residents and African Americans), depending on access and previous experiences of investigators. There are sufficient similarities in these venues (attended by individuals of modest means; host conventional, biomedical health programs; often, health-care providers) to expect that recruitment from these sites would not bias results.

Although we did not gather income data, several factors suggest income insufficiency among the study sample. First, 37%, 36%, 39%, and 24% of African American, Mexican American, Native American and rural older adults in the Kentucky county from which the samples were drawn, respectively, live near or below the poverty level (KY State Data Center 2003; Lamison-White 1997). In addition, our recruitment sites are likely to have captured a lower income population; university-affiliated or public health-care clinics generally serve low-income populations, and clients of senior centers have lower incomes

Table 3.1. Selected Characteristics of Study Participants (N = 80)

CHARACTERISTICS	AFRICAN AMERICANS (N = 20)	MEXICAN AMERICANS (N = 20)	GREAT LAKES INDIANS (N = 20)	WHITES (N = 20)	TOTAL (N = 80)
Mean age in years (s.d.)	69.3 (12.2)	69.6 (9.0)	66.2 (5.9)	65.5 (8.4)	67.6 (9.2)
Gender					
Female (%)	70.0	68.4	60.0	64.7	65.8
Male (%)	30.0	31.6	40.0	35.3	34.2
Marital Status					
Married (%)	50.0	45.0	40.0	40.0	43.8
Divorced (%)	15.0	5.0	20.0	10.0	12.5
Widowed (%)	25.0	45.0	35.0	50.0	38.8
Other (separated/ never married) (%)	10.0	5.0	5.0	—	5.0
Education° (years completed)	11.7 (3.7)	5.5 (5.0)	12.1 (2.5)	7.8 (3.1)	9.3 (4.5)
Employment Status					
Retired	55.0%	55.5%	63.2%	35.0%	51.9%
Employed	15.0%	10.0%	26.3%	10.0%	15.2%
Disabled	25.0%	20.0%	5.3%	35.0%	21.5%
Other	5.0%	15.0%	5.3%	20.0%	11.4%
[a]Health Status°°					
Mean (s.d.)	3.1 (1.0)	3.4 (1.0)	3.0 (1.2)	3.9 (1.0)	3.3 (1.1)

° p < .000

°° p < .041

[a]Self-reported, on scale from 1 to 5, where 1 = excellent, 2 = very good, 3 = good, 4 = fair, and 5 = poor.

than the general older adult population (Krout, Cutler, and Coward 1990). Finally, since only 15% of participants are currently employed, income earning potential is limited.

At each site, we were assisted by a gatekeeper who either had access to medical charts to confirm a diagnosis of diabetes or were acquainted with the individuals well enough to know about the diagnosis of diabetes in them (Arcury and Quandt 1999; Schoenberg and Drew 2002). Potential participants were asked if they would be interested in being interviewed about diabetes. If, after being approached by the gatekeeper or investigator, the potential partici-pant expressed interest in joining the study, a mutually convenient time and location for interview was arranged.

Interviewer Training and Research Protocols

We hired local interviewers, all of whom had extensive experience in inter-viewing and were either from the same background as or very familiar with the groups they interviewed. Interview sessions with Mexican American elders were conducted either in Spanish or English, depending on the participant's preference. To ensure that all sites followed consistent research protocols, we used professional training procedures, including the use of standard manuals, training sessions, and quality assurance measures, involving the investigators in listening to the first few tapes at each site and providing extensive feedback to the interviewers.

Upon completion of human subjects protocols, participants were asked structured and semi-structured questions on demographics, health history, and diabetes, the latter of which involved a modified Kleinman explanatory model (EM) framework (Kleinman 1988). This framework focuses on the cause of the illness, timing (why it started when it did, the duration of the illness), symptoms associated with diabetes, and possible treatments and their efficacy. Interviewers did not inquire about stress; rather, the fundamental place of stress within lay narratives on diabetes emerged as a central thematic con-struct during analytic procedures. Unless requested otherwise (no one did), all interviews were tape-recorded, allowing interviewers to focus on culling rich insights rather than on note taking. Interviews generally lasted between 45 and 90 minutes and informants were provided with a $15 honorarium to compensate them for their time.

Analysis

Upon completion of the transcription of the tape-recorded sessions, we under-took analysis in two stages (Strauss and Corbin 1990). First, five qualitative researchers coded (broke data down into manageable segments) each line of the transcripts, using the interview guide as a template to help organize responses. To ensure consistency in the coding process, we developed a codebook, essentially a long and comprehensive list of the codes with definitions. The researchers refined the codebooks by comparing and discussing interpretation of the codes (Bernard 1995). Second, researchers drew out examples of salient narratives and verbatim statements related to these codes (Spradley 1979).

Diabetes Narratives

A key finding of this study was the prevailing perspective, regardless of ethnicity or residential background, that (1) stress can cause or precipitate the onset of diabetes; (2) stress may directly affect or exacerbate DM; (3) stress may undermine optimal DM self-care practices; and (4) stress serves as both a precursor to and a consequence of complications due to diabetes. A fifth result, one that was threaded throughout the other sections, was how descriptions of inadequate resources and stress-inducing environments were implicated in the onset, exacerbation, and management challenges of diabetes. The narratives presented subsequently elaborate on these findings.

"My Tears Was Sweet": Narratives on Stressful Life Circumstances and the Development of Diabetes

Stress as an etiological factor in the onset of diabetes was described in one of several ways—as a proximate or distal factor and as a sudden versus protracted factor in the onset of diabetes. The distinction among these descriptors concerns *cause* (with proximate or distal referring to the direct versus indirect or mediating position of the factor relative to disease onset) and *timing* (with sudden versus protracted referring to whether the disease onset was swift or prolonged) of diabetes etiology.

Sudden and Proximate Factor. Diabetes could be immediately brought on by one or more direct stress-inducing and, therefore diabetes-inducing, events. In the terse words of a 65-year-old rural White woman, "My mother told me that she thought I was shocked into diabetes. My brother-in-law was murdered by my son." An immediate and direct attribution of stress to diabetes is also provided by a 52-year-old African American woman in the following narrative.

> Yeah I went for a biopsy and I was in the car, after the biopsy, and I got so thirsty and they brought me some orange juice and that didn't get it and I couldn't hold my water and stuff, you know ... and my lips were all white and that's how I knew. I called my doctor and I went up to there and they took my blood sugar and gave

me some insulin immediately, I take insulin three times. I think I was so scared of going for that biopsy, the stress, it brought it on out.

This narrative also suggests that diabetes may be latently residing in one's body and may be triggered suddenly by stressful events. Diabetes was "brought on out" by the stressor directly (i.e., without reference to any mediating variables) and suddenly (i.e., in the car right after the biopsy).

Protracted and Proximate Factor. Other informants described a protracted period of time over which they experienced stressful circumstances to be directly responsible for the onset of their diabetes. The experience described by a 57-year-old Mexican American man encapsulates many perspectives that difficult experiences bring about stress, which in turn, causes diabetes. His narrative reveals how, as a new immigrant, he was faced with stress-inducing circumstances, including lack of health insurance and questionable roommates, which ultimately wore down his health and directly caused his diabetes.

> I remember that I was going through a lot of stress, I mean extremes … like when you're very desperate, you know, like anxiety and desperate for some solution. For some reason, I don't know, I just got so depressed and I look back and that's what I believe that maybe really triggered the diabetes … I was here only, maybe five months and I had my son with me. My son was only, he just turned two years old and I didn't know anybody and I was having problems coping. I didn't want my son to get sick, you know, because it was during October, November, you know, the cold weather. I didn't have any insurance and he didn't have any insurance and we were living with some people and I was just under a lot of stress and then that's when I noticed that I was urinating a lot, then after awhile I started seeing blurred and then I just felt so tired and I could barely see. I ended up at T. Hospital; they put me on a stretcher. They drew blood. Well, they gave me the bad news, I have diabetes.

Other high-stress environments and circumstances described by informants included stressful workplaces, resource deficiencies, or other family challenges.

Sudden and Distal Factor. Sudden or distal narratives, such as that of the 64-year-old African American woman here, focused on a swift onset of their diabetes; however, they often referred to a long-term exposure to stress as the etiologic agent responsible for increasing their body's susceptibility to diabetes. Although the events that lead up to the onset of her diabetes might be construed as a protracted onset of diabetes, the informant's emphasis on the punctuated event (her grandson's murder) that served as the final blow to her health suggests a rapid onset.

> Well I was married and now I've been married for over forty years now and he passed and everything went down then, just like, downhill, I haven't been no

where else since I've taken care of him like for ten years, I think about ten years. ... He had small cell lung cancer and the doctors gave him six months to live and he lived ten years. ... And then I heard this ... my grandson got killed, he got killed over by X. And so, I cried and, and uh, you know, with my husband being as ill as he is, was, and I couldn't ... I couldn't just wipe my face and have tears run down ... and then that, it was sweet. My tears was sweet. Yes. And so I went to the doctor, I told him about it so, I told him to test me for diabetes and he did and I have it.

Protracted and Distal Factor. An example of how stress may be secondarily related to the onset of diabetes is provided through the narrative of a 76-year-old African American woman who connects the onset of her diabetes with the stress brought on by the death of her mother, which catapulted her into managing a series of stress-inducing responsibilities. As she recalls, she coped with this demanding series of responsibilities by engaging in problematic eating behaviors. Thus, the informant implicates stress as mediated though eating patterns, in the onset of her diabetes.

> PARTICIPANT: I'd always been high-normal or pre-diabetic because I have it in family. Both my mother's family and my father's family there was diabetes and we had diabetics in the family. So I knew that but after my mother's death, and I was the executrix for her estate and, well as I said, we, we're a very, very close family and although I handled her death very well I know I ate all the wrong things. And I eat lots of things, the scales tipped over.
> INTERVIEWER: Why did diabetes come on at that time?
> PARTICIPANT: My mother's death. She had just died recently. There were friends and relatives who brought lots of good food and cakes and all those good things and I ate like it was going out of style. It was emotional thing. I think personality enters into it to. I am stressed. I have a tendency to worry.

These narratives linking stress to the onset of diabetes reveal the fluidity and overlapping nature of etiologically ascribed stressors. Participants appear to place both timing and cause on intersecting continua with specific stressors spilling over and not necessarily confined to one timing–cause linkage. The death of a spouse, for example, might be viewed as either causing a sudden stressor or causing a protracted series of stressors leading to diabetes.

"The Worry Itself over Having it Would Cause You to Be Sick": Narratives on How Stress or Stress-Linked Emotions Exacerbate Existing Diabetes

In addition to attributing stress to diabetes onset, many described how stress or stress-linked emotions (anxiety, frustration, or anger) experienced in daily life or work directly exacerbate existing diabetes. A 78-year-old Mexican American man described the connection between his stressful living environment and higher BG levels as "Because with me living with a guy that is a drug addict, I been having a hard time with that son-of-a-gun. I mean he's always ... drugged up, you know. He makes me so mad. That's when my sugar was up a lot. When I get mad it's dangerous, dangerous."

Some informants specified the connection between one's attitude or mental coping strategies, and the ability to keep BG levels within manageable limits. One 63-year-old rural White woman explained,

> You have a stressful day and it's hard ... It's like blood pressure, it will go right up. I just try to keep it out of my mind, that is the main thing, is learning to live with it, accept it, and not be afraid, do what you're supposed to do, for yourself and the diabetes but not let it be part of you're life, not let it overrule.

Narratives suggest not only that emotional stress can raise or lower BG levels, ultimately exacerbating diabetes, but also that positive coping strategies are important in the midst of difficult life and work situations. As one 75-year-old rural White man summarized, "I guess the worry itself over having it would cause you to be sick. It'd do more damage to you than any other thing and I don't want it affecting me that way."

"When I Got Too Much Tension, Too Much Worry About Something ... I Start Eating": Narratives on the Role of Stress in Undermining Optimal Self-Care Practices

In addition to linking stress directly to BG levels, several informants also described how stress at home and at work compromised their ability to engage in optimal self-care practices. A 60-year-old Mexican American woman explains,

> Well, I guess I overworked myself because I have a full time and two part time jobs. I have to take care of my kids and I have the bills and me and my kids always they eat home-made cooked food. They don't eat McDonald's so I have to buy groceries. I sleep. ... not too much sleep and I working sometimes and when I work in other place, you know, I work some days 12, 14 hours a day and later sleep a little bit. Take my kids to school and later come back and got to the other job and later go back and cook something. Well, when I got too much tension, too much worry about something and I start eating, like I say, things I don't have to and I love breads.

This narrative demonstrates that given the stressful life and work situations of these diabetic individuals, the inability to comply with standard diet and exercise regimens is not just a simple disregard for the regimen, but rather a contextually mediated response shaped by stress. However, the influence of stress on self-care is not only limited to diet, but also serves to undermine recommended self-care practices. As a 61-year-old Great Lakes Indian man describes, the recognition of being under stress reminded him to monitor his BG.

> My ex-mother-in-law had diabetes ... she controlled it by shot twice a day. She used to fluctuate how many cc's she was getting. She'd raise or lower the cc level depending on how she felt that day. And the doctor used to get upset with her but she didn't care. And I think a lot of that had to do with stress that she was under. ... I know there are certain days when, if I have stressful days, yeah, I test my blood ... and well I should do it regularly everyday but I don't, I'll do it maybe once a week. On certain days I will do it because, depending upon my stress level. And on those days it's been high. ... What I find happening is, I get tense with the amount of tension placed on me. I am in a very stressful job to begin with, which doesn't help matters any.

"I'm So Afraid ... Losing My Limbs 'Cause Those Are First to Go": Narratives on How Stress Operates As a Precursor to and a Consequence of Diabetes Complications

A final way in which informants linked diabetes and stress was through their awareness of the potentially devastating complications associated with diabetes. Some informants simply, in almost a matter-of-fact tone, discussed the possibility of deteriorating eye sight, organ failure, limb loss, and even death resulting from diabetes, whereas other informants framed such a discussion in terms of "fears," "dread," "troubles," "worries," and being "scared to death."

Many suggested a great breadth of awareness of the wide array of possible complications from diabetes that worried them, and some, like this 63-year-old African American woman discussed them in avoidance priority order:

> I don't wanna go on no, any dialysis. Every time I go to the doctor, I say check my kidney and see how my kidney now but he said everything is ok. I would rather have a amputation. I don't wanna be, my leg to be amputated, that's how come I walk, but if I have to choose between amputation and being on the dialysis, I'd take amputation anytime because I can have me some kind of life. I see people out there with wheelchairs going on but that dialysis, I don't want go on that. And another thing, I don't wanna go blind, either so I keep going to the eye doctor so I can have the laser surgery. He said it can't turn back the clock but it'll keep me from going, cause I do love to read. Even going blind, I wouldn't wanna do that but my main fear is that dialysis. I don't wanna go on that.

One African American woman discussed her diabetes education where films were shown on the possible complications from diabetes. Although it is uncertain whether these films had the desired effect of blood glucose regulation, the informant clearly articulated her feeling of being frightened or worried over the possibility of complications:

> (T)hey start telling you the scary part of diabetes, how you can lose your limbs. You know you can lose, lose your feet, first they cut your feet, pretty soon its going up and they cut below the knee and then they can cut all the way up to the hip and then it goes from one side to the other one. Once they start, once they start cutting you and I have known it, once they start cutting people for diabetes it always goes to the other side. If they cut you on one foot then pretty soon it's that other part of your leg, then it may go to the other one, then they gotta cut that foot off … .

Adding to the existing sensation of stress about the possibility of complications was a lack of certainty about how such complications might manifest themselves, as highlighted in the case of a 60-year-old Great Lakes Indian man:

> INTERVIEWER: Is there anything else about how it (diabetes) might have changed your life or about how you think it may change your life in the future?
> PARTICIPANT: Well, if I get all those other terrible things that diabetes brings on, God only knows what it'll be like. Maybe I will need help somewhere down the road. Maybe neuropathy and maybe your eyes or …. Never know what's tomorrow going to bring. I don't know.

A 58-year-old Mexican American woman explained that she is constantly kept on guard because her diabetes team "told me that was kind of like a death sentence in a way. That's how I took it and I just couldn't believe it. Well, by that I mean you'll always have it. You'll never … you can't get any better. You can only get worse."

Many informants provided detailed descriptions of kin whose lives have been compromised by loss of limbs, organ function, vision, and more, including a rural White 65-year-old woman who noted, "Well … my grandfather is a diabetic and it cost him a leg and then the other toes, the other foot had started turning dark when he died with gangrene. My mother lost her left leg almost up to the hip with it. And her clogged artery, then they operated and it set into gangrene and they took her leg off."

The Stress in Diabetes

From our analysis of these narratives, we formulate three primary interpretations regarding the nexus between diabetes and stress: (1) a sizable divide exists between lay and biomedical perspectives on the place of stress in diabetes, potentially undermining the appropriate provision of care; (2) informants contextualize the experience of stress, drawing on both specific events in their autobiographies and life circumstances that expose them to demanding conditions and environments; and (3) frequent references to these stressful settings compel us to examine the connections between larger sociopolitical forces, stress, and the disease process and management of diabetes.

The Lay–Biomedical Divide

First, these narratives add to the extant anthropological discussions by attending to the contrast between a narrower biomedical purview and the expansive lay perspectives on the nexus between diabetes and stress. Since we did not interview health-care providers, we are limited in our ability to state that informants' providers and possibly other members of the medical community share identical perspectives to those espoused in most medical text books, research priorities, and patient education pamphlets (Havel and Taborsky 2003; NIDDK 2002). However, careful examinations of the narratives provided by our informants and by current clinical texts suggest that biomedical perspectives are less attentive to the salience of stress than people with diabetes, as exemplified by the four specific ways our informants note that stress interfaces with diabetes.

One of these four ways—stress as an etiologic agent for diabetes—has been explored fruitfully by others (Cohen et al. 1994; Loewe and Freeman 2000; Mercado-Martinez and Ramos-Herrera 2002; Weller et al. 1999). The narrative in which stress over a biopsy serves as a catalyst to elicit a latent case of diabetes typifies the complex integration of biomedical knowledge, personal biography, and, in Mattingly's words, "small dramas, rituals of the everyday world of Western biomedicine" (2000:181). In these emergent narratives, the biographer attempts to weave together personal history, "a complex repertoire of cultural resources" (Mattingly 2000:205), and authoritative knowledge based in the clinical encounter to rectify biographical disruption and provide an explanatory framework (Bury 1997).

The narratives demonstrate not only this complex integration including the strong influence of biomedical professional interactions, but also some resistance to biomedical authority, as illustrated by a 55-year-old rural White man:

> INTERVIEWER: Why do you think it (diabetes) came at that particular time in your life?
> PARTICIPANT: Stress. Peggy was given, was diagnosed with emphysema. I think stress has a lot to do with diabetes. Though I asked my doctor and he said not really, but I just don't think in my case that was ... I just didn't believe what he said.

This description of the medical encounter as mutually dismissive, with both parties (patient and physician) remaining stalwart in their own perspectives, raises concerns about the implications of such divergences. Can we assume that health outcomes will improve when the two parties operate on distinct and only occasionally intersecting planes? With power and privilege primarily vested in the physician's authority, it is likely that such disjuncture in self-care orientation will take a subversive path, similar to Ferzacca's (2000) and Broom and Whittaker's (2004:2379) informants, some of whom "concealed their transgressions" by falsifying blood glucose records or manipulating medication.

Contextualizing Stress

In the absence of an explicit and biomedically sanctioned recognition that stress intrudes into the lives of people with diabetes in numerous ways, clinicians and public health officials who disregard stress in people's lives may unwittingly undermine their own advice for warding off complications. For example, the film described by a participant that admonishingly informs about the slow and steady devastation of a life with diabetes may actually add to the anxiety of dealing with a lifelong illness. Such warnings may be unnecessarily excessive in populations where diabetes makes its presence well known to loved ones, many of whom suffer visible complications.

It has been suggested that inadequate knowledge on the part of public health and health-care professionals of how individuals actually perceive a disease, and how they operate as "people" rather than as "patients," may undermine the ability of such professionals to suitably address optimal management (Cohen et al. 1994). Indeed, it is no accident that patients who share the fewest common life features with their physicians are members of the same groups disproportionately burdened by diabetes and have been shown to have poor results from medical management (Cook et al. 2001; Schoenberg, Amey, and Coward 1998). As Hunt and Arar (2001) found in their examination of the divergent perspectives of patients and providers on diabetes management, providers often disregard the life worlds of patients that constrain and shape management and, instead, interpret noncompliance as a lack of information or simple unwillingness to change. Providers adhering to the reductionism of conventional biomedicine run the risk of oversimplifying (Kleinman 1995:29).

In part, this essentialism derives from providers' limited collection of patient information (both extent and type), generally focused on strictly clinical parameters. Such restricted parameters necessarily overlook the patient's knowledge repertoire and/or accumulated life history and current social, economic, and health circumstances, all of which play a well-documented role in health and health behavior (Chavez, McMullin, Mishra, and Hubbell 2001). Moreover, what may be perceived on the part of biomedical practitioners as medically indicated and advantageous, may conflict with the life world activities and constraints of individual sufferers.

The Political Economy of Diabetes

The experiences shared by our informants lead us to advocate for a comprehensive view of illness management that considers how individuals make decisions on the basis of their own particular setting and conditions that (1) empower or disempower them to follow standard biomedical regimens, (2) place them at greater risk for encountering multiple forms of stress, and (3) do not provide adequate "resistance resources" (Antonovsky 1979; Dressler 1991)—psychological, physical, or material. Without any predetermined prompting about stress and irrespective of cultural group, most informants highlighted how inadequate resources, stressful life events, and deleterious environments played a role in their diabetes. Such a finding among the four populations examined in this study refutes relegating the stress–diabetes linkage to a culture-specific folk model.

Research on diabetes management most often focuses either on patients, isolating individual predictors of nonadherence, or on practitioners, blaming poor patient outcomes on inappropriate and authoritative biomedical practice. Although such research may be useful in creating interventions to improve patient–provider interaction and to reduce patient barriers to effective management, informants' discussions of environments where close family members get murdered, or where you live in fear of losing the minimum wage job that supports five family members, or where you share a kitchen and bathroom with a person who is "always drugged up" oblige us to move beyond the everyday world of providers and their patients to consider the larger political-economic context in which health and disease develop.

As expressed through many informant narratives, stress that derives from these taxing circumstances, including exposure to deleterious environments and exclusion from participation in a sustainable, meaningful, and secure economic, social, and political structure, relegates people to a persistent lack of resources. As we saw with the 57-year-old man recalling his experiences as a recently arriving immigrant struggling to safeguard his child from illness since they lacked health insurance, absence of participation in a socioeconomically secure existence often exposes people to substandard medical care (Mullings 1997; Schoenberg and Drew 2002). This inadequate care, in combination with and sometimes originating from dangerous environments, results in chronic stress and deprivation that corrodes a healthy existence (Krieger 2000; Morsy 1996). Informants' description of the insidious nature of stressful circumstances that ultimately lead to the onset, exacerbation, or complications of diabetes give credence to Broom and Whittaker's (2004: 2376) suggestion that diabetes is a "metaphoric time bomb," and stress its incendiary device.

Studies that examine the effects of the larger political economy on health (Donahue and McGuire 1995; Doyal 1995; Dressler 1993; Dyson 1998; Farmer

1997; Scheper-Hughes 1992) have highlighted the multiple ways in which inequalities based on social relations (formal and informal hierarchies of power based on social location) constitute forms of "structural violence" in which "persons are socially and culturally marginalized in ways that deny them the opportunity for emotional and physical well-being" (Anglin 1998:147), or what David White (1998:795) refers to as the "pathogenic role of social inequalities". The problem is further compounded when behaviorists solely target individual choice as the root of risky behaviors with detrimental health outcomes (Farmer 1997; Loewe and Freeman 2000). Providers' acknowledgment of the struggles faced by persons with diabetes, however, will not resolve the problems flowing from "up stream"—that is, stress-producing conditions that ultimately can be traced to broader socioeconomic or political economic structures that create or perpetuate stressful lives.

Conclusion

Anthropological approaches have the potential to elucidate significant contributions of the social environment to disease causation without dismissing the biological dimensions of human suffering. Ethnographic methods, including elicitation of lay narratives through in-depth interviewing, can reveal how patients make decisions about illness management in the context of their physical suffering and social inequities. In their detailed treatment of the etiology of DM among Native Americans (2001), Benyshek, Martin, and Johnson (2001:52) admonish anthropologists and others against ignoring the unique interaction between "complex biological responses (adaptations) ... and larger social disruptions." Indeed, this sentiment is affirmed in the recent statement of the Commission on Social Determinants of Health (World Health Organization 2007:4), in which the authors focus on the "causes of the causes"—"the fundamental structures of social hierarchy and the socially determined conditions these structures create in which people grow, live, work and age—the social determinants of health."

Sociopolitical forces shaping diabetes worldwide certainly warrant multiple approaches to mitigate the stress-producing conditions, ranging from more appropriate and effective clinical encounters to existing supportive institutions and practices, to improving an individual's ability to cope with or reduce the threat of developing diabetes. In their introduction to *Indigenous Peoples and Diabetes: Community Empowerment and Wellness* (2006), a volume that includes anthropological examinations in the United States, Canada, Australia, and South Asia, editors Ferreira and Lang (2006:7) echo this call for "research and clinical practice to take into consideration a much wider range of variables, including the common history of dispossession, trauma, inequality and emotional suffering".

The limitations of viewing patients as empty vessels in need of only biomedical information are well established. To address the diabetes epidemic worldwide, the next steps for the public health and anthropological communities must involve creating and sustaining institutions, structures, policies, and programs that meet the needs of those suffering continuous threats to well-being. In this chapter, we have given a voice to participants attempting to maintain their health in environments that present numerous obstacles to well-being. These narratives provide stunning evidence to practitioners and policy makers that solutions to vexing public health problems require integrating the perspectives of those who experience the day-to-day struggles and victories over demanding chronic health conditions.

References

Anglin M (1998) Feminist perspectives on structural violence. *Identities* 5(2):145–151.

Antonovsky A (1979) *Health, Stress, and Coping.* San Francisco, CA: Jossey-Bass.

Arcury TA, Quandt SA (1999) Participant recruitment for qualitative research: A site-based approach to community research in complex societies. *Human Organization* 58:128–133.

Benyshek DC, Martin JF, Johnson CS (2001) A reconsideration of the origins of the Type 2 diabetes epidemic among Native Americans and the implications for intervention policy. *Medical Anthropology* 20:25–64.

Bernard HR (1995) *Research Methods in Anthropology.* 2nd edition. Walnut Creek, CA: AltaMira Press.

Boyle JP, Horeycutt A, Narayan V, Hoerger T, Geiss L, Chen H, et al. (2001) Projection of diabetes burden through 2050. *Diabetes Care* 24:1936–1940.

Broom D, Whittaker A (2004) Controlling diabetes, controlling diabetics: Moral language in the management of diabetes Type 2. *Social Science and Medicine* 58:2371–2382.

Bury M (1997) *Health and Illness in a Changing Society.* London: Routledge.

Centers for Disease Control and Prevention (2002) National diabetes fact sheet. www.cdc.gov/diabetes/pubs/estimates.htm#prev. Accessed June 1, 2003.

Chapleski EE, Lichtenberg PA, Dwyer JW, Youngblade LM, Tsai PF (1997) Morbidity and comorbidity among Great Lakes American Indians: Predictors of functional ability. *The Gerontologist* 37(5):588–597.

Chavez LR, McMullin JM, Mishra SI, Hubbell FA (2001) Beliefs matter: Cultural beliefs and the use of cervical cancer-screening tests. *American Anthropologist* 103(4):1114–1129.

Cohen MZ, Tripp-Reimer T, Smith C, Sorofman B, Lively S (1994) Explanatory models of diabetes: Patient practitioner variation. *Social Science and Medicine* 38(1):59–66.

Cook CB, Lyles RH, El-Kebbi I, Ziemer DC, Gallina D, Dunbar V, et al. (2001) The potentially poor response to outpatient diabetes care in urban African Americans. *Diabetes Care* 24:209–215.

Cox DJ, Gonder-Frederick L (1992) Major developments in diabetes research. *Journal of Consulting and Clinical Psychology* 60(4):628–638.

Donahue JM, McGuire MB (1995) The political economy of responsibility in health and illness. *Social Science and Medicine* 40:47–53.

Doyal L (1995) *What Makes Women Sick: Gender and the Political Economy of Health*. New Brunswick, NJ: Rutgers University Press.

Dressler WW (1991) *Stress and Adaptation in the Context of Culture: Depression in a Southern Black Community*. Albany, NY: State University of New York Press.

Dressler WW (1993) Health in the African American community: Accounting for health inequalities. *Medical Anthropology Quarterly* 7:325–345.

Dyson S (1998) Race, ethnicity and haemoglobin disorders. *Social Science and Medicine* 47:121–131.

Farmer P (1997) "On Suffering and Structural Violence: A View from Below." In: *Social Suffering*. A Kleinman, V Das, and M Lock, eds. Berkeley, CA: University of California Press, pp. 261–283.

Ferreira ML, Lang GC (2006) *Indigenous Peoples and Diabetes: Community Empowerment and Wellness*. Durham, NC: Carolina Academic Press.

Ferzacca S (2000) "Actually, I don't feel that bad": Managing diabetes and the clinical encounter. *Medical Anthropology Quarterly* 14(1):28–50.

Garro LC (1995) Individual or societal responsibility? Explanations of diabetes in an Anishinaabe (Ojibway) community. *Social Science and Medicine* 40(1):37–46.

Harris MI (2001) Racial and ethnic differences in health care access and health outcomes for adults with Type 2 diabetes. *Diabetes Care* 24:454–467.

Havel P, Taborsky G (2003) "Stress-Induced Activation of the Neuroendocrine System and its Effects on Carbohydrate Metabolism." In: *Ellenberg and Rifkin's Diabetes Mellitus*. 6th edition. D Porte, RS Sherwin, and A Baron, eds. New York: McGraw-Hill, Medical Publishing Division.

Helz JW, Templeton B (1990) Evidence of the role of psychosocial factors in diabetes mellitus: A review. *American Journal of Psychiatry* 147(10):1275–1282.

Hinkle LE, Wolf S (1952) Importance of life stress in course and management of diabetes mellitus. *Journal of the American Medical Association* 148:513–520.

Hunt LM, Arar NH (2001) An analytic framework for contrasting patient and provider views of the process of chronic disease management. *Medical Anthropology Quarterly* 15(3):347–367.

Hunt LM, Valenzuela M, Pugh J (1998) Porque me toco a mi? Mexican American diabetes patients' causal stories and their relationship to treatment behaviors. *Social Science and Medicine* 46(8):959–969.

Kentucky State Data Center (2003) Poverty Rates for Seniors. www.ksdc.louisville.edu. Accessed April 10, 2004.

Kleinman A (1980) *Patients and Healers in the Context of Culture*. Berkeley, CA: University of California Press.

Kleinman A (1988) *The Illness Narratives: Suffering, Healing, and the Human Condition*. New York: Basic Books.

Kleinman A (1995) *Writing at the Margin: Discourse Between Anthropology and Medicine*. Berkeley, CA: University of California Press.

Krieger N (2000) "Discrimination and Health." In: *Social Epidemiology*. LF Berkman and I Kawachi, eds. Oxford, UK: Oxford University Press, pp. 36–75.

Krout J, Cutler SJ, Coward RT (1990) Correlates of senior center participation: A national analysis. *The Gerontologist* 30:72–79.

Lamison-White L (1997) Poverty in the United States. U.S. Bureau of the Census, Current Population Report, Series P60–198. Washington, DC: U.S. Government Printing Office.

Loewe R, Freeman J (2000) Interpreting diabetes mellitus: Differences between patient and provider models of disease and their implications for clinical practice. *Culture, Medicine and Psychiatry* 24(4):379–401.

Mattingly C (2000) "Emergent Narratives." In: *Narrative and the Cultural Construction of Illness and Healing.* C Mattingly, LC Garro, eds. Berkeley, CA: University of California Press, pp. 181–211.

Mercado-Martinez FJ, Ramos-Herrera IM (2002) Diabetes: The layperson's theories of causality. *Qualitative Health Research* 12(6):792–806.

Morsy SA (1996) "Political Economy in Medical Anthropology." In: *Medical Anthropology: Contemporary Theory and Method.* CF Sargent, TM Johnson, eds. Westport, CT: Praeger, pp. 21–40.

Moss N, Krieger N (1995) Measuring social inequalities in health: Report on the conference of the National Institutes of Health. *Public Health Reports* 110:302–306.

Mullings L (1997) *On Our Own Terms: Race, Class, and Gender in the Lives of African-American Women.* New York: Routledge.

National Institute of Diabetes and Digestive and Kidney Disease (2002) National Diabetes Statistics Fact Sheet, 2000. Bethesda, MD: U.S. Department of Health and Human Services, National Institutes of Health.

Peyrot M, McMurry JF, Kruger DF (1999) A biopsychosocial model of glycemic control in diabetes stress, coping, and regimen adherence. *Journal of Health and Social Behavior* 40(2):141–158.

Poss J, Jezewski MA (2002) The role and meaning of susto in Mexican Americans' explanatory Model of Type 2 diabetes. *Medical Anthropology Quarterly* 16(3):360–377.

Rock M (2003) Sweet blood and social suffering: Rethinking cause-effect relationships in diabetes, distress, and duress. *Medical Anthropology* 22:131–174.

Scheder JC (1988) A sickly-sweet harvest: Farmworker diabetes and social inequality. *Medical Anthropology Quarterly* 2(3):251–277.

Scheper-Hughes N (1992) *Death without Weeping: The Violence of Everyday Life in Brazil.* Berkeley, CA: University of California Press.

Schoenberg NE, Amey CH, Coward RT (1998) Stories of meaning: Lay perspectives on the origin and management of non-insulin dependent diabetes mellitus among older women in the United States with diabetes. *Social Science and Medicine* 47:2113–2125.

Schoenberg NE, Drew EM (2002) Articulating silences: Experiential and biomedical constructions of hypertension symptomatology. *Medical Anthropology Quarterly* 16(4):458–475.

Spradley JP (1979) *The Ethnographic Interview.* New York: Holt, Rinehart and Winston.

Strauss A, Corbin J (1990) *Basics of Qualitative Research: Grounded Theory Procedures and Techniques.* Newbury Park, CA: Sage.

Walrath D (2003) Social and biological facts in diabetes treatment failure. Paper presented at the Annual Meeting of the Society for Applied Anthropology, Portland, March 20.

Weller SC, Baer RD, Pachter L, Trotter R, Glazer M, Garcia de Alba JG, et al (1999) Latino beliefs about diabetes. *Diabetes Care* 22(5):722–728.

Whites DG (1998) Third World medicine in first world cities: Capital accumulation, uneven development and public health. *Social Science and Medicine* 47(6):795–808.

World Health Organization (2007) Interim Report. Commission on Social Determinants of Health. www.who.int/social_determinants/en/. Accessed September 30, 2007.

4

Understanding Pregnancy in a Population of Inner-City Women in New Orleans—Results of Qualitative Research

CARL KENDALL, AIMEE AFABLE-MUNSUZ,
ILENE SPEIZER, ALEXIS AVERY, NORINE SCHMIDT,
AND JOHN SANTELLI

Introduction

Unintended pregnancies are defined as births that are either unwanted or mistimed or those that end in abortion (Brown and Eisenberg 1995; Finer and Henshaw 2006). Almost half (49%) of the pregnancies in the United States in 2001 were unintended and almost half of unintended pregnancies ended in abortion (Finer and Henshaw 2006). Longitudinal studies of women in Europe who had their abortion requests denied have found severe negative effects on the children's long-term psychosocial development including effects on schooling, social adjustment, alcohol and drug abuse, criminal activity, and employment (Kubicka et al. 1995; Myhrman, Olsen, Rantakallio, and Laara 1995). Where abortion is illegal and unsafe, unintended pregnancy is a major contributor to maternal morbidity and mortality (Bernstein and Rosenfield 1998; Daulaire, Leidl, Mackin, Murpy, and Stark 2002). Although the unfavorable consequences of unintended pregnancy are well delineated, unintended pregnancy itself is less well defined.

Clearly a serious health problem, unintended pregnancy is a difficult problem to address as well. The apparent ambivalence seen in reports of women asked whether a pregnancy was intended, such as in statements that they did not want to get pregnant but were either not using contraception or using it irregularly, calls into question the idea that intendedness can be routinely and easily inferred from survey research. Correspondingly, it is not possible to simply assume that either intentionality or future intentions directly affect decisions to use contraception. The problem is that many factors, structural and individual, affect women's preferences and ability to postpone a pregnancy or to use contraception effectively.

Unintended pregnancy, although an apparently commonsense notion, has spawned considerable debate about its meaning and measurement. In demography, the term is used to describe the sum of pregnancies that were either mistimed (a pregnancy that was wanted but not at that time) or unwanted (a pregnancy that was not desired at any time) or a pregnancy resulting in abortion. In discussions about unintended pregnancy, simplistic notions about the relationship between intention and behavior have been questioned by demographers, anthropologists, and health-care providers (see Barrett and Wellings 2002; Luker 1975; Moos, Petersen, Meadows, Melvin, and Spitz 1997; Santelli et al. 2003; Trussell et al 1999; Ward 1990).

The relationship between measures of intention to perform a behavior and performing the behavior is rarely straightforward. An example is the relationship between intending to use a condom and self-report or use of condoms. Although many studies report a correlation between intention to use a condom and condom use, both report of intention to use and use are moderated by many individual and community factors (Jemmott, Jemmott, and Villarruel 2002; Jemmott and Jemmott 1990) and the correlation may be low (Molla, Astrøm, and Brehane 2007). To account for this, behavior change specialists have sought to build theory that sets intent and use within a broader framework of structural and individual characteristics such as availability and cost, community and peer standards, gender power and roles, and social psychological constructs such as self-efficacy (Hornik 1991).

Theories of behavior have not been involved in discussions of pregnancy intendedness; instead the notion of intention is seen as a practical measurement tool in family planning. For example, rates of unintended pregnancies have been used to demonstrate an unmet need for family planning services. But as the following discussion makes clear, changing demographics and community norms about sex, marriage, and contraception, as well as improvements in social research demand that the intendedness of pregnancy be reexamined from a more comprehensive multidimensional and structural perspective, that is, an anthropological perspective.

One difficulty with exploring the notion of intendedness in pregnancy is that it overlaps contested domains of gender: female individual and legal autonomy, female sexuality, female adolescence, gender power, religion, and ethnicity. These domains freight the discussion with topics and issues that need to be considered beyond any simple operational definition of "intendedness." As noted above, diverse group of academics and health-care providers have already questioned its utility and its meaningfulness to women (see Barrett and Wellings 2002; Luker 1975; Moos et al. 1997; Santelli et al. 2003; Trussell, Vaughan, and Stanford 1999; Ward 1990). A comprehensive exploration demands a comprehensive approach, combining qualitative and quantitative methods.

It is not unreasonable that a single measure, a small number of measures, or even a series of algorithms for measuring pregnancy intendedness should fail to reflect complex circumstances and desires. Understanding the meaning of intendedness was the primary motivation behind this ethnographic study. The areas we explored included life and career expectations, perceptions and experiences with sex, values associated with childbearing and motherhood, perception of family and local community support for early childbearing, adult and juvenile identities, relationships with partners, experiences with contraception, and attitudes toward abortion. We explore these areas as only an ethnographic study can in a sample of inner-city, low-income, predominantly African American women attending public clinics in New Orleans, Louisiana.

Our respondents present a complex story to support their pregnancy decisions: idealized expectations set against poverty and poor career opportunities; gaming with the chance of conception in the heat of the moment; community notions of sex and sexuality and the inevitability of early intercourse; the high prevalence of teen pregnancy and acquiescence to teens getting pregnant after the fact; the volatility of relationships and marriage; imperfect contraceptive practice and knowledge; and the rejection of abortion as an alternative to contraception. These concerns combine to explain the difference between general intentions—perhaps formed in retrospect—reported in surveys and the intentionality of pregnancy at the time of conception.

Studying unintended pregnancy in New Orleans provides key insights for other poor urban environments, given its sociodemographic composition and fertility patterns. It needs to be noted that although the study reported here was conducted before Hurricanes Katrina and Rita devastated the city and the surrounding coast, we use the present tense to describe New Orleans. About 28% of individuals in New Orleans live in poverty (Census 2000), compared with about 17% in all of Louisiana (Proctor Dalaker 2003) and 12.4% in the United States as a whole (Census 2000). In Louisiana, poverty is strongly associated with reported levels of unintended pregnancy. Overall, slightly more than half of live births to all women in Louisiana are reported as unintended (Louisiana Department of Health and Hospitals 2000). Moreover, among births to women who used Medicaid to pay for health care before and during pregnancy, almost 70% are reported as unintended, as compared with 31% among births to women who reported other sources of payment (Louisiana

Department of Health and Hospitals 2000). Nationally, reported unintended pregnancy increases with the poverty level of the population. For example, of the births to women with household incomes of less than 100% of the federal poverty level, almost 45% were reported as unintended, compared with 21% of the births to women with household incomes greater than or equal to 200% of the federal poverty level (Henshaw 1998).

Teen births also contribute to elevated unintended pregnancy rates in New Orleans. Over 17% of births in New Orleans were to women aged between 15 and 19 years in 2001 (Louisiana Department of Health and Hospitals 2003). This percentage is higher than the national average; about 13% of births in the United States are to teens (AGI 1999). Furthermore, over 77% of live births that occur to women under 20 in Louisiana are reported as unintended (Louisiana Department of Health and Hospitals 2000). This estimate is also high in comparison to the national average. According to the latest estimates at the national level, about 66% of live births to women 15 to 19 years of age are unintended (Henshaw 1998). These data suggest that poor and young women in New Orleans are at higher risk of unintended pregnancy, in comparison to the general U.S. population.

This research attempts to provide a more in-depth look at adolescent and unintended pregnancy in a high-risk population and explores the meanings of pregnancy planning and intendedness within this context. We believe that a qualitative study like this, in a context such as New Orleans, can contribute to the national discussion on unintended pregnancy, particularly since, as noted above, the overwhelming majority of adolescent pregnancies are reported as unintended (Henshaw 1998) and adolescent pregnancies contribute to high rates of unintended childbearing in the United States.

Designing the Study

This chapter reports on The Determinants of Unintended Pregnancy Risk in New Orleans study. The study, funded by the U.S. Centers for Disease Control and Prevention (CDC), had qualitative and quantitative components. The overall goals of this study were to (1) determine what pregnancy planning means in the study community, (2) examine the perceived consequences of unintended pregnancy in this community, (3) assess factors that differentiate women with intended pregnancies from women with unintended pregnancies, (4) determine factors that differentiate effective from less effective contraceptive users, and (5) develop better measures for the multiple dimensions of pregnancy intention that may be useful in research and surveillance. Two sites were used: a public prenatal clinic and a public family planning clinic. In the prenatal clinic, we interviewed currently pregnant women attending their first prenatal screening appointment. In the family planning clinic, we interviewed new and continuing users of family planning. This chapter reports the results of the qualitative phase of the study, specifically to inform goals 1 and 2.

The Field Guide

Many research guides were developed by senior members of a research team and then modified during field testing. We set out to have a collaborative design process with all members of the research team from the beginning. Although this was more time consuming, it gave members of the team an opportunity to work together before data collection started and positions in the project solidified. The time was used to explore and articulate the goals for the study and share knowledge of the subject and expectations for the research. The research team—Ilene Speizer, director of the quantitative study, Carl Kendall, director of this study, John Santelli, CDC project officer, and field-workers Aimee Afable-Munsuz, Alexis Avery, and Norine Schmidt—collectively developed the field (interview) guide that was used for the qualitative phase of the study. The field-workers had substantial prior experience working with the target population on family planning issues.

First, the team talked about their experiences working on these research projects and their general opinions about adolescent knowledge and attitudes toward sex, contraception, and pregnancy among adolescents in New Orleans. Then we reviewed the proposal and available questionnaires from the quantitative study. The demographer on the team, Ilene Speizer, reviewed the findings from the NTFS, the national survey conducted about women's fertility behavior. Following this, the team collectively identified factors that they felt influenced adolescent sexual behavior. We call these domains or themes. These domains served to organize the research guide. The domains and content area were derived both from the published literature and from personal experience with the target population. For example, we identified a domain of contraception that we called family planning (that was how the population referred to contraception). The team then identified a range of topics within the domains, and specified information to be collected about each topic. For example, within the family planning domain we wanted to know which methods were familiar to the young women, which ones were used, how they were used, and the drawbacks and benefits associated with each method. We wanted to know this both from the personal experience of these women and from a community perspective. At this stage the team did not worry about the length of the interview; what was important was participation in the process.

Next, the team focused on designing the questionnaire. Since we were collecting a mix of responses to closed and open-ended questions, and since we were using three interviewers, we selected a rapid assessment design for the questionnaire. Rapid assessment procedures in anthropology began with Scrimshaw and Hurtado's early efforts to involve health workers in conducting qualitative research on local understanding of health and illness (Scrimshaw and Hurtado 1987) and have become a very common approach for qualitative data collection in many fields. They mix open-ended questions that are suggested to the respondents with suggestions for probes and follow-ups, with a few close-ended questions. The interviewer is not required to read the question as written, but to focus on the underlying concepts and issues. This is facilitated by the participation of the interviewers in the development of the study and the guide. Items did not need to be presented in the order they occur in the guide, but the order was suggested. This kind of research instrument is called a semi-structured guide.

During the development of the guide, some of the discussion focused on what respondents would and would not feel comfortable talking about in the clinic setting and under the limited conditions of rapport established in single interviews. Here, we suggested that the interviewers depersonalize questions and ask about others—such as friends or community members. We also asked respondents to comment on hypothetical scenarios that we presented. The guide was repeatedly tested in the field for salience, ability to engender discussion, and duration. The final guide contained 115 open- and close-ended items. Open-ended items predominated and the instrument included free lists and responses to extended hypothetical scenarios. Free lists are a spontaneous listing of a response to a question. The only legal probe is "what else?" An example would be "list all the forms of birth control you know." The scenarios detailed the travails of two teenagers in love, and choices when they started having sex and when they got pregnant. Respondents could provide their own conclusions for the short scenarios, or select from options and justify their choices. Among the close-ended items were dates and timing of pregnancies, and tables documenting contraceptive use.

The guide was developed to elicit women's perceptions of community standards as well as their own expectations and experiences. The guide was long, but a culling of questions took place after saturation was reached on items. Saturation refers to the point when questions elicit no new information. For example, after sufficient information on community standards was elicited and no new information was being obtained, the sections assessing these standards were eliminated from subsequent interviews. This procedure is disconcerting for quantitative researchers, since it generates "missing information" for some informants, and questions by themselves may provoke ways of responding to other questions. We certainly wanted to avoid the latter effect, and the kind of "missing information" was of the general community knowledge sort. It is easy to test that the information already collected is generally shared by the population by asking questions such as "Is it true that people around here think that ..." in subsequent interviews.

The guide consisted of eleven sections: two of them collected basic demographic information, four elicited information on community standards, and the remaining five included a scenario, and questions about individual behavior as described in the following text. The sections on community standards covered general attitudes toward childbearing and contraceptive use, perspectives on pregnancy planning and contraceptive practices of the women's friends and acquaintances, and attitudes toward sexual practices and the different motivations of boys and girls for sex (data were relatively uniform across respondents, became quickly repetitive and these sections were dropped from later interviews). The seventh section used a scenario approach to elicit respondent attitudes about abortion, marriage, sex, and adolescent childbearing. In the scenarios, Tanya, a 16-year-old high school girl, must make decisions about an unintended pregnancy with her 21-year-old boyfriend, James.

Sections eight through eleven dealt with the respondents' own history of experiences and relationships. First, we gathered information about the age, residence, education, and occupation of current boyfriends, fiancés, and husbands, along with information about their partners' goals and interactions with the interviewees. Specifically, we explored communication and power dynamics between the women and their partners. Second, we assessed women's contraceptive history and asked a series of questions about pregnancy and childbearing and the impact of these pregnancies on relationships and plans for the future from a woman's point of view. We did not interview their male partners for several reasons. It would have been very difficult to arrange logistically, but more importantly, we felt that our respondents would be more open and frank if their partners were not involved. Third, women were asked about their personal sexual histories, including the age at which they had sex for the first time, and their concerns about sexually transmitted diseases (STDs). Finally, women were asked about their experience with reproductive health services.

No names or patient numbers were collected, but because adolescents were included in the sampled population, the interviews were not treated as exempt from institutional ethical review procedures. The complete field guide and the consent procedures were approved by the institutional review boards (IRB) of the Tulane University Health Sciences Center, CDC, and the collaborating clinics. The interviews were conducted between February and August of 2001. No reimbursement was provided for participating in the study.

Fieldworkers

As mentioned above, three female fieldworkers with masters of public health degrees and experience conducting qualitative research in inner-city New

Orleans communities were selected for the study. All the interviewers were non–African American; two were White and one was Asian. All were in their late 20s and early 30s. We selected the interviewers based on their skill and experience, as well as dedication to the topic. One fieldworker was the graduate assistant on the overall project, and would use the data for her dissertation. A second fieldworker was also a doctoral student at the time of the study.

Although taping and transcribing field notes are rapidly becoming standard for many qualitative inquiries, we decided not to do this. Taping and transcribing interviews would permit detailed content and linguistic analyses and provide a check of the performance of our interviewers. However, the clinics where the interviews were conducted were noisy, which would have required the informant to hold an intrusive and conspicuous tape recorder or microphone to the respondents' faces. In addition, we felt that tape recorders would be viewed with suspicion. Further, recording and transcription adds substantial time and costs to the process. Given the instrument, confidence in the interviewers, the relatively large number of interviews, and the expectation that much of the content of each interview would be either short answer or redundant, we opted not to record the interviews. We taped a small number of interviews (approximately six, two for each interviewer) for interview quality control, but for all interviews, the fieldworkers transcribed responses in notebooks as the interview was being conducted. Later that day, they retyped and expanded those notes into electronic field notes using the research guide as a template. The field notes were reviewed for content and completeness by project staff and returned to the interviewers for revision when appropriate. During the first few days of the study, we attempted to provide daily feedback. This close supervision, especially during the first dozen or so interviews, is critical to the success of rapid assessment procedures or other qualitative data collection methods that use interviewers. Final versions were collated into the project database. Normally, an interviewer completed two interviews each day. The three fieldworkers transcribed verbatim as well as paraphrased responses, a method that guarantees both content relevance and the alertness of the interviewer.

Each week, fieldworkers met with the rest of the research team and were asked to provide summaries, including composite results, unusual cases, and to ask any questions that they had about the interviews. These meetings also provided a forum for the discussion of problems and challenges encountered during the interviews. At these meetings, interviewers would indicate if they thought that a particular informant was open and forthcoming. For the most part, the interviewers felt that their interviews and interaction with the women went well. They noticed that the women talked candidly about sex, and appeared quite eager to talk about topics that they admitted they might not discuss freely with friends or family. These findings were fairly consistent across informants and inspired confidence in the veracity of the reported histories. After all the data had been collected, the interviewers participated in summarizing, analyzing, writing reports, and preparing this chapter.

Recruiting Clients

At the prenatal clinic, fieldworkers recruited clients at their first prenatal screening appointment to avoid interviewing the same women twice. Most of the screening patients were in the early stages of pregnancy, although some were pregnant for 6 months or longer. In the family planning clinic, fieldworkers kept a list of women who had been interviewed to avoid duplication. This log was maintained separately from the interviews themselves, and was destroyed after the completion of data collection to preserve confidentiality. In both clinics, women 3 or 4 places back on the appointment calendar were recruited because they had the best chance of completing the interview that took between 45 minutes and 1 hour without interruption. Women were not selected by age, race, marital status, and childbearing status, but fieldworkers occasionally looked for women in certain age ranges to compensate for under-representation in the total sample. No inclusion or exclusion criteria were used to screen prenatal or family planning clients into the sample. The interviews took place in private, non-examination rooms of the clinics.

Data Management and Analysis

A project database was created to archive interviews. The weekly summary meetings provided a forum to discuss themes relating to the research domains in the original research guide and to identify new, emerging themes. Quantifiable responses from the few close-ended questions in the guide were coded and summarized with SPSS®. The interviews were entered into MS Word® and indexed and searched with dtSearch® 5.25. User thesauri, a list of related terms were developed and potential relationships among terms explored. For example, condoms might be recorded in the notes as condom, rubber(s), or protection. A user thesaurus would search for all four terms at once with a single entry {condoms}. The final dimensions analyzed in this chapter were chosen based on findings that emerged from research meetings where we discussed results of interviews and preliminary analyses of terms and themes in the data. In the regular weekly meetings, we asked the field-workers to summarize each question in the guide across all their interviews, highlighting anything new that might have emerged that week. In these meetings, various terms or themes would emerge. After discussion, we would decide to pursue some of these themes in subsequent interviews. We also developed a spreadsheet for the interviews to track sociodemographic characteristics of the sample and responses to both closed and some open-ended questions. This allowed us to check how frequently certain responses were found, and to informally explore associations. Thus, we had two kinds of data: impressionistic accounts of the way respondents answered our questions and how those accounts knitted together, and a database with "quasi-statistical" information about frequencies of responses and correlations. Neither source of information was treated as definitive by itself. Both the terms explored and the conclusions drawn were based on independent agreement among the entire research team including co-investigators, fieldworkers, and the project coordinator. Of course, some findings emerged as versions of this chapter were written. These findings were illustrated with quotes from the interviews. These quotes were selected because they either characterized the main positions shared by women in the sample, or they effectively linked apparently divergent positions.

Findings

Seventy-seven interviews were completed, 37 in the prenatal clinic and 40 in the family planning clinic. The age of respondents ranged from 14 to 38 years. Half of the women were 19 years of age or younger, with the average at 21 years. Seventy-three women were African American, 3 were Hispanic, and 1 was White. Fifty-three were Baptist, 7 Catholic, 5 "other," and 12 reported no religion or did not respond to this question. We measured degree of religiosity by asking the women whether they felt themselves to be "not," "somewhat," "very," or "extremely" religious. A little over half said they were "somewhat religious," 15 said "not religious," and 12 described themselves as "very" religious. Only one woman answered she was "extremely" religious.

About a quarter of the sample were attending high school, and 17 women were attending or had completed college. Twenty-nine were not attending college but had completed high school. Ten women had dropped out of high school.

Among women aged 20 and above, 14 were unemployed and 23 were employed. Exactly half of the 22 women between 18 and 19 years were employed, as were 5 of the 11 between 16 and 17 years, but none of the 3 between 14 and 15 years were employed. Most of the employed women worked in the retail, restaurant, and tourism sectors or in administrative support positions.

Nine of the women reported they were not currently in a relationship. Forty-nine reported having boyfriends, nine were engaged, and nine were married. Some of the women with boyfriends reported that they were planning to marry in the near future but did not consider themselves "engaged."

Age at first sex ranged from 12 to 22 years, with a median of 16. Among those who had ever given birth, age at first birth ranged from 13 to 28 years, with the median at 21 (mean 18.5) years. Of the 64 women who reported at least one pregnancy, 37 reported using a contraceptive method at the time of conception. Of the 97 first or last pregnancies with detailed information, 45 took place while the woman reported using a contraceptive method. The frequency of contraceptive use at the time of pregnancy corresponds closely to the frequency of reported use in the year before the pregnancy in the quantitative data generated in the survey component of the study (see Speizer et al. 2004 for details of the quantitative data).

The classification of pregnancies as intended, mistimed, or unwanted was a difficult task. Our examination reveals the relevance of the multiple domains we identified, as illustrated in the account of this 26-year old single mother (family planning client):

> When I got pregnant when I was 17, I had an abortion. I wanted to graduate high school and go off to college. I found out I was pregnant 2 weeks before graduation. That was messed up. I wanted to get an abortion, was too young to have a child, could have gone to college even with a baby but it would have been too hard. The second time I got pregnant when I was 24 and felt like I was old enough to have that baby. I was in school and didn't think it would change things too much. I was in a bad relationship with that baby's father so I knew I would have to have it by myself but I wanted her. Even though I didn't plan on getting pregnant I wanted her once I did. It was different than the first time. I wasn't using birth control and so I knew it was possible I would get pregnant, that's why I was taking pregnancy tests every month. With me, I didn't plan on getting pregnant and did, but it was because I wasn't using birth control so I knew it was possible and it happened, so I didn't really plan it but I didn't really prevent it either.

The interview demonstrates how important contextual issues are for decision making about fertility. Timing and the difference between her expectation of ideal age for pregnancy and her actual age seem critical reasons for her initial abortion. With respect to her second pregnancy, a bad relationship with her boyfriend and being in college seemed plausible reasons for this woman to avoid pregnancy, but she did not use birth control. Although she did not plan to become pregnant, once she did, that became the reason to want the pregnancy, reversing our expectations of the sequence of planning. A conventional approach to determining whether this woman was experiencing unintended pregnancies would classify the second pregnancy as unintended. Yet, the account provides evidence to support the opposite conclusion as well. The woman in question, as did many others in the study, seemed to take risks with pregnancy that she manifestly—if somewhat ambivalently—claims to be avoiding, a phenomenon that perplexes many researchers in this field. Clearly, a complex web of motivations underlies her decision. The present study addresses only part of this paradox by providing insight into the cultural and social context in which key events and decisions take place. The following sections will explore the multiple conceptual domains that shape women's sexual risk-taking behavior and desires for pregnancy in the study population.

Sex

Initiation of sexual intercourse, generally during adolescence, places a young woman at immediate risk of pregnancy, but motivation to initiate sex is often unrelated to a desire to have children. Our respondents are clear about what constitutes sex. Sex is penile–vaginal sex and it occurs soon after girls start dating. Dating means spending time alone with a partner. Sex often begins within the year after a girl starts dating, and a third of the sample population reported getting pregnant in the first year after they first had sex. Because dating starts at around age 14, this pattern contributes enormously to teen pregnancy. The women often treated sex as unavoidable and seemed unconcerned about the possible pregnancy and STD risks they were taking when engaging in sex. Although some women reported having discussed sex with their boyfriends before it happened, having sex was generally described as something expected and rather uneventful. The following passage illustrates this perspective:

> (18-year-old, family planning client, 1 child)
> I had first sex at 13, had sex for a year before I got pregnant. I didn't use birth control. I didn't worry about pregnancy or STDs. I did it just to do it, don't even know why. Like, my cousin and him [first sex partner] was best friends, and my cousin was telling me that he [the friend] wanted to just do it, so I just did it.

Our respondents had a difficult time explaining why they had sex at an early age and often blamed it on the boys. One respondent remarked:

> (17-year-old, family planning client, no children)
> It feels good, they like it, they're freaky, if you are young and the boy keeps bucking his head against you then you might do it for him, it's like drugs, once you start you keep doing it, you have a weak mind, you should be thinking of other things. Don't know really why girls do, don't get it, I don't even really like kissing.

Many responded with "don't know" when asked why girls have sex. Others gave "disinterested" reasons: "[Reasons to have sex] just to do something, to feel important, just because other girls did it already."

Informants were also asked to give reasons why boys have sex. According to some, sex for boys is a "need" or "urge." According to many, boys are obsessed with how reports of their sexual activity boost their reputation. They reported that boys have sex to impress their friends or "be macho," and to feel like men. Yet, sexual curiosity, feeling accepted among peers, and occasionally being in love were sentiments reported to be shared by both girls and boys. Further, the ways in which sex asserts adulthood was a common theme, as illustrated in the following accounts:

> (23-year-old, family planning client, 2 children)
> Some boys think having sex makes them a man, some boys think having babies make them a man. They just trying to be big like that.

> (22-year-old, prenatal client, on third pregnancy)
> Make them [girls] feel grown, they want babies, most when they start having sex that young it's because their fathers weren't in the picture, or didn't give them enough attention, so they need attention from another man.

Eventually women developed a justification for sex. Sex for these young women was reported to fill an emotional void. Sex can secure the attentions and affections of boys, and ultimately can bring a child, described by most women as one of the only reciprocated loves in a woman's life. All in all, the picture these young women paint of sex and sexuality is an emotionally logical and coherent one. It legitimizes intercourse, rather than alternative forms of sex, and justifies it for its potential outcome as a life-giving event rather than as a self-indulgent act. The link between sex for reproduction—a sexuality that publicly denies or even condemns pleasure—and the idea that any pregnancy intention is real, but not straightforward, bespeaks an ambiguity that characterizes intentions.

> (25-year-old, prenatal client, no children)
> It just happens—it's one of those things that happen. It's gonna happen.
> You want one of your own—after you take care of other kids soon you want one too.
> You can trick a guy and have one—girls do this cause they think the guys will stick around for them, some guys do and some don't. Girls think it's worth the try.

Thus, early sexual play and first sex exposes young women to the risk of an unintended pregnancy, especially because contraception is often not used.

Childbearing and Motherhood

Respondents were asked at several points in the interview about their perceptions of childbearing and motherhood. A theme that emerged was that the women's ideal childbearing goals seemed incongruent with their lived reality, in which early childbearing was a key feature. In fact, women in our study reported two different responses when confronted with an early pregnancy: an ideal one in which teen pregnancy was frowned upon, and an alternate one in which teen pregnancy was accepted and eventually supported by families and friends, one that sometimes brought greater intimacy and communication with family.

The Ideal Reproductive Life Course. When asked about the "best" or "ideal" time to have a baby, many responded that it was preferable to wait until after school was finished and a steady job was found and the woman felt prepared to raise a child or was more or less "established":

(18-year-old, family planning client, no children)
(Ideal time to have child) I think 24 or 25. I want to finish school. I want to have more to offer to my child when I have one. I'm here today worrying about my pregnancy test, so it's funny to tell you this. But I do want to wait until I get established before I have children. I think you should stop when you are 30. After that you are old to be having kids. I don't want to be 35 having a little baby, when your child is a teenager you'll be too old to enjoy it. I think I want my baby before 30. If I don't have one by then maybe I'll change my mind.

Another common theme that emerged from the discussion was that a woman is not ready to have a baby if she lacks responsibility or cannot take care of herself. An interesting observation here is that this negative was not age related. Older women and younger women were considered equally able or unable to fulfill these criteria.

(18-year-old, family planning client, no children)
If you're not ready for the responsibility, can't take care of yourself, no job, if you got no goals as far as school, people that like to go out a lot can't take care of a baby and do that at the same time.

(23-year-old, family planning client, 2 children)
You should be financially stable, emotionally stable, able to take care of the kids, finish high school. It isn't really about age.

Reasons not to have a baby included schooling and valuing yourself:

(17-year-old, family planning client)
So you can finish school, education is important and you should concentrate on school. So you put yourself first, the boy should not be, he should be last and you should be concentrating on yourself. If you are too young; if you are in school you need to worry about the new LEAP test (Louisiana Educational Assessment Program, a standardized educational achievement test) so that you can graduate. You can't do that if you are caring for a baby; your boyfriend is not serious about having kids.

Although many women consistently reported ideal expectations about pregnancy, they often found themselves living a different life. This situation was a source of anxiety for many young women, like this 20-year-old mother (family planning client) of a 4-month-old son, who reflected on how she was unable to live up to her father's expectations:

My dad, he's a minister and it took him some time [to accept the pregnancy]. He found out when he saw my navel popping out, I was 7 months pregnant. I was scared to tell him. He was disappointed. My older sister got pregnant at 16. I was his baby. He didn't think I would get pregnant without being married. Even though I was in school and older, it still was hard for him. I was a good girl to him, his little girl. Then they treated me differently. I made the choice to be an adult. I was not the baby any more. They wanted me to move out and get a job and take care of myself like an adult. It was stressful.

These initial feelings of surprise and confusion expressed by the women and their families were later tempered with the unconditional support of family and friends, as discussed in the next section. As these women lived out their own reproductive careers, they described their own norms and values as an alternative to the ideal.

An Alternative Reproductive Life Course. Many young women—after espousing the ideal life course—also described an alternative one. The goal of this alternative life course is to complete fertility at a very early age. According to one young woman, desiring to complete fertility in the early 20s seemed to be pretty common among her peers:

> (17-year-old, family planning client, no children)
> They want to have their family soon, not worried about much after graduating high school. Some act like they want to go to college but they don't really want to, if they had a baby they'd be fine. Most of my friends do want to finish [high] school first. They think they should have all their babies by the time they are 22. Get it all done with. The school I go to has about 1100 kids and lots of the girls are pregnant. In the graduating class maybe there is 200 boys and 100 girls and maybe 30 of those girls are pregnant. Some in my class are already working on their second child. Now they talk about finishing school but it is so hard for them to really do it, how would they have the time?

In fact, many younger respondents spoke about the benefits that having a baby at a young age could bring. They revealed that a baby was an opportunity to have someone to love, to receive love back, and to receive attention either from a boyfriend, other friends, or parents. Many of the younger respondents stated that pregnancy was a way to restore a young woman's self-confidence. This young prenatal client reflects some of these issues in the following quote:

> (15-year-old prenatal client pregnant with second child, first pregnancy at 13 years of age)
> They really give me a lot with these babies, I got a lot of new attention when before they really didn't. They are making sure I'm ok, buying lots of things, didn't buy me anything the whole time [prior to first pregnancy].

Older women were more likely to mention starting a family and settling down as reasons for having a baby (ideal expectations). Still, they also articulated feelings similar to their younger counterparts, even hostility toward their parents. A 29-year-old pregnant woman listed the following reasons for having a baby: "Makes you feel important, to get attention, to get at your parents."

Furthermore, although women acknowledged potential obstacles in the future, there was a general sense of acceptance of an unplanned pregnancy by them and their community and little apprehension about the long-term impact. Surprisingly, many women reported that their first pregnancy had little or no effect on their dreams or goals. Of those who admitted their goals would have to be put on hold, many did not seem too disappointed about the unexpected turn of events. In fact, some women perceived an early pregnancy as something that brought meaning into their lives, indicating that it made them more motivated and more diligent about achieving their goals:

> (20-year-old family planning client talking about her four-month old first child) My life is more meaningful now. I'm not trying to get the guy anymore, wasting my time. Now I'm trying to get through my classes. I'm more focused. I've got to support my baby.

To summarize, although women report an ideal time to have children, they also accept an alternative life course that permits variation in the timing of these events. Whether this acceptance is because of alternative or changing ideals or reflects acceptance of the reality of mistimed or unwanted pregnancies can be further enlightened by examining factors that affect women's motivation and control over pregnancy timing including relationships, contraception, and abortion.

Marriage and Partner Relationships

First pregnancy had a special meaning in women's romantic lives. Many young respondents believed their first pregnancy affected their relationship with their boyfriend in a positive way. They felt that the pregnancy made them grow closer. When asked how their first pregnancies affected their relationships, two young women responded:

> (21-year-old prenatal client pregnant for first time)
> It brought us closer together. It's like we got a bond now.
> (17-year-old prenatal client pregnant for first time): Well, he [is] closer now. He just be doing different things. Every time he comes over, he touches my stomach. He rubs my stomach and asks me if I feel alright.

These positive sentiments were not always long lived. As the demands of motherhood became more real and more taxing, so did the demands on the relationship, often ending it. In fact, most women no longer had a relationship with the father of their first baby. Many women in the sample reported a general sense of scepticism about men, relationships, and marriage.

Unstable relationships characterized many of these women's lives, and many had to face a reality that foreshadowed life as a single mother. Generally, the women were determined to raise their children without the support of the men in their lives, as articulated by this 26-year-old single mother of a 2-year-old girl (family planning client, who had an abortion at 17):

> I didn't think he would care so little for the baby. I thought it would be ok with him but even if he left I wanted to have that baby. My girl could care less about him now. Most girls are daddy's girls and love their father, but my girl could care less about him.

Furthermore, many women, despite their age, did not foresee marriage at all. Just as the goal of "being established" before getting pregnant was some-what "idealistic," so was the goal of being married. In some cases, marriage was even viewed as undesirable because it changed relationships in a negative way. Ironically, for advocates of marriage, it was perceived as burdensome and signaled an even greater commitment than parenthood, as this young woman explains:

> (15-year-old prenatal client, currently pregnant with second child from a father different than that of the first child)
> Yeah, it's serious. We're having this baby together. I ain't marrying him. I'm not ready for that, wait until I get older. I'm not worried about being married. My momma isn't married, she's staying with my brother's daddy. Getting married isn't important really, as long as you are together. If you have a baby then that's one thing. You don't need the papers. Being married is different, it changes your life. (More than having a baby with someone?) Yeah, it's different, it's another person, adult in your life. Boyfriends get all unruly and then they can go, not when you're married.

Many of the women we interviewed recognized that the father would not necessarily be in the picture for the long term, even if the pregnancy was being used to "keep" the man. Women knew and accepted that pregnancy is associated with the risk of being a single parent.

Contraception

All respondents had experience using birth control. A common scenario in this community is illustrated with the following comment:

> (20-year-old, family planning client, 1 child)
> I was using condoms only when I first started having sex and then decided to get pills my freshman year of college. I took them for a year and a half. They were giving me

headaches and making me have worse cramps but that's not why I stopped taking them, just didn't like taking them. I was using condoms after that and now after my baby I'm on Depo. It has made me bleed a lot, but that's been my only side effect. I can't tell if it's making me gain weight because I just had my baby.

Misconceptions about use and effects of methods seemed to drive method switching. When women switch methods they may be more vulnerable to pregnancy. Many women switched because the effectiveness of methods was suspect. They were also uncertain about the plausibility of planning a pregnancy:

(38-year-old, family planning client, mother of 3 children)
You know, I was using pills when I got pregnant with my last 2 children and I still got pregnant, so I don't know. Sometimes I wonder if God's got plans for me that I don't know about. With my last pregnancy I wanted to get my tubes tied and something happened with my delivery and they couldn't do it then. Must be something with me, keep having these kids at this time in my life. I was not planning to but it happened anyway. I think we can do what we can do but sometimes things just happen to us that we aren't planning.

In these cases, the women's uncertainty about contraception was related to (1) misinformation about hormonal methods and experience with a wide range of side effects; (2) poor experience with condoms; and (3) the fact that there was very little discussion about contraception between the women and their partners. We cannot rule out difficulties with the quality of care these women received or poor patient–provider communication. We elaborate briefly on the first three areas.

Hormonal Methods: Side Effects, Misperceptions, Misinformation, Limited Access. "The pill" and "the shot" (Depo-Provera) were the methods most commonly used, yet women reported a range of serious side effects with these two methods. Irregular bleeding, weight gain, nausea, leg pain, varicose veins, and mood swings were reported by women on the pill. Prolonged or breakthrough bleeding, headaches, and weight gain/loss were reported by women on the shot. Additionally, fatigue, migraine headaches, calcium depletion, and links to cancer were side effects that women reported to be associated with the shot. According to several women, the side effects often became so unbearable they had no choice but to discontinue the method they were using. These respondents both got pregnant almost as soon as they stopped contracepting.

(26-year-old, family planning client, 1 child)
I went on pills after my abortion until I was 21. I went on Depo after that for a couple of years but then started having side effects. I was bloating and had enlarged breasts and then having break-through bleeding. I thought I was pregnant so didn't get my next shot. I kept asking the nurses here why I was all of

a sudden getting these side effects and all they could say were they were side effects and it was ok but that wasn't good enough so I stopped the shots.

Similar to side effects, which concerned many women, misperceptions and misinformation about contraception served as potential barriers to effective method use. Women who had used or were using the pill or the shot often reported missing pills, failing to return to the clinic for a new pill prescription, or failing to return to the clinic for their trimonthly injection, both because of their imperfect knowledge of the mechanism of action of these birth control methods and because of financial difficulties:

> (23-year-old, family planning client, children)
> I got on the pill at 15, before I was sexually active. It was a birthday present from my Aunt and Grandmother. I was seeing a boy and they brought me for pills. Then I got big on the pills so I stopped them. I was using condoms on and off and got pregnant at 18. After my son was born I got on Depo, it was good, no side effects, I liked it. I lost my Medicaid and couldn't afford to get the shot at my doctors, it was $60 a visit and $20 a shot. So I got off it. They told me there that I wouldn't get pregnant for a year after stopping, but 6 months later I got pregnant.

Women had many misperceptions about contraception, including the injection's duration of effectiveness, as mentioned earlier. Other concerns included the risk of infertility and cancer from hormonal contraception and misinformation on how to take pills correctly. Women reported that they needed to "rest" their body from birth control, particularly hormonal methods. We could not discover the source of this information, although a few women mentioned learning about this from their family planning providers. Side effects of hormonal methods and misperceptions about method use led women to cycle these methods on and off, resulting in periods of pregnancy risk, unless condoms were used in the interim. The next section discusses condom use and perceptions among the women interviewed.

Condoms. Almost all women reported having used condoms, often called protection. When used, they were often employed temporarily or as a default method during the transition between two hormonal methods. Respondents generally had little faith in the effectiveness of condoms. Many reported having condoms pop or fail, although some admitted it was the condom slipping off and not tearing or ripping that was responsible for pregnancy. Seven women even contended that men poke holes in condoms on purpose so they can get the woman pregnant. According to one family planning client:

> (19-year-old, 1 child)
> I used condoms when I was having sex at first. I would bring 'em. I didn't want him to use his 'cause who knows what kind they were, if they were old or something. We used condoms but one popped and I got pregnant. (How did it pop?)

It just did, after we were done it was popped. I check 'em too. I make sure there ain't no holes in 'em. So I got pregnant. (Did that only happen once, that the condom popped?) Yeah. After my son [was born] I went on Depo in the hospital and that's what I use still.

Another common reason mentioned for not using condoms consistently was that the women did not always have them around. Also, women reported that requesting a partner to use a condom can undermine the trust in the relationship. When describing the first time she had sex, one woman expressed her reluctance to insist on using condoms because she feared that it would jeopardize her relationship with her first boyfriend:

(20-year-old, family planning client, no children)
(When did you first have sex?) My senior year when I was 18. His name was Harry. We went to 2 different schools but we were in this program where we went to Delgado [a community college] in the morning. He was the first person I was talking to in the 9th grade, my first boyfriend or relationship. We always talked about it [having sex] because he always brought the subject up. I was scared. He didn't use a condom. I asked him but he talked about, "Oh I trust you and you should trust me."

Men are presented in these interviews as playing an intentional role in contraception often through sabotage or manipulation. This situation is exacerbated by the general lack of discussion about contraception between women and their partners.

Discussing Contraception with Partners. Women usually took it upon themselves to initiate a contraceptive method, because they reported that men generally responded apathetically when the topic was introduced. Even though women were cognizant of the potential risks to which they were exposed, they were reluctant to confront their partners about condom use (even if they suspected STDs) or other contraceptive methods, often leading to an unanticipated pregnancy.

(20-year-old, prenatal client, children)
After my first son I went on Depo and then on pills. It was my decision. We don't talk about it much. He knows I wouldn't sleep around and I think he doesn't. I should know better because he goes away. If he brings back something (STD) I would just die but I just don't do anything about it.

(26-year-old, family planning client, child)
We use condoms, not every time but most of the time. He don't really worry about it at all, I'm the one who's here getting the shot. I decide on it. He would use nothing if it was up to him. He doesn't really like condoms. He doesn't like to use them.

Women were using contraception based on their own initiative to avoid an unintended pregnancy. In more challenging situations, however, such as having sex with someone for the first time or when the partner disapproves of birth control, many women seem more willing to risk pregnancy than to confront their partners.

Abortion

To generate an understanding of unintended adolescent pregnancy and abortion, the questionnaire included several hypothetical scenarios describing a 16-year-old high school student named Tanya and her 21-year-old boyfriend James. In response to a scenario in which Tanya gets pregnant accidentally, there seemed to be a strong sentiment that the right thing to do was to keep and raise the baby even if the boyfriend was not willing to assume the role of father or if it interfered with Tanya's career plans. Respondents generally assumed that Tanya's family would help out, that she could "get the boy on child support," get a job herself, or get help from the government, and that things would work out one way or another.

In addition, some respondents seemed to suggest that Tanya's decision to keep the baby signaled greater self-confidence, responsibility, and maturity, a possible indication of her passage into adulthood. In contrast, when respondents raised the issue of abortion spontaneously, they portrayed it as less admirable because it allowed young women to duck the inevitable responsibility of motherhood.

Of the 72 women who responded to the scenario questions, 47 were opposed to abortion for any reason. Women commonly referred to abortion as "killing the baby." Many of them expressed feelings about abortion similar to those expressed by this 15-year-old prenatal client, pregnant for the first time:

> SCENARIO: Tanya and James talked about it (the unintended pregnancy). James is really worried about making enough money to support Tanya and the baby. Tanya wants to have an abortion. What should she do?
> R: She shouldn't have the abortion, her mama didn't kill her, why should she kill the child? He'll make some money, and save it.

Twenty-five of the 77 women felt that abortion was an acceptable option. A 22-year-old pregnant mother of three (on her fourth pregnancy) expressed the following:

> R: If she wants it (the abortion), she should have it no matter what he say. Because sooner or later he's gonna be gone.

Women's personal experience with abortion coincided with these attitudes. Abortion was used rarely in this sample. Six women had a total of seven abortions in this group. The perceived immorality of abortion, combined with the women's perceptions of and experience with contraception, restricted the women's choices as articulated by this young woman:

> (18-year-old prenatal client, 5-month-old child)
> All the ones that take the shot, none of them get pregnant. But most of the ones who take the pill got pregnant. I knew that condoms break. I should have expected it (pregnancy) to happen. I don't mind having children. I want children, I love babies. I was the only child. It's not like I tried to get pregnant. But I feel if it does happen, I would accept, I would never get an abortion.

Ambivalence toward contraception, rejection of abortion, and acceptance of pregnancy created a different spectrum of choices than might be thought for these women, one which excluded pregnancy termination and treated pregnancy as the inevitable consequence of sexual intercourse, no matter the woman's intent.

Discussion

It is important to emphasize, as Luker (1999) does, that the discourse of "unintended pregnancy" today refers to a different set of issues than when it was introduced in the past. As discussed earlier, a study on unintended pregnancy conducted in the 1960s might have interviewed mothers in their 30s or 40s with large families to explore unwanted pregnancies at the end of their childbearing period. But the bulk of unintended pregnancies today are early (mistimed) pregnancies (Brown and Eisenberg 1995). Certainly different factors are involved in the intentionality of pregnancy measured at these two separate times. Our findings generally characterize women's preferences at the beginning of their reproductive careers, as opposed to women's or couples' views of how long to extend childbearing.

To plan a pregnancy, a woman would have to feel in control of many of the factors—both personal and structural—we outlined earlier. This study suggests that in the lives of the women we studied, having control over these factors is not a realistic expectation. In these circumstances women's report of the intendedness of pregnancy often seems more like a rationalization after discovering that they are pregnant rather than the outcome of a deliberate choice. The notion that planning pregnancy is irrelevant for certain women is not a new one. Moos et al. (1997), who conducted focus groups with 18 African American and White women in North Carolina, suggest that the concept of planning a pregnancy might not be salient in lower-income groups. However, Barrett and Wellings (2002), who conducted in-depth interviews among different ethnic groups in London, England, provide a cross-cultural perspective among a more diverse audience. Of the 47 women interviewed, 18 were not born in the United Kingdom and the pool represented great ethnic diversity. Their data suggest that the act of deliberately planning a pregnancy is foreign to many women, despite their socioeconomic status and/or ethnic origin. In their study a "planned" pregnancy had to meet four criteria: intending to become pregnant, stopping contraception, partner agreement, and reaching the right time in terms of lifestyle/life stage. They conclude that women tend not to use terms like "planned" and "intended" spontaneously, and that there is variation in women's understanding of these terms. They also leave open for discussion the findings that the "adoption of planning behavior some of the time suggest that pregnancy planning is an available choice" and that "not planning may have particular advantages in certain contexts and needs further investigation" (Barrett and Wellings 2002:555).

Our study sheds light on the applicability of the concept of "planning" or "intending" pregnancy. The study illustrates that the elements we explore in our domains—knowledge, access, and support for use of contraception, the value of pregnancy timing, and supportive relationships with partners—that might make planning pregnancy relevant are either absent, under transformation, or not perceived as under women's own control.

When discussing their first sex and first pregnancies, many of the women in our study described inadequate preparation for sex and contraception. Contraception as understood in this community has unpredictable consequences and is loaded with economic, physical, and psychological costs. Hormonal methods are perceived to take a physical toll on women's bodies, and continued use is easily disrupted by missed appointments and/or the inability to make payments. The effectiveness of the methods themselves is suspect, knowledge and use of them is inadequate, and reported condom failure is high. Women's partners are often able to manipulate or sabotage the use or nonuse of contraception.

These factors—side effects, negative knowledge and attitudes, and lack of partner support—that make contraception difficult to adhere to are reported by women in other studies (Miller 1986; Sable and Libbus 1998). Further, reports of condom breakage and/or slippage are consistent with findings of several clinic-based studies, although the magnitude varies according to the population studied (Crosby, Sanders, Yarber, Graham 2003; Macaluso et al. 1999; Spruyt et al. 1998). According to the most recent of these studies, which sampled both men and women in a university setting, reports of condom slippage/breakage reached 28% among those who had reported they used a condom in the last 3 months (Crosby et al. 2003). Within this climate of family planning uncertainty, choosing to keep a pregnancy may be seen as a feasible and responsible action, while controlling conception may not. The family planning choice appears to be between abortion and pregnancy, not between pregnancy and nonpregnancy, and abortion is not an option for many women in this sample.

Additional family and community factors influence pregnancy. For example, the negative consequences of early pregnancy seem less relevant to this population of women. Educational and career opportunities are often lacking; fathers of the babies are often not present; and marriage is viewed as a burden to women and sometimes an even greater commitment than motherhood itself. Zabin (1999:2) makes a similar point when she refers to the "weakness of couples' timing intentions" in the context of unstable relationships. She argues that women who expect to marry in the future may place more value on avoiding pregnancy with a casual partner than women in similar relationships who do not foresee marriage at all. As suggested by several studies (Miller 1986; Schoen, Astone, Kim, and Nathanson 1999; Stevens-Simon, Beach, and Klerman 2001; Zabin, Astone, and Emerson 1993), effective planning or behaviors necessary to avoid conception occur only when there exist strong motivations and a supportive environment to remain nonpregnant. Our study finds that the women in our sample express these motivations, but they also describe conditions that might make pregnancy, or even an unplanned pregnancy, an option valued in this community.

Our study also suggests that the desire to assert adulthood, develop both natal and conjugal family stability, and attain greater intimacy with partners are possibly more powerful motivations for pregnancy than idealized scripts for career and marriage are for postponing pregnancy. These findings are consistent with the earlier literature on adolescent childbearing in poor African American communities (Anderson 1994; Burton 1990; Geronimus 2003, 1991, 1996). Much of this literature suggests that the idealized and conventional female life course that is promoted in higher-income groups—one that prescribes the sequence of educational achievement, career fulfillment, and then family formation—needs to be reconsidered. Anderson's (1994) ethnographic work in inner-city Philadelphia suggests that as urban poverty persists, the conventionalized family constituted by love, marriage, and career loses its meaning. In this context, early pregnancy is a consequence of young women's search to fulfill normal developmental and emotional goals, such as the search for identity and love (Anderson 1994). Burton's (1990) work in a poor suburban Northeastern community also characterizes an accelerated family timetable, which she ascribes to perceptions of early mortality and the low probability of marriage, and gives rise to early childbearing.

In line with our critique of the concept of pregnancy planning, Geronimus (1996, 2003) urges public health policy analysts and researchers to reconsider how they have come to understand and frame the public health issue of early childbearing in poor African American contexts. She reminds us that fertility norms are culturally and socially defined, and demonstrates this notion with empirical evidence of differential age-at-first-birth distributions in several US contexts (Geronimus 2003). She argues that in the case of poor, urban, African

American populations, an early fertility timing norm is a collective strategy in response to poverty and the rapid deterioration of poor women's health (Geronimus 2001, 2003). She claims that "poor women may attempt to fulfill their multiple roles and obligations in a sequence that fits the realities of different social circumstance and health-risk profile than those familiar to many researchers and policy analysts" (Geronimus 1991:466). From this perspective, it is reasonable to conclude that the material, gender, and other socioeconomic realities of the women in our study give rise to a world in which planning pregnancy, in the traditional sense, or from the majority's perspective, loses its force. This reality shapes, and to some extent, makes uncertain, the elements—sexual experience, contraception, timing of motherhood, relationships with partners—of women's lives that make pregnancy planning salient.

Given that this study reports on a small sample of 77 women recruited purposively from publicly funded reproductive health clinics in New Orleans, we cannot make substantiated claims for the generalizeability of the findings presented here. However, as discussed, many of the themes that emerged in this study are consistent with the unintended pregnancy literature and with the literature on adolescent childbearing in poor African-American communities. While these findings may not be strictly generalizeable beyond our sample, to the extent that poverty and socioeconomic disadvantage shape personal motivations and the traditional institutions that make pregnancy planning salient, the themes presented here are relevant to other populations (see Anderson 1994).

Conclusion

The portrait of young men and women faced with poverty and reduced schooling and/or job opportunities, in an environment of unstable and impermanent relationships and early sexuality is certainly not unique to the women in this study, New Orleans, or even the United States. To the extent that this chapter contributes to understanding the interplay of reduced opportunities, sexuality and fertility, and community and individual response, it contributes to more universal concerns.

As we have presented in this chapter, women's decision making about sexual risk taking and childbearing is multifaceted. Our respondents present complex stories to support their childbearing decisions:

- idealized expectations set against poverty and poor career opportunities;
- gaming with the chance of conception in the heat of the moment;
- conventional notions of sexuality and the inevitability of early intercourse;
- a community with a high prevalence of teen pregnancy and acquiescence to it after the fact;
- the volatility of relationships and marriage;

- imperfect contraceptive practice and knowledge; and
- the rejection of abortion as an alternative to contraception.

These concerns combine to explain the difference between general intentions—perhaps formed in retrospect—reported in surveys and the intentionality of pregnancy at the time of conception.

Returning to the theme that began this chapter, the simple statistical indicator of unintended pregnancy itself is a poor proxy for the rich social, cultural, and health information that surrounds this concept. While perhaps useful for advocacy, it provides little insight for developing health programs, or understanding the complex web of social determinants that define health and ill health and create healthy outcomes. As public health moves to understand how social and economic conditions produce health and illness and to redress health disparities as a primary role, the unpacking of popular indicators, and the detailing of the multidimensional web of social, cultural, political, and economic determinants of health will continue to be an important role for medical anthropology.

References

AGI (1999) *Teenage Pregnancy: Overall Trends and State-by-State Information.* New York: AGI.

Anderson E (1994) "Sex Codes among Inner-City Youth." In: *Sexuality, Poverty, and the Inner City.* J Garrison, MD Smith, DJ Besharov, eds., pp. 1–36. Menlo Park, CA: Henry J. Kaiser Family Foundation.

Bachrach CA, Newcomer S (1999) Intended pregnancies and unintended pregnancies: Distinct categories or opposite ends of a continuum? *Family Planning Perspectives* 31(5):251–252.

Barrett G, Wellings K (2002) What is planned pregnancy? Empirical data from a British study. *Social Science and Medicine* 55(4):545–557.

Bell DC, Trevino RA, Atkinson JS, Carlson JW (2003) Motivations for condom use and nonuse. *Clinical Laboratory Science* 16(1):20.

Bernstein PS, Rosenfield A (1998) Abortion and maternal health. *International Journal of Gynecology and Obstetrics* 63:S115–S122.

Brown S, Eisenberg L, eds. (1995) *The Best Intentions: Unintended Pregnancy and the Well-being of Children and Families.* Washington, DC: National Academy Press.

Burton LM (1990) Teenage childbearing as an alternative life-course strategy in multigeneration black families. *Human Nature* 1(2):123–143.

Campbell AA, Mosher WD (2000) A history of the measurement of unintended pregnancies and births. *Maternal and Child Health Journal* 4(3):163–169.

Census (2000) Sample demographic profiles. Table DP-3, U.S. Census Bureau, HHES/PHSB.

Crosby R, Sanders S, Yarber WL, Graham CA (2003) Condom-use errors and problems: A neglected aspect of studies assessing condom effectiveness. *American Journal of Preventive Medicine* 24(4):367–370.

Daulaire N, Leidl P, Mackin L, Murpy C, Stark L (2002) *Promises to Keep: The Toll of Unintended Pregnancies on Women's Lives in the Developing World.* Washington, DC: Global Health Council.

Finer LB, Henshaw SK (2006) Disparities in the rates of unintended pregnancy in the United States, 1994 and 2001. *Perspectives in Sexual and Reproductive Health* 38(2):90–96.

Geronimus AT (1991) Teenage childbearing and social and reproductive disadvantage: The evolution of complex questions and the demise of simple answers. *Family Relations* 40(4):463–471.

Geronimus AT (1996) What teen mothers know. *Human Nature* 7(4):323–352.

Geronimus AT (2001) Understanding and eliminating racial inequalities in women's health in the United States: The role of the weathering conceptual framework. *Journal of the American Medical Women's Association* 56:1–5.

Geronimus AT (2003). Damned if you do: Culture, identity, privilege, and teenage childbearing in the United States. *Social Science and Medicine* 57(5):881–893.

Giddens A (1986) *The Constitution of Society: Outline of the Theory of Structuration.* Berkeley, CA: University of California Press.

Ginsburg F (1998) *Contested Lives: The Abortion Debate in an American Community.* Berkeley, CA: University of California Press.

Ginsburg F, Rapp R (1995) *Conceiving the New World Order: The Global Politics of Reproduction.* Berkeley, CA: University of California Press.

Glenn EN, Chang C, Forcey LR (1994) *Mothering: Ideology, Experience and Agency.* New York: Routledge.

Henshaw S (1998) Unintended pregnancy in the United States. *Family Planning Perspectives* 30(1):24–29, 46.

Hornik R (1991) "Alternative Models of Behavior Change." In: *Research Issues in Human Behavior and Sexually Transmitted Diseases in the AIDS Era.* JN Wasserheit, SO Aral, KK Holmes, eds., pp. 201–218. Washington, DC: American Society for Microbiology.

Jemmott L, Jemmott J (1990) Sexual knowledge, attitudes, and risky sexual behaviour among inner-city black male adolescents. *Journal of Adolescent Research* 5(3):346–369.

Jemmott L, Jemmott J, Villarruel AM (2002) Predicting intentions and condom use among Latino college students. *Journal of the Association of Nurses in AIDS Care* 13(2):59–69.

Joffe C (1986) *The Regulation of Sexuality.* Philadelphia, PA: Temple University Press.

Kubicka L, Matejcek Z, David HP, Dytrych Z, Miller WB, Roth Z (1995) Children from unwanted pregnancies in Prague, Czech Republic revisited at age thirty. *Acta Psychiatrica Scandinavia* 91:361–369.

Louisiana Department of Health and Hospitals Office of Public Health (2000) LA PRAMS Datebook. http://oph.dhh.state.la.us/maternalchild/laprams/pagecd21.html?page=537

Louisiana Department of Health and Hospitals Office of Public Health (2003) 2003 Louisiana health report card. New Orleans, LA: LA State Medical Center, Auxiliary Enterprises, Duplicating, Printing and Graphics.

Luker KC (1975) *Taking Chances: Abortion and the Decision Not to Contracept.* Berkeley, CA: University of California Press.

Luker KC (1999) A reminder that human behavior frequently refuses to conform to models created by researchers. *Family Planning Perspectives* 31(5):248–249.

Macaluso M, Keleghan J, Artz L, Austin H, Fleenor M, Hook EW, et al. (1999) Mechanical failure of the latex condom in a cohort of women at high STD risk. *Sexually Transmitted Diseases* 26:450–457.

Miller WB (1986) Why some women fail to use their contraceptive method: Psychological investigation. *Family Planning Perspectives* 18(1):27–32.

Molla M, Aström AN, Brehane Y (2007) Applicability of the theory of planned behavior to intended and self-reported condom use in a rural Ethiopian population. *AIDS Care* 19(3):425–431.

Moos MK, Petersen R, Meadows K, Melvin CL, Spitz AM (1997) Pregnant women's perspectives on intendedness of pregnancy. *Women's Health Issues* 7(6):385–392.

Mukhopadhyay CC, Higgins PJ (1988) Anthropological studies of women's status revisited: 1977–87. *Annual Reviews in Anthropology* 17:461–495.

Myhrman A, Olsen P, Rantakallio P, Laara E (1995) Does the wantedness of a pregnancy predict a child's educational attainment? *Family Planning Perspectives* 27:116–119.

Petchesky RP, Judd K (1998) *Negotiating Reproductive Rights: Women's Perspectives Across Countries and Cultures.* London: Zed Press.

Proctor BD, Dalaker J (2003) *U.S. Census Bureau, Current Population Reports, P60-222, Poverty in the United States: 2002.* Washington, DC: U.S. Government Printing Office.

Russell A, Sobo E, Thompson M (2000) *Contraception across Cultures: Technologies, Choices, Constraints.* Oxford UK: Berg.

Sable NR, Libbus MK (1998) Beliefs concerning contraceptive acquisition and use among low-income women. *Journal of Health Care for the Poor and Under-served* 9(3):262–275.

Santelli J, Rochat R, Hatfield-Timajchy K, Gilbert, BC, Curtis K, Cabral R, et al. (2003) The measurement and meaning of unintended pregnancy: A review and critique. *Perspectives on Sexual and Reproductive Health* 35(2):94–101.

Scrimshaw SCM, Hurtado E (1987) *Rapid Assessment Procedures for Nutrition and Primary Health Care.* Los Angeles: UCLA Latin American Center Publications.

Schoen R, Astone NM, Kim YJ, Nathanson CA (1999) Do fertility intentions affect fertility behavior? *Journal of Marriage and Family* 61:790–799.

Speizer I, Santelli J, Afable-Munsuz A, Kendall C (2004) Measuring factors underlying intendedness of women's first and later pregnancies. *Perspectives on Sexual and Reproductive Health* 36(5):198–205.

Spruyt A, Steiner MJ, Joanis C, Glover LH, Piedrahita C, Alvarado G, et al. (1998) Identifying condom users at risk for breakage and slippage: Findings from three international sites. *American Journal of Public Health* 88:239–244.

Stanford JB, Hobbs R, Jameson P, DeWitt MJ, Fischer RC (2000) Defining dimensions of pregnancy intendedness. *Maternal and Child Health Journal* 4(3):183–189.

Stevens-Simon C, Beach RK, Klerman LV (2001) To be rather than not to be—that is the problem with the questions we ask adolescents about their childbearing intentions. *Archives of Pediatrics and Adolescent Medicine* 155(12):1298–1300.

Trussell J, Vaughan B, Stanford J (1999) Are all contraceptive failures unintended pregnancies? Evidence from the 1995 National Survey of Family Growth. *Family Planning Perspectives* 31(5):246–247.

Ward MC (1990) "The Politics of Adolescent Pregnancy: Turf and Teens in Louisiana." In *Births and Power: Social Change and the Politics of Reproduction.* W. Penn Handewerker, ed., pp. 147–164. Boulder, CO: Westview Press.

Zabin LS (1999) Ambivalent feelings about parenthood may lead to inconsistent contraceptive use and pregnancy. *Family Planning Perspectives* 31(5):250–251.

Zabin LS, Astone NM, Emerson MR (1993) Do adolescents want babies? The relationship between attitudes and behavior. *Journal on Research on Adolescents* 3(1):67–86.

5

The Limits of "Heterosexual AIDS": Ethnographic Research on Tourism and Male Sexual Labor in the Dominican Republic

MARK B. PADILLA

Ricardo's Story

"Ricardo,"[1] a well-respected and charismatic *bugarrón* (a local term for male sex worker) in Santo Domingo, Dominican Republic, had 20 years of experience in the tourism and sex industries when I met him in 1999. In an interview for my ethnographic research on Dominican male prostitution,[2] he described how he began engaging in sex-for-money exchanges after relocating to Santo Domingo in his early teens to escape the bleak economic prospects he faced in his rural home. The move had required him to live with his aunt in a sprawling *barrio* of the capital city while he completed high school, a period during which he got involved with "bad people," began using drugs, and was "seduced" by the allure of urban night life. His first contact with the possibility of sex work occurred when, at age 15, a friend—also a *bugarrón*—took him to a gay disco frequented by many foreign tourists. Ricardo recalled:

> The person who took me explained to me, "Look, a lot of American guys come here. Here they pay you. You have a good piece [*pedazo*, meaning penis] between your legs. With that you can make a lot of money." So, he educated me in what "the search" [*la busqueda*, roughly, sex work] is, because he had been in that environment and he knew how things worked there ... [In friend's voice:] "I'm going to take you to a place like this and like that, where you're going to be able to get

money easily, things that you like, and you're not going to have to do anything disgusting either."

With this introduction, Ricardo began regularly engaging in sex-for-money exchanges, specializing in providing sexual services to foreigners, both men and women. His friendships with business owners and wealthy foreign clients, combined with his charismatic personality, also placed him in an ideal position from which to broker contacts between local men and gay tourists, and to thereby acquire commissions. As he describes, his growing awareness of his social position in the world of international sex work convinced him to begin what he called an "agency" of *bugarrones* specializing in serving foreign gay visitors. He conducted much of his professional business out of his home, which he shared with his wife and infant daughter. Ricardo explains:

> Well, the American queens [*las locas americanas*, meaning gay men] started to visit me at my house. They began with the *bugarrones* that I know from my generation, and from the disco [a gay bar that closed in 1999]. They have the ability to get the expensive tennis shoes, the jewelry, the clothes ... And so [the *bugarrones*] come to me and they say, "Look, are you Ricardo? I'm so-and-so, I go to such-and-such gym, I don't drink, I don't use drugs, I'm in the university, things are really hard, I *like* doing this. Help me." So I think, I look at the economic situation like it is ... and the idea occurs to me, I say, "Well, these boys who look good, young, and look good, that don't have vices, and the queens come to me because they trust me, so why don't I start an agency?" And so through one I got another, and through that one another, and I got 25 guys ... And if I had my way I'd have 75 or 100 sex workers here right now.

While Ricardo had benefited economically from his years of work in the tourism and sex industries, he did believe this was potentially risky, and as with many sex workers, HIV was prominent in his mind. In his simple, eloquent style, he described in his interview how witnessing the death of many friends was directly related to his personal commitment to use condoms every time with clients, as well as his insistence that his "boys" do the same:

> I've lost many coworkers [*compañeros de trabajo*], I mean, lots of sex workers [*trabajadores sexuales*]. I've seen them die. I've seen them in terminal phase. And I've suffered. I've seen them sick in bed. I've lost true friends, dear friends [*amigos de corazón*], because of craziness ... In an alcoholic amnesia, they've erased [everything] and don't think about the condom. Others say to me that with the condom, they couldn't get it erect [*no se les paraba bien*], and that they don't want to be embarrassed, because if you don't get it erect, they don't pay you. So, I've seen all this that's happened, and all my true friends that I've lost. So because of those guys, because of those guys, thank God, I've gotten a little bit of knowledge. I've never let myself get lost in that, in the issue about work. I'm obsessive about protection.

Introduction

In the contemporary Dominican Republic, as in most Caribbean countries today, tourism has become the fastest growing industry and the lifeblood of the state's economic development strategy. After nearly four decades of incentives to foreign investment in tourism infrastructure, the country, with a population of 9.3 million, now receives approximately 3 million tourists a year to one of the largest hotel infrastructures in the Caribbean. These macroeconomic changes have had ripple effects that can be discerned throughout Dominican society, as the local culture has become increasingly immersed in the global tourism industry. Nostalgic Dominicans sometimes talk about a time not long ago when the virgin areas of Caribbean coastline were not inundated with five-star, all-inclusive hotels and resorts. Public service announcements remind Dominicans to proudly display their *"sonrisa Dominicana"* (Dominican smile) to their foreign guests, and previously quiet fishing towns, such as the coastal village of *Las Terrenas*, are quickly being transformed into transnational spaces complete with internet cafes, European cuisine, and New York-style *discotecas*. Between bouts of sunbathing, red-faced tourists browse through the numerous souvenir shops and food stands, or hire a tour guide for a trip to Santo Domingo's historic *Zona Colonial* (colonial zone), before stumbling back onto the cruise liner or into the numerous walled-in resort complexes. As in other Caribbean countries recently "invaded" by foreign pleasure seekers, the social consequences of tourism dependence have occasionally spurred debate regarding the influence of foreign vices on the moral foundation of society. Perhaps nowhere is this debate more evident than in the case of gay sex tourism. In 1984, as the volume of gay tourists entering the country was reaching its peak, a Dominican journalist wrote (translation by author):

> As part of the accelerated disintegration that Dominican society is undergoing, we are confronted by a growing phenomenon: homosexuality in its phase of male prostitution. Go to any area of the Zona Colonial and you will find scenes that don't permit uncertainty and explain why one North American tour company has promoted the Dominican Republic as a "paradise for homosexuals." And this advertisement isn't the fault of that company, which, imbued with an excess of liberalism as is possible in the United States, has simply conducted promotion based on the observed realities of our country (Cepeda 1984).

Three years later, Koenig et al. (1987) published an analysis of HIV sero-prevalence that analyzed blood samples from 1500 individuals, including "homosexuals/bisexuals," collected between 1983 and 1985. The epidemiological evidence led the authors to conclude that "tourists ... were the most likely source of virus transmission to Dominicans, because contact occurs frequently between tourists (e.g., male homosexuals) and Dominicans" (quoted in Farmer 2001:119). Importantly, Koenig et al. took their interpretation a step further, concluding that men who consider themselves "heterosexual" and who exchange sex for money with gay tourists were at the highest risk for infection. They describe these men as follows:

> Persons who engage in homosexual acts only to earn money usually consider themselves heterosexual. This situation, public health workers have indicated, is particularly prevalent in the tourist areas with young adolescents. It could explain our finding of three positive serum samples in schoolchildren from Santo Domingo (Koenig et al. 1987)

Given these epidemiological trends, it may seem somewhat paradoxical that 20 years later there have still been no sustained HIV prevention interventions oriented toward Dominican male sex workers, and the country's AIDS epidemic is now labeled—as in the Caribbean more generally—predominantly "heterosexual" by public health officials (Bond, Kreniske, Susser, and Vincent 1997; Cáceres et al. 1998; Garris et al. 1991; Pérez 1992; PROCETS 1994; UNAIDS 2002). The Caribbean now shows prevalence rates second only to those found in sub-Saharan Africa, with adult prevalence rates of HIV infection highest in Haiti (3.8%), the Bahamas (3.3%), Trinidad and Tobago (2.6%), Barbados (1.5%), Jamaica (1.5%), and the Dominican Republic (1.1%) (UNAIDS 2006). Because the Dominican Republic and Haiti have among the highest population sizes in the region, more than three-fourths of the Caribbean's AIDS cases are found on the single island of Hispaniola, which contains both of these high-prevalence countries (UNAIDS 2007).

Drawing on ethnographic evidence, this chapter seeks to interrogate more deeply the assumptions implicit in the idea of a heterosexual Caribbean epidemic by examining the political economy of sex tourism and the ways that heterosexually identified Dominican men use their sexual transactions with both male and female tourists to make ends meet in an increasingly difficult world. It is argued that the dynamics of HIV risk cannot be fully understood without consideration of the political economy of tourism in the country, as well as the gender-specific social practices that systematically veil sexual–economic transactions between local men and foreign tourists. The fact that the vast majority of the sex workers described in this study did not identify themselves as gay or homosexual, were simultaneously involved in intimate relationships with women, and avoided open communication about their same-sex behaviors further calls into question the unqualified assertion of a "heterosexual epidemic"—a designation that has come to dominate public health interpretations of HIV/AIDS in the Dominican Republic despite the fact that it generally fails to capture the nuances of same-sex transactions in the country's expanding tourism industry. Given these observations, a framework that considers the social and structural dimensions of AIDS among Dominican male sex workers is examined.

Methodology

This research involved 3 years of multisited ethnographic fieldwork between January 1999 and December 2001. My access to the study population and data collection were greatly facilitated by my research association with the staff at *Amigos Siempre Amigos* (ASA), a nongovernmental organization, the primary donor support for which comes from the United States Agency for International Development and which has nearly 20 years of experience conducting HIV prevention interventions among gay-identified men. The methodology was both qualitative and quantitative, involving continuous ethnographic observation throughout the duration of the project as well as three distinct phases of data collection as follows.

First, the primary areas and social spaces in which male sex work occurs in the two study sites of Santo Domingo and Boca Chica were identified, described, and mapped. This exploratory phase also included three focus groups with male sex workers in Santo Domingo to examine issues related to self-identification practices, to catalogue local terms and definitions for types of male sex workers, and to check the maps of sex work sites against sex workers' lived experience.

Second, quantitative surveys were conducted with 200 sex workers in both research sites. Surveys include measures of sociodemographic profile (e.g., various measures of socioeconomic status, household composition, marital and extra-marital history, patterns of spousal support, education, occupation, and income); self-identifications (e.g., as *"bugarrón,"* as *"trabajador sexual,"* as *"sanky panky"*; social norms about sex work (e.g., preferred types of clients, perceived behavior of social peers); sexual behaviors and condom use with clients (both male and female) as well as with girlfriends, wives, or intimate partners; affective and emotional bonds with clients; substance use history; frequency of internal and transnational migration experiences; and numerous relatively standardized measures of "co-factors" of HIV and STD risk (e.g., access to condoms, perception of risk, knowledge of HIV, and social support).

In the third stage of the research, audio-taped semi-structured interviews were conducted with 98 sex workers, exploring issues such as childhood experiences and traumas; current and past relations with parents and siblings; stigma management techniques; initiation into sex work; relationships with girlfriends, spouses, and children; stories of worst and best clients; beliefs and fears about HIV/AIDS; and future aspirations.

Ethnographic techniques—most importantly participant observation, informal interviewing, and ethnographic note-taking—were used throughout the research. This involved many hours of socializing with male sex workers and clients in various contexts, at first largely in sex work areas—such as bars, discos, parks, restaurants, and streets—and later in more private settings, including sex workers' homes. The ethnographic data continually informed the emerging results from the more formal methodologies, allowing for triangulation and verification of data as well as the cultural contextualization of particular findings. This was especially important in the case of the surveys, since simple frequencies of responses can be misleading when interpreted without reference to sociocultural or political–economic context. This research thus utilized a self-consciously mixed-methods approach within an overall ethnographic design.

Research Subjects and Sexual Identities

Participants were recruited through social networks that were gradually expanded through contacts made in the course of ethnographic observations, such that the team established initial contacts and gained rapport through informal interviewing in sex work venues during the first phase of the study, met additional sex workers through these contacts, established rapport with these new associations, met new network members, and so on. Over 3 years of ethnographic research by multiple ethnographers, this led to a wide and complex network of male sex workers with whom we ultimately established a considerable degree of rapport, through which we were able to obtain large numbers of participants, despite the largely clandestine nature of the activities under consideration.

The local terms *"bugarrón"* and *"sanky panky"* generally correspond to the categories of self-identity used by the male sex workers described here, although not all of the men who participated in this study used these terms as forms of self-reference. As described in prior studies (De Moya, García, Fadul, and Herold 1992; De Moya and Garcia 1998), the *sanky panky* identity—based on a linguistic Dominicanization of the English phrase "hanky panky"—emerged in the 1970s and 1980s in response to the growing presence of young, well-built Dominican men who made a modest living by hustling foreign men and women in heavily touristed beach areas. The term therefore connotes both a particular masculine style—including, for example, the small dreadlocks often mentioned by sex workers as a signature feature of the classic *sanky panky*—and a specific location, that is, the beach. The spatial specificity of the *sanky panky* identity explains its more common self-attribution among sex workers in Boca Chica, a beach town and a primary tourist destination on the country's southern coast.

The word *bugarrón*, which De Moya and García (1998) argue takes its root from the French *bougre*, has a deeper history in the Dominican Republic and, consequently, does not have the same connection to the development of the tourism industry as *sanky panky*. Rather, *bugarrón* was a preexisting identity that was subsequently incorporated into, and commodified by, gay sex tourism in the Caribbean. As an ideal type, *bugarrón* refers to a man who engages in *activo* (insertive) anal sex with other men, often for money or other noneconomic benefits (such as clothing, tennis shoes, and gifts from abroad), but who in other domains of life may not be noticeably different from "normal" men.[3] Neither the *bugarrón* nor the *sanky panky* identity is socially ascribed in a way that is analogous to the public self-ascription practices typical of many gay-identified men in the contemporary Euro-American sexual system, and these terms are therefore best understood as situational identities that are generally veiled in public, and especially familial, social contexts.

Thus, it is important to recognize that these identities are more fluid in actual social practice. This is illustrated by the fact that the research revealed several cases of specific men who identified themselves differently depending on the social context, and many self-identified "*bugarrones*" became "*sanky pankies*" when they relocated to the beach to look for clients. This demonstrates the importance of an ethnographic perspective on these sexual identities, since observations of behavior as it occurs in practice can reveal the dynamic nature of social categories that may appear artificially static when examined using quantitative data alone.

The Political Economy of Sex Tourism in the Dominican Republic

To understand the historical growth in sexual–economic transactions between Dominican men and foreign tourists, we must first consider the large-scale structural changes that have altered patterns of male labor and the global demand for their sexual services in the last three decades. Since at least the early 1980s, the informal sector has employed more men than any other sector of the economy, and the country represents one of the rare cases in which men and women have approximately equal rates of informal sector employment (Safa 1995:107). In the Dominican Republic, the rapid informalization of male work is rooted in several parallel processes, including the expansion of the tourism sector; the privatization of major state-owned industries; a reduced emphasis on agricultural exports (most importantly sugar); and the proliferation of free trade zones employing mostly women. These macroeconomic trends have been spurred by 30 years of political hegemony by former President Joaquín Balaguer, a layover from Rafael Trujillo's dictatorial regime,

whose policies favored opening the Dominican economy to foreign investment, principally in the areas of tourism and free trade zones (Betances 1995).
Indeed, as Barry, Wood, and Preusch (1984) have pointed out, Balaguer's rise
to power in 1966, with backing by the United States, was concurrent with
the country's transition to a tourism-based economy, and was followed by a
regime that was, in the words of anthropologist Amalia Cabezas, "heavily subsidized, sanctioned, and guided by the United States, the United Nations, the
World Bank, and the Organization of American States in its effort to develop
an investment climate favorable for the development of international tourism"
(Cabezas 1999:96).[4]

Thus, in recent years the Dominican economy has made an historic shift
from a colonial economic model based primarily on agricultural exports to a
service sector economy that depends on the influx of foreign exchange through
tourism and free trade zones, and on the ability to sell cheap local labor that is
affordable to multinational investors. Tourism is now the principal industry of
the Dominican economy (ASONAHORES 1995), and since 1982 it has been
the country's main source of foreign exchange (Freitag 1996:231). In 1994,
according to Cabezas (1999:96), "close to 150,000 persons were [formally]
employed in the tourism sector, making it the largest source of employment
in the Dominican Republic". Nevertheless, estimates of the number of
Dominicans formally employed by tourist-oriented businesses overlook entirely
the extent to which local Dominicans depend on informal sector labor within
the tourism economy. More significantly for the current discussion, figures of
tourism sector employment do not account for the thousands of individuals
involved—either full time or intermittently—in sexual–economic exchanges
with tourists.

A significant industry based on gay sex tourism began in the Dominican
Republic during the 1970s, following a pattern similar to that described by
Farmer (1992, 1996) for the country's neighbor to the west, Haiti. While
there are no formal statistics on the extent of gay tourism to the Dominican
Republic, foreign tourists are prominent, if impermanent, fixtures in many gay
social spaces. Indeed, in many ways gay life in Santo Domingo rises and falls
with fluctuations in the tourism sector. Owners of gay businesses, despair-
ing the lower profits during the hot summer months of *la temporada baja*
(the low tourist season), wait impatiently for the first signs of winter in the
United States and Europe that inevitably precede a surge in foreign clients
with cash in hand. A travel agency specifically oriented toward gay tourists
to the Dominican Republic is currently operating out of New York, providing
personalized vacation packages and travel advice to gay travelers. And there
are now several active internet sites for gay tourists to the country that provide
information on local gay businesses and opportunities to arrange social or sexual encounters with Dominicans.

Many gay tourists come to the Dominican Republic solely or primarily for sex tourism. At least one local gay business in Santo Domingo, which I call "Charlie's," resembles an all-male brothel and caters almost entirely to a foreign clientele of primarily middle-aged clients from the United States. In all gay bars and discos, foreign sex tourists can be regularly seen, often accompanied by the *bugarrones* who frequent most gay businesses or nearby public areas where they meet potential clients. Gay tourists generally fit into two broad categories: one-time vacationers and regular, repeat travelers. Regular travelers, including Dominican gays residing abroad, often develop social relationships with local gays and establishment owners, facilitating the transmission of privileged gay knowledge and the shaping of Dominican gay culture. Some of these regular travelers develop long-term relationships with sex workers, frequently sending them regular remittances from abroad—a phenomenon I have described as the "Western Union Daddy" (Padilla 2007a, 2007b).

While De Moya and García (1998) have shown that gay sex tourism to the Dominican Republic tapered in the late 1980s and 1990s, probably in response to the growing fear of AIDS, there are nevertheless a significant number of studies showing that contact with gay tourists continues to be quite common among Dominican men who have sex with men. In Ramah, Pareja, and Hasbun's (1992) "KABP" (Knowledge Attitudes, Beliefs, and Practices) survey among Dominican "homosexuals" and "bisexuals," for example, one-third of the study population had had sex with a tourist in the previous 6 months—a very significant finding given that the study population was not of sex workers, but a diverse sample of men with same-sex sexual experiences. A more recent KABP study virtually replicated these results, finding that 30% of the youngest Men Who Have Sex with Men (MSM) in the sample had had sex with male tourists (CESDEM 1999). Studies among male sex workers, including this one, have reported even higher frequencies of contact with tourists, with most sex workers indicating that tourists are their preferred clients (De Moya et al. 1992; De Moya and García 1998; Padilla 2007a, 2007b; Silvestre, Rijo, and Bogaert 1994). In Silvestre et al.'s (1994) study in five Dominican cities with a sample of 412 male and female adolescent street children who marginally subsisted through prostitution, most indicated that they catered specifically to foreign tourists. Similarly, Vásquez, Ruiz, and De Moya (1991) report that in their study of 30 adolescent male prostitutes in Santo Domingo, 85% had had sex with a mean of 11 foreign gay clients.

In their exchanges with male clients, the *bugarrones* and *sanky pankies* in the present study showed a strong preference for foreigners, often alluding to the fact that such clients represent *"dinero fácil"* (easy money) in the context of an otherwise difficult economic environment. This assessment must be understood in the context of the poverty and lack of options these men generally confront, and the relatively greater pay that is possible to negotiate in the

Table 5.1. Preferred Male Clients[a]

CATEGORY	NUMBER (%)
Foreign tourist	96 (57.8%)
Local tourist	4 (2.4%)
Foreign executive	18 (10.8%)
Local executive	18 (10.8%)
Married man	3 (1.8%)
Travesti	2 (1.2%)
Gay man	16 (9.6%)
No response	9 (5.4%)
Total	166

[a]Only those respondents with experience with male clients are included (*n* = 166).

informal tourism market. Martín, a 33 year-old *bugarrón* in Santo Domingo, for example, explained in an interview the reasons he prefers tourists as clients:

> I've gone for about 10 or 12 years without work. So, you know, here in the Dominican Republic things are really hard, so since there are some opportunities with some guys who come from abroad, and they offer you money or something to be with them, you grab it, you understand? It's the easiest way to get money. That's what's going on.

This preference for foreign clients is also evident in the survey data on preferred clients, as summarized in Table 5.1, which shows an overwhelming bias toward foreign tourists.

The fact that most *bugarrones* and *sanky pankies* do not self-identify as gay and are frequently involved in sexual relationships with women presents a number of analytical questions regarding the ways that these men manage their same-sex exchanges within spousal and familial contexts. The following section addresses these questions through an analysis of the elaborate techniques that sex workers use to evade suspicion despite their regular engagement in same-sex transactions with tourists.

Stigma Management

On a late night in July 2001, I was drinking with Orlando across the street from *Tropicalia*, a gay disco on Santo Domingo's *malecón* (boardwalk) where sex workers frequently make contacts with clients. Figure 5.1 shows a late-night image of a stretch of the *malecón* where negotiations occasionally occur.

Orlando, while only 27, had considerable experience in the sex trade, and was well-known and friendly with most of the *bugarrones* in the area—

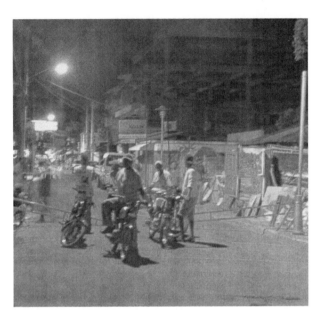

Figure 5.1. Motorcycle taxi drivers in a sex work area of Boca Chica, Dominican Republic. (Photo by Mark Padilla)

qualities that would serve him well as he approached an age at which his networking skills, rather than his direct sexual exchanges, would be his primary economic resource. He had joked with me on several previous occasions about the *"lío"* (big problem) that had developed as a result of his involvement with two women, as well as his somewhat ineffective attempts to prevent his sister, with whom he was then living, from learning about his sexual exchanges with men. Since we had chatted before, I asked him if I could audio-tape our conversation, to which he agreed. During the course of our conversation, we had the following exchange, which I quote here at length because of its vivid illustration of the cover *bugarrones* struggle to preserve amidst the surveillance of their wives, girlfriends, family, and clients:

MP: Do your girlfriends know that you "look for it" [*te la buscas*] with men?

ORLANDO: No, because maybe if they knew they wouldn't be with me.

MP: You think they'd react badly?

ORLANDO: Yeah, because—Also if my friends [regular clients] knew that I had others, for example my friend the doctor, if he knew that I had others, he'd dump me [*me botaría*]. Or if he knew that I have a girlfriend, he'd think the same.

MP: He'd dump you?

ORLANDO: Yeah, because he says he would.

MP: So, is that difficult for you, to have, like, two lives, because you have your life with your girlfriend, and she doesn't know that you—

ORLANDO: No.

MP: And the doctor doesn't know anything either.

ORLANDO: No.

MP: Is that difficult for you?

ORLANDO: [No response]

MP: Do you feel bad that you have to tell lies sometimes?

ORLANDO: No.

MP: No?

ORLANDO: I sometimes have to tell little lies [*mentiritas*].

MP: What kinds of lies?

ORLANDO: Well, sometimes I even have to tell them [regular clients] that I have an uncle that's been feeling bad, that I have to go for a week to the country, but it's a lie because it's to be with my girlfriend. And sometimes I tell my girlfriends that I—I have a job, that I'm painting a house really far away and that I won't be back until really late, so I won't be able to go by their house, but it's a lie, since that's when I'm with my friends, right?

MP: But that doesn't bother you, to tell those lies?

ORLANDO: No.

MP: Is it easy?

ORLANDO: [Laughing] Yeah, because since the lie was invented, it hasn't betrayed anyone [*desde que se inventó la mentira, ya nadie queda mal*].

MP: [Laughing] Oh! So they don't suspect anything?

ORLANDO: No.

MP: Are you a good liar?

ORLANDO: [Long pause] No, because sometimes I make mistakes.

MP: Give me an example of a mistake you've made.

ORLANDO: Like, the other day I told the doctor that I was going to the country for a week, and the next day, or like two days later, he called my sister's house and it was me who answered the phone. But it was because I wanted to see my girlfriend, or to divide my time between my girlfriends.

MP: And the doctor? What did he say when you answered?

ORLANDO: Nothing. He came right over to my sister's house. He said, 'Let's go drink some beers', and that's when we started to argue.

MP: Did he get mad? What did he say?

ORLANDO: [Laughing] Yeah! He was furious!

MP: And you argued?

ORLANDO: Yeah, of course. We had a bad argument, and he went like four days without calling, and later he called and said that he wanted to talk to me, and I said that I know I shouldn't have lied to him but that I did it because I wanted to hang out and relax at my sister's. He didn't know about my girlfriend.

MP: What did he say? Did he believe that? Did he believe you?

ORLANDO: I don't know if he believed it. I did it so he would relax [laughing]. I don't know if he believed it.

MP: Sometimes they find out, and sometimes they have suspicions, I imagine.

ORLANDO: I guess so. Sometimes he even calls my sister's house and he asks her about me, and sometimes I think that even my sister suspects.

MP: Really?

ORLANDO: Yeah.

MP: But she never asks you anything?

ORLANDO: No.

MP: Why do you think she suspects then?

ORLANDO: Because guys call me in the morning, in the afternoon, every day. She has a right to suspect something. And there are times when I'm not there and he [the doctor] just shows up at my sister's.

MP: Really? He drives by in his car, or what?

ORLANDO: No, there's an alley by my house, so he leaves the car around the corner and comes through the alley to my sister's.

MP: How often does he do that?

ORLANDO: Sometimes—almost every day.

MP: Really? Oh, I can understand why your sister might suspect something.

ORLANDO: Yeah, she might be suspecting something.

MP: So, when you're at your sister's and he shows up, you go out with him then?

ORLANDO: Yeah, because he's not obvious [*no se le nota nada*].

MP: And do the neighbors have—Do they bother you or gossip in the neighborhood or anything?

ORLANDO: No.

MP: No?

ORLANDO: No, because the neighbors have always seen me with lots of women.

MP: Okay, so they don't have any idea—

ORLANDO: No, and I sometimes—Like every once in a while I go by to, as they say, to "kill the bad thoughts" [*matar la mala mente*], or kill the bad tongues of the neighbors. I go to my sister's house with my girlfriend.

MP: To avoid gossip [*evitar los chismes*].

ORLANDO: Yeah. Because a few months ago my sister said to me, "Listen, you always used to bring girlfriends here, almost weekly, and now you're—it's been a long time since you introduced me to a girlfriend," and I said, "I have a girlfriend, but I didn't think you'd want me to bring women here." So later I showed up with my girlfriend.

Orlando's narrative is, in many respects, an apt example of the complex techniques that *bugarrones* and *sankies* employ to manage information about their extra-relational sexual activities—including, but not limited to, their sexual–economic exchanges—with their wives, girlfriends, and clients. In many cases, these strategies are consciously employed to create the illusion of fidelity or to diffuse questions about involvement with men. Some are used primarily to justify one's physical absence, as in Orlando's "little lie" to his girlfriend about a painting job that requires him to work until late at night. Others, such as his taking a girlfriend to his sister's house in order to "kill the bad thoughts" of the neighbors, are intended to dispel any suspicions about engagement in potentially stigmatizing homosexual behavior. In both of these examples, the strategies employed are premeditated in that they involve planning and coordination to create a convincing "scene." This is most dramatically illustrated by cases in which other sex workers or persons in-the-know are paid to buttress a particular alibi, usually by vouching for one's presence in a non-incriminating location. These techniques are therefore highly demanding, requiring a continuous awareness of potential reactions and a talent for eliciting desired impressions.

The constant preoccupation with evasive techniques demonstrates that sex workers are not only engaged in a passive game of mutual pretense with their partners and families but are also actively trying to deflect curiosity through the use of deception and "little lies"—described in Erving Goffman's (1963:42) theory as *stigma management techniques*. Goffman has explained as follows the quandary faced by the stigmatized individual in his social relations: "The issue is not that of managing tension generated during social contacts, but rather that of managing information about his failing. To display or not to display; to tell or not to tell; to let on or not to let on; to lie or not to lie; and in each case to whom, how, when, and where". This sociological theory draws attention to the numerous behavioral influences of stigma on marginalized individuals as they attempt to reduce the social impact of what Goffman describes as their "spoiled identity"—the aspect of the stigmatized person's social location that results in the perception by others that they are somehow less than fully human.

The centrality of stigma management techniques for sex workers' psychosocial lives is perhaps best explained by the great lengths at which they spoke with me about them, sometimes resulting in highly emotional conversations about anxieties related to wives and girlfriends. This is because for many sex workers, the ethnographic interview was the first time they had talked extensively about the various lives they were struggling to keep in balance, usually quite precariously, and often causing significant emotional stress about the potentially damaging consequences of their work for their intimate relationships with women. For example, Hector, 27, became visibly anxious when I asked him about how his wife would feel if she knew about his sex work with men. "That's why I want to leave this [sex work] forever," he explained. "Because, you know, I have my woman now, you see? If my woman realizes that I have sex with men, maybe she'll leave me, you understand?" Similarly, Edgar, 19, described how he had hurled rocks at his neighbor for spreading rumors about his involvement with *maricones* (gay men), and later described to me his fears about the fallout from this very public conflict: "My girlfriend will dump me, of course, because she's going to think that I don't love her and I don't respect her, and I can infect her with some strange disease. She loves me and she wants to marry me, and I'd like to marry her too, but if she finds out about this she's going to look for something—something better."

It is important to emphasize that sex workers' strategies for stigma management are often supported to a certain degree by their families' emphasis on discretion—rather than direct communication—regarding male sexual deviance. Whereas female sexuality in the Dominican Republic is relatively more guarded and controlled, male sexuality is not similarly subject to public surveillance. In this regard, Dominican masculinity allows for particular freedoms that mitigate the stigmatizing effects of sex work. The relative permissiveness toward male sexuality and the gender-specific expectation of men's philandering assist *bugarrones* and *sankies* in evading detection. Further, the emphasis on discretion regarding men's sexual transgressions, as distinct from sexual restraint, means that men are unlikely to be confronted by family members unless there is a relatively public breach of social/sexual decorum. To prevent such a breach, many sex workers attempt to divide their lives, separating their familial and spousal relations from the world of their sexual exchanges.

Reading "Heterosexual AIDS" from the Perspective of the Sex Tourism Economy

In their analysis of the epidemiology of HIV/AIDS among female sex workers in the Dominican Republic, Fadul, De Moya, García, and Herold (1992) have noted: "The pervasive sexual interaction of Dominican FSWs [female sex workers] with foreign male tourists during their vacations is a breeding ground for HIV/STD transmission between local women and North American and European males in the Caribbean." This assessment is supported by the evidence of a national HIV prevalence among female sex workers between 6% and 7%, with regional rates as high as 10% in some areas (Kerrigan, Moreno, Rosario, and Sweat 2001). Similar patterns may also be operative among male sex workers, yet data are more limited for this population, and the potential for transmission between foreign gay tourists and Dominican men has been largely obscured by the designation of the country's AIDS epidemic as predominantly "heterosexual." This section seeks to interrogate the gaps in epidemiological interpretation that may result from a neglect of the dynamics of risk in the tourism economy, as well as the ways that sex workers' stigma management techniques may contribute to a persistent underestimation of same-sex transmission of HIV in the sex tourism industry.

The most important seroprevalence study of HIV among Dominican MSM was conducted by Tabet et al. (1996:202) with 354 men recruited during November and December, 1994, through venue-based sampling at "a wide variety of settings where MSM meet." Because true randomization was not possible through these means, results cannot be presumed to represent a larger population, and should therefore be regarded as suggestive trends. Participants were categorized into five sexual identities—*cross dressers, homosexuals, gigolos, bisexuals,* and *heterosexuals*—with the *gigolo* category roughly corresponding to the category *sanky panky* described in the present study. The authors note that "[g]igolos are a previously described distinct group of CSW [commercial sex workers] from the beach areas of Santo Domingo (Boca Chica) and Puerto Plata who accept money and gifts from female tourists, yet will also engage in sex trade with male tourists" (Tabet et al. 1996:204). It is likely that those men categorized by the authors as *bisexuals* and *heterosexuals* also included many self-defined *bugarrones*, although neither this term nor any other Spanish identity term is mentioned in their report. The study reported HIV prevalence rates of 34.4% for *cross dressers*, 11.7% for *homosexuals*, 6.5% for *gigolos*, 6.1% for *bisexuals*, and 8.2% for *heterosexuals*.

Notably, while *cross dressers*—most likely corresponding to the identity *travesti* in Dominican Spanish—and *homosexuals* had significantly higher HIV prevalence rates and were more likely to report engaging in receptive anal and oral sex, the authors found a few patterns across all identity categories. First, most of the sample of MSM self-identified as *heterosexual*, and this category accounted for half of participants. Second, sex with women was very commonly reported among all groups, with nearly all *heterosexuals*, *bisexuals*, and *gigolos* reporting sex with women, as well as more than half of the self-defined *homosexuals* (55.8%) and a third of *cross dressers* (31.3%). The importance of these results is underlined by the authors' finding—paralleling other studies discussed in the following section—that rates of consistent condom use with female partners were significantly lower than with male partners, practiced by only 14% of men who reported having sex with women. Third, one of the only statistical associations that the authors found between HIV seropositivity and various sociodemographic measures was reported as "ever having been in at least one of the four local brothels" between 1975 and 1985 (Tabet et al. 1996:205). Given that these "brothels" often cater to tourists, this provides strong epidemiological evidence of a continuing association between sex tourism and HIV prevalence among MSM, particularly those who have had sexual contact with tourists.

Importantly, Tabet et al.'s analysis emphasizes the need to place sex workers' same-sex encounters within the entire behavioral context of their lives. Indeed, it is when their sexual relationships with women are brought into focus that the larger public health implications of these behavioral patterns become clear. Sex workers in the present study frequently expressed fear about passing HIV or other STDs along to their unsuspecting wives and girlfriends. Nevertheless, they often rejected the idea of using condoms with their female partners, feeling that this would be unnatural, shameful, or would raise suspicion. More than a decade ago, Ramah, Pareja, and Hasbun (1992) found that only one-fourth (24%) of Dominican MSM who reported having female partners had used a condom during sex with women in the previous year. Similarly, in the present study, less than a third (31%) of survey participants felt that it is necessary to use a condom with one's wife or girlfriend, despite the fact that many of these men engaged in unprotected sex with clients (Padilla 2007a). An even lower proportion (24%) believed that their fellow sex workers used condoms consistently with their wives or girlfriends, demonstrating a perception of very low social support for condom use among their peers.

Humberto, a *bugarrón* in Santo Domingo, typifies this somewhat paradoxical juxtaposition of concern about infecting female partners and a categorical refusal to use condoms with them. At the time of our interview, his wife was pregnant and Humberto explained that this had convinced him to behave more safely with clients, to protect his wife and unborn child:

MP: So, you use condoms with your clients?

H: [Nodding] To prevent any disease, because like I said, my wife is pregnant ['*ta preñada*] and I don't want any disease for her or for my son.

MP: Okay. And when was the last time you didn't use a condom with [your last regular client]?

H: Always. I've always used condoms with him. And there are times that he says no, but I say yes, or otherwise we don't do it.

MP: So, you prefer to use condoms always with him?

H: With him, yes. But with my wife, no, because it would be a shame [*un bochorno*] with my wife.

MP: Have you ever been afraid of infecting your wife with an *enfermedad de la calle* [STD]?

H: Of course! Because of the gays.

MP: "Because of the gays." In what way "because of the gays"?

H: I mean, I use condoms with them [gays] because I'm afraid of making my wife sick.

Here, Humberto articulates a model of selective condom use that was common among sex workers: condoms are seen as a means to shelter the family and the domestic sphere from diseases *de la calle* (from the street), but are not considered appropriate for use with wives or steady girlfriends. The fact that many of these men are exposed to other risks for HIV infection outside of the home, and the fact that some of them do not consistently use condoms with their sex work clients, apparently did not influence their decision to forego condoms in their intimate relationships with women. Condoms are construed as something that one does outside of heterosexual marriage and intimacy, partly as a means to protect the sanctity of that institution, and partly because condom use in marriage symbolizes infidelity and mistrust. The inappropriateness of condoms for the marital context is underlined by Humberto's comment that it would be a *"bochorno"* (shame or embarrassment) to use them with his wife, a feeling which he reiterated several times during the interview. Other sex workers expressed similar sentiments, some of them mentioning in addition their desire to have children, which further diminished their receptivity to the use of condoms with their wives.

The fact that condom use within heterosexual partnerships was not even considered an option by most sex workers, even when fear about infecting wives was quite high, demonstrates the power of the association between condoms and street behavior. This bifurcation of risk contexts into the discrete domains of the home and the street is consistent with dominant Dominican gender models that associate feminine purity with the domestic sphere and masculine impurity with the public sphere. In this framework, condoms are not only perceived as unnecessary within the home but are also symbolic of the moral impurity of the outside world, and may in fact spoil the sanctity of the heterosexual marital bond. Such an interpretation is consistent with sex workers' expressions of shame in response to the prospect of using condoms with their wives.

This moral–spatial bifurcation of the erotic universe is probably more pronounced in the case of male sex workers because homosexuality is seen as highly impure—both by the larger society and by most sex workers themselves—and as a behavior associated with the degeneracy of the street. To the degree that condoms are conceptually associated with impurity and the outside, then, they are seen as much more appropriate for exchanges with men than with women. This explains why even those men who expressed a very strong conviction to use condoms consistently with their male partners—such as Humberto, quoted earlier—did not feel they were appropriate to use with their wives. Further, the permissiveness toward male infidelity and philandering within the gender system reinforces men's perceived right to place women at risk without communicating about outside behaviors. While some sex workers feared placing their female partners at potential risk, they rarely initiated condom use with them to protect them from infection. These decisions were made *for* women, rather than with them, and their potential implications for women's risk were often regarded—when they were considered at all—with a kind of abstract or diffuse fear, rather than a sense of responsibility to take action to reduce their partners' risk.

Tabet et al. make an important statement in the conclusion of their analysis that is worth highlighting here, particularly since it reflects an attention to the accuracy of quantitative behavioral data collected among MSM:

> We hypothesize that the strong social stigma against MSM influences bisexual individuals to self-identify as heterosexual. This bias undoubtedly could contribute to an underestimation in the proportion of HIV-positive men reported to be infected by homosexual transmission if risk behaviors are not carefully and appropriately defined (Tabet et al. 1996:205).

While the authors do not elaborate on the potentially profound epistemological consequences of this fact, it is important to reiterate that—as already described for the Caribbean region as a whole—the Dominican AIDS epidemic has been defined by government personnel and public health agencies as "heterosexual," with only 10% of cases officially attributed to "homo/ bisexual" contact (PAHO 1998:232). Given the historical associations between seropositivity and contact with sex tourists, as well as the very high proportion of MSM and sex workers who report sex with both men and women, the uncritical designation of the Dominican AIDS epidemic as heterosexual may obscure more than it reveals. Behavioral assessments of risk behavior, condom use, and other potential HIV co-factors—as well as ethnographic evidence from this and other studies—further suggest that a significant domain of HIV transmission continues to be neglected by most epidemiological depictions of the Dominican AIDS epidemic. The reasons for this neglect call our attention to large-scale structural dynamics that are rarely considered in epidemiological models, and to the social processes of stigma and shame that systematically veil these linkages.

Conclusion

For nearly two decades, the AIDS epidemic in the Caribbean—now showing HIV prevalence rates that are second only to Sub-Saharan Africa—has been officially described in public health and epidemiological reports as "heterosexual." During this same period, most of the island nations in the region have witnessed a dramatic structural shift from colonial economic models of dependence on cash crops to economies based primarily on tourism, leading to unprecedented historical shifts in the organization of gender and work. This chapter draws on 3 years of ethnographic research in two cities in the Dominican Republic among men involved in informal tourism employment, and considers how men's experiences of informal sexual–economic exchanges with tourists problematizes static public health labels such as "the heterosexual epidemic." Ethnographic and interview material with these men demonstrates how men's personal experiences of the broad political–economic exchanges in the region resulting from the expansion of tourism have created new challenges for them as they seek to *"buscarse la vida"* (look for life), a local phrase used to explain the increasingly ad hoc, informal sector strategies employed to make ends meet. These challenges, compounded by the loss of traditional sources of male labor, have led to broad changes in gender and work that have been almost entirely neglected by prevailing public health interpretations of and prevention programs for HIV/AIDS among heterosexually identified men. Ethnographic and interview data reveal the complicated dilemmas created by these dynamics for men involved in informal sexual labor in the tourism industry. While the dual stigmas of homosexuality and sex work motivate men's use of numerous strategies for ensuring discretion with wives, partners, and community members as a means of maintaining one's status as *"un hombre normal"* (a normal man), traditional public health approaches are largely incapable of capturing these nuances of men's intimate experiences or the ways that their risk behavior is shaped by large-scale transformations in gender, sexuality, and work.

These findings not only demonstrate that the AIDS epidemic follows the contours of global processes—a quintessential example of what some medical anthropologists have described as the structural determinants of health and disease (Farmer 2001; Singer 1998)—but also challenges epidemiological depictions of Caribbean AIDS that have often failed to capture the ongoing linkages between sex tourism, tourism dependence, and patterns of HIV risk behavior. The blind spots created by facile categorizations of regional epidemics, in conjunction with largely imported public health models and funding priorities that focus almost exclusively on gay-identified men, have led to a troubling wholesale neglect of men's sexual labor in the tourism sector. The ethnographic analysis presented here aims to refocus public health attention to men's narratives of sexual labor that do not fit within dominant public health categories, and urges epidemiologists and public health practitioners to formulate new models that are consistent with political–economic shifts and the social context of tourism areas.

To date, interventions among the population of men who exchange sex for money with tourists have been neglected, and may be an important means by which to reduce HIV transmission to women who are likely to be unaware of their partners' same-sex activities. Yet this study also suggests that traditional behavioral interventions focused exclusively on individual factors such as HIV-related knowledge and self-efficacy are unlikely to be effective in altering many of the factors that may be driving HIV transmission. Instead, interventions should be comprehensive and multilevel, extending beyond the population of "men who have sex with men" and involving broad-based stigma reduction initiatives, policy changes to protect sex workers from discrimination, and the creation of community interventions to improve men's skills for risk communication, social support, and a sense of collective responsibility. Finally, the interconnections between sex work, social stigma, the expanding tourism industry, and the HIV epidemic urgently require attention by the public health system, tourism developers, and civil society, in an effort to alleviate the structural conditions that contribute to vulnerability among sex workers. Global HIV/AIDS research should contribute to this effort by moving beyond the simplified categories such as "heterosexual" and "homosexual" that have dominated research, permitting a more nuanced understanding of how HIV risk behavior is shaped by the social norms, cultural meanings, and hierarchical power structures that individuals encounter in their daily lives.

Notes

1. All proper names used in this paper are pseudonyms. All specific place names have been changed, except when referencing larger geographical areas or *barrios*.

2. This research was conducted under the auspices of the doctoral program in anthropology at Emory University, with financial support from the Wenner-Gren Foundation for Anthropological Research, the National Science Foundation, Fulbright IIE, the Fogarty AIDS Training and Research Program, and the *AcciónSIDA* project in Santo Domingo (USAID). See Padilla (2007a).

3. Indeed, as discussed in Padilla (2007a), traditional constructions of Dominican homoeroticism blur the boundaries between *bugarrones* and "normal" men, since gender normativity is defined in relation to sexual positionality rather than sexual object choice. Similar arguments have been made in other Latin American and Caribbean contexts (Carrier 1995; Kulick 1998; Lancaster 1992; Lumsden 1996; Murray 1995; Parker 1991, 1999).

4. For other discussions of the impact of structural adjustments and Balaguer's economic reforms on the Dominican economy, see Bray (1984, 1987), Deere et al. (1990), Freitag (1996), Silié and Colón (1994), and Wiarda (1995). Tracing the relationships between these structural changes and their numerous social and economic consequences, several authors have drawn attention to the connections between structural adjustment programs and the practices of offshore banking, money laundering, drug trafficking, informal commercial trading, information processing, and export manufacturing in the Caribbean (Block and Klausner 1987; Kempadoo 1999; Maingot 1993; Watson 1994).

References

ASONAHORES (1995) *Estadísticas Seleccionadas del Sector Turístico.* Santo Domingo: Asociación Nacional de Hoteles y Restaurantes, Inc.

Barry T, Wood B, Preusch D (1984) *The Other Side of Paradise.* New York: Grove Press.

Betances E (1995) *State and Society in the Dominican Republic.* Boulder, CO: Westview Press.

Block AA, Klausner P (1987) Masters of Paradise Island: Organized crime, neo-liberalism and the Bahamas. *Dialectical Anthropology* 24:85–102.

Bond GC, Kreniske J, Susser I, Vincent J, eds. (1997) *AIDS in Africa and the Caribbean.* Boulder, CO: Westview.

Bray D (1984) Economic development: The middle class and international migration in the Dominican Republic. *International Migration Review* 18(2):217–236.

Bray D (1987) "Industrialization, Labor Migration, and Employment Crises: A Comparison of Jamaica and the Dominican Republic." In: *Crises in the Caribbean Basin.* R Tardanico, ed. Newbury Park, CA: Sage, pp. 79–93.

Cabezas AL (1999) "Women's Work Is Never Done: Sex Tourism in Sosúa, the Dominican Republic." In: *Sun, Sex, and Gold: Tourism and Sex Work in the Caribbean.* K Kempadoo, ed. Boulder, CO: Rowman and Littlefield, pp. 93–123.

Cáceres FI, Duarte I, De Moya EA, Perez-Then E, Hasbún J, Tapia M (1998) *Análisis de la Situación y la Respuesta al VIH/SIDA en República Dominicana.* Santo Domingo: PROFAMILIA.

Carrier J (1995) *De Los Otros: Intimacy and Homosexuality among Mexican Men.* New York: Columbia University Press.

Cepeda C (1984) Falta de Legislación Impide Detener Auge de la Prostitución Homosexual. *La Noticia* April 2:12–13.

CESDEM (1999) *Informe de resultados: Encuesta sobre conocimientos, creencias, actitudes y prácticas acerca del VIH/SIDA en hombres que tienen sexo con hombres.* Santo Domingo: AcciónSIDA.

De Moya EA, García R (1998) "Three Decades of Male Sex Work in Santo Domingo." In: *Men Who Sell Sex: International Perspectives on Male Prostitution and AIDS.* P Aggleton, ed. London: Taylor & Francis, pp. 127–140.

De Moya EA, García R, Fadul R, Herold E (1992) *Sosúa Sanky-Pankies and Female Sex Workers: An Exploratory Study.* Santo Domingo: La Universidad Autónoma de Santo Domingo.

Deere CD, Antrobus P, Bolles L, Melendez E, Phillips P, Rivera M, et al. (1990) *In the Shadow of the Sun: Caribbean Development Alternatives and U.S. Policy.* Boulder, CO: Westview Press.

Fadul R, De Moya EA, García R, Herold E (1992) Sexual interaction and HIV/STD risk between female sex workers and foreign tourists. *International Conference on AIDS* 8(2):D492, abstract no. PoD 5618.

Farmer P (1992) *AIDS and Accusation: Haiti and the Geography of Blame.* Berkeley, CA: University of California Press.

Farmer P (1996) Social inequalities and emerging infectious diseases. *Emerging Infectious Diseases* 2(4):259–269.

Farmer P (2001) *Infections and Inequalities: The Modern Plagues.* Berkeley, CA: University of California Press.

Freitag TG (1996) Tourism and the transformation of a Dominican Coastal Community. *Urban Anthropology and Studies of Cultural Systems and World Economic Development* 25(Fall):225–258.

Garris I, Rodríguez EM, De Moya EA, Gomez E, Puello E, Weissenbacher M, et al. (1991) Predominance of heterosexual transmission of HIV in Dominican Republic: AIDS surveillance data from 1983–1990. *International Conference on AIDS* 7(1):365, abstract no. M.C.3270.

Goffman E (1963) *Stigma: Notes on the Management of Spoiled Identity.* New York: Simon & Schuster.

Kempadoo K (1999) "Continuities and Change: Five Centuries of Prostitution in the Caribbean." In: *Sun, Sex, and Gold: Tourism and Sex Work in the Caribbean.* K Kempadoo, ed. New York: Rowman & Littlefield, pp. 3–33.

Kerrigan D, Moreno L, Rosario S, Sweat M (2001) Adapting the Thai 100% condom programme: Developing a culturally appropriate model for the Dominican Republic. *Culture, Health and Sexuality* 3(2):221–240.

Koenig E, Pittaluga J, Bogart M, Castro M, Nuñez F, Vilorio I, et al. (1987) Prevalence of antibodies to the human immunodeficiency virus in Dominicans and Haitians in the Dominican Republic. *Journal of the American Medical Association* 257(5):631–634.

Kulick D (1998) *Travestí: Sex, Gender and Culture among Brazilian Transgendered Prostitutes.* Chicago, IL: University of Chicago Press.

Lancaster RN (1992) *Life is Hard: Machismo, Danger, and the Intimacy of Power in Latin America.* Berkeley, CA: University of California Press.

Lumsden I (1996) *Machos, Maricones, and Gays: Cuba and Homosexuality.* Philadelphia, PA: Temple University Press.

Maingot AP (1993) "The Offshore Caribbean." In: *Modern Caribbean Politics.* A Payne, P Sutton, eds. Kingston: Ian Randle Publishers, pp. 259–276.

Murray SO (1995) *Latin American Male Homosexualities.* Albuquerque, NM: University of New Mexico Press.

Padilla M (2007a) *Caribbean Pleasure Industry: Tourism, Sexuality, and AIDS in the Dominican Republic.* Chicago, IL: University of Chicago Press.

Padilla M (2007b) Western Union daddies and their quest for authenticity: An ethnographic study of the Dominican gay sex tourism industry. *Journal of Homosexuality* 53(1/2):241–275.

PAHO (1998) *Health in the Americas.* Pan American Health Organization Report.

Parker R (1991) *Bodies, Pleasures, and Passions: Sexual Culture in Contemporary Brazil.* Boston, MA: Beacon Press.

Parker R (1999) *Beneath the Equator: Cultures of Desire, Male Homosexuality, and Emerging Gay Communities in Brazil.* New York: Routledge.

Pérez J (1992) Situation and trend analysis of AIDS epidemic in the Dominican Republic. *International Conference on AIDS* 8(2):C254, abstract no. PoC 4055.

PROCETS (1994) *El SIDA y la Infección VIH en República Dominicana.* Santo Domingo: Programa Control de Enfermedades de Transmisión Sexual y SIDA.

Ramah M, Pareja R, Hasbun J (1992) *Lifestyles and Sexual Practices. Results of KABP Conducted among Homosexual and Bisexual Men.* Santo Domingo: AIDSCOM.

Safa HI (1995) *The Myth of the Male Breadwinner: Women and Industrialization in the Caribbean.* Boulder, CO: Westview Press.

Silié R, Colón M (1994) "Ajuste Estructural y Modelo Neoliberal en República Dominicana." In: *Los Pequeños Países de América Latina en la Hora Neoliberal.* G de Sierra, ed. Ciudad de Mexico: Editorial Nueva Sociedad.

Silvestre E, Rijo J, Bogaert H (1994) *La Neo-prostitucion Infantil en Republica Dominicana.* Santo Domingo: UNICEF.

Singer M, ed. (1998) *The Political Economy of AIDS.* Amityville, NY: Baywood.

Tabet SR, De Moya EA, Holmes KK, Krone MR, de Quiñones MR, de Lister MB, et al. (1996) Sexual behaviors and risk factors for HIV infection among men who have sex with men in the Dominican Republic. *AIDS* 10(2):201–206.

UNAIDS (2002) Epidemiological Fact Sheet on HIV/AIDS and STIs, Dominican Republic. UNAIDS/UNICEF/PAHO/WHO.

UNAIDS (2006) Report on the global AIDS epidemic. Joint United Nations Programme on HIV/AIDS.

UNAIDS (2007) Key facts by region—2007 AIDS Epidemic Update. Joint United Nations Programme on HIV/AIDS.

Vásquez RE, Ruiz C, De Moya EA (1991) AIDS prevention motivation and condom use among Dominican male street kid sex workers, Santo Domingo. *International Conference on AIDS* 7(2):71, abstract no. TH.D.61.

Watson HA, ed. (1994) *The Caribbean in the Global Political Economy.* Boulder, CO: Lynne Rienner Publishers.

Wiarda HJ (1995) *Democracy and Its Discontents: Development, Interdependence, and U.S. Policy in Latin America.* New York: Rowman and Littlefield.

6

Male Infertility and Consanguinity in Lebanon: The Power of Ethnographic Epidemiology

MARCIA C. INHORN, LOULOU KOBEISSI, ANTOINE
A. ABU-MUSA, JOHNNY AWWAD, MICHAEL H. FAKIH,
NAJWA HAMMOUD, ANTOINE B. HANNOUN,
DA'AD LAKKIS, AND ZAHER NASSAR

This problem changed my mind, my life, my prayers. I asked God, "Don't leave me to be like this, never to have children." It broke my life. I want to have my own children too much.

An infertile Lebanese man

Introduction

Infertility, classically defined as the inability to conceive after a year or more of trying and resulting in involuntary childlessness, is a problem of global proportions, affecting more than 80 million individuals of reproductive age worldwide (Vayena, Rowe, and Griffin 2002). Recent estimates suggest that 14% to 17% of all couples may be unable to conceive at some point in their reproductive lives (Campbell and Irvine 2000; Fishel, Dowell, and Thornton 2000). In some societies, however—particularly those in the "infertility belt" of central and southern Africa—as many as one-third of all couples are infertile (Bentley and Mascie-Taylor 2000; Boerma and Mgalla 2001; Larsen 1994, 2000; Vayena et al. 2002). Factors causing high rates of infertility in parts of the non-Western world are varied. Tubal infertility due to sexually transmitted infections and postpartum, postabortive, and iatrogenic infections, as well as pelvic tuberculosis and pelvic schistosomiasis, is widely regarded as the primary form of preventable infertility in the world today (Sciarra 1994, 1997; Vayena et al. 2002). As noted in a recent World Health Organization report, tubal blockage is responsible for about two-thirds of all cases of infertility among women in sub-Saharan Africa, and about one-third of all cases of infertility among women in the developing world (Vayena et al. 2002). Prevention of reproductive tract infections (RTIs) is therefore imperative, especially in the context of scarce health resources to overcome infertility in most non-Western countries (Inhorn 2003a; Sundby 2002; Vayena et al. 2002).

Male Infertility

Not all infertility is preventable. Male infertility is a neglected reproductive health problem, yet it contributes to at least half of all cases of subfertility worldwide (Chan 2007; Kim 2001). Male infertility is often "idiopathic," or of unknown cause; hence, it is recalcitrant to prevention, and is among the most difficult forms of infertility to treat (Carrell, De Jonge, and Lamb 2006; Devroey, Vandervorst, Nagy, and Van Steirteghem 1998; Irvine 1998; Kamischke and Nieschlag 1998). So-called male factors in infertility include low sperm count (oligospermia), poor sperm motility (asthenospermia), defects of sperm morphology (teratozoospermia), and total absence of sperm in the ejaculate (azoospermia), the latter sometimes due to infection-induced obstructions of the epididymis.

Male infertility is a health and social problem that remains deeply hidden, even in the West. Studies have shown male infertility to be among the most stigmatizing of all male health conditions (Becker 2000, 2002; Gannon, Glover, and Abel 2004; Greil 1991; Inhorn 2004; Lloyd 1996; Upton 2002). Such stigmatization is clearly related to issues of sexuality. Male infertility is popularly, although usually mistakenly, conflated with impotency, as both disrupt a man's ability to impregnate a woman and to prove one's virility, paternity, and manhood (Inhorn 2002, 2003a, 2003b, 2004; Upton 2002; Webb and Daniluk 1999). Although little is known about the experience of male infertility worldwide, scattered reports from Egypt, Israel, and Botswana show that male infertility, like female infertility, has profound effects on personhood, marriage, and community relations, particularly in pronatalist settings where all adults are expected to marry and produce offspring (Carmeli and Birenbaum-Carmeli 1994, 2000; Inhorn 2002, 2003b, 2004; Upton 2002). Thus, male infertility is often a cause of profound human suffering, particularly in high-fertility societies where all men are expected to father offspring. For this reason alone, it is a global reproductive health problem of considerable significance.

The New Genetics of Male Infertility and Consanguinity

Unfortunately, in at least 45% of men with abnormal sperm production, a well-defined cause cannot be established (Chan 2007; Maduro and Lamb 2002). However, because of advances in the field of genetics, it is now realized that a significant percentage of male infertility cases, particularly those that are severe, are due to genetic abnormalities. Indeed, "a virtual explosion in the identification of genes affecting spermatogenesis has occurred" in recent years (Maduro and Lamb 2002: 2197). A variety of abnormalities in both the Y and X chromosomes, as well as genetic abnormalities of the hypothalamic–pituitary–gonadal axis involved in the production of reproductive hormones, are now well-established causes of male infertility (Maduro and Lamb 2002; Maduro, Lo, Chuang, and Lamb 2003).

Probably the most frequent molecular genetic cause of infertility in men involves microdeletions of the long arm of the Y chromosome, which are associated with spermatogenic failure (Chan 2007; Krausz, Forti, and McElreavey 2003). In men with such deletions, these genetic alterations are incurable and will be present throughout a man's lifetime (Baccetti et al. 2001). Such deletions are manifest in a variety of sperm defects, including defects of the sperm head (e.g., round heads, heads with craters) and sperm tail (e.g., stunted, immotile, or detached tails) (Baccetti et al. 2001).

A growing literature suggests that such genetic sperm defects cluster in families, for example, among sterile brothers, and may be linked to ancestral consanguinity. Consanguinity (known as "cousin marriage" in popular parlance) is usually defined as the intermarriage of two individuals who have at least one ancestor in common, the ancestor being no more distant than a great-great grandparent. The progeny of such consanguineous marriages are usually referred to as inbred (Gunaid, Hummad, and Tamim 2004). Recent studies by Baccetti et al. (2001) and Latini and colleagues in Italy (2004) suggest that consanguinity is highly correlated with rare genetic sperm defects. These include a range of syndromes that impact sperm morphology (shape) and motility (movement) and may be transmissible to the male offspring. Consequently, male infertility may be heritable, and may cluster in families and communities, depending upon the level of consanguineous marriages in the general population.

Consanguinity in the Middle East

Within the Middle East, the rates of consanguineous marriages are quite high, ranging from 16% to 78%. For example, the following rates of consanguineous marriages have been recently reported across the Middle Eastern region: Algeria, 36.4%; Bahrain, 32%; Egypt, 29% to 39%; Iran, 23% to 78%; Jordan, 51.3%; Kuwait, 35% to 54.3%; Lebanon—29.6% for Muslims and 16.5% for Christians; Libya, 46.5%; Mauritania, 60.1%; Oman, 54%; Qatar, 46%; Saudi Arabia, 54% to 57%; Sudan, 65%; Syria, 38%; Tunisia, 40.2%; Turkey, 21.2%; and United Arab Emirates, 50% to 54%. Between 8% and 30% of these marriages are first-cousin marriages, the closest form. For example, first-cousin marriage rates have been recorded for a number of Middle Eastern countries as follows: Egypt, 11.4%; Jordan, 32%; Kuwait, 26% to 30.2%; Lebanon—17.3%

among Muslims and 7.9% among Christians; Oman, 34%; Saudi Arabia 31.4% to 41.4%; United Arab Emirates, 30%; and Yemen, 32%. Furthermore, in several of these countries, rates of first-cousin marriages are increasing (e.g., Yemen, United Arab Emirates), while the rates are either stable (e.g., Oman) or declining (e.g., Jordan, Lebanon, Kuwait, Syria) in other Middle Eastern countries where media may have played a role in discouraging cousin unions (Al-Gazali et al. 1997; Gunaid et al. 2004; Hamamy, Jamhawi, Al-Darawsheh, and Ajlouni 2005; Jurdi and Saxena 2003; Saadat, Ansari-Lari, and Farhud 2004; Abbasi-Shavazi, McDonald, and Hosseini-Chavoshi [in press]; Sueyoshi and Ohtsuka 2003).

According to a recent overview of mutation research, Mediterranean, and Muslim Mediterranean populations in particular, rank highest in the world in terms of increased frequency of congenital malformations and recessive disorders linked to consanguinity (Birenbaum-Carmeli 2004). Indeed, as shown in the seminal volume on *Genetic Disorders among Arab Populations* (Teebi and Farag 1996), Arab populations have high frequencies of autosomal recessive disorders, homozygosity of autosomal and X-linked traits, and a plethora of new genetic syndromes and variants, the majority of them autosomal recessive. In clinical settings in the Arab world, consanguinity manifests itself in congenital malformations, mental retardation, blindness and deafness, sickle cell anemia and thalassemia, cystic fibrosis, congenital hydrocephalus, Down syndrome, and specific metabolic diseases (Rajab and Patton 2000; Zlotogora 1997). Recent studies have also linked consanguinity to a range of poor child health outcomes, including neonatal diabetes mellitus, low birth weight, and apnea (cessation of breathing) associated with prematurity (Mumtaz et al. 2007; Tamim, Khogali, Beydoun, Melki, and Yunis 2003).

Although consanguinity has never been definitively linked to male infertility in the Middle East, it is striking to observe that male infertility cases are highly prevalent in Middle Eastern infertility clinics, often making up between 60% and 90% of the patient caseload in in vitro fertilization (IVF) centers (Inhorn 2004). In addition, many infertile Middle Eastern men present with severe oligo-, astheno-, and teratozoospermia, as well as azoospermia of nonobstructive origin. It is widely speculated within the Middle Eastern assisted reproductive community that these severe forms of male infertility are attributable to genetic causes. However, with the exception of Kuwait (Alkhalaf, Verghese, and Mhuarib 2002; Mohammed et al. 2007), genetic studies of male infertility have yet to emerge from the Middle Eastern region. To our knowledge, no studies have attempted to examine the association between male infertility and consanguineous marriage practices.

To that end, this chapter presents a novel attempt to determine whether consanguinity is related to male infertility in the Middle Eastern nation of Lebanon. We conducted a study that combined epidemiological and ethnographic approaches to the study of male infertility, in the hopes of shedding light on this troubling male reproductive health condition. We argue that "ethnographic epidemiology," involving a case–control research design and mixed-methods approach, is a powerful means to achieve understanding of a variety of important public health problems. In the next section, we briefly describe what we mean by this concept, before turning our attention to the study, its methodology, and results.

The Power of Ethnographic Epidemiology

In recent years, anthropologists have pointed to the overlapping nature of anthropological and epidemiological interests and have sung the praises of collaborative research, especially that focusing on the health consequences of human behavior (Dunn and Janes 1986; Fleck and Ianni 1958; Hahn 1995; Inhorn 1995; Inhorn and Buss 1994; Trostle 2005; True 1996). Books have been written on the need for interdisciplinary, anthropological–epidemiological approaches to the study of health and disease (Janes, Stall, and Gifford 1986; Trostle 2005). Sessions at national meetings have been devoted to this theme, and editorials in major journals have deemed the "integration of epidemiological and ethnographic research methods" to be necessary for the continued maturation of the field of medical anthropology (Brown 1992). Nevertheless, as noted by Trostle (1986a, 1986b, 2005), the history of such collaboration has been one of "benign neglect" and "missed opportunities," and some observers have even pointed to an active "schism" or "divergences" between the anthropological and epidemiological communities (Inhorn 1995; Rubinstein and Perloff 1986).

Nonetheless, as highlighted in Trostle's (2005) recent book on *Epidemiology and Culture*, a new field of "cultural epidemiology" is emerging, one that focuses attention on culturally defined categories of disease classification, meaning, risk, and behavior, in addition to the more commonly employed "social variables," such as income, marital status, and occupation (Trostle 2005). Trostle urges the integration of both qualitative (textual) and quantitative (statistical) methods to improve the understanding of disease problems. He provides many relevant examples of "productive collaboration" between the disciplines of anthropology and epidemiology, with regard to health problems such as epilepsy, cholera, and adolescent smoking.

Like Trostle, we argue that anthropology and epidemiology "need each other." Epidemiology, as a methodologically exacting discipline, is devoted to the discovery of disease prevalence and incidence rates and to the statistical assessment of causal associations between risk factors and disease outcomes in human populations. However, what epidemiology possesses in terms of methodological rigor, it often lacks in contextual understanding of *why* certain human groups are at risk of problems such as infertility at particular historical moments, in specific places, and within particular political, economic, legal, and religious contexts (Turshen 1984). This lack of contextual understanding has led one critic to point to epidemiology's methodological *"rigor* mortis" (Nations 1986). Ultimately, epidemiology needs to understand and utilize anthropology's ethnographic methods and forms of qualitative data analysis to understand the range of possible culture-specific behavioral patterns requiring assessment as disease risk factors. Once these risk factors are assessed, anthropology can help to explain why such culturally embedded risk practices persist and may be resistant to change for sociocultural and political–economic reasons.

Anthropology also needs to understand and utilize epidemiological methods and forms of quantitative data analysis. Through ethnography, anthropologists are able to identify myriad, potentially health-demoting environmental risk factors and behavioral practices. Yet, to assess *which* of the many factors identified through ethnographic research place people, usually unwittingly, at risk of problems such as infertility, a formal epidemiological approach to risk assessment is also necessary.

Methodologically, anthropology and epidemiology converge in more ways than one. The vast majority of epidemiological studies are "observational" (Kelsey, Thompson, and Evans 1986), just as anthropological studies are "participant observational." In fact, perhaps the most common method of data collection employed in epidemiology is the same one that is employed in anthropology, that is, talking with people. Epidemiologists gather data through communicating with research subjects, just as medical anthropologists do. Although the interviewing techniques of epidemiology tend to be more formal than those of anthropology, since they rely on standardized interview schedules, they nevertheless may be quite in-depth.

If anthropology and epidemiology do differ methodologically, the difference may be one of scope rather than kind. Anthropologists tend to have a greater variety of methods to choose from than do epidemiologists, and are much less concerned than most epidemiologists in establishing normative methodological standards (Rubinstein and Perloff 1986). However, all of the methods used by epidemiologists, including interviewing, archival research, and record review, are also components of the anthropological tool kit. Conversely, epidemiologists tend to deal with larger sample sizes than do anthropologists and to work with people who do not view themselves as necessarily connected in any way (Dunn and Janes 1986). Yet, some epidemiological studies, especially those in genetic epidemiology, may work with very small sample sizes of individuals who are often related. Thus, there are no fixed rules that divide the epidemiological and anthropological enterprises on a methodological basis, and it could be argued that their similarities are perhaps greater than their differences (Hahn 1995; Inhorn 1995).

Within anthropology, a movement is afoot to examine the ethnographic enterprise itself, in terms of both methodological rigor and reflexivity. Recent calls to reassess the ethnographic toolkit have pointed to the improved validity achieved by using multiple, or "mixed" methods in one study, rather than relying on the ethnographic standbys of participant observation and/or interviews with key informants (Bernard 2005). The use of multiple methods is considered to be one form of *triangulation*, a term referring to the process of cross-checking data that is being used within the social sciences, including anthropology (Fetterman 1998).

It is no wonder, then, that more and more medical anthropologists have begun to conduct synthetic ethnographic–epidemiological studies, in which both ethnographic and epidemiological research designs, methods of data collection and analysis, and interpretive insights are employed in order to understand more clearly the factors underlying a variety of public health problems. This is particularly true of those who have received training in both disciplines (including the first author of this chapter and several other authors in this volume). For example, in Inhorn's earlier study of male infertility in Egypt (Inhorn 1994; Inhorn and Buss 1994), both ethnographic and epidemiological approaches were employed, showing that the culturally embedded practice of male water pipe smoking increased the risk of male infertility outcomes.

Unfortunately, few other integrative studies of this kind have been conducted in the Middle East. Nonetheless, the literature on the potential health effects of consanguinity in the Middle East is burgeoning[1] because of the high prevalence of both consanguinity and genetic disorders across the region, as well as concerns over the need to initiate culturally sensitive genetic counseling programs (Al-Gazali 2005; Panter-Brick 1991; Raz, Atar, Rodnay, Shohan-Vardi, and Carmi 2003).

Given this background, our goal in this study was to assess whether consanguinity is a possible risk factor for male infertility in Lebanon, whether Lebanese men are concerned about this possibility, and why the practice of consanguineous marriage is socially and culturally supported. To that end, an ethnographic–epidemiological study was undertaken in Lebanon in 2003 to determine possible risk factors for male infertility, including men's own causal assessments of their male infertility problems (Inhorn 2004). Male infertility clearly troubles Lebanese men, who, in their concerted attempts to overcome the problem, pose the question, "Why me?" Although men rarely link consanguinity directly to their infertility problems, they are concerned that male infertility may "run in the family." As our study will show, these men are probably right: Male infertility *does* cluster within families, particularly families characterized by intergenerational patterns of consanguinity. Thus, consanguinity may be linked to male infertility in Lebanon, even though the rates of consanguinity in that country are the lowest in the region.

In this chapter, we will describe the research setting and methodology, present the results of our epidemiological research on consanguinity and male infertility, and then provide an ethnographic analysis of why consanguinity is a deeply embedded cultural practice in Lebanon as elsewhere in the Middle East. We include two case studies of infertile Lebanese men who are deeply troubled by their infertility and the family and child health problems that have ensued. In the end, we suggest that consanguinity, male infertility, and genetic disorders are understudied public health issues that deserve increased attention. We believe that anthropologists working in public health are ideally situated to address these problems, given anthropology's long history of research on cousin marriages cross-culturally (Carsten 2004; Dumont and Parkin 2006; Fox 1984; Holy 1996; Westermarck 2003), as well as the recent anthropological interest in new forms of genetic testing (Finkler 2000; Franklin and Roberts 2006).

Research Setting and Methods

Lebanon (population, 4.3 million) is a small, Middle Eastern nation on the Eastern Mediterranean, bordered by Israel on the South and Syria on the North and East. Lebanon is the most religiously diverse nation in the Middle East, with 18 officially recognized religious sects. Unfortunately, intersectarian tensions and ongoing disputes with both Israel and Syria have plunged Lebanon into more than 30 years of ceaseless violence, including a 15-year civil war (1975–1990), numerous political assassinations, and a summer war between Israel and Lebanon's Hizbullah in 2006. Thus, this war-torn country has experienced considerable death and destruction. Not surprisingly, many infertile Lebanese men who lived through the war years attribute their reproductive health problems to *il harb*, "the war" (Inhorn 2004), which is a likely risk factor for male infertility in the country (Kobeissi et al. in press).

This study was conducted in 2003, a relatively "quiet" year, despite the initiation of the U.S.-led war in Iraq, which led to several acts of violence against American and British interests in Lebanon. During 2003, the first author (Inhorn) joined with a group of six Lebanese physicians (Abu-Musa, Awwad, Fakih, Hannoun, Lakkis, Nassar) to undertake a combined ethnographic–epidemiological study of male infertility in the capital city, Beirut. The study, supported by the National Science Foundation and the U.S. Department of Education Fulbright-Hays Faculty Abroad Program, was designed to accomplish both epidemiological and ethnographic goals. On the epidemiological side, the study attempted to assess a number of behavioral and environmental risk factors for male infertility in Lebanon, including the effects of the Lebanese civil war. On the ethnographic side, the study attempted to assess Lebanese men's subjective experiences of male infertility, which were characterized in the ethnographic study design as consisting of "four M's": masculinity, marriage, morality, and medical treatment-seeking.

To accomplish both these epidemiological and ethnographic goals, a classic epidemiological case–control study design was utilized, drawing upon the infertile patient populations in two of the busiest and most successful IVF clinics in central Beirut. One of these was located in a large, private university-based teaching hospital, the American University of Beirut Medical Center (AUBMC), and catered to a religiously mixed patient population of both Sunni and Shia Muslims, Christians of various sects, Druze (a minority Muslim sect), and various immigrant and refugee populations, including Palestinian refugees living in Lebanon. The other clinic, FIRST IVF, was a private, stand-alone center catering primarily to southern Lebanese Shia patients, but also to Christian and Sunni Muslim patients coming from both Lebanon and neighboring Syria.

Between these two clinics, 220 married men, who had been unable to conceive a child with their wives during at least the 12 months before the study, were recruited as research subjects by the physicians and the AUBMC IVF unit head nurse (Hammoud). The patients were divided into two groups according to their fertility status based on their semen analyses. The cases included 120 men who were considered infertile because of repeated abnormal semen analyses. The control group included 100 men with repeated normal semen analyses, but who were seeking fertility treatment because of female factor infertility, including tubal, polycystic ovary syndrome (PCOS), unexplained, or endometriosis-related infertility. Subjects underwent semen analysis at the time of the study, generally on the day of study recruitment at the IVF center to confirm the results of previous analyses. Semen analysis was reliable and standardized to reflect current World Health Organization guidelines (World Health Organization 1999). Semen analysis results were important to this study, as they clearly distinguished infertile cases from fertile controls. This epidemiological case–control design also served important ethnographic purposes; it allowed the anthropologist leading the study to understand the experiences and perspectives of infertile men, as well as men who were not infertile but who were experiencing childless marriages.

Following informed consent, interviews were conducted by the anthropologist with all of the men in the study. The interviews took place in a private room in the clinics, where the study was explained and assurances of confidentiality were reiterated through both verbal and written informed consent. About half of the interviews were conducted in Arabic and half in English, depending on the preference and ability of informants (many of whom were well educated and spoke excellent English). Although tape-recording was presented as an option on the informed consent form, most of the men were uncomfortable with being tape-recorded, declining this option.[2] In most cases, the anthropologist conducted interviews alone, but a research assistant was present during some of the Arabic interviews, especially in the initial stages of the research when the first author was learning a new and distinct dialect of Levantine Arabic.

A large amount of data was collected during an 8-month study period (January–June 2003), given that multiple epidemiological and ethnographic methods were utilized. Reproductive history and epidemiological semi-structured interviews were used to collect baseline information on demographics (age, religion, place of residence, education, income) and reproductive and sexual history (age at first sexual intercourse, number of sexual partners, age at marriage, number of marriages, pregnancies and births). Detailed questions were asked about consanguineous marriage practices between spouses (first cousin, second cousin, distant relative), between the research subject's parents (i.e. first-degree consanguinity) and grandparents (i.e., second-degree consanguinity, of maternal or paternal relatives or both). In addition, questions were posed about other known cases of male infertility in the immediate family (i.e., brothers, cousins, uncles, fathers). Other reproductive risk factors were also assessed through the semi-structured interview, including various reproductive illnesses, presence of chronic diseases, lifestyle factors (especially tobacco and caffeine consumption), and occupational and war exposures. As noted earlier, this epidemiological data collection strategy was coupled with laboratory-based semen analysis, generally carried out at the time of the reproductive interview in the clinic-based IVF laboratories. In addition, more than 200 men in the study agreed to have blood samples drawn for the purposes of later toxic metal analysis at the University of Michigan (Inhorn et al. 2008).

The ethnographic portion of the study consisted of both in-depth, open-ended interviews and participant observation in the clinics. Once the reproductive history and epidemiological interviews were completed, most of the men in the study agreed to speak about their lives more generally, and, in some cases, wives joined these discussions. These interviews focused on men's experiences of male infertility and the "four M's" (masculinity, marriage, morality, medical treatment-seeking) and generated 1200 pages of qualitative interview transcripts, which were then coded and analyzed for salient themes. Case study reports were also written immediately after each interview, to summarize the stories and topics that men chose to discuss with the anthropologist.

In addition, the anthropologist conducted both formal and informal interviews with staff at both clinics, including physicians, nurses, and embryologists. Participant observation and conversations held in clinic waiting areas, laboratories, and doctors' offices were recorded in detailed field notes, 550 pages of which were also coded and later analyzed.

The epidemiological data were also coded and entered by one of the authors (Kobeissi), a Lebanese graduate of both American University of Beirut and University of Michigan (UM), who analyzed the data for her doctoral thesis at UM's School of Public Health. Data were analyzed using the Statistical Package for Social Sciences (SPSS Version 12). Univariate analysis consisted of frequency and percentage distributions for the different categorical variables in the study. Means, standard deviations, and ranges were computed for the different continuous variables, with checking for normality and outliers.

Bivariate analysis mainly utilized Chi-Square-Fisher's exact test to test the association between the main outcome variable (male infertility) and the various exposure and confounding variables. The purpose of this analysis was to examine crude associations and to check for potential confounders and effect modification.

Multivariate analysis involved a backward logistic regression model, where analysis included the different exposure and confounding variables that yielded significant results during bivariate analysis. Odds ratios, P-values, and confidence intervals were computed at a type I error (alpha) of 5%. The final model incorporated the exposure and confounding variables that displayed the most significant odds ratios.

The Epidemiology of Consanguinity

As shown in Table 6.1, there were no significant differences between cases and controls in terms of sociodemographic background. The average age in both groups was 39, and most subjects had completed high school. The average monthly income in both groups was around US$ 1800. The majority of cases and controls resided in Beirut (46% versus 35%, respectively). The religious backgrounds of cases and controls were comparably heterogeneous; approximately one-quarter of the cases and controls were Christians and three-quarters were Muslims. Controls were slightly more likely to be white-collar professionals; however, the professional background of both groups was relatively similar. Reflecting Lebanon's high educational levels, around 60% of cases and controls held professional sector jobs, including as physicians, engineers, professors, and businessmen.

As shown in Table 6.2, 16% of cases and 24% of controls reported consanguineous marriage to a related spouse, a difference that was not statistically significant. The cases were more likely than controls to report first-degree (parental) and second-degree (grandparental) consanguinity; but the difference (46% cases versus 37% controls) was also not statistically significant. The socioeconomic and educational backgrounds did not differ significantly between

Table 6.1. Distribution of Sociodemographic Factors among Cases and Controls

VARIABLES	MALE INFERTILITY STATUS	
	CASES[a]	CONTROLS[b]
Age (y), mean (SD)	38.5 (6.6)	39.4 (6.1)
	P-value = .901	
Years of education (y), mean (SD)	13.7 (4.2)	14.2 (5.5)
	P-value = .606	
Salary (US$ monthly), mean (SD)	1768 (2500)	1829 (2130)
	P-value = .541	
Current residence, n (%)		
Beirut	43 (35.8)	45 (45.0)
South Lebanon	25 (20.8)	8 (8.0)
Mount Lebanon	16 (13.3)	8 (8.0)
Elsewhere in Lebanon	12 (10.0)	10 (10.0)
Outside Lebanon	24 (20.0)	29 (29.0)
	P-value = .034	
Religion, n (%)		
Christian	32 (26.7)	27 (27.0)
Muslim	84 (70.0)	68 (68.0)
Druze (Muslim sect)	4 (3.3)	5 (5.0)
	P-value = .721	
Profession, n (%)		
Blue collar	17 (14.2)	6 (6.0)
Clerical	18 (15.0)	22 (22.0)
Business/teaching	40 (33.3)	40 (40.0)
Doctor/lawyer/diplomat/professor	31 (25.8)	26 (26.0)
Government employee	14 (11.7)	6 (6.0)
	P-value = .151	

[a] Cases are those in whom infertility is present.
[b] Controls are those in whom infertility is absent.

those who reported first- and second-degree consanguinity in the parental and grandparental generations and those in the study who did not report such consanguineous backgrounds. Both groups were equally likely to have married a related wife (i.e., paternal or maternal cousin), suggesting that consanguineous marriage practices in Lebanon are continuing over the generations.

As shown in Table 6.3, those who reported first- or second-degree consanguinity (or both) were more likely to be Muslims or Druze (83%) than

Table 6.2. Bivariate Analysis of Consanguinity among Cases and Controls

VARIABLES	MALE INFERTILITY	
	CASES N (%)	CONTROLS N (%)
Consanguineous marriage to wife		
Wife is a relative (maternal or paternal cousin)	19 (15.8)	24 (24.0)
Wife is not a relative	101 (84.2)	73 (73.0)
Relationship unknown	0 (0)	3 (3.0)
	P-value = *.102*	
Type of consanguineous marriage		
Wife: maternal cousin	8 (6.7)	16 (16)
Wife: paternal cousin	10 (8.3)	7 (7)
Wife: both paternal and maternal cousin	1 (0.8)	1 (1)
Wife: unspecified cousin	3 (2.5)	0 (0)
Wife is not related	98 (81.6)	76 (76)
	P-value = *.107*	
Consanguineous marriage between parents and/or grandparents		
None are related	64 (53.4)	60 (60.0)
Parents or grandparents are related	34 (28.3)	29 (28.0)
Both parents and grandparents are related	22 (18.3)	8 (8.0)
Relationship unknown	0 (0)	3 (3.0)
	P-value = *.113*	
Reported male infertility problems in immediate family		
Yes	52 (42.6)	14 (14.0)
None	68 (57.4)	85 (85.0)
Unknown	0 (0)	1 (1)
	P-value < *.001*	

Christians (17%). Reflecting intersectarian socioeconomic differences, they also had lower average monthly reported incomes (US$ 1723) than those who did not report consanguineous backgrounds (US$ 1925).

As noted above, cases were more likely than controls to report first- or second-degree consanguinity or both (46% versus 37%), suggesting that infertility in men may be the product of consanguineous marriage practices in previous generations. However, this difference was not found to be statistically significant, as shown in Table 6.2.

Table 6.3. Distribution of Socioeconomic Background by Consanguinity Status

VARIABLES	FIRST OR SECOND CONSANGUINITY STATUS	
	PRESENT	ABSENT
Age at marriage (y), mean (SD)	32.1 (6.1)	32.4 (6.8)
	P-value = .725	
Wife's age at marriage (y), mean (SD)	26.3 (5.5)	26.8 (6.3)
	P-value = .577	
Years of education (y), mean (SD)	14.2 (5.6)	13.8 (4.1)
	P-value = .384	
Monthly salary (US$), mean (SD)	1723 (1847)	1925 (2921)
	P-value = .539	
Kinship to wife, n (%)		
Wife related	21 (50.0)	21 (50)
Wife not related	68 (39.3)	105 (39.3)
	P-value = .207	
Religion, n (%)		
Christian	18 (17.3)	6 (6.6)
Druze	2 (1.9)	6 (6.6)
Muslim	84 (80.8)	67 (73.6)
	P-value = .207	

However, a clear family clustering of male infertility cases was detected in this study. Controlling for other risk factors, the odds of reported infertility problems among immediate family members, particularly brothers, male cousins, uncles, and, in some cases, fathers, was 2.58 times as high among cases as in controls ($P < 0.057$), as shown in the multivariate logistic regression analysis in Table 6.4.

In addition, when only azoospermic and severely oligospermic men (<1 million sperm/mL^3) were separated from the rest of the male infertility cases, the consanguinity and family clustering effects were amplified. Exactly 50% of these infertile men reported first- and/or second-degree consanguinity, and nearly 40% reported known male infertility problems among close male relatives, as shown in Table 6.5. In other words, half of the most severely infertile Lebanese men in this study came from consanguineous families.

Table 6.4. Multivariate Logistic Regression Analysis of Consanguinity and Family Clustering of Male Infertility

VARIABLE	ADJUSTED ODDS RATIO	P-VALUE (95% CI)
Male infertility problems in immediate family (yes/no)	2.58	0.057 (0.971–6.8)
Consanguineous marriage between parents and/or grandparents (yes/no)	0.865	0.756 (0.34–2.17)

Table 6.5. Consanguinity and Family Clustering of Male Infertility among Men with Severe Oligospermia and Azoospermia

VARIABLES	MEN WITH SEVERE OLIGOSPERMIA AND AZOOSPERMIA	
	N	%
Distribution of first- or second-degree consanguinity		
None	33	50.8
First or second degree	19	29.2
Both First and second degree	13	20.0
Distribution of infertility problems in immediate family		
None	38	58.5
Male factor	25	38.4
Female factor	2	3.1

Male infertility clustered among the men in these families, suggesting a strong genetic component to their sperm defects.

To summarize, although first- and second-degree consanguinity did not prove to be significantly associated with male infertility outcomes overall, two findings of this study are of possible significance. First, male infertility clearly clustered in families among cases in this study; nearly 40% of these men could identify other known cases of male infertility in the immediate family, particularly among brothers, first cousins, uncles, and, in some cases, fathers. Second, among the "most infertile" subset of Lebanese men in this study—those with either azoospermia or severe oligospermia—half were the offspring of consanguineous unions among the parental or grandparental generations (or both). These findings suggest a genetic predisposition to male infertility in Lebanon.

Clearly, more epidemiological work needs to be done to ascertain the underlying mechanisms of genetic male infertility, including whether consanguinity can lead to the propagation of male infertility among future generations (Al Abdulkareem and Ballal 1998; Al-Gazali et al. 1997). Moreover, molecular genetic testing to search for Y chromosome microdeletions is also necessary, and represents one of the major limitations of our own study. However, because of the availability of standardized semen analysis, objective evidence of azoospermia and severe oligospermia was provided in this study, allowing us to determine frequencies of consanguinity and family clustering of male infertility cases among the most severely affected infertile men. Furthermore, the quality of the measures in this study was high, because of the use of multiple validation techniques (i.e., in-depth reproductive history and risk factor interviews, coupled with the results of semen analysis). Semen analysis of both cases and controls was possible in this study, because of the recruitment of infertility clinic–based research subjects; clinic-based research samples are common in infertility studies, despite the potential for selection bias when fertile controls are not drawn from the general population. No major problems existed in terms of adjusting for missing and nonresponse data, and the size of the sample approximated required statistical "power." Although the study relied on self-report of consanguinity and infertility among family members, research subjects usually had no difficulty providing this information. Some men even volunteered to sketch their family genealogy, marking the relevant infertility cases at the time of the interview.

The Ethnography of Consanguinity

Given these epidemiological findings, two major questions of anthropological interest may be posed. *Why* do men marry their cousins in Lebanon and other parts of the Middle East? And, do men recognize that consanguinity may be a risk factor for male infertility in the region? It is important to begin with some context—namely, consanguineous marriage is a socially supported institution throughout much of the non-Western world, not only the Middle East. For example, in the primarily Hindu states of South India, marriages between close relatives occur in 20% to 45% of all cases, with uncle–niece and first-cousin marriages, usually mother's brother's daughter (MBD), the preferred form (Bittles, Manson, Green, and Rao 1991; Bittles, Grant, Sullivan, and Hussain 2002). Before World War II, MBD first-cousin marriages were also quite common among the Han of China, who make up about 90% of the total population. Similarly, Buddhists, Christians, Jews, Parsees, and Druze living in Asian countries frequently marry their kin. Anthropological and ethnographic surveys have also reported cousin marriage rates of 35% to 50% across sub-Saharan Africa (Bittles et al. 1991, 2002). Although contemporary Westerners have been prohibited religiously and legally from entering into consanguineous marriages, particularly with first cousins, it should be noted that (1) 0.5% of North Americans and Western Europeans are reported to marry their cousins (Bittles et al. 1991), and (2) legal statutes in many U.S. states disallow first-cousin marriages but allow consanguineous unions with other relatives of varying degrees (Ottenheimer 1996).

Consanguinity receives particularly strong expression in the various regions of the Muslim world, including North and Sub-Saharan Africa, the Middle East, and Central, South, and Southeast Asia (Hussain and Bittles 1999, 2004). Among the world religions, consanguineous marriage finds it highest level of support within Islam, with the Prophet Muhammad having married his daughter Fatima to his first-cousin Ali. In Middle Eastern Muslim societies, first-cousin marriages—especially patrilateral parallel, that is, father's brother's daughter (FBD) marriages (*bint 'amm*)—are the preferred form (a preference that is unique to the Middle East), with partners having at least one set of grandparents in common, and sometimes two (Bittles et al. 1991; Eickelman 2001). In the Muslim world, 20% to 55% of all marital unions are consanguineous, with even higher rates (>75%) in some regions of the Middle East (Abbasi-Shavazi et al. in press).

Why are consanguineous marriages so commonly practiced in the contemporary Muslim Middle East? A wide range of deeply rooted historical, sociocultural, economic, and religious rationales support consanguinity in these societies. It is often believed that consanguineous marriages offer a range of social and economic advantages, including better compatibility between husband and wife and their respective families (who are known to each other rather than being "strangers," often within the context of arranged marriages); maintenance of wealth, property, and inheritance within the family; superior prenuptial negotiations vis a vis reduced bridewealth payments; reinforcement of familial and tribal affiliations; strengthened affective ties between the relatives who marry their children to each other; and fewer of the complications and uncertainties inherent in marriages with nonrelatives (Bittles et al. 1991; El-Hazmi et al. 1995; Gunaid et al. 2004; Jurdi and Saxena 2003; Rajab and Patton 2000; Shah 2004; Tremayne 2006). Furthermore, it is believed that the family is the main source of personal identity and security; thus, only through endogamy (within-family marriage) can a family's strength and family members' personal security be assured. For women in particular, marrying a cousin facilitates the transition of a wife to a husband's family in a "soft" manner, without the disruption of existing family bonds or even household arrangements (Gunaid et al. 2004).

In addition, as shown in Inhorn's research (1996), cousin marriages may serve as a buffer against divorce in cases of marital infertility. Familial loyalty seems to play a role in securing such marriages, since male cousins often tend to feel protective toward their female cousins in general, and female cousins often feel an obligation to "take care of their husband's name" (i.e., to protect his and the family's reputation) in cases of male infertility. In addition, it is widely believed that fertility may be *enhanced* in cousin marriages, because of the salubrious mixing of the "same blood." In a pronatalist setting, the belief that cousin marriages produce more and better offspring may be a major impetus for perpetuation of this practice.

In Inhorn's (1996) Egyptian study, where 35% of marriages were between cousins, consanguineous marriages tended to occur among nonworking women of lower educational backgrounds, a finding that is true across the Middle Eastern region as a whole (Bittles et al. 2002; Hussain and Bittles 2004). However, among men in many communities, the higher the educational–occupational status, the higher the rate of consanguineous unions. One plausible explanation for this pattern is that the "best males" are pressured to remain "within" the family by marrying a cousin. Such males, especially eldest sons, are regarded as valuable assets, who should be conserved within sociofamilial boundaries. This "best males" hypothesis has been forwarded in studies conducted in Yemen and Jordan, but has been questioned as a cause of cousin marriage in studies conducted in Lebanon, Kuwait, and Saudi Arabia (Al Abdulkareem and Ballal 1998; Gunaid et al. 2004; Jurdi and Saxena 2003; Shah 2004).

The educational and literacy levels in Lebanon, the focus of this study, are among the highest in the Middle Eastern region, but the rates of consanguineous marriage are among the lowest. Nonetheless, the level of consanguinity there may be increasing as well (Gunaid et al. 2004). The importance of kinship as manifested in consanguineous marriage in Lebanon remains strong, a powerful means to ensure patrilineal solidarity and property in a society that has been fractured by years of civil war and ongoing political violence (Joseph 1993; 2001). Indeed, 15 years of civil war (1975–1990) resulted in the death of 7% of the Lebanese population, serious injuries in 10% of the population, displacement of up to 24% of the population, and emigration of up to 30% of the population (Inhorn et al. 2008). Many demographic disruptions occurred in Lebanon as a result of the civil war, including most significantly, delayed age at first marriage; decreased family size; an increased proportion of unmarried adult women as a result of high male outward migration and mortality; reduced employment opportunities; and shortages of safe, affordable housing. Because of the dearth of wage-earning males, Lebanese women increased their levels of educational attainment and involvement in the labor force. The influence of higher educational attainment among women has further affected their postwar lives, resulting in what has generally been referred to as a "celibacy trap"—namely, the postponement of marriage to the late 20s, coupled with the dearth of marriageable Lebanese men, has resulted in an increased lifetime expectancy of celibacy (what used to be known as "spinsterhood") for many Lebanese women (Saxena, Kulczyck, and Jurdi 2004; Jabbra 2004). As a result, Lebanese women have become more tolerant of less socially desirable marriages, including to either younger or much older men, men with lower educational levels, and cousins whom they might not have preferred to marry otherwise.

Current figures demonstrate that nearly one-third of all Lebanese Muslims and nearly 17% of Lebanese Christians marry consanguineoustly, even though many Christian sects technically forbid close kinship in marriage. In our study of both Muslim and Christian men, approximately one-fifth of all men in the study (16% of cases, 25% of controls) were currently married to their cousins indicating the persistence of consanguineous marriage in this population over time. In addition, fully two-thirds of Muslim men in the study were the product of either first- or second-degree consanguinity, as were one-fifth of the Christian men, indicating the prevalence of consanguinity in previous generations.

To illustrate some of these issues, it is useful to turn to the cases of two infertile Lebanese men, whom we will call "Abbass" and "Hussain." Both volunteered to participate in the study after reading an advertisement placed by the authors in the clinic waiting area. Both offered compelling accounts of their severe male infertility problems, although neither attributed these problems to consanguinity per se.

The Case of Abbass

Abbass was the first man to volunteer for the study, perhaps because he had lived in the United States for 7 years, felt favorably toward the U.S., and wanted to practice his English skills with the American anthropologist. He was a tall, robust, sandy-haired man with a large moustache, which, along with his weathered skin, made him look much older than his 34 years. In the interview, which took place in both Arabic and broken English, Abbass proved to be a lively, even jolly interlocutor, who nonetheless wanted to share his deep heartache over aspects of his life that were beyond his control.

A Shia Muslim from a tiny, tobacco-producing village in southern Lebanon, Abbass came from a family of 11 children, as had his father before him. Abbass considered the latter fact quite remarkable, given that his grandfather was missing a testicle but had still managed to produce 11 healthy children.

Abbass and his siblings never intended to move from their hometown. But the Lebanese civil war broke out, and Abbass, still a high school student, was drafted into the Lebanese marines. He was lucky to survive his 2-year period of conscription, and when he was released from the military, he was able to take refuge in Cyprus, and then in America, where he worked at odd jobs in New York City.

As a tall, blond Lebanese man, Abbass found many young American women who were willing to help him with his English and to explore his as yet untapped sexuality. Abbass bragged that he had many girlfriends in *"Amrika,"* but he was careful to use condoms to prevent an unplanned pregnancy. Meanwhile, through messages sent back to Lebanon, he began to court a respectable young woman, Fatima, his *bint 'amm*, or his FBD. Although she represented the ideal form of cousin marriage, Fatima was also Abbass' love interest, and he was happy that his affections were reciprocated.

After spending 7 years in the United States, Abbass returned to Lebanon, where he married Fatima. When no pregnancy had occurred after 2 years of marriage, the young couple consulted several gynecologists, who deemed Fatima to be healthy and fertile. Abbass, meanwhile, was shown to be azoospermic, that is, there were no spermatozoa in his ejaculate.

Multiple, painful testicular biopsies proved that Abbass was producing sperm in his testicles. But the sperm were trapped inside, because Abbass was lacking a vas deferens, the testicular vessel involved in sperm transport. Abbass described how he felt when he learned this shocking news:

> We asked the doctor about what I can do, and he explained to me that there's nothing I can do. Everything else is okay, wonderful. I have sperm inside, and I "come" [ejaculate] when I make love with my wife and it's wonderful. It's "the line" [vas] I don't have. It's not only me; it's my brother and one cousin. I asked the doctor why this happened. The doctor explained to me, "It's biology. It's coming from your mother and father. It's coming to the men in your family."
>
> This problem changed my mind, my life, my prayers. I asked God, "Don't leave me to be like this, never to have children." It broke my life. I want to have my own children too much. I thought about divorce many times. My brain "moved" a lot [he motioned to his head, circling his hand around it]. I thought about my life, my wife, and it was a very, very dangerous period [i.e., he suggests that he was suicidal].
>
> But the first and last is my God. He sees everything. And I decided to leave that to God. If he wants to help, he'll help, but I can't do anything. It's not between your hands or in your brain. This is God's will. I prayed to my God, and I stayed to myself [during this period], even though my wife and I talked and talked, all night some times.
>
> Nobody can know how I felt … you don't know how I was feeling inside. Anybody who has this problem, he can feel it. [Addressing the anthropologist] You're a doctor, so you can feel it. But other people have no idea how it feels [to be faced with this problem].
>
> About myself, about me, I'm okay now. I looked to my God, and this is what happened to me. I realized that there was not anything wrong with me. I was born with this. Not from a disease. There was nothing I did wrong, and nothing I can do. I am Abbass. I don't need it [a vas deferens] or children. You have to believe in yourself. You have to take care of that first. When you feel like this, then nobody will act differently toward you. I realized that it's not my problem if I don't have the "line." All my family knows [about his medical problem]. I can't keep it from them. Everybody was crying with me when I told them. Everybody thought about this problem and tried to help me. We sold land, 2,000 meters, and I spent all of that for treatment.

Indeed, Abbass was fortunate to have met a knowledgable urologist, who encouraged Abbass to try intracytoplasmic sperm injection (ICSI), saying, "You can't stop here." ICSI can create children for men such as Abbass with a congenital absence of the vas, through extraction of sperm directly from the testis. Nonetheless, ICSI can also perpetuate genetic disorders into the next generation, particularly among male offspring. Congenital absence of the vas is a definitive marker of the autosomal recessive cystic fibrosis gene, which Abbass, his brother, and cousin all carry. If their wives, who are relatives, carry this familial gene as well, then their children face the threat of cystic fibrosis, a deadly pulmonary condition that debilitates children and kills them by the time they are young adults. For his part, Abbass was never told about his cystic fibrosis carrier status, or if he was counseled, he failed to understand the seriousness of this genetic threat to his future offspring.

With the help of ICSI, Abbass and his wife were able to bear a son, who was 9 months old at the time of the interview. Abbass proudly described him as a "special boy," highly intelligent even though he was still too young to talk. Furthermore, when I met Abbass at the in vitro fertilization (IVF) clinic, he was in the process of helping his younger brother, now a resident of the Netherlands, to obtain ICSI in Lebanon. Abbass was profoundly grateful to the Beirut IVF clinic for giving him the gift of an ICSI son, and he wanted to share this blessing with his younger brother (Figure 6.1). Yet, Abbass was not aware of the debates surrounding ICSI, a technology that

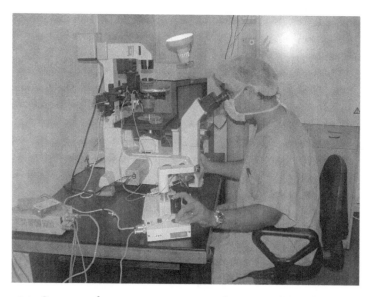

Figure 6.1. Intracytoplasmic sperm injection being performed in an in vitro fertilization clinic in Beirut, Lebanon. (Photo by Marcia C. Inhorn.)

"assists" reproduction, while at the same time "reproducing" genetic defects in the next generation (Bittles and Matson 2000; Chan 2007; Kurinczuk 2003; Ola et al. 2001).

If both Abbass and his brother are lucky, their ICSI offspring will be spared from painful deaths via cystic fibrosis. However, their sons will share the genetic destiny of their fathers, namely, serious male infertility, linked to cystic fibrosis, the likely consequence of generations of consanguinity.

The Case of Hussain

Like Abbass, Hussain was one of the few infertile men who volunteered to participate in the study, without being asked by a clinic staff member. A hulking Lebanese Army commando with tobacco-stained teeth, he was dressed on the day of the interview in camouflage gear and army boots, with a closely shaved head and massive arm muscles bulging out of his uniform. He would not shake the anthropologist's hand when she extended it.[3] Nonetheless, he was amazingly candid and forthcoming during the interview, perhaps experiencing some catharsis through the telling of his painful story.

Hussain was a 37-year-old Shia Muslim, who had spent a 20-year career in the Lebanese Army. As a soldier, he had spent a full 15 years "on the front line" in the civil war, experiencing "everything," including participation in combat and living through periods of intense bombing. He does not attribute his male infertility problems to the stresses of the civil war, as many other Lebanese men in this study did. In fact, although he saw many frightening scenes of war and carnage, he said that he never felt fear while participating in actual combat.

Hussain has been married twice. His first marriage occurred when he was only a teen (aged 17), and did not produce any children. His mother-in-law blamed him for the infertility, and so he went to a doctor for a semen analysis. According to Hussain, the semen analysis was normal, so he took the report to his mother-in-law, telling her "The problem is not from me." Although the lack of pregnancy was not the ultimate cause for the divorce, the marriage dissolved before Hussain could prove his fertility. He now doubts the accuracy of his initial semen test.

In his second marriage, Hussain took the safer route by marrying his double first cousin, who was both his FBD and MBD. Hussain himself is the product of multiple generations of consanguinity. His grandparents on both sides were cousins, and both sets of grandparents were related to each other (i.e., the grandfathers were brothers). His mother and father are first cousins (FBD). Hussain has never considered consanguinity as an important factor in his life or health, since cousin marriage is "normal" in his Shia Muslim community in southern Lebanon. He said that his marriage to a tall, attractive, veiled woman is "happy enough," and that they will stay together, even if they do not have children.

However, Hussain went on to relate a painful 17-year history of male infertility punctuated by hundreds of semen analyses, multiple hormonal injections, four unsuccessful intrauterine insemination attempts (using his sperm), and an unwarranted testicular surgery called varicocelectomy, which is commonly performed in Lebanon as a money-making venture by unscrupulous urologists. Hussain said that "only God knows" why he is infertile in his second marriage. To his knowledge, there are no other known cases of male infertility in his family, as all of his five brothers (and six sisters) have children. As he explained, "I went to all *good* doctors, specialists and professors in Beirut, but not one of them said, 'You have *this* problem that causes your infertility.'"

Finally, through a loan from the army in the year 2000, Hussain gathered together enough money to undergo one trial of ICSI. The ICSI procedure was performed, but Hussain lamented that "the doctor, he didn't do his best for us." Hussain was elated to learn that his wife was pregnant for the first time after 10 years of marriage. But his happiness lasted only through the delivery, when the nurse came to tell him that a baby son had been born. Minutes later, the nurse reappeared and, according to Hussain, "told me he is a Mongol" (i.e., a baby with Down Syndrome).

"I had a strong shock, and I threw up," Hussain recalled. "I stayed for one month crying. My wife also felt so bad. But I believe in God, and this is what God wants. So *hamdu-lillah* [praise be to God]. If he had lived, we would have raised him. But I felt so bad when he died [8 months later, from a heart defect]. I cried and cried. He was so intelligent. Even though he was a Mongol, it wasn't a 'strong case.'"

Although Down Syndrome is one of the genetic disorders attributable to consanguinity in the Middle East, Hussain has not considered this possibility and is instead trying to mobilize the financial resources for a second ICSI trial. His father is helping him to pay for treatment, but has not been informed about the ICSI, which Hussain and his wife are keeping "top secret." They believe that an IVF or ICSI child would be ridiculed in their conservative Muslim community. "Because all my family have children, perhaps in the future they'll say to my child, 'You are an in vitro child.' Not all people understand IVF, what it means. Perhaps they will think bad things about it, like that we've used other people's sperm [which is forbidden in most of the Muslim world]."

As Hussain explained at the end of the interview,

> The child, he completes the family, and no marriage is completed without the child. Because they are fun, children make for a nice family life, with happiness and humor. We must have children to be happy. No couple is happy without them. My wife and I are happy now, but to complete our happiness, we must have children.

Given his history of long-term, severe male infertility, and the birth of a child who died from a serious genetic disorder, Hussain and his wife are ideal candidates for genetic counseling. Repeating ICSI may not be advisable, as ICSI is known to perpetuate serious genetic defects into the next generation. However, genetic screening and genetic counseling are not well-developed specialties in Lebanon, or in other parts of the Middle East. Therefore, Hussain and his wife will probably not receive wise counsel about their chances for conceiving a future healthy child. At the time of the interview, they were visiting the IVF clinic in the hope of beginning their second round of ICSI.

Conclusion

Given these stories and the overall findings of this study, counseling infertile Middle Eastern couples about possible genetic problems relating to male infertility seems necessary, especially in the light of the rapid expansion of ICSI in this region. For example, in Lebanon, a relatively small country of only 10,452 km^2 area and 4.3 million people, nearly 20 IVF centers serve the population, one of the highest numbers per capita in the world. The use of ICSI in this population may be inadvertently perpetuating genetic disorders into future generations in a significantly consanguineous population with limited comprehension of the basic principles of genetics or risks of consanguinity.

Indeed, in Lebanon, as in other regions of the Middle East, religion is often invoked to explain genetic diseases as manifestations of God's will, as seen in both cases above. Furthermore, consanguineous marriages are common, while genetic conditions are relatively uncommon. Thus, community members are often unwilling to link consanguinity to genetic disorders, particularly when there are strong religious, sociocultural, and economic incentives for marrying cousins (Hussain 1999, 2002).

A significant percentage of Lebanese couples—30% of Muslims and 17% of Christians in the general population, and 20% of the men in our study—continue to marry consanguineously. Even though educational levels are relatively high in Lebanon, many men have never studied reproductive biology or basic genetics in their high school or university curricula. In general, "genetic thinking" is not part of the cultural milieu in Lebanon or other parts of the Middle East. Genetic testing and genetic counseling are also quite rare, even in university-based medical settings. Thus, few Lebanese men question the potential genetic consequences of marrying their close female relatives, particularly when cousin marriages are highly valued for a variety of reasons.

In Lebanon, one of the consequences of cousin marriages may be male infertility among the offspring of consanguineous unions. As our study has revealed, relatively high levels of consanguinity over multiple generations in Lebanon may be leading to family clustering of genetically based male infertility cases, particularly among Lebanese men with the most severe forms of infertility.

Anthropologists have spent more than a century studying kinship patterns and practices of cousin marriage across the globe (Fox 1984; Holy 1996; Westermarck [1903] 2005). Thus, they bring special insights and sensitivity to the study of a practice that "makes sense" in the lives of the men and women around the world who enter into these unions, often because of tradition and family arrangement, but sometimes out of desire and love for one another. Consanguineous marriage is not a practice to be condemned as "backward" or "dangerous." Rather, it is a practice with elevated genetic risks that need to be thoroughly explained to susceptible populations through culturally tailored messages that are neither frightening nor offensive. Revealing the relationships between consanguinity and genetic disorders, including those that cause male infertility, will require not only basic medical and epidemiological research, but also comprehensive religious, governmental, and media-based intervention programs, which set in place the basic groundwork for effective public health preventive measures (Panter-Brick 1991). Epidemiologists and anthropologists working together can help shed light on the health risks of consanguinity among the populations who support this practice for a variety of important reasons. Their ethnographic findings may lead to the development of culturally sensitive public health education messages, ones that support genetic counseling and risk management, without condemning consanguineous marriage practices per se.

Acknowledgments

The authors thank the National Science Foundation (BCS 0549264) and U.S. Department of Education Fulbright-Hays Faculty Research Abroad Program for financial support of this study. The first author thanks the men in Lebanon who made this study possible by speaking candidly about their infertility and reproductive lives. Thanks also go to Abbass Fakih, Mary Ghanem, Azhar Ismail, Hanady Sharara, and Khaled Sakhel for research assistance.

Notes

1. Since the year 2000, numerous peer-reviewed journal articles on this topic have been published, as shown in our bibliography: Al-Gazali (2005); Alkhalaf et al. (2002); Gunaid et al. (2004); Hamamy et al. (2005); Hussain (2002); Jurdi and Saxena (2003);

Mohammed et al. (2007); Mumtaz et al. (2007); Rajab and Patton (2000); Raz et al. (2003); Saadat et al. (2004); Shavazi et al. (2006); Sueyoshi and Ohtsuka (2003); and Tamim et al. (2003).

2. The option to be tape-recorded was presented to each informant on the written informed consent form. Most informants asked about this, and when told that it was not necessary to tape-record the interview, they uniformly declined, usually with visible relief. This "tape-record-less" strategy, which the first author has used in most interviews in Egypt and Lebanon, requires her to take verbatim shorthand notes, which she learned through a previous career as a medical journalist.

3. Many conservative Muslim men will not physically touch a woman other than their wives or close female relatives. Shaking hands across genders is replaced by holding one's outstretched hand over the heart, as a gesture of greeting and good will.

References

Abbasi-Shavazi MJ, McDonald P, Hosseini-Chavoshi M (in press) Modernization or cultural maintenance: The practice of consanguineous marriage in Iran. *Journal of Biosocial Sciences.*

Al Abdulkareem A, Ballal SG (1998) Consanguineous marriage in an urban area of Saudi Arabia: Rates and adverse health effects on the offspring. *Journal of Community Health* 23:75–83.

Al-Gazali LI (2005) Attitudes toward genetic counseling in the United Arab Emirates. *Community Genetics* 8:48–51.

Al-Gazali LI, Bener A, Abdulrazzaq YM, Micallef R, Al-Khayat AI, Gaber T (1997) Consanguineous marriages in the United Arab Emirates. *Journal of Biosocial Sciences* 29:491–497.

Alkhalaf M, Verghese L, Mhuarib N (2002) A cytogenetic study of Kuwaiti couples with infertility and reproductive disorders: Short arm deletion of chromosome 21 is associated with male infertility. *Annales de Genetique* 45:147–149.

Baccetti B, Capitani S, Collodel G, Cairano G, Gambera L, Moretti E et al. (2001) Genetic sperm defects and consanguinity. *Human Reproduction* 16:1365–1371.

Becker G (2000) *The Elusive Embryo: How Women and Men Approach New Reproductive Technologies.* Berkeley, CA: University of California Press.

Becker G (2002) "Deciding whether to tell children about donor insemination: An unresolved question in the United States." In: *Infertility around the Globe: New Thinking on Childlessness, Gender, and Reproductive Technologies.* MC Inhorn, F van Balen, eds. Berkeley, CA: University of California Press, pp. 119–133.

Bentley GR, Mascie-Taylor, eds. (2000) *Infertility in the Modern World: Present and Future Prospects.* Cambridge, UK: Cambridge University Press.

Bernard HR (2005) *Research Methods in Anthropology: Qualitative and Quantitative Approaches*, 4th ed. Lanham, MD: AltaMira.

Birenbaum-Carmeli D (2004) Increased prevalence of Mediterranean and Muslim populations in mutation-related research literature. *Community Genetics* 279:1–5.

Bittles AH, Matson PL (2000) "Genetic Influences on Human Infertility." In: *Infertility in the Modern World: Present and Future Prospects.* GR Bentley, CG Mascie-Taylor, eds. Cambridge, UK: Cambridge University Press, pp. 46–81.

Bittles AH, Grant JC, Sullivan SG, Hussain R (2002) Does inbreeding lead to decreased human fertility? *Annals of Human Biology* 29:111–130.

Bittles A, Manson W, Greene J, Rao NA (1991) Reproductive behavior and health in consanguineous marriages. *Science* 252:789–794.

Boerma JT, Mgalla Z, eds. (2001) *Women and Infertility in Sub-Saharan Africa: A Multi-Disciplinary Perspective*. Amsterdam: KIT Publishers.

Brown PJ (1992) Challenges for medical anthropology: Notes from the new editor in chief. *Medical Anthropology* 15:1.

Campbell AJ, Irvine DS (2000) Male infertility and intracytoplasmic sperm injection (ICSI). *British Medical Bulletin* 56:616–629.

Carmeli YS, Birenbaum-Carmeli D (1994) The predicament of masculinity: Towards understanding the male's experience of infertility treatments. *Sex Roles* 30:663–677.

Carmeli YS, Birenbaum-Carmeli D (2000) Ritualizing the "natural family": Secrecy in Israeli donor insemination. *Science as Culture* 9:301–324.

Carrell DT, De Jonge C, Lamb, DJ (2006) The genetics of male infertility: A field of study whose time is now. *Archives of Andrology* 52:269–274.

Carsten J (2004) *After Kinship*. Cambridge, UK: Cambridge University Press.

Chan P (2007) Practical genetic issues in male infertility management. Paper presented at American Society for Reproductive Medicine, October 13.

Devroey P, Vandervorst M, Nagy P, Van Steirteghem A (1998) Do we treat the male or his gamete? *Human Reproduction* 13(Suppl 1):178–185.

Dumont L, Parkin R (2006) *An Introduction to Two Theories of Social Anthropology: Descent Groups and Marriage Alliance*. Oxford, UK: Berghahn Books.

Dunn FL, Janes CR (1986) "Introduction: Medical Anthropology and Epidemiology." In: *Anthropology and Epidemiology: Interdisciplinary Approaches to the Study of Health and Disease*. CR Janes, R Stall, SM Gifford, eds. Dordrecht, Netherlands: D. Reidel, pp. 3–34.

Eickelman DF (2001) *The Middle East and Central Asia: An Anthropological Approach*, 4th ed. Englewood Cliffs, NJ: Prentice-Hall.

El-Hazmi MA, Al-Swailem AR, Warsy AS, Al-Swailem AM, Sulaimani R, Al-Meshari A (1995) Consanguinity among the Saudi Arabian population. *Journal of Medical Genetics* 32:623–626.

Fetterman DM (1998) *Ethnography: Step by Step (Applied Social Research Methods)*. Thousand Oaks, CA: Sage.

Finkler K (2000) *Experiencing the New Genetics: Family and Kinship on the Medical Frontier*. Philadelphia, PA: University of Pennsylvania Press.

Fishel S, Dowell K, Thornton S (2000) "Reproductive Possibilities for Infertile Couples: Present and Future." In: *Infertility in the Modern World: Present and Future Prospects*. GR Bentley, CGN Mascie-Taylor, eds. Cambridge, UK: Cambridge University Press, pp. 17–45.

Fleck A, Ianni FAJ (1958) Epidemiology and anthropology: Some Suggested affinities in theory and method. *Human Organization* 16:38–40.

Fox R (1984) *Kinship and Marriage: An Anthropological Perspective*. Cambridge, UK: Cambridge University Press.

Franklin S, Roberts C (2006) *Born and Made: An Ethnography of Preimplantation Genetic Diagnosis*. Princeton, NJ: Princeton University Press.

Gannon K, Glover L, Abel P (2004) Masculinity, infertility, stigma and media reports. *Social Science and Medicine* 59:1169–1175.

Greil AL (1991) *Not Yet Pregnant: Infertile Couples in Contemporary America*. New Brunswick, NJ: Rutgers University Press.

Gunaid A, Hummad N, Tamim K (2004) Consanguinity marriage in the capital city Sana'a, Yemen. *Journal of Biosocial Sciences* 36:111–121.

Hahn RA (1995) "Anthropology and Epidemiology: Two Logics or One?" In: *Sickness and Healing: An Anthropological Perspective*. New Haven, CT: Yale University Press.

Hamamy H, Jamhawi L, Al-Darawsheh J, Ajlouni K (2005) Consanguineous marriages in Jordan: Why is the rate changing with time? *Clinical Genetics* 67:511–516.

Holy L (1996) *Anthropological Perspectives on Kinship*. London: Pluto Press.

Hussain R (1999) Community perceptions of reasons for preference for consanguineous marriages in Pakistan. *Journal of Biosocial Sciences* 31:449–461.

Hussain R (2002) Lay perceptions of genetic risks attributable to inbreeding in Pakistan. *American Journal of Human Biology* 14:264–274.

Hussain R, Bittles AH (1999) Consanguineous marriage and differentials in age at marriage, contraceptive use and fertility in Pakistan. *Journal of Biosocial Sciences* 31:121–138.

Hussain R, Bittles AH (2004) Assessment of association between consanguinity and fertility in Asian populations. *Journal of Health, Population and Nutrition* 22:1–12.

Inhorn MC (1994) *Quest for Conception: Gender, Infertility, and Egyptian Medical Traditions*. Philadelphia, PA: University of Pennsylvania Press.

Inhorn MC (1995) Medical anthropology and epidemiology: Divergences or convergences? *Social Science and Medicine* 40:285–290.

Inhorn MC (1996) *Infertility and Patriarchy: The Cultural Politics of Gender and Family Life in Egypt*. Philadelphia, PA: University of Pennsylvania Press.

Inhorn MC (2002) Sexuality, masculinity, and infertility in Egypt: Potent troubles in the marital and medical encounters. *Journal of Men's Studies* 10:343–359.

Inhorn MC (2003a) Global infertility and the globalization of new reproductive technologies: Illustrations from Egypt. *Social Science and Medicine* 56:1837–1851.

Inhorn MC (2003b) *Local Babies, Global Science: Gender, Religion, and In Vitro Fertilization in Egypt*. New York: Routledge.

Inhorn MC (2004) Middle Eastern masculinities in the age of new reproductive technologies: Male infertility and stigma in Egypt and Lebanon. *Medical Anthropology Quarterly* 18:162–182.

Inhorn MC, Buss KA (1994) Ethnography, epidemiology, and infertility in Egypt. *Social Science and Medicine* 39:671–686.

Inhorn MC, King L, Nriagu JO, Kobeissi L, Hammoud N, Awwad J et al. (2008) Occupational and environmental exposure to heavy metals: Risk factors for male infertility in Lebanon? *Reproductive Toxicology* 25:203–212.

Irvine DS (1998) Epidemiology and aetiology of male infertility. *Human Reproduction* 13(Suppl 1):33–44.

Jabbra N (2004) Family change in Lebanon's Biqa valley: What are the results of the civil war? *Journal of Comparative Family Studies* 35:259–270.

Janes CR, Stall R, Gifford SM, eds. (1986) *Anthropology and Epidemiology: Interdisciplinary Approaches to the Study of Health and Disease*. Dordrecht, Netherlands: D. Reidel.

Joseph S (1993) Connectivity and patriarchy among urban working-class Arab families in Lebanon. *Ethos* 21:452–484.

Joseph S (2001) Among brothers: Patriarchal connective mirroring and brotherly deference in Lebanon. *Cairo Papers in Social Science* 24:165–179.

Jurdi R, Saxena C (2003) The prevalence and correlates of consanguineous marriages in Yemen: Similarities and contrasts with other Arab countries. *Journal of Biosocial Sciences* 35:1–13.

Kamischke A, Nieschlag E (1998) Conventional treatments of male infertility in the age of evidence-based andrology. *Human Reproduction* 13(Suppl 1):62–75.

Kelsey JL, Thompson WE, Evans AS (1986) *Methods in Observational Epidemiology.* New York: Oxford University Press.

Kim ED (2001) An overview of male infertility in the era of intracytoplasmic sperm injection. *Chinese Medical Journal* 64:71–83.

Kobeissi L, Inhorn MC, Hannoun AB, Hammoud N, Awwad J, Abu-Musa AA (in press) Civil war and male infertility in Lebanon. *Fertility and Sterility.*

Krausz C, Forti G, McElreavey K (2003) The Y chromosome and male fertility and infertility. *International Journal of Andrology* 26:570–575.

Kurinczuk JJ (2003) Safety issues in assisted reproduction technology: From theory to reality—just what are the data telling us about ICSI offspring health and future fertility and should we be concerned? *Human Reproduction* 18:925–931.

Larsen U (1994) Sterility in sub-Saharan Africa. *Population Studies* 48:459–474.

Larsen U (2000) Primary and secondary infertility in sub-Saharan Africa. *International Journal of Epidemiology* 29:285–291.

Latini M, Gandini L, Lenzi A, Romanelli F (2004) Sperm tail agenesis in a case of consanguinity. *Fertility and Sterility* 81:1688–1691.

Lloyd M (1996) Condemned to be meaningful: Non-response in studies of men and infertility. *Sociology of Health and Illness* 18:433–454.

Maduro MR, Lamb DJ (2002) Understanding the new genetics of male infertility. *Journal of Urology* 168:2197–2205.

Maduro MR, Lo KC, Chuang WW, Lamb DJ (2003) Genes and male infertility: What can go wrong? *Journal of Andrology* 24:485–493.

Mohammed F, Al-Yatama F, Al-Bader M, Tayel SM, Gouda S, Naguib KK (2007) Primary male infertility in Kuwait: A cytogenetic and molecular study of 289 infertile Kuwaiti patients. *Andrologia* 39:87–92.

Mumtaz G, Tamim H, Kanaan M, Khawaja M, Khogali M, Wakim G, et al. (2007) Effect of consanguinity on birth weight for gestational age in a developing country. *American Journal of Epidemiology* 165:742–752.

Nations MK (1986) "Epidemiological Research on Infectious Disease: Quantitative Rigor or Rigormortis? Insights from Ethnomedicine." In: *Anthropology and Epidemiology: Interdisciplinary Approaches to the Study of Health and Disease.* CR Janes, R Stall, SM Gifford, eds. Dordrecht, Netherlands: D. Reidel, pp. 97–123.

Ola B, Afnan M, Sharif K, Papaioannou S, Hammadieh N, Barratt CLR (2001) Should ICSI be the treatment of choice for all cases of in-vitro conception? Considerations of fertilization and embryo development, cost effectiveness and safety. *Human Reproduction* 16:2485–2490.

Ottenheimer M (1996) *Forbidden Relatives: The American Myth of Cousin Marriage.* Champaign, IL: University of Illinois Press.

Panter-Brick C (1991) Parental responses to consanguinity and genetic disease in Saudi Arabia. *Social Science and Medicine* 33:1295–1302.

Rajab A, Patton MA (2000) A study of consanguinity in the sultanate of Oman. *Annals of Human Biology* 27:321–326.

Raz AE, Atar M, Rodnay M, Shohan-Vardi I, Carmi R (2003) Between acculturation and ambivalence: Knowledge of genetics and attitudes towards genetic testing in a consanguineous Bedouin community. *Community Genetics* 6:88–95.

Rubinstein RA, Perloff JD (1986) "Identifying Psychosocial Disorders in Children: On Integrating Epidemiological and Anthropological Understandings." In: *Anthropology and Epidemiology: Interdisciplinary Approaches to the Study of Health and Disease*. CR Janes, R Stall, SM Gifford, eds. Dordrecht, Netherlands: D. Reidel, pp. 303–332.

Saadat M, Ansari-Lari M, Farhud DD (2004) Consanguineous marriage in Iran. *Annals of Human Biology* 2:263–269.

Saxena C, Kulczyck A, Jurdi R (2004) Nuptiality transition and marriage squeeze in Lebanon: Consequences of sixteen years of civil war. *Journal of Comparative Family Studies* 35:241–258.

Sciarra J (1994) Infertility: An international health problem. *International Journal of Gynecology and Obstetrics* 46:155–163.

Sciarra J (1997) Sexually transmitted diseases: Global importance. *International Journal of Gynecology and Obstetrics* 46:765–767.

Shah N (2004) Women's socio-economic characteristics and marital patterns in rapidly developing Muslim society, Kuwait. *Journal of Comparative Family Studies* 35:163–183.

Sueyoshi S, Ohtsuka R (2003) Effects of polygyny and consanguinity on high fertility in the rural Arab population in South Jordan. *Journal of Biososocial Sciences* 35:513–526.

Sundby J (2002) "Infertility and Health Care in Countries with Less Resources: Case Studies from Sub-Saharan Africa." In: *Infertility around the Globe: New Thinking on Childlessness, Gender, and Reproductive Technologies*. MC Inhorn, F van Balen, eds. Berkeley, CA: University of California Press, pp. 247–259.

Tamim H, Khogali M, Beydoun H, Melki I, Yunis K (2003) Consanguinity and apnea of prematurity. *American Journal of Epidemiology* 158:942–946.

Teebi AS, Farag TI, eds. (1996) *Genetic Disorders among Arab Populations*. Oxford, UK: Oxford University Press.

Tremayne S (2006) Modernity and early marriage in Iran: A view from within. *Journal of Middle East Women's Studies* 2:65–94.

Trostle JA (1986a) "Early Work in Anthropology and Epidemiology: From Social Medicine to the Germ Theory, 1840 to 1920." In: *Anthropology and Epidemiology: Interdisciplinary Approaches to the Study of Health and Disease*. CR Janes, R Stall, SM Gifford, eds. Dordrecht, Netherlands: D. Reidel, pp. 25–57.

Trostle JA (1986b) "Anthropology and Epidemiology in the Twentieth Century: A Selective History of Collaborative Projects and Theoretical Affinities, 1920–1970." In: *Anthropology and Epidemiology: Interdisciplinary Approaches to the Study of Health and Disease*. CR Janes, R Stall, SM Gifford, eds. Dordrecht, Netherlands: D. Reidel, pp. 59–94.

Trostle JA (2005) *Epidemiology and Culture*. Cambridge, UK: Cambridge University Press.

True WR (1996) "Epidemiology and Medical Anthropology." In: *Medical Anthropology: Contemporary Theory and Method*, Revised Edition. CF Sargent, TM Johnson, eds. Westport, CT: Praeger, pp. 325–346.

Turshen M (1984) *The Political Ecology of Disease in Tanzania*. New Brunswick, NJ: Rutgers University Press.

Upton RL (2002) Perceptions of and attitudes towards male infertility in Northern Botswana: Some implications for family planning and AIDS prevention policies. *African Journal of Reproductive Health* 3:103–111.

Vayena E, Rowe PJ, Griffin PD, eds. (2002) *Current Practices and Controversies in Assisted Reproduction*. Geneva: World Health Organization.

Webb RE, Daniluk JC (1999) The end of the line: Infertile men's experiences of being unable to produce a child. *Men and Masculinities* 2:6–25.

Westermarck EA ([1903] 2005) *The History of Human Marriage*. Boston: Adamant Media.

World Health Organization (1999) *WHO Laboratory Manual for the Examination of Human Semen and Sperm-Cervical Mucus Interaction*, 4th ed. Cambridge, UK: Cambridge University Press.

Zlotogora J (1997) Genetic disorders among Palestinian Arabs. *American Journal of Medical Genetics* 68:472–475.

7

Structural Violence, Political Violence, and the Health Costs of Civil Conflict: A Case Study from Peru

TOM LEATHERMAN AND R. BROOKE THOMAS

Introduction

An estimated 225 armed conflicts have been recorded since World War II, and 115 between 1989 and 2001 (Gleditsch, Wallenstein, Eriksson, Sollenberg, and Strand 2002). These conflicts have claimed millions of lives and have left many millions more prone to hunger, malnutrition, disease, psychological trauma, and the chronic effects of living displaced and disrupted lives in disrupted environments, economies, and societies. Hence, armed conflict is a political-economic, environmental, and major public health issue. Yet, the interrelationship between conflict and health has not been historically a central focus of conflict research, or in training public health professionals (Levy and Sidel 1997). This is certainly changing, and over the past several decades there has been a steady increase in publications focusing on health effects of armed conflicts (e.g., Ghobarah, Huth, and Russett 2004; Inhorn and Kobeissi 2006; Levy and Sidel 1997; Pedersen 2002; Zwi and Ugalde 1989). Also, agencies tasked to respond to crises with nutrition and disease components (e.g., World Health Organization, Centers for Disease Control and Prevention, World Food Program) are beginning training programs for emergency response in wars and other disasters.

Because of the difficulty in researching the health effects of war (see Nordstrom and Robben 1995), little information is gathered *in situ* during

196

conflicts, and thus, much of the published research is in the form of case studies using countrywide or regional survey data, and interviews with affected populations carried out at a later time and place. In a recent analysis of postwar health effects of civil conflicts, Ghobarah et al. (2004) argue for the need to move beyond country and regional case studies toward comparative analyses, because the immediate and long-term health effects of conflict vary across wars, environments, and populations. While comparative analyses *are* essential, we argue here for greater attention to the other end of the spectrum, i.e., for more ethnographically informed longitudinal analyses that can link historical antecedents of conflict to postconflict conditions, and can better understand people's vulnerability and resilience to political violence in local sociocultural, political-economic, and environmental contexts (Pedersen 2002; Summerfield 1999). Such analyses might better capture how the complex interrelationship between "structural violence" and "political violence" affects health and well-being.

Structural violence refers to the violence of poverty, social and political marginalization, racism, sexism, and other forms of structured inequalities and their effects on people's lives, health, and agency (Farmer 2003, 2004). Within medical anthropology, it highlights the ways inequalities promote malnutrition and disease, and increase the vulnerabilities to their effects. Political violence is "targeted physical violence and terror administered by official authorities and those opposing it, such as military repression, police torture, and armed resistance" (Bourgois 2001:3). In this sense, structural violence provides an important context for political violence, which may, in turn, exacerbate, alleviate or otherwise reshape key elements of structural violence. Thus, a challenge to war and public health research is to ascertain how postconflict measures of health and well-being are influenced by the violence of conflict, antecedents to conflict, or the complex intersection of both. Longitudinal observations in local contexts of violence are key to this effort.

In this chapter, we offer local-level observations on one conflict in one specific area, the 20-year civil war in Peru initiated by the PCP-SL, Communist Party of Peru-*Sendero Luminoso* ("Shining Path"). We examine how the conflict played out in the District of Nuñoa in the Department of Puno, in the southern highlands, where we had conducted research in the mid-1980s, and have returned briefly since. We will advance three central points based on the Peruvian case study, but argue that these are broadly applicable across many instances of global conflict.

1. The consequences of structural violence (e.g., extreme poverty, food insecurity, undernutrition, and illness) are important catalysts for violent conflict, and conflict, in turn, reshapes the conditions of poverty and poor health.

2. In assessing the health and human costs of conflict and postconflict environments, changes in food security, social cohesiveness, and political power are relevant and potentially important measures of public health outcomes, along with mortality, morbidity, and psychosocial stress.

3. Violent conflict has many negative effects on individuals and the social environment, but individuals and communities experience these effects with varying degrees of vulnerability and resilience, depending in part on their position within the larger society and economy. Hence, the effects of conflict are uneven in terms of short- and long-term food security and health.

We first discuss briefly some of the public health impacts of armed conflict worldwide, and then turn to the recent civil war in Peru. The majority of the chapter discusses the pre- and postconflict situation in Nuñoa, and offers preliminary observations on some of the apparent and potential consequences of civil war on this region and people.

Public Health Costs of War

The public health costs of war can and should be viewed broadly (see Ghobarah et al. 2004; Inhorn and Kobeissi 2006; Pedersen 2002; WHO 2002). Following "The Declaration of Alma-Ata" (WHO 1989), we view health as "a state of complete physical, mental, and social well-being, not merely the absence of disease or infirmity," and review the public health costs of conflict in terms of physical health, infrastructure, social and psychosocial well-being, and environments and food security.

Physical Costs: Morbidity and Mortality

One of the most obvious costs of war is in human life—of military participants especially, and increasingly, of civilians. An estimated 2.5 million civilians lost their lives during wartime in the Democratic Republic of Congo (1998–2001), up to 200,000 in Bosnia, and perhaps between 500,000 and 800,000 during the 1994 Rwandan genocide (Waldman 2005). Ghobarah et al. (2004), using WHO data, report that about 269,000 people died because of the direct effects of all wars in 1999 alone, and this amounted to a loss of 8.44 million years of healthy life (DALYs). Moreover, they estimate that as many as 15 million additional lives were lost in 1999 because of death and disability from disease and the chronic effects of previous years of civil war.

Most of the victims in mortality estimates (perhaps 90%) (SIPRI 2002) are civilians, and most of the deaths occur away from the battlefield. The majority are refugees and the internally displaced, especially women, children, and the elderly, who are particularly vulnerable to psychological trauma, malnutrition, disease, violence, and sexual abuse in crowded, unhygienic, and often unsafe conditions of emergency camps (Guha-Sapir and Gijsbert 2004; Pedersen 2002; Pieterse and Ismail 2003; Ager 1999; Messer, Cohen, and D'Costa 1998; Kalipeni and Oppong 1998). Those living in refugee camps are prone to disease outbreaks from relatively common problems such as diarrhea, to more severe infectious diseases such as cholera, dysentery, acute respiratory infections, and measles, and to new and reemergent diseases, such as HIV-AIDS and TB (Ghobarah et al. 2004; Kalipeni and Oppong 1998; Pedersen 2002; Waldman 2005). The presence of landmines in conflict areas extends the risk of death and disability for years into the future. There are between 60 and 119 million mines in 70 countries, and land mines kill or maim 2000 people every month (Messer et al. 1998). One in every 236 persons in Cambodia is an amputee because of mine-related injury (Messer et al. 1998).

Social and Psychosocial Costs

The long-term mental heath costs of the social and psychological trauma experienced during violent conflict is perhaps the area of health and conflict most frequently studied. Levels of suicide and interpersonal violence often increase in postwar societies, and post-traumatic stress disorder (PTSD) is a common diagnosis for those suffering from anxiety, sleep disorders, nightmares, depression, dissociation, alcoholism, and a range of other psychological and physical symptoms (e.g., Cervantes, Salgado, and Padilla 1989; Hollifield et al. 2002). Yet, while PTSD has become synonymous with "trauma", most individuals in conflict situations (75%) do not develop PTSD, and show varying degrees of resistance and resilience (Pedersen 2002).

Conventional means of assessing trauma on the basis of PTSD scales may be far from adequate when applied across the multiple cultural and social contexts in which conflicts occur (Bracken, Giller, and Summerfield 1995; Pedersen 2002; Summerfield 1999). The application of traditional western notions of psychosis, which is heavily personalized, misses the very important point that trauma is interpreted within cultural frameworks, and is experienced and felt socially as much as personally in many cultural settings (Summerfield 1999). Prescribing drugs and individual one-to-one talk therapy is often not appropriate in the cultural contexts where trauma appears, yet remains a common curative approach. This means that it is important to study trauma in local cultural contexts, as opposed to the more common practice of interviewing victims far removed from the environments, communities, and social contexts in which trauma occurred (Pedersen, Gamarra, Planas, and Errazuriz 2001; Summerfield and Toser 1991).

It is also clear that levels of trust, cooperation, and social support are all diminished during and following conflict. In a recent review of *Anthropology and Militarism*, Gusterson (2007:161–162) discusses how "fear as a way of life" leads to uncertainties over when one might be killed, mistrust of friends and neighbors, and diminished hopes for a better future; and, citing Green (1994:231), how "routinization allows people to live in a chronic state of fear with a facade of normalcy, while the terror, at the same time, permeates and shreds the social fabric" (see also Scheper-Hughes and Bourgois 2004). This is an understudied but critical area of concern because an in-tact social fabric is critical for resilience and hope in the future, both of which directly affect health outcomes and contribute to rebuilding social structures and infrastructures that promote food security and health.

Environments and Food Security

Armed conflicts not only take a toll in lives and property and promote massive population displacement, but also degrade environments and disrupt food production and the distribution of food and medicine (Cohen and Pinstrup-Anderson 1999; Food and Agriculture Organization of the United Nations [FAO] 2002; Leatherman 2005; Messer et al. 1998; Teodosijevic 2003; WHO 2002). Conflicts were cited as major causes in one-third of the 44 countries that suffered extreme food emergencies in 2001–2002 (FAO 2002), and comparative analyses across multiple countries and wars have found average reductions in food production of 10% to 12% during years of conflict (Messer et al. 1998; Teodosijevic 2003).

The most obvious way in which conflict leads to food insecurity and hunger is through the deliberate use of hunger as a weapon (Macrae and Zwi 1994; Messer et al. 1998). Armies starve opponents, steal produce, destroy food supplies, livestock, and other means of production, cut off markets, and impede or divert food relief. Decline in farming populations, and hence production, results from attacks, terror, enslavement, forced recruitment, malnutrition, illness, and death. Livestock raiding, which often increases during conflicts, is potentially devastating to livelihoods and slows the recovery from conflicts and other disasters such as droughts and famines (Hendrickson, Armon, and Mearns 1998). Moreover, combat destroys environments and, in the case of landmines, makes them dangerous for years to come (a buried landmine can stay active for 50 years).

Disrupted food security leads to hunger and malnutrition, and significantly increases the risk of mortality and morbidity for displaced populations. In such contexts, even relatively rare micronutritional diseases have occurred—scurvy (vitamin C deficiency) in Afghanistan, pellagra (niacin deficiency) among Mozambican refugees in Malawi, and beri-beri (thiamine deficiency) among Bhutanese refugees in Nepal (Waldman 2005).

Infrastructure Costs

Destruction to health care infrastructures and reduced government support of social, education, and health sectors during conflicts constitutes another form of attack on health (Cervantes et al. 1989; Lundgren and Lang 1989; Zwi and Ugalde 1989). In many instances, health centers and health workers are directly targeted (Summerfield and Toser 1991; Pedersen 2002), but in other cases, health programs might be allowed to continue and health indicators might even improve. During war years of the 1980s and early 1990s in El Salvador, infant mortality, rates of immunization, and some other common health indicators remained steady or improved slightly. This was in part due to relief efforts from the World Food Program and others, and apparent efforts by warring factions to spare hospitals and to allow immunization campaigns to proceed (Ugalde, Selva-Sutter, Castillo, Paz, and Canas 2000).

In most countries experiencing armed conflict, increased military spending is necessarily paired with a concurrent reduction in expenditures in health, education, food, and other basic needs. Between 1960 and 1994, the developing world imported US$775 billion worth of military supplies. According to Martin Donahue (2003:580), "three hours of world-wide military spending is equal to the WHO's annual budget. Three weeks of world arms spending could provide primary health care for all individuals in poor countries including water and hygiene." Health systems are also affected by structural adjustment programs of the International Monetary Fund (IMF) and World Bank that link much needed international loans to open markets and reductions in the public sector, price subsidies, assistance programs, and other safety nets. Debt and structural adjustment burdens correlate with conflict. Smith (1994) found that 50 of 71 countries receiving structural adjustment loans were experiencing armed conflict, and that 22 of the top 25 developing country debtors were in conflict, including Argentina, Honduras, Mexico, Peru, the Philippines, and many African countries.

Summary: Reproducing Contexts and Consequences of Conflict

Armed conflict directly and indirectly heightens mortality and morbidity, promotes psychosocial distress and social disruption, degrades environments, diminishes food security, and reduces infrastructures and investments critical to public health. These multiple effects do not occur in isolation but carry the added likelihood that each might synergistically amplify the effects of the other. The effects of political violence, in turn, may well reproduce and intensify the negative effects of structural violence, and negatively impact livelihoods and health into the future. In the remainder of the chapter, we examine how these interrelationships played out in one conflict, the recent civil war in Peru (1980–2000), and in one specific region, the District of Nuñoa in the southern Peruvian highlands (1986–1992).

Armed Conflict in Peru: The Case of *Sendero Luminoso*

Beginning in 1980 and extending well into the 1990s, the Communist Party of Peru-*Sendero Luminoso* ("Shining Path") waged war against the Peruvian state and all factions who threatened their potential control of the countryside, including leftist groups advocating peasant rights. The war began in the impoverished Department of Ayacucho in the Andean highlands, under the leadership of philosophy professor Abimael Guzman and his followers, and from this epicenter, sought to expand its base especially into areas that provided an opportunity for gaining recruits and resources that could help finance the revolution: cities, the tropical forest (particularly coca-growing areas), and impoverished peasant communities of the central and southern highlands (McClintock 1989; Poole and Renique 1992; Stern 1988). Once the war began in Ayacucho, a slow initial government response was followed by repressive military actions, a "dirty war," in which atrocities on both sides led to death and displacement of residents in many *campesino* (peasant) communities (Poole and Renique 1992).

There is a consensus that the seeds of revolt were sown in deep poverty, neglect, political marginalization, and little hope that future generations would fare any better (McClintock 1984; Poole and Renique 1992). The history of the central and southern highlands is one of repeated exploitation, from the Spanish conquest and colonization, postcolonial domination of indigenous populations by a landed oligarchy, and a failed agrarian reform, to a series of more recent economic shocks and crises in the decades leading up to the revolution. Between 1970 and 1990, the Peruvian population grew by 60%, but the economy did not. In 1980, the rate of growth in GDP was negative (UN 1996). Salaries dropped, unemployment and underemployment rose, inflation reached triple digits, real incomes were less than 50% of 1973 levels (Reid 1985), and the poor became poorer. By 1990, the inflation rate was over 7000% (Poole and Renique 1992; Sheahan 1999).

These economic shocks overlay extreme inequalities that especially disadvantaged the rural highlands. Infant mortality rates in the southern Andes in the early 1980s were between 110 and 129 per thousand live births, more than twice as high as in Lima (Sheahan 1999). Sixty percent of the population was in extreme poverty, and levels of growth stunting, indicative of chronic undernutrition, were equally high. Medical care was limited (less than 1 physician per 10,000 residents in the central and southern highlands; Poole and Renique 1992), and illiteracy rates were five to nine times higher than in Lima (Sheahan 1999). Moreover, government economic policies that favored urban industrial growth and neglected the rural sector, as well as a severe and sustained drought, led to the stagnation of agriculture in rural highlands. An ineffective agrarian reform implemented by the early 1970s placed much of the appropriated land in the hands of large state-controlled cooperatives, and not indigenous communities. This further deepened the sense of hopelessness and anger at the state and its agents.

Public Health Costs of Conflict

A report of the "Truth and Reconciliation Commission" estimated that 70,000 died and 1 million people were displaced during the 20 years of internal conflict, which is twice the earlier Peruvian government estimates for death and displacement (Ball, Asher, Sulmont, and Manrique 2003; UN 1996). Material losses due to conflict are estimated at US$21 billion, a figure equivalent to Peru's entire foreign debt (UN 1996). Although hyperinflation was down to 15% in the mid-1990s, per capita GDP was at 1961 levels. Absolute poverty increased between 1985 and 1991 and fell slightly between 1991 and 1996 (FAO 2002). These levels of poverty and food insecurity at the national level during the civil war were reflected in changing levels of chronic undernutrition, estimated by FAO (2002) as 28% in 1980, 40% in 1991, and 11% in 1996.

The vast majority of deaths, and an estimated 70% of those displaced, were from rural indigenous communities, especially in the central and southern highlands. The epicenter of the conflict was in the Department of Ayacucho where an estimated 10,000 were killed or disappeared, and another 180,000 (36% of the population) were displaced in the 10-year period between 1983 and 1992 (Pedersen et al. 2001). Massive displacement depopulated the countryside, left communities and households without support networks, and threatened livelihoods by disruption of local production. Population displacement, burning of fields, killing of animals, and loss of tools meant that there were severe reductions in the production of basic foodstuffs, and this in turn contributed to severe food insecurity for many households (Pedersen et al. 2001). Moreover, the fear of attacks disrupted patterns of temporary outmigration for wage work, a common livelihood strategy in most Andean populations; fear also disrupted historically traditional patterns of working fields in distinct (and sometimes distant) ecozones to enhance crop diversity and lower risk to crop loss in any one zone. Hence, a rural household's ability to secure its live-lihood and meet basic household needs through wage work and subsistence production was severely curtailed. Between 55% and 65% of children living in rural zones and the rural highlands suffered from chronic undernutrition (indicated by stunting or low height for age) in the 1980s through the early 1990s, but these rates dropped to 40% by 1996 (FAO 2002). In some cases up to 80% of the displaced indigenous and native communities still suffers from malnutrition, and insufficient health care has led to persistence or increase of cholera, TB, and other infectious and parasitic diseases (UN 1996).

Social and psychological trauma (e.g., depression, nightmares, fear, distrust) may be the most widespread but unmeasured effect in rural areas. In addi-tion, reports from displaced and returnee communities note that poverty and landlessness are increasingly associated with alcoholism and interpersonal and domestic violence, and the "extremely aggressive" behavior of minors who had been forcibly recruited by *Sendero* or the *Rondas campesinos* (UN 1996).

Duncan Pedersen et al. (2001) conducted systematic surveys of psychoso-cial trauma in the central highlands, the epicenter of violence. One in four adults from the five communities they studied reported symptoms that met the criteria of PTSD. Because "trauma" had no equivalent in Quechua language and culture, they focused on terms of suffering and sadness (*nakary* and *llaki*) that better evoked the experience of trauma. Evocations of distress (i.e., suffer-ing and sadness) and accompanying somatic symptoms (e.g., headaches, body aches, weakness, dizziness, etc.) also referred to the hardship and suffering of everyday life and persistent poverty. Levels of traumatic stress associated with exposure to extreme violence were mediated by income, gender, displacement status, and coping strategies. Thus, it was critical to understand patterns and meanings of distress, vulnerability, and resilience in local cultural contexts to better understand the psychosocial impacts of violence and conflict on indi-viduals and broader social groups.

Contexts and Consequences of Conflict in Nuñoa: A Case Study

In this section, we offer some local-level observations on the civil war in the District of Nuñoa (Province of Melgar, Department of Puno) in the southern highlands. We summarize conditions in Nuñoa before the civil war, and present preliminary information on real and potential public health consequences of the civil war and its aftermath. The objectives are threefold:

1. to begin to document the biography of conflict in this region, and the impacts it had on people's lives and livelihood;

2. to illustrate how specific antecedent conditions of structural violence provided the foundation from which conflict emerged, and how conflict reshaped these conditions and hence real and potential effects on health; and

3. to demonstrate that for this area (and we expect in other sites of conflict) the impacts of armed conflict on food security, health, and livelihoods are experienced unevenly by the local population, and with different implications for the future.

In considering effects of "low intensity" conflicts such as those that occurred in Nuñoa, where fear and uncertainty were persistent but deaths were few, there may be relatively few measurable effects in mortality or morbidity. However, the social and psychosocial costs, and changes to social and economic infrastructure, access to land, and political power are important effects that may impact food security and health well into the future.

Research Objectives and Methods

The observations presented here are based on a 3-year project carried out from 1983 to 1985, on the eve of heightened activity of *Sendero Luminoso*, and on three brief research trips to Nuñoa between 2003 and 2006. This region is a high-altitude zone (4000 meters) comprised of many small-scale farming and herding families. Farming is primarily of potatoes, other tubers, and grains (wheat, barley, oats, and two Andean cultigens *quinoa* and *cañihua*). Herd animals are primarily sheep, llamas, alpacas, and cattle. The objective of the project from the 1980s was to detail consequences and responses to illness among small-scale farmers and herders in three communities that were differentially affected by the agrarian reform and growth of rural capitalism in the district (e.g., Thomas, Leatherman, Leatherman 1998; Carey 1990). The team of American and Peruvian researchers conducted surveys of over 140 households, and gathered information on household demography and economy, diet, nutrition, health, food production, and coping responses to illness (Carey 1990; Leatherman 1996; Leonard and Thomas 1988; Luerssen 1994). We supplemented these surveys with anthropometric studies of child growth and nutrition in schools, time allocation studies of a sample of 40 households, and unstructured interviews and participant observation. Our analyses pointed to the precarious position of many households socially, economically, and in terms of diminished health. It was clear at the time that the revolutionary movement was growing, and would soon impact this part of the southern Andes. It also appeared logical that *Sendero Luminoso* might find support among the most vulnerable communities in the district (Figure 7.1).

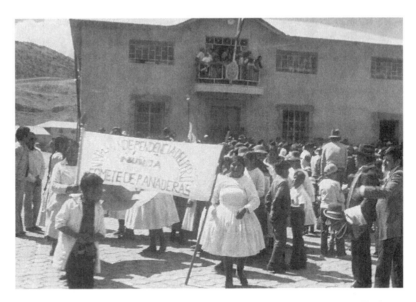

Figure 7.1. Protest by local bread makers over government-controlled prices in the early 1980s. In the background is the town hall that *Sendero Luminoso* blew up in a raid during the late 1980s. (Photo by Tom Leatherman)

We have returned to Nuñoa and the region on three separate occasions (2003, 2005, 2006) to begin documenting the timeline of conflict in the district, memories of the conflict and perceptions of its effects, and consequences on changing levels of community infrastructure, land tenure, production systems, and health. Preliminary data on the conflict and its effects come from archival research, semi-structured interviews with 12 key informants, and 10 shorter interviews with public officials, health professionals, schoolteachers, priests, store owners, and members of newly formed indigenous communities (*communidades campesinos*). The key informants were individuals we knew well from earlier research, and others (e.g., NGO staff) who had firsthand knowledge of the conflict and postconflict era in Nuñoa and surrounding areas. The semi-structured interviews were used to establish a timeline and chronicle of the years of conflict, and to assess the changes in livelihoods, food security, health, and social structures that coincided with the conflict and immediate postconflict periods. The information presented here is primarily from these interviews, and to a lesser extent archival data. The archival data were primarily limited to regional census data; there are no available health records for the war years.

Local Contexts: Antecedents to the Revolution

The broader context for crisis in Nuñoa was a combination of historic poverty, severe and persistent drought, and especially a feeling of disillusionment and disenfranchisement over what was seen as a failed agrarian reform. This region of northern Puno was the site of many of the largest wool-producing haciendas in Peru. While most of the former haciendas had been expropriated during the agrarian reform, most of the land was converted into large state-run herding cooperatives, which employed some of the workers from the original haciendas but left many in the rural countryside without access to land. In the District of Nuñoa before the reform, 2% of the landholders controlled 61% of the land base. After the reform, three cooperatives controlled 60% of the land and employed only about 25% of the rural population (Luerssen 1994). Many rural households formerly linked to large holders through sharecropping and other informal arrangements became landless and moved into the larger town in search of work. Only three *communidades campesinos* (peasant communities) were registered and their holdings were relatively small.

We worked in three sites: a semi-urban town of about 5000 residents, a small *ayllu* (one of the three *communidades campesinos*) of 25 households, and an alpaca herding cooperative of 25 households. Those experiencing land reform and rural capitalism positively (herders on cooperatives, waged workers with steady jobs) had higher and more stable incomes, and better health and nutrition (Leatherman 1998). Others, such as landless or near-landless people in the town, and many members of the *ayllu*, experienced heightened food insecurity, more extreme levels of chronic undernutrition, and constant illness. Infant mortality in the District of Nuñoa was 128/1000 live births, one of the highest in the rural highlands, and a rough estimate of infant mortality from the *ayllu* was closer to 200/1000 (20%). Seventy-three percent of children from the *ayllu* were considered chronically undernourished (stunted) compared to 54% from the cooperative and town (Leatherman 1998). Similarly, more individuals reported higher levels of illness (more cases and symptoms), and more work disruption due to illness in the *ayllu* than in the town or cooperative. Annual estimates of work lost due to illness suggest that households from the *ayllu* lost about 75 days of adult labor each year, which was almost twice that of town households and three times that of the cooperative.

Throughout the district, the poorest households reported the highest levels of illness, more work disruption due to illness, and the greatest impact of illness on agricultural production, and hence further diminished food security, nutrition, and health. In part, this was because the poorest households not only suffered illness of greater severity and duration but also had the weakest coping capacities to deal with illness and its effects on work and production. In particular, households without the social networks or cash to replace lost family labor were often left with no other recourse but to plant fewer crops, or employ labor-saving but less productive farming techniques. Thus, they experienced the most negative effects of illness on farming production and their household economy. This reproduction of poverty and poor health sent those most vulnerable into a spiral of household disintegration and desperation, with little hope for improvement (Leatherman 1998).

Thus, health as "a state of complete physical, mental, and social well-being" (WHO 1989) was in an interdependent relationship with levels of poverty, economic strategies, and coping capacities of rural households. It follows that changing access to land, economic opportunities, political power, and networks of social support and cooperation are all relevant to understanding real and potential health outcomes of conflict. It also means that the structural violence that shapes vulnerability and resilience before conflict mediates the experience of conflict, individual and social responses to conflict, and hence the health outcomes of conflict.

Biography of Conflict

In this context, *Sendero Luminoso* became a major force in Nuñoa from the mid-1980s until the early 1990s. By 1986 *Sendero* was on the offensive, with two to three columns of about 50 combatants each and with perhaps 200 local people recruited as logistical support—operating primarily in the provinces of Azangaro and Melgar in northern Puno. In 1986, the first of several well-organized and orchestrated raids on cooperatives and larger landowners led to the loss of perhaps 1000 animals (mostly sheep and cattle). Also, cooperative buildings and the homes of land owners were vandalized and looted. It is unclear if these raids were carried out by *Sendero*, or by others taking advantage of the social unrest. Soon *Sendero* made their presence very clear through the torture and assassination of a veterinarian from the largest cooperative in the area. Local understanding is that the attack was a case of mistaken identity—the intended victim was the director of the cooperative. The body was left tied to a tree in the town center. The display not only communicated the brutality of the movement, and hence ever-present fear, but also the seeming arbitrariness of victims (that potentially anyone was at risk). In subsequent raids over the next 5 years, the town hall was demolished, elected leaders assassinated, and police stations were attacked and robbed of their weapons. Most of these raids also entailed very public displays in the town center (a strategy to enhance local fear and *Sendero's* control). Retaliation by specialized antiterrorist police (*Sinchis*) placed the area under siege by a second force, leaving most of the population feeling caught in the middle. By 1990, there was no permanent police force or local government authority, and the district was declared a "liberated zone" by *Sendero*. During those years, *Sendero* moved in and out of town at will and thus became a constant presence, sometimes on the streets and always in the minds of the residents. Army troops were stationed permanently in the district in 1991, following a visit by President Alberto Fujimori. By 1992, most of the overt violence and large-scale theft of animal herds had abated.

In September 1992, Abimael Guzman was captured in Lima, and this marked a steady decline in *Sendero's* activities throughout much of Peru.

As we have begun to address the impacts of conflict in Nuñoa, it has been important to remember that livelihood and health in conflict and postconflict conditions were influenced by a combination of

1. the structural violence that shaped people's lives before and after the revolution;
2. the experience of conflict; and
3. other changes in the economy and society that may be linked directly or indirectly (or not at all) to the civil war.

Since the early to mid-1990s, changes in local and regional infrastructure have developed in several ways. Many roads throughout the region were paved, facilitating the transportation of people and products. The number of small stores increased, and they carried a broader range of commodities and foods that had been scarce (e.g., meat, cheese, eggs) before and during the conflict. By the late 1990s, 72% of town residents (17% of the District) had electricity, 79% (26% of the District) had potable water, and five new rural health posts had been built (Nuñoa 2001). Some of these changes are attributed to the Fujimori government, which increased expenditures by 800% in the Department of Puno in an effort to bolster dwindling political support (Graham and Kane 1998). Increases in public spending in the mid-to-late 1990s throughout Peru may have eased what would otherwise have been lingering and exacerbating effects of *Sendero Luminoso* (Sheahan 1999) and the structural adjustment policies of the Fujimori regime that reduced public assistance in other sectors.

Impacts on Livelihood and Food Security

By all accounts, the years of civil war were a time of increased food insecurity in Nuñoa and the region, and are reflected in department-level data for the 1990s. Documented acts of violence were reduced by 74% between 1990 and 1993 at the height of conflict and 1994 through 1996 in immediate postconflict years. This shift to postconflict conditions coincided with a 37% increase of land area in potato cultivation, and 34% larger cattle herds. In Nuñoa, constant rustling had decimated herds and led many larger landowners to sell herds to meat buyers at a considerable loss. Because most of the meat was shipped out to larger cities, little was available locally. The frequent raids on animal herds did not discriminate between high-quality breed stock and other animals, and the quality of herds in this area (known especially for its fine alpaca stock) was further diminished. Farmers limited the amount of land put into cultivation in fear that crops might be destroyed or stolen.

They planted only those fields close to home, and abandoned herds in distant pastures or paid others to tend them.

Government efforts to reallocate land from cooperatives to indigenous communities began in the mid-1980s in part as a response to the spread of *Sendero* and also in response to the demands of peasant organizations and elements of the Catholic Church. Under constant threat of attack, all but one cooperative was abandoned. Thus, production on the largest landholdings dropped precipitously. By the mid-1990s, ten new *communidades campesinos* arose on the abandoned and repatriated cooperative land. For the most part, these households consume what they produce, and the shift in land tenure has not led to an increase in local foods in the market. What members of these communities said about their newly gained access to land was that conditions had not improved drastically, and poverty and hunger were still prevalent, but that now they had a means of survival where before they had nothing.

In addition to diminished food production during the civil war, local stores could not be restocked with goods and weekly markets were disrupted because the roads were considered unsafe for travel. Indeed, *Sendero* practiced a strategy of preventing the flow of goods throughout the region, especially between city and countryside. Many stores shut down or were abandoned out of fear of being robbed by *Sendero* (or by counterterrorist forces), and because there were few products to sell and even fewer customers with money to spend. Moreover, inflation led to higher prices, and this further accentuated food insecurity in the region.

The short- and long-term nutritional and health effects of the combination of these events in Nuñoa are unclear. Levels of chronic undernutrition (as indicated by stunting or low height for age) in the late 1990s remained unchanged from the 1980s, while other regions showed significant improvements in child growth (Pawson, Huicho, Muro, and Pacheco 2001). Records from clinics and health posts in 2005 suggest that undernutrition remains a leading cause of morbidity for children in Nuñoa between the ages of 5 and 15, accounting for perhaps 15% of reported morbidity (Centro de Salud Nuñoa 2005).

These findings suggest that significant improvements in nutrition have not occurred, in accord with the views of local officials and residents. Despite the greater availability of food, the consensus is that undernutrition remains a major problem in the countryside and in the town. The town population has grown with an influx of rural residents during and after the civil war. While the economy is expanding, there are still few opportunities for steady waged employment. Officials and residents report that rural poverty is still acute, and that alcoholism, violence, and crime have increased. This is consistent with many reports from postconflict zones.

In short, food security was clearly affected by conflict and has been slow to recover despite infrastructural changes in the area. Nutritional indicators of health remain stagnant and lag behind other highland regions. Yet, those most marginalized in the past have some hope for the future. The best example of such shifts is in the *ayllu* where we worked in the 1980s (with 70% chronic undernutrition and an IMR of close to 200). Members of this community were widely suspected to have been leaders of raids on the herds of land-owners and cooperatives and also collaborating with *Sendero Luminoso*. The role they may have played is uncertain, but most community households have doubled their landholdings, and more importantly, their pastures for herding. The cooperative land they now occupy is the site of a thriving dairy industry supplying mozzarella cheese to pizzerias in Cuzco's tourist economy. They may be responsible for the 31% increase in milk production in the district between 1995 and 2000 (Municipalidad Distrital de Nuñoa 2001). They also have the only secondary school in the district outside of the main town, and one of the better-staffed rural health clinics. This community has therefore substantially improved its economic situation in the past 20 years, and this should translate into greater food security and improved nutrition and health.

Physical and Psychosocial Health Impacts of Conflict

In interviews with informants and local health professionals, none noted specific health outcomes of the conflict. The infant mortality rate in 1993 at the end of violence was 111.9, down somewhat from that in the early 1980s, but still among the highest in Puno and in all of Peru. By 1996, infant mortal-ity was down to 104 deaths per 1000, and had dropped to around 90 per 1000 by 2001, which is still higher than in most areas in the southern Andes. The reports of local health workers noting few changes in health during the civil war make sense from two vantage points. The first is that health status was so poor before conflict that it is unlikely they would see a noticeable increase in morbidity despite heightened food insecurity. Also, Nuñoa was not the site of many violent battles but more the site of a campaign of fear and control by *Sendero*. Hence, likely effects on morbidity would relate to the somatization of anxiety and distress (e.g., local illness categories of *nervios*, related to anxiety, worry, and depression, or *susto*, attributed to fright and soul loss), and these are not problems treatable in the clinic.

No systematic surveys of the sort carried out by Pedersen et al. in the cen-tral highlands have been attempted in Nuñoa, but interviews with a sample of 12 informants illustrate a range of social and psychosocial effects, and the unevenness of these effects on individuals and communities. The period between 1989 and 1992 was clearly a time of fear. Common practice was to lock the doors and turn off the lights in one's home as soon as night fell, and hope for no knocks at the door or other disturbances. Many fled the area and have not returned. We heard accounts of persistent nightmares, *"ataques de nervios*" (intense anxiety), and of youths now in their late teens and 20s who still are disturbed by the sounds of gunfire on TV. One informant told us that people became afraid; many became quiet, almost mute, and others became agitated and even violent in their interpersonal interactions, especially teens and young adults. The son of a relatively wealthy rancher talked about how his whole family turned inward, stopped communicating with each other, and were quick to anger.

Yet, even here, it was hard to predict how the effects changed individuals' character; we can see this in the experience of two friends from the 1980s. The first, Ramiro, took pride in his classically stoic nature and ability to deal with anything. He recounted how in the late 1980s he was threatened to either leave his teaching post and the town or be killed. He slept in hiding and on guard most nights, but after repeated threats and almost being caught on the streets during the night of an invasion and assassination, he moved several hours away. Fifteen years later, he speaks of these events with sadness and bitterness, and is firm in his decision that he can never return to his birth home for any reason (though other family members have returned). Another friend, Antonio, was a quiet, timid man with an almost subservient manner about him. He had a low-paying but steady job working in the town hall, and served as a secretary to several peasant organizations. First, at the behest of his family, he quit his job with the town government after three death threats by *Sendero*—threats to anyone who worked for a government office. But later, he was detained, interrogated, beaten, and almost killed by counterinsurgency forces suspicious of his work with peasant communities. He also recounted sleeping in different houses or out in the countryside most nights over a 3-year period. The ultimate event for him was a battle between *Sendero* and the police outside the door of the house he rented; four police were killed and he and another friend dragged the bodies from the street to his house. After this, he says that he was no longer afraid of anyone; for him the events were strangely empowering. As he said "I was *muy callado y timido* (quiet and timid), but now I am *muy rebelde* (more assertive)." He currently works to organize his barrio and seems to take pleasure in being an occasional thorn in the side of local officials.

While an analysis based on these findings is still premature, it would appear in the case of these two individuals that higher status, and even ethnicity, might have worked to intensify a sense of fear and loss. Ramiro was not wealthy but was linked by kinship to former landowners in the region, and had an established life and profession as a teacher and a well-planned future that was forcibly and radically altered. Antonio went through an equally radical transformation but although he lost his job and experienced threats to his life, he had little to lose economically, identified more strongly with indigenous peasant communities, and in fact now has permanent holdings in one of those communities. He is still poor but feels empowered, demands respect, and, one expects, has a stronger sense of well-being. These stories suggest that the impacts of trauma are uneven and unpredictable, and their understanding requires systematic exploration of local contexts and local idioms of distress, as Pedersen et al. have suggested.

Social Relations and Work

All informants have told us that the social structure and broader social relations have shifted in Nuñoa, again in uneven ways and with ambiguous consequences. For many townspeople, the period of *Sendero's* dominance (1989–1992) established an atmosphere of fear and uncertainty, which is still felt and manifests in a reportedly heightened aura of wariness and distrust of other townspeople. Informants spoke of the "1000 eyes and ears" of *Sendero* that disciplined their speech and activities then, and to a lesser degree, now. The consensus is that people are moving on with their lives, but with a heightened distrust, lack of confidence, and consequently, a diminished set of cooperative social relations, which Andean peoples have long used to meet work and production tasks and other social needs. The potential impact here can be evaluated relative to our previous work that illustrated the importance of social relations (especially in the absence of secure incomes) in coping with illness or other sources of work disruption in order to complete production tasks in a timely manner. In some cases, where illness affected the household labor force (and hence work potential) and households were not able to replace the lost labor (through family, social networks, or hiring workers), we saw diminished production, heightened food insecurity, and the persistence of poverty, undernutrition, and illness (Leatherman 1996, 1998). Diminished levels of trust, cooperation, and social networks can only add to this negative dialectic of poverty and poor health.

On the other hand, the most dramatic shift in social relations over the past 20 years is that they favor indigenous groups previously marginalized and disenfranchised. The economy and politics of Nuñoa in the 1980s were dominated by ex-*hacendado* families (who still owned the largest ranches), their friends and *compadres*, and teachers. Now, the town leaders are primarily middle class and indigenous, and the majority of store owners are also indigenous. One individual, formerly landless, but now part of a newly formed *campesino* community, stated that "it's not as if conditions have improved much, and there is still a lack of equality and justice, but at least now we are treated with a little respect—not like animals as before." There is clearly a much greater sense of empowerment among these poor small-scale farmers, and this can only contribute to a greater sense of hope and well-being, and perhaps ultimately to improved food security, nutrition, and health.

Conclusion: Examining the Public Health Costs of War and Conflict in Peru

In this example from Peru, we have argued that the preconflict conditions of structural violence were important precursors to the civil war instigated by the PCP-SL. In Nuñoa, away from the frontlines of intense conflict, the civil war appears to have most affected food security, individual and collective trust, and psychosocial health and well-being. While there are few data available on physical health during and immediately after the civil war, the information from residents and health workers suggests that the major effects on morbidity, nutrition, and infant mortality was "business as usual"—a continuation of earlier patterns of very poor health and nutrition. In this case, it is hard to distinguish between the health effects of structural violence, political violence, or some complex interaction of both. We suspect that this may be the case in other sites of low intensity conflict during civil wars—currently the most common, if not the most publicized, forms of conflict confronting populations around the globe.

The effects of civil war in Nuñoa are perhaps clearer for food security and social and psychological distress, though both await systematic study. The experience and expectation of violence and loss negatively affected lives, livelihoods, psychosocial well-being, and community social relations. However, the effects were uneven. Food insecurity persists, but those who were the most disadvantaged and food insecure (i.e., landless or near-landless peasants and members of the poor farming *ayllu*) now control more land than they did before the civil war, which could lead to greater food security in the future. All of our informants communicated a clear expression of the various ways in which the civil war produced a sense of loss, regret, and diminished lives. Yet, some emerged empowered and others more deeply disturbed. This appears to reflect results in other zones of conflict, where many prove to be more or less vulnerable and resilient to the experience of conflict (Pedersen et al. 2001; Summerfield and Toser 1991). Yet, to begin to understand why and how this takes place, it is essential that more research involves local-level ethnography, using idioms of distress that are culturally salient.

A key concern for anthropologists and public health workers is how armed conflict shapes health and well-being well into the future. Given the uneven effects of conflict on health, and social, economic, and political structures that influence health, this can be extremely difficult. In Nuñoa, there are clearly possibilities for future health effects due to the chronic nature of psychosocial distress experienced during conflicts. The broad impacts on diminished social cooperation and trust can affect community function, social support networks, and even access to labor, and these can affect food security and health in important ways. It is also hard to ignore that two objectives of social

movements over the past two centuries—to reclaim land for indigenous peasant communities, and to increase political representation and decrease marginalization among indigenous populations—have been realized in part, however
incomplete and tentative at the moment. This empowerment and greater
access to basic resources could significantly improve livelihoods, health, and
well-being in the future. In this sense, it is an important public health outcome
of the war.

In sum, the political violence of armed conflict is underlain by structural
violence that robs people of access to resources, creates food insecurities, and
strengthens the reciprocal synergism of poverty and poor health. The costs of
conflict, in turn, help reproduce and intensify the very conditions that create
crisis and desperation, and prompt violence as an option for social change.
Thus, measuring the health costs of conflict and violence entails knowledge
of both preexisting contexts and myriad responses to conflict at both local
and national levels. It requires a sense of the lived histories of individuals
and communities that shape their vulnerability and resilience when faced with
violent environments. Thus, the need for more longitudinal and community-
based ethnographic research on the public health costs of conflicts emerges as
a challenge for both anthropology and public health.

References

Ager A, ed. (1999) *Refugees: Perspectives on the Experience of Forced Migration.*
New York: Pinter.
Ball P, Asher J, Sulmont D, Manrique D (2003) How Many Peruvians Have
Died? Human Rights Data Analysis Group of the American Association for
the Advancement of Science as Part of the Report of the Peruvian Truth and
Reconciliation Commission. Washington: AAAS.
Bourgois P (2001) The power of violence in war and peace: Post Cold-War lessons from
El Salvador. *Ethnography* 2(1):5–34.
Bracken P, Giller J, Summerfield D (1995) Psychological responses to war and
atrocity: The limitations of current concepts. *Social Science and Medicine*
40(8):1073–1082.
Carey J (1990) Social system effects on local level morbidity and adaptation in the rural
Peruvian Andes. *Medical Anthropology Quarterly* 4:266–295.
Centro de Salud Nuñoa (2005) Reporte annual de actividades: Micro red Nuñoa.
Ministerio de Salud.
Cervantes RC, Salgado VN, Padilla AM (1989) Posttraumatic stress in immi-
grants from Central America and Mexico. *Hospital and Community Psychiatry*
40(6):615–619.
Cohen MJ, Pinstrup-Andersen P (1999) Food security and conflict. *Social Research*
66(1):375–416.
Donahue M (2003) Causes and health consequences of environmental degradation and
social injustice. *Social Science and Medicine* 56:573–587.
FAO (2002) The State of Food Insecurity in the World, 2002. Rome: FAO.

Farmer P (2003) *Pathologies of Power: Health, Human Rights, and the New War on the Poor.* Berkeley, CA: University of California Press.

Farmer P (2004) Sidney W. Mintz lecture for 2001: An anthropology of structural violence. *Current Anthropology* 45(3):305–325.

Gleditsch NP, Wallenstein P, Eriksson M, Sollenberg M, Strand H (2002) Armed conflict 1946–2001: A new dataset. *Journal of Peace Research* 39(5):615–637.

Ghobarah HA, Huth P, Russett B (2004) The post-war public health effects of civil conflict. *Social Science and Medicine* 59:869–884.

Graham C, Kane C (1998) Opportunistic government or sustaining reform: Electoral trends and public-expenditure patterns in Peru, 1990–1995. *Latin American Research Review* 33(1):67–104.

Green L (1994) Fear as a way of life. *Cultural Anthropology* 9(2):227–256.

Guha-Sapir D, Gijsbert W (2004) Conflict-related mortality: An analysis of 37 datasets. *Disasters* 28(4):418–428.

Gusterson H (2007) Militarism and anthropology. *Annual Review of Anthropology* 36:155–175.

Hendrickson D, Armon J, Mearns R (1998) The changing nature of conflict and famine vulnerability: The case of livestock raiding in Turkana District, Kenya. *Disasters* 22(3):185–199.

Hollifield M, Warner TD, Lian N, Krakow B, Jenkins JH, Kesler J, et al (2002) Review: Measuring trauma and health status in refugees. *Journal of the American Medical Association* 288(5):611–621.

Inhorn MC, Kobeissi L (2006) The public health costs of war in Iraq: Lessons from post-war Lebanon. *Journal of Social Affairs* 23:13–47.

Kalipeni E, Oppong J (1998) The refugee crisis in Africa and implications for health and disease: A political ecology approach. *Social Science and Medicine* 46(12):1637–1653.

Leatherman TL (1996) A biocultural perspective on health and household economy in southern Peru. *Medical Anthropology Quarterly* 10(4):476–495.

Leatherman TL (1998) "Illness, Social Relations, and Household Production and Reproduction in the Andes of Southern Peru." In: *Building a New Biocultural Synthesis: Political-economic Perspectives on Human Biology.* A Goodman, T Leatherman, eds. Ann Arbor, MI: University of Michigan Press, pp. 245–268.

Leatherman TL (2005) "Poverty and Violence, Hunger and Health: A Political Violence of Armed Conflict". In: *Globalization, Health and the Environment: An Integrated Perspective.* G Guest, ed. New York: AltaMira Press, pp. 55–80.

Leonard WR, Thomas RB (1988) Changing dietary patterns in the Peruvian Andes. *Ecology of Food and Nutrition* 21:245–263.

Levy BS, Sidel VW (1997) *War and Public Health.* New York: Oxford University Press.

Luerssen S (1994) Landlessness, health, and the failures of reform in the Peruvian highlands. *Human Organization* 53(4):380–387.

Lundgren RI, Lang R (1989) "There is no sea, only fish": Effects of United States policy on the health of the displaced in El Salvador. *Social Science and Medicine* 28(7):697–706.

Macrae J, Zwi A (1994) "Famine, Complex Emergencies, and International Policy in Africa." In: *War and Hunger: Rethinking International Responses to Complex Emergencies.* J Macrae, A Zwi, eds. London: Zed Books, pp. 6–36.

McClintock C (1984) Why peasants rebel: The case of Peru's Sendero Luminoso. *World Politics* 37:48–84.

McClintock C (1989) "Peru's Sendero Luminoso Rebellion: Origins and Trajectory". In: *Power and Popular Protest: Latin American Social Movements*. S Eckstein, ed. Berkeley, CA: University of California Press, pp. 61–101.

Messer E, Cohen MJ, D'Costa J (1998) Food from peace: Breaking the links between conflict and hunger. Food, Agriculture, and the Environment. Discussion Paper 24. Washington: IFPRI.

Municipalidad Distrital de Nuñoa (2001) Plan Estrategico Desarrollo 2002–2011: Distrito de Nuñoa. Nuñoa (Puno) Peru: Municipalidad Distrital de Nuñoa.

Nordstrom C, Robben A (1995) *Fieldwork under Fire: Contemporary Studies of Violence and Survival*. Berkeley, CA: University of California Press.

Pawson IG, Huicho L, Muro M, Pacheco A (2001) Growth of children in two economically diverse Peruvian high-altitude communities. *American Journal of Human Biology* 13:323–340.

Pedersen D (2002) Political violence, ethnic conflict, and contemporary wars: Broad implications for health and social well-being. *Social Science and Medicine* 55(2):175–190.

Pedersen D, Gamarra J, Planas M, Errazuriz C (2001) Violencia political y salud en las communidades alto-andinas de Ayacucho, Peru. Memorias del VI Congreso Latinoamericano de Ciencias Sociales y Salud. Lima, Peru, June 10–13.

Pieterse S, Ismali S (2003) Nutritional risk factors for older refugees. *Disasters* 27(1):16–36.

Poole D, Rénique G (1992) *Peru: Time of Fear*. London: Latin American Bureau Limited.

Reid M (1985) *Peru: Paths to Poverty*. London: Latin American Bureau Limited.

Scheper-Hughes N, Bourgois P, eds. (2004) *Violence in War and Peace: An Anthology*. Oxford, UK: Blackwell Publishing.

Sheahan J (1999) *Searching for a Better Society: The Peruvian Economy from 1950*. University Park, PA: Pennsylvania State University Press.

SIPRI (2002) *SIPRI Yearbook 2002*. Stockholm: Stockholm International Peace Research Institute.

Smith D (1994) War, Peace and Third World Development. Occasional Paper No. 16, Human Development Report Office. New York: United Nations Development Programme.

Stern S, ed. (1998) *Shining and Other Paths: War and Society in Peru, 1980–1995*. Durham, NC: Duke University Press.

Summerfield D (1999) A critique of seven assumptions behind psychological trauma programmes in war-affected areas. *Social Science and Medicine* 48:1449–1462.

Summerfield D, Toser L (1991) "Low intensity" war and mental trauma in Nicaragua: A study in a rural community. *Medicine and War* 7:84–99.

Teodosijevic S (2003) Armed conflicts and food security. ESA Working Paper No.03–11, Agricultural and Development Economics Division. Rome: FAO.

Thomas RB, Leatherman TL, Carey JW, Haas JD (1988) "Consequences and Responses to Illness among Small-Scale Farmers: A Research Design". In: *Capacity for Work in the Tropics*. KJ Collins, DF Roberts, eds. New York: Cambridge University Press, pp. 249–276.

Ugalde A, Selva-Sutter E, Castillo C, Paz C, Canas S (2000) The health costs of war: Can they be measured? Lessons from El Salvador. *British Medical Journal* 321:169–172.

UN (1996) Profiles in Displacement: Peru. Report to Commission on Human Rights. Geneva, Switzerland: UN Commission on Human Rights.

Waldman R (2005) Public health in war. *International Health* 27(1):1–4.

WHO (1989) "The Declaration of Alma-Ata". www.who.int/hpr/NPH/docs/declaration_almaata.

WHO (2002) "Collective violence". In: *World Report on Violence and Health*. WHO, ed. Geneva: WHO, pp. 214–239.

Zwi A, Ugalde A (1989) Towards an epidemiology of political violence in the Third World. *Social Science and Medicine* 28:633–642.

Part II

ANTHROPOLOGICAL DESIGN OF PUBLIC HEALTH INTERVENTIONS

8

Bridges between Mental Health Care and Religious Healing in Puerto Rico: The Outcomes of an Early Experiment

JOAN D. KOSS-CHIOINO

Introduction

Following more than a century of distrust of religious healing by medical professionals in the United States, the incorporation of spirituality and religion into health and mental health care is beginning to acquire creditability. Studies that demonstrate positive associations between health/mental health and spirituality and/or religion have increased exponentially in the last 3 decades (Koenig 2007). A subgroup of these publications focuses on the importance of clinician and patient satisfaction with clinical applications that include spirituality in patient care (Miller and Thoresen 2003; Puchalski 2006). As a result, greater acceptance of the clinical relevance of religion in mental health care has begun to emerge (Boehnlein 2006; Lake and Spiegel 2007).

A large body of anthropological literature describes how many persons and communities outside of the medical trend-setting United States continue widespread use of various forms of spirit healing (associated with diverse belief systems), which I label (for want of a better term) *popular medicine*. These healing practices are also fairly widespread in the United States, mostly among ethnic minority and immigrant communities, but also in some mainstream communities. Until the last two decades, they have been almost invisible to the general public and medical institutions, given the lack of knowledge about ethnic communities and the lack of openness to understanding them. By recognizing popular medicine embedded within folk and communitarian religions, the ways of life and cultures of these communities are revealed. In addition, interest in the health of ethnic minority communities has become important to public health care providers in the last decade. They have been pressured by national health interests in the United States and Europe to facilitate utilization and availability of health and mental health care services for minority and immigrant communities.

The question of whether religiosity or spirituality have an effect on mental illness beyond a possible increased sense of well-being (life satisfaction, happiness, positive affect, and better morale) might be raised. Can there also be negative effects, as suggested by Pargament (1997)? The problem is complex, and the studies do not show causal relationships. However, they do show that higher levels of religious involvement are positively associated with less depression, fewer suicidal thoughts, and recovery from alcohol and substance abuse (Moreira-Almeida, Lotufo, and Koeing 2006). A group of studies shows decreased risk for depressed mood and fewer symptoms in those elderly patients and troubled, older adolescents who regularly participate in religious practices (Koenig 1998; Koenig, McCullough, and Larson 2000). One generalization that seems to hold and provide a reasonable hypothesis is that religion is used to cope with all kinds of life crises; it particularly helps persons in highly stressful situations (Pargament 1997). A specific question asked is whether spiritual or religious practices can or should be integrated into community mental health care.

On the international scene, almost 30 years ago, the World Health Organization (WHO) made a commitment to a collaborative program aimed at increasing the role of traditional healers in the provision of primary health care (WHO-UNICEF 1978). This commitment was renewed not long ago (Ramsey 2002; WHO 2002) as a "global strategy" for traditional medicine, largely focused on the HIV/AIDS epidemic. However, although small pilot programs integrating traditional healers and public health care have been carried out, they have not been replicated on a national scale. There is abundant descriptive material on traditional medicine, medical pluralism, and mental illness, but few reports of collaborative projects in this area are available (Kiesser, McFadden, and Belliard 2006; Ravi Shankar, Sarvanan, and Jacob 2006). Reports on mental illness treated by traditional healers do not frame them as religious practices or view them within the newer perspective on integrating religion and spirituality into mental health care.

The Birth of an Innovative Project

On the initial cusp of a change in attitudes toward religion in mental health care in the mid-1970s (mainly focused on minority communities), I was invited by the National Institute of Mental Health (NIMH) to submit a proposal for a project in Puerto Rico that would incorporate Spiritist healing practices as a community mental health resource. The Division of Mental Health of the Department of Health of Puerto Rico had been reorganized as a community mental health program in accordance with the U.S. Community Mental Health Act (1963), and agreed to sponsor the project as part of its community mandate. (It might be noted that my employer at the time, the Department of Sociology and Anthropology at the University of Puerto Rico, refused to be involved in such "superstitions"!) The sponsorship of the proposal (and subsequently, the training/research project) by the health department of Puerto Rico reflected the widespread knowledge of Spiritism among persons from all social classes in Puerto Rico, including many health and mental health professionals who had grown up in families that subscribed to Spiritist practices.

The initial idea to develop a bridge between popular ("traditional") healing and mental health care delivery in the community was not entirely new in 1974, when I wrote the proposal. There were at least 3 precedents. First, there was an NIMH-funded project for Navajos in the American Southwest, called the School for Medicine Men, directed by a psychiatrist, Robert Bergman (1973). Projects in New York, New Jersey, and Miami had also been planned that included a focus on Spiritism and other popular healing systems, such as *Vodun* among Haitians, and *Santería* among Cubans (Garrison 1977; Koss-Chioino 2000). A limited experiment at Lincoln Hospital in New York City, which experimented with integrating Puerto Rican Spiritist mediums as attendants in a psychiatric hospital ward, was short lived (Ruiz and Langrod 1976). The Spiritists hired as attendants in the psychiatric wards were coopted by the medical system and did not appear to have actively carried out Spiritist ritual practices with patients. (Personal communications with other Puerto Rican Spiritists who have worked in mental health settings indicate that they feel stigmatized bringing Spiritist beliefs and practices into a hospital in the United States.)

A second precedent can also be found in the interest of international health institutions, as mentioned previously. In response to regulations passed in 1977 by the Thirtieth World Health Assembly and resolutions made by the WHO's meeting "Promotion and Development of Traditional Medicine," the WHO decided to promote traditional medicine as a complement to biomedical health care (MacLean and Bannerman 1982). This was viewed as a way to ensure more appropriate referrals for severe or special cases, opportunities for traditional healers to increase their skills, and low-cost expansion of public health care. The Aro Project in Nigeria pioneered the attempt to relate traditional healing and mental health-care delivery (Ademuwagun, Ayoade, Harrison, and Warren 1979; Lambo 1978; Bibeau [1985] describes some later projects).

A third precedent comes from early literature in cross-cultural psychiatry that describes traditional healing in many parts of the world (for reviews see Gaines 1992; Csordas and Lewton 1998). A number of studies have since documented informal referrals between mental health care providers and traditional healers in Africa and Latin America (Ezeji and Sarvela 1992; Koss 1980, among others). Complex interchanges between biomedicine and traditional healing have taken place for more than 130 years in Brazil, where Spiritists have established mental hospitals and set up cooperative arrangements between Spiritist mediums and mental health care providers in both Spiritist and government institutions (Hess 1991).

The program in Puerto Rico was named the Therapist–Spiritist Training Project, in part to call attention to its main theme, an exchange of knowledge and training across the mental health care and Spiritist healing systems. The idea of "training" came from the NIMH section that supported the proposal. For example, they supported the Navajo project, the School for Medicine Men. Its chief aim was pedagogical, leading to better understanding of both the medical and Navajo healing systems of health and mental health care across the systems. In developing the program in Puerto Rico, the goal of sociability and friendship between the mental health professionals and Spiritist mediums was also considered important to enhance relatedness among 2 very different types of healing systems and healers. In the project in Puerto Rico, everyone was referred to as "healers" regardless of whether they were medically or spiritually trained. This was deemed necessary in order to level differences in social status and create a shared forum.

I will first briefly describe the political, social, medical, and religious contexts of the Therapist–Spiritist Training Project in Puerto Rico (1976–1980), including both positive and negative conditions for its inception and adoption. This project was focused on mental health in 3 health regions of Puerto Rico and officially became a special part of the community mental health initiative of the sub-secretariat for mental health of the Department of Health of Puerto Rico at that time. The design of the project and its methods will be very briefly described, including some ideas that grounded the project, on the basis of my early studies of Spiritism in Puerto Rico. The project, conducted 30 years ago, was unique among the relatively few projects in the world that aimed to integrate conventional and popular alternative types of mental health care. It is now part of the history of health and mental health care in Puerto Rico. I will briefly examine some major societal trends in that history over the last three decades in order to describe changes in the current situation of medical pluralism, and also consider the role of religion in dealing with emotional distress in recent years. This discussion includes information on trends in integrating both popular and alternative medicines into health care—one aspect of the larger picture of community-based mental health care in Puerto Rico.

Background: The Social, Political, and Religious Context of Popular Healing and Mental Health Care in Puerto Rico

Puerto Ricans are heirs to 2 equally popular but competing worldviews from the nineteenth century, the "scientific" and the "spiritual." Examples of this conundrum are the persistence, since the late nineteenth century, of the widespread religious/healing cult "Spiritism" (*Espiritismo*) and the ready reception of the Cuban cult, *Santería*, since the mid-twentieth century. Spiritist ritual is focused on "working" with spirits in small household-based *centros* (and a few larger temples) staffed mostly by female mediums, who hold 2 or more weekly sessions with the participation of 25 to 40 people. The mediums become possessed by spirits, and/or experience visions in order to heal (*sanar*) supplicants, who bring a wide range of health and social problems (Garrison 1977; Harwood 1977; Koss 1975; Rogler and Hollingshead 1961). Variations on this form of popular religious healing (found throughout Latin America and many European and some Asian countries) have developed over the last 3 decades; *Santería*, a Cuban import based on West African religious beliefs and rituals, gained in popularity until the 1990s, but currently appears to be waning. There are also other religious groups with healing practices that have steadily increased in popularity, such as hundreds of Evangelical and Pentecostal churches. What we now call "comprehensive and alternative" medicine (CAM) has been increasingly popular in this mix of popular healing systems over the last 3 decades, and includes some spiritually based healing disciplines.

In the mid-1970s, almost all Spiritist centers followed the teachings of spirits, as codified by Allan Kardec (pen name of French scholar Hippolyte Denizarth Leon Rivail, 1803–1869), who published 7 books and a journal translated into Spanish. A few centers in Puerto Rico followed the revised doctrines of an Argentinian, Joaquin Trincado. A few temples, composed mainly of middle-class Spiritists, strictly followed the doctrines of Kardec (an increasing number still do), eschewing the incorporation of Afro-Caribbean and folk Catholic popular healing practices that preceded Spiritism on the island.

History of Spiritism and Community Mental Health in Puerto Rico

Although there is evidence of Spiritism in Puerto Rico since at least 1873, until very recently, its practice has met varying degrees of opposition from both the Catholic Church and the biomedical establishment (Koss 1976). Spiritism was introduced into Puerto Rico as the new "psychological" science—as it had been hailed by French scholars of that time—by intellectual elites who had studied in France and Spain. It almost immediately met opposition from the medical boards established by Spain in its colonies. In the latter part of the nineteenth century and the early years of the twentieth century, however, some fervent Spiritists held political power and were also associated with the anti-theological Masonic movement (Koss 1976). With more extensive medical accul-turation due to North American subsidies and imported programs, and ongoing modernization of public health institutions, Spiritism went underground in terms of public visibility, and yet maintained its large base of adherents among both the poor and the elites (including some government officials). That seems to be changing, given the expanding popularity of integrative medicine and greater receptivity on the part of medical doctors—which is described later.

One side of the neocolonial coin in Puerto Rico in the 1960s was the growing popularity in the United States of the community mental health movement, destined like many other public health programs to be adopted—with spon-sorship from the U.S. Public Health Service—in Puerto Rico. Ideas about the causes of mental illness had expanded at this time to include a broad focus on interpersonal relations, family influences, emotional traumas, and other psy-chosocial phenomena. New psychotropic medications were so promising that patients with severe mental illness could be expected to have long periods of remission from dysfunctional cognitive and behavioral states. Before the 1960s, as in most states, severe mental illness was treated in long-term residen-tial care hospitals, most of which were established and run by the state. After the community mental health act, community-based institutions, such as day hospitals, 24-hour emergency services, and halfway houses, were designed to permit persons with severe mental illness to leave psychiatric hospitals. Eleven community mental health centers, with a variety of outpatient care services, were thus established in Puerto Rico during the 1960s and 1970s to serve ambulatory patients.

Community mental health assessments in Puerto Rico frequently noted that Spiritist centers were a widespread healing resource upon which many persons depended for mental illness crises or when treatment at the mental health centers was not adequate for their perceived needs. Aspects of the relationship between Spiritism and persons with severe psychiatric illness are described by Rogler and Hollingshead (1961, 1965), who view Spiritism as an important source of support for the mentally ill and their families, as well as a means to explain etiology and the course of illness within an indigenous frame of reference.

Method and Design of the Project: Understanding
Two Systems in Contact

Following almost 5 years of part-time research into Spiritism in Puerto Rico and a consultancy with the mental health division of the Puerto Rican

Department of Health, I designed a project that would bridge Spiritist healing practices in the community with the Department of Health's division of mental health programs.

From 1968 to 1974, I carried out a series of ethnographic studies in the extended San Juan metropolitan area, in different types of Spiritist centers. This ethnographic research was the basis for decisions about the bridging project. Several facts from these studies were important to planning the project. It was clear, for example, that all of the small centers as well as the larger temples were autonomous, although several attempts had been made for some to join into a loose alliance. Each center or temple relied on 1 or 2 mediums (usually the president and a close associate) to carry out organizational duties, such as scheduling and holding meetings. In the small centers, sessions were held at the president's home (most commonly a structure attached to the house and built for that purpose). Many centers were victims of divisiveness when someone from among the mediums challenged the president's capacity to protect those assembled—especially the mediums—from the influences of the negative spirits (Koss 1977). The larger temples had endured over decades (i.e., *Circulo Lumen* in Ponce has been active for more than 125 years) but many of the smaller centers closed when the president's hegemony was challenged, she suffered from serious illness, or died. This meant that we had to separately recruit the presidents and then seek their recommendations regarding which of the mediums at their centers to invite. A survey of the centers and temples on the island yielded a small group of presidents very interested in the project who later acted as advisors to the project. Several of these women, well known among Spiritists, became lecturers in the project's programs.

I began to understand Spiritism as an ethnomedical system through 2 studies carried out in the early 1970s. The first was a survey utilizing the Cornell Medical Index (Brodman, Erdmann, and Wolf 1956; Koss 1975) and open-ended questions regarding help seeking. My students conducted household interviews in the *barrios* near the university. Because they collected data during the daytime, almost all the respondents were women. They reported a very large number of complaints, far more than considered "normal" by the designers of the index. The distress reported by these women was taken to Spiritist mediums, priests, and older women relatives significantly more frequently than to mental health professionals or medical doctors. It appeared that particular symptoms were associated with particular sources of help, and help-seeking paths were influenced by prior successes or failures. Later, data from the Spiritist–Therapist Project documented the types of complaints taken to the Spiritists as compared with those brought to the mental health system (Koss-Chioino 1992). These data showed a clear division of labor; nonserious emotional and bodily distresses were more often brought to the Spiritists, and severe emotional distress (diagnosable as mental illness) was most often seen by mental health professionals. However, many persons used the 2 systems consecutively according to the amount of relief each was expected to provide, or because of dissatisfaction with the interventions.

The second set of observations was collected in the years just before the project's inception. As a consultant to the mental health program of the department of health, I discussed patient cases with mental health professionals who made clear their recognition of the many contradictions between psychotherapeutic methods and spirit healing. These professionals most often came from families of Spiritist mediums or believers. In a similar vein, Spiritists interviewed in the early studies clearly voiced their interest in biomedical approaches to mental health care—particularly, neurophysiology and psychotropic medications. This interest stemmed not only from their desire to eclectically incorporate knowledge of treatment techniques, but also from the need to know how to refer clients who spirits could not help.

At the beginning of the project, when designing the content of the seminars, we acknowledged that the 2 systems and their "healers" were very different, but chose to focus on the parallels when possible. We designed the seminars to give equal time to each system and promoted an approach that conferred equal status on the participants.

Designing an Integrated Project

The general goals of the Therapist–Spiritist Training Project were to establish a forum for the meaningful mutual exchange of information between Spiritist mediums and mental health professionals (primary-care medical doctors in training were later added); to offer a training curriculum to transfer knowledge and skills across the 2 healing systems; and to develop new psychotherapeutic approaches from a synthesis of the most relevant and effective healing techniques in both systems. It was decided to run the same program in 3 different communities each year for 3 years, to explore possible differences in community response and conditions for replication.

The original plan was for groups of Spiritists and mental health professionals to meet once per week at health department facilities for 9 months in each of the 3 different communities. A second weekly meeting was planned to take place in the *centro* of a Spiritist participant, rotating each week among different *centros* that volunteered. However, the first important change in plans came with the difficulty of meeting weekly at the Spiritist centers, in part for reasons of logistics; also, the therapist (health department) participants found that plan untenable because it did not accord with the idea that they were participating in continuing medical education courses. It became immediately apparent that the hoped-for leveling of the large gap in social status between the health professionals and Spiritists would not be easy to achieve. However, from the perspective of the lower-status Spiritists, there was compensation by the legitimizing effect of attending seminars in a public mental health facility or a hospital.

Although the project proved workable, the face-to-face interactions between people from 2 very different healing worlds led to a number of unexpected events, some quite negative, others positive. A few are detailed in the section on participant responses.

Project Organization

The program of the Spiritist–Therapist Training Project had the following specific objectives: to augment the therapeutic skills of practitioners from both systems; augment knowledge of the psychological basis of behavioral disorders for both groups; develop formal referral networks between the 2 systems; develop a general training model that included all practitioners from both systems; provide practitioners with a guided training experience that would increase clinical effectiveness; provide trainees with information about community health resources and the lifestyles and typical patterns of interpersonal relationships among patients and Spiritist clients; promote attitudinal changes toward mutual understanding and cooperation between therapists and Spiritists; and encourage use of community mental health services by the Spiritists and outreach activities by the therapists.

Balance in participation between therapists and Spiritists was very important to the structure of the seminar programs; the didactic seminar sessions were equally divided between health professionals, academic lecturers, and Spiritist lecturers. Dual perspectives were discussed on each topic. Although the Spiritists were accustomed to volunteering their time and expertise because they considered healing an avocation, they were paid to lecture according to the same schedule as the health professionals (which included medical doctors and PhDs).

The project proposal outlined 3 evaluation measures and added others as the project progressed: (1) gauge changes in the attitudes and notions of participants regarding beliefs and understandings about mental health, using a questionnaire based on Spiritism and fundamental knowledge of psychopathology and psychotherapy; (2) collect responses to questionnaires about expectations and outcomes of each type of treatment from 100 new patients/clients, with at least 1 patient of each core participant in the project; and (3) assess changes in management and treatment, and collect case histories of each new patient/client of each core participant at baseline and posttreatment follow-up. In addition, we videotaped sessions with Community Mental Health Center (CMHC) patients of participants, as well as Spiritist sessions in centers where participants worked with spirits. The project programs were also videotaped, and an 11-item questionnaire was developed to measure response to the lectures and case review sessions. We also held informal discussions about the project's program, which were followed by socializing (parties) at the halfway point and end of each project year. In addition, once per year, 3 outside consultants from the United States and 2 from Puerto Rico (4 medical doctors and an anthropologist) worked with the CMHC unit directors at our site centers to review the materials and program sessions, and meet participants. Consultants produced detailed evaluation reports each year.

Over the 3 years, dossiers (life histories, personality profiles, treatment histories of client cases, profiles of beliefs) were collected on core participants (although many more Spiritists and mental health professionals attended 1 or several seminars). These participants included 35 women and 13 male Spiritists; 17 women and 11 male mental health professionals; and 7 women and 20 male medical doctors, two-thirds of whom were medical residents.

Community Reactions

Shortly after the health department's public announcement of the project (before the initiation of the project), the most popular daily paper in San Juan ran an article entitled *"Escuela de Curanderos en Salud."* It featured a cartoon in which an African-looking medicine man is showing a chicken's claw and a small glass of a (supposed) herbal infusion to a medical doctor as a prescription for a rather brutish-looking (mental) patient. The burlesque tone of the article speaks to the lack of belief that the health department would sponsor a project involving folk healers. This reaction was balanced somewhat by several supportive letters addressed to the sub-secretary for mental health by prominent Spiritists who sent copies of articles from Spiritist media about "psychic therapy" as analogous to spirit healing, thus attempting to explain the relationship of spirit healing to mental health treatment. These persons offered their time to work with the project, and noted the international provinence of Spiritism as reported in the major Spiritist newsletter, *La Aurora del Pueblo* (Sifre Lajara 1974). Some months later, an article in a prestigious newspaper, *El Mundo*, provided a more even-handed account. Over the following 5 years, several newspapers ran multipage articles on Spiritism, describing aspects of the project and Spiritism's importance as a healing resource.

Initial Reactions of Participants

A few examples of the kinds of problems that arose are instructive. In the first year Spiritists expressed considerable distress over the proximity of severely mentally ill persons (we met regularly in a conference room at the CMHC), whom they could see through a window in a locked ward in the passageway that led to the seminar room. (For them this meant that the patients were "obsessed"—that is, taken over by a bad spirit—and had not been treated.) This was countered by a Spiritist lecturer's presentation on how to practice Spiritism in a hospital. She described such practices as very different from those at a Spiritist center, and suggested that hospital practice required more "control" (appeals to protector spirits) in the absence of the "table" and water container (spirit fluids) common in Spiritist practice. This was received with considerable heated discussion, and some Spiritists dropped out. Another example was that a rumor circulated that we intended to establish a Spiritist center within the CMHC or at the regional hospital next door. We assured the group that this was not a goal of the project, and most of the original participants settled into the seminars for the remainder of the year.

Outcomes

The most salient outcome was that Spiritists and therapists began to refer themselves to the opposite healing system for help; they later began referring a few patients. The possibility of formalizing referrals was realized when a mental health technician participating in the project, who had experience with Spiritism while seeking help for her schizophrenic mother, made a suicidal gesture. She was found by her boyfriend, who took her to a health center in a town they were visiting. The attending physician had been at the project seminars and agreed with her plea that she not be referred to mental health services. Instead, she self-referred to a well-known Spiritist medium who participated in the project. She told the physician that she was afraid she would lose her job if treated in a mental health setting. He also felt that she might get better care (i.e., protection against another attempt) from the Spiritists, because he was dissatisfied with the lack of attention given to another of his patients at the CMHC emergency service. When the crisis had passed the therapist called a meeting of her colleagues and her supervisor at the home of the Spiritist who had cared for her and whose sessions she was still attending. Under the thin disguise of an anonymous recording as a "training" vehicle, she told the story of her psychological crisis. As the Spiritists had diagnosed her as "obsessed," she could claim lack of awareness for her actions and lack of responsibility; therefore, she did not expect negative sanctions. Her plan worked. It illuminated the dilemma faced by mental health professionals who feel they cannot seek help for emotional crises from their colleagues. This led to the establishment of a referral unit at the CMHC, where we held the program during the second year.

The referral unit had its beginnings in the very first year of the project's programs when 4 therapists and 8 other CMHC staff participants consulted

Spiritists about their anonymous patients. In the second and third years, a few referrals by Spiritist participants, of their relatives or themselves to mental health professionals, and referrals by therapists to Spiritists, also occurred. We documented this process for 4 mental health workers and 6 medical doctors; in addition, 4 Spiritists consulted mental health professionals for their own problems. Once they had acquired more knowledge about mental illness, the Spiritists developed a new etiological category, "psychic cause," an addition to the usual dichotomy into material and spiritual causes.

We were able to follow up 10 cross-referrals among Spiritists and therapists (going in both directions) before the establishment of the referral unit in the third year. Organization of the referral unit was facilitated by the director (a psychologist) of the CMHC, where we held the second year's program (see Koss 1980 for more details). Nine Spiritist healers volunteered to staff the unit and the director of the outpatient unit and several members of her staff also volunteered to take part. Twenty-six patients were enrolled in response to a governing committee composed of Spiritists and therapists, who reviewed each case for treatment strategies and evaluated whether Spiritist treatment was indicated (with patient consent). These cases were followed up and outcomes assessed, depending upon how quickly the patient returned to pre-episode levels of functioning. Success was measured in part by whether these patients did not have to have temporary or continued hospitalization. It is to be noted that all but 2 of the latter group were sent home subsequent to their treatment in the referral unit. This subprogram of the project was an example of extensive cooperation between therapists and Spiritists who had participated together during 1 training year.

Two cases illustrate the way referrals were made and some of the reasons involved. In one case, a therapist was treating a 6-year-old girl for speech delay and incontinence (bladder and bowel, which she said was due to fear of using the toilet). After about a year of monthly visits, the therapist became aware that the parents were Spiritist believers. They shared with him that a Spiritist had told them that a spirit had imposed the fear on the child when she had once been left alone. The therapist then invited one of the project's Spiritists to join him in the case. The medium then located the spirit cause of the child's fear—a woman who had died by hanging. She then worked on the child during the therapy session. The little girl was partly helped but remained bowel incontinent. However, the parents were then able to put her into a head-start program, where she received special psychological services.

A young man of 17 years was very short in stature (5'2"), and had a severe case of acne scars, a pervasive feeling of loneliness, headaches, and severe difficulties and anxiety regarding his studies. He had regularly been attending a Spiritist session for 2 months (his family were believers), believing that it was helping him stay in high school despite a very low grade average.

He interpreted his difficulties as a spiritual test. The Spiritist medium referred him to neurological services (having attended lectures on neurology in the project). She thought that he might have either epilepsy or migraine headaches, which were affecting his ability to learn. After a number of tests the results were negative. The medium then declared that he was developing his faculties to become a medium and should continue to attend sessions to support this development.

The success of the referral unit was due in part to the therapists' discomfort over sending some patients into long-term residential treatment. In response to these successes, the Department of Health promised to fund permanent positions in the referral unit. The CMHC director appointed a psychologist to take charge of the unit, and it continued over the following year (until 1981). However, the division heads of the health department changed after that year's island election, and the referral unit never received its staff positions. Despite the failure of the referral unit to officially continue its mission, we heard occasional reports of referrals on both sides over the next 5 years.

Some Lessons and Limitations

In reviewing the model for linkage and possible integration of the 2 very different healing systems developed in the Puerto Rican experiment, the following approaches appeared successful: (1) the rule of flexibility that permitted response to the views and suggestions of the participants about how to proceed and the directions to take on important issues; (2) the scheduled opportunity to interchange views informally and form friendships through socializing; (3) the opportunity for discussion in an environment as free of judgment as possible, in which ideological differences could be transcended; (4) the opportunity, especially for the therapists, to admit to supporting (or having) beliefs considered suspect by many health professionals (but that they had often acquired in childhood), and were sometimes labeled "craziness," superstition, or black magic; and (5) the pedagogical framework that provided a structure (and idiom) for the leveling of status differences, which in turn facilitated (and was crucial to) the interchange of ideas.

The last of our 3 main goals was not met; treatments and/or diagnostic techniques synthesized from both healing systems into new psychotherapeutic approaches were never formalized or tested. The Spiritist healers did not enter into intense interchanges of ideas and techniques with the therapists. Whether their reactions reflected the difficulties of decreasing the not inconsiderable ideological and social distance between them, it seemed that the Spiritists continued to feel subordinate to the therapists. The healers appeared reluctant to openly share their most closely held ideas and techniques, perhaps in fear of cooptation. Suspicion about the effect of giving up secrets (a deeply rooted aspect of Spiritism) is an inheritance from their earlier prosecution and a response to ongoing discrimination (Koss 1977).

There is little doubt that, in the first years following the project, there was a new consciousness in the health care community, as well as greater acceptance of Spiritism as a healing system by those who had experienced it. However, this has not continued to increase, I suggest, because of the growing popularity of other healing alternatives in Puerto Rico, such as complementary and alternative medicine and consciousness transformation movements. In addition, community mental health services have undergone far-reaching change; the practice of Spiritism has also changed, as will be described in the next section.

Community Mental Health in Puerto Rico over the Last Decades

Puerto Rican society has become increasingly turbulent since 1980. Several statistics could be cited, such as the high rates of HIV/AIDS and crime. Moreover, Puerto Rico was designated as a place of high-intensity drug trafficking in 2001 (National Drug Intelligence Center 2003). In 1998, a household survey of people from the ages of 15 to 64 found that 5.6% of the population needed treatment for substance abuse (Colon, Canino, Robles, Lopez, and Orraca 1998). The rate of homicide is one per 100,000, which places Puerto Rico the sixth highest in the world (and the other 5 countries are at war; Gonzalez 2007). The drug-related homicide rate is 3 times that in the United States. Homicide is the leading cause of death in youth 15 to 19 years of age, which accounts for 50% of death in this age-group (Hansen 2004).

Although some substance abusers presented to Spiritist healers in past years, they were mostly seen in public health addiction treatment programs. Since the reform of the community mental health system by the Puerto Rican government in 1994, and the establishment of a managed care system, available substance abuse treatment is mostly carried out in crowded, faith-based treatment programs by evangelical Protestant churches, some of which are supported by the government (Hansen 2004).

A September 2, 2007 article in *El Dia*, one of the 2 largest newspapers in Puerto Rico, entitled "*Ecosicología*," describes how poverty (currently over 60%), high incidence of psychiatric illness (25%, according to the WHO in 2002–2003), and addiction disorders contribute to creating an environment of very high stress, which perpetuates widespread emotional distress. This very difficult social environment leads to greater appreciation and utilization of nonconventional medical alternatives, such as complementary and alternative treatments in addition to popular religious healing, such as

Spiritism, Catholic charismatic healing, and personal devotion to the saints. Before considering the availability and use of these alternatives, it is useful to briefly review the state of the current public community mental health program, which is mandated to deal with the increasing burden of emotional disorders.

In an attempt to cover more of the uninsured population, in 1994 the Puerto Rican health department dramatically changed the overburdened health care system that had served about half of the population—those who fell below the poverty line—since the 1960s. Dividing the island into 10 health regions, public health care facilities were privatized, and a managed health care system that included both health and mental health care was established (Alegria et al. 2001). One goal of this drastic institutional change was to provide care for the uninsured who fell into the category just above the poverty line. This followed trends in the United States, in which private insurers proposed health care packages at a fixed capitation rate. Eligibility was based on residence and income limits (now expanded), as well as veteran status and employment in the police force. These changes were phased in gradually, in 2 regions each year. Most of the mental health care was provided by U.S. behavioral health companies who staffed mental health centers and detoxification programs with counselors, psychiatric nurses, and B.A.-level therapists. Only one company offered a contract for the care of chronically ill patients.

A study comparing reformed with the unreformed regions showed an increase in use of the specialty services by the nonpoor, and a level or slight decrease in utilization by the poor in the reformed regions (Alegria et al. 2001). The researchers suggest that the nonpoor had more experience in dealing with private practitioners and knew how to utilize specialty services, and that the poor simply substituted public for private practitioners, given the lack of experience with private mental health care. One might also speculate that the poor in the reformed regions increased their use of community alternatives (i.e., popular healers, elderly relatives, alternative medicine), to which they had always resorted. This increase in utilization of popular medicine and CAM may not reflect less accessibility but a perception of poorer quality of care.

The larger question is what affects utilization of public mental health care in a medically pluralistic society, particularly in relation to chronically distressed persons. The deficits of managed mental health care, particularly for serious mental illness, seem to have become apparent. In the past year, the health department of Puerto Rico has decided to reestablish a community mental health program, starting with the western region of the island. Three new community mental health centers have been opened in Mayaquez, Moca, and Arecibo, and 2 more are in the planning stage. However, resources have continued to be limited for the health department (it went bankrupt 2 years ago), although the need for mental health-care services may be growing, given reports of increasing societal violence.

Complementary and Alternative Medicine

The use of CAM in many developed societies has increased significantly in the last 3 decades (Lake and Spiegel 2007). This is similar for Puerto Ricans, who seem to have become somewhat disillusioned by the complex and invasive technology and bureaucracy of biomedicine and greater formality in the physician–patient relationship, frustrating the expectation of *confianza* (familiarity) in therapeutic relationships. Moreover, they have traditionally resorted to the use of various, alternative types of health and mental health care available to them (such as religious healing, including Spiritism and *Santería*). It has been suggested that this belief in using whatever help is available is the legacy of the relative lack of modern medical care—especially mental health-care services—for most of the urban and rural poor in the first part of the twentieth century. My observations as a resident from the 1960s to the 1980s were that dual (and even triple) use of biomedical and CAM alternatives for the same complaints, especially for emotional distress, was generally considered wise and necessary behavior (Koss-Chioino 1992).

Although studies of utilization patterns of CAM in Puerto Rico by researchers in the Puerto Rico Health Services Research Institute are reported to be in process, a search for published data was fruitless. CAM's recent popularity is evidenced by a free, independent newspaper (*La Era Ahora*), published from 1996 to 2005, with a circulation of 8000. It ran articles and advertised events and services that covered all of the CAM alternatives (herbal and mineral preparations of Asia and other origins, lectures and seminars by local and imported health gurus, naturopathic doctors, massage therapists, acupuncturists, and so forth), including meditation and new-age spiritual teachers. This newspaper has been replaced by a widely distributed, consumer-oriented magazine that does not cover most of the spiritually oriented events. Much of CAM in Puerto Rico comes from the United States, but some originates from other Latin American countries, such as the establishment of 2 "adaptogenic medical centers" by a group from Venezuela. The Adaptogenic group advertises "evidence-based CAM" treatments, based mainly on research into herbal medicines.

There are no data from Puerto Rico on the extent to which CAM serves to alleviate emotional distress or help with psychiatric illness. Stores that sell herbal medicines and mineral preparations are very popular; for example, they sell Omega-3 products, which are claimed to alleviate depression and some psychotic symptoms (Lake 2007). Many medical doctors in Puerto Rico now practice integrative medicine, having studied acupuncture or homeopathy. There are a few centers of learning where CAM practitioners are trained; the main one for medical doctors is a program attached to 1 of the 4 medical schools in Puerto Rico, the *Universidad del Caribe*, in Bayamon. This institution offers its medical students electives given by physicians who have a CAM skill. The program also offers a range of CAM health care services, including chiropractic, massage, and acupuncture, by licensed and certified practitioners, several of whom are medical doctors. I was recently told that about 5 out of 60 students take these electives each year. A physician–acupuncturist from this program estimated that about 50 doctors practice integrative medicine on the island. In addition, the College of Physicians and Surgeons offers courses and conferences that focus on CAM, in which doctors can receive continuing medical education credits.

It appears that increasingly for many, especially those in the expanding educated middle class, CAM is a viable treatment alternative, often utilized because of dissatisfaction with care from the conventional medical system. A study among "Hispanic" (culture unspecified) women in New York City showed that commonly used alternative remedies were teas and herbs, vitamins and nutritional supplements, prayer, spiritual healing, and relaxation techniques (Cushman, Wade, Factor-Litvak, Kronenberg, and Firester 1999). As popular medicine in Latin American countries also uses teas and herbs, and prayer is ubiquitous, there seems to be little that is very new in these practices. The women in New York frequently saw chiropractors, herbalists, and acupuncturists. Use of alternative remedies and practitioners was more frequent among those over 40 years of age; this age-group was less skeptical about alternative health care than younger women.

In Puerto Rico, it appears that CAM has partially supplanted popular healing alternatives, such as Spiritism and *Santería*. Its increasing popularity may be due to its being endorsed and adopted by some medical doctors. The College of Physicians has backed the licensing of acupuncturists and is contemplating other licenses. Given the opportunistic nature of care seeking in conjunction with less availability of mental health care and the higher incidence of stress-related emotional disorders, CAM has provided more choice of medical alternatives so that the buffet of healing possibilities is richer.

With the increase in CAM, it appears that the type of Spiritism of the project is not as widely practiced as it was 20 years ago. Many of the prominent mediums who participated in the project have "passed over" into the spirit world. A few of the larger centers no longer exist, and there seem to be fewer small centers in the mediums' homes. Of interest, however, is the growing number of new centers and meetings in urban settings among educated, middle-class people. These practices more strictly follow Kardec's teachings than the centers in the project described previously. They focus mainly on personal well-being and moral and philosophical themes; the mediums in these groups are somewhat less ecstatic and less active in incorporating spirits. This expansion of Spiritist practice may be a response to a general search for spiritual experience related to personal coping in a stressful and often chaotic society. Although they continue to offer healing rituals, healing is only one aspect of their practice, which aims to promulgate a worldview that focuses on the progressive evolution of spirit and teaches karmic principles.

Spiritist Medical Doctors in Puerto Rico: An Emergent Bridge

Over the initial 10 years (1969–1979) of research into Spiritism in Puerto Rico, I came across 5 medical doctors who were reputed to be practicing Spiritist mediums. I did not interview them in a systematic way, but they were known to the Spiritists who participated in our project. Over the last year, however, I collected the names of over 40 qualified (almost all board certified) medical doctors in the greater San Juan metropolitan area who are reputed to be involved in Spiritist practices either as believers or as practicing mediums. The actual number may be higher because many medical doctors are still reluctant to be identified by the public as Spiritist mediums.

It might be noted that this phenomenon is fairly widespread in parts of Brazil (Hess 1991). A Spiritist medical association was founded in São Paulo more than 20 years ago and now has branches in Rio and several other cities. This association held its first U.S. congress, in suburban Washington, DC, in 2006. It was attended by approximately 300 medical doctors and other health professionals, most of whom were living in the United States, with origins from all of the countries in Latin America. Although Spiritism is as much an import (mainly from Europe) as biomedicine or as complementary and alternative medical techniques, there seems to be a view in Latin American societies that spiritism is integral to Latin culture, an essential part of the threads of a group-constructed, "traditional" culture. It is also the case that Brazil and other countries have their African-derived rituals and religious healing systems, such as *Candomblé* and *Umbanda*, but most of the educated classes view these beliefs and practices with ambivalence, if considered part of their cultural identity. African-derived elements of popular ritual practice in Spiritism appear to be disappearing from Puerto Rico, perhaps because of accelerating acculturation to U.S. values and ways of seeing the world.

Preliminary analysis of 12 interviews of medical doctors who are also Spiritist practitioners yielded descriptions of the ways in which they relate to Spiritism in their clinical practices. Some report their awareness of spirit presences in hospitals or in their offices, and say it is necessary to support patients and other health care professionals who are frightened by experiences with spirits.

One doctor told us about near-death experiences during his tenure as a resident in a regional hospital.

> I had a patient there who went flat line about 3 times (signaling death on the cardiograph) and I was with my friend who was an internist. She (the patient) had come out of this condition in the past, and she was always very afraid. This last time I had been working on her for about 11 minutes, and I was finally able to bring her back, but we really did not expect her to last too long. When she came out she was completely peaceful and even smiled. So we said, "Why don't we ask her? She came out so peaceful." We said, "Maria, can you finally tell us? You were out for a long time. This time you came back very peaceful, you were smiling. Can you tell us what happened, what did you see?" She told us, "You'll see," and she smiled. The dirty dog did not even tell us; we were dying of curiosity.

Since practicing Spiritists have psychic abilities (*videncias*), by which they see, hear, or feel something within the bodies of other persons, the doctors involved in Spiritism acknowledge their unusual abilities to diagnose patients when the patients have not verbalized a particular symptom or condition. These visions and inner feelings often come as a surprise to the doctors, who then use their medical skills to check on the spirit-derived information. In several cases, doctors reported that patients recovered from their illnesses when all that the doctors had done was to lay hands on them. One physician actually reported his surprise to his patient that a "cure" had been achieved without any medical intervention. He said that he had not given the patient any medicine or other type of intervention, but the patient indicated that he fully recovered.

Some of the doctors also have mediumistic faculties and report that 1 of their personal spirit guides may appear in their clinics when they are treating patients who believe in spirits. Some of their patients also see these spirits and acknowledge them. Those who incorporate spirits report that they are unexpectedly given previously hidden information about patients' illnesses. One doctor who gradually developed extensive mediumistic faculties and then began to heal in Spiritist centers had his cases anonymously reported at a medical conference:

> A friend of mine presented some of my cases at a medical congress here in Puerto Rico, "Alternative Medicine by Doctor X," and the hall was packed. There were a lot of physicians that really wanted to know about this stuff, but when he showed all of this evidence there was a big roar, to the point that I left. I was in another room and I realized what was going on, and I said, "I'll leave before somebody says he's in the other room." I thought, no, there are many physicians who send their patients to me; it's a question of teaching them.

It was a huge surprise when last year (27 years after the project ended) Spiritists in Ponce told me that the project had been mentioned on the radio!

On a recent visit I encountered 3 people who knew about the project and asked when such a project might be repeated. At the time of the project, and for several years after, we received media notice and mostly positive comment. The outstanding feature that created a legacy, I believe, was the health department's sponsorship and integration into its community mental health programs, thus initiating a process of legitimization of Spiritism. However, many doctors who are Spiritists still do not want that aspect of their lives to be known by other doctors or the general public. Most are not attendees or members of a Spiritist center, but some are. I have been able to establish a few direct links between the project and doctors who believe in Spiritism. For example, one of our participants during the second year, a (then) young neurologist who chaired the Department of Public Health at the medical school in that region, still talks about the project. At the time he attended our seminars and gave some lectures on neurology, he also privately consulted 1 of our leading mediums for his own problems. He recently confirmed that the experience of Spiritism through the project "changed my life." As he said joyfully, "My life then made sense to me. It also changed my way of looking at my patients, who were no longer bundles of neurons and electrochemical properties." This doctor continues to practice neurology and study Spiritism, but only discusses his beliefs with close friends. In another case, a doctor who was the medical director of a hospital where the project was based during 1 year has continued to be involved with Spiritism and attends a center. This doctor currently offers integrative medicine in her private practice.

It appears that the project's aim to build a bridge between a popular religious healing system and medical and mental health care has been achieved in a way that not even the spirits could have predicted.

Conclusion

I suggest that healing with spirits, in various culturally patterned ritual forms, will probably continue over the twenty-first century, and perhaps beyond. The opening wedge for greater legitimization is that spirituality is now being seriously considered a part of the therapeutic tool-kit by some medical doctors and psychiatrists as well as allied mental health care professionals in the United States and Western Europe (Koenig 2007; West 2004). Some health care professionals (medical doctors and psychologists) are discussing how to integrate traditional healing practices into primary health care and psychotherapy (Moodley and West 2005; Pulchalski 2006). It appears that new bridges between healing alternatives, including Spiritism, have emerged in the last 3 decades in Puerto Rico, as elsewhere. These bridges are mainly within the individual practices of medical and other mental health care practitioners such as psychologists rather than community oriented and based on referrals between alternative healing systems. The larger question now is whether these alternatives should be integrated into public mental health care services as viable preventive or ameliorative interventions for emotional distress or disorder, given their current status as individual practice alternatives. It could be argued that increasing awareness (and even practices) related to alternative healing systems by the dominant biomedical system makes the case for inclusion in the public mental health care system even more compelling. It also leads to research and expanded understanding of these alternative healing systems.

Responding to the WHO initiative for collaboration between modern and traditional health sectors in relation to HIV/AIDS care, a recent study of community perspectives in Zambia identified three key areas: protection of traditional medicine and just compensation of the healers; improvement in the healers' preparation; and education of groups of providers and enhanced community involvement (Kaboru et al. 2006).

These kinds of studies illustrate the importance of an anthropological approach to health policy, one that seeks to discover the degree of awareness and participation of healers endorsed by the community. Regarding mental health care policy, studies such as that by Ravi Shankar et al. (2006) illustrate the anthropological approach when they seek to understand how "common mental disorders" are explained by traditional healers in a non-Western culture (in this case, south India). The message is clear that not only is there a new appreciation of the role of spirituality and religion in mental health and health care, but medical pluralism is now being seen by health policy makers as important to serving local communities in an optimal way. This is not only related to developing societies. For example, Kiesser et al. (2006), referring to Mexican Americans, assert that biomedicine and traditional CAM are not opposed health care systems if their practitioners learn to dialogue and understand how each system might be integrated into the practices of the other system. This was exactly what the Therapist–Spiritist Project in Puerto Rico did 30 years ago. There have been small, local experiments in many communities across the world over the past decades, but the pluralistic approach to mental health care policy has yet to take hold in an official way. The Puerto Rican experience and the Navajo medicine man project (Bergman 1973) were mere seedlings of an idea that is still searching for fulfillment across the world.

Acknowledgments

Four studies were funded by the National Institute of Mental Health (NIMH) and sponsored by the Department of Health of Puerto Rico: 1968–1969, Social and psychological aspects of Spiritism in Puerto Rico, NIMH (MH-14246–01);

1969–1970, Social and psychological aspects of Spiritism in Puerto Rico, NIMH (MH-17997–01); 1976–1979, Therapist–Spiritist Training Project in Puerto Rico, NIMH (MH-14310–03), Health Department of Puerto Rico, Rio Piedras, Puerto Rico; and 1979–1980, Therapist–Spiritist Training Project in Puerto Rico, NIMH (MH-15992–01), Health Department of Puerto Rico, Rio Piedras, Puerto Rico. See Koss-Chioino (1980, 1992) for details on the projects and the subject. I acknowledge my appreciation to the Department of Health of Puerto Rico, which sponsored the projects, and to the National Institute of Mental Health, which funded them. I also acknowledge a few of the many wonderful persons who assisted in these studies: Hector Rivera Lopez, Fredeswinda Roman, Edgardo Rivera Saez, don Jorge Quevedo (now deceased), Doña Clara Millan (now deceased), Dr. Michael Woodbury, Jose Gomez, and many others—researchers, mental health professionals, and Spiritists—too numerous to mention (some of whom have passed over but are still with me in spirit). These institutions and persons are not responsible for what I report, however.

References

Ademuwagun ZA, Ayoade, JA, Harrison I, Warren M, eds. (1979) *African Therapeutic Systems*. Waltham, MA: Crossroads Press.

Alegria M, McGuire T, Vera M, Canino G, Matias L, Calderon J (2001) Changes in access to mental health care among the poor and the nonpoor: Results from the health care reform in Puerto Rico. *American Journal of Public Health* 91(9):1431–1434.

Bergman RL (1973) A school for medicine men. *American Journal of Psychiatry* 130(6):663–666.

Bibeau G (1985) From China to Africa: The same impossible synthesis between traditional and Western medicines. *Social Science and Medicine* 21:937–943.

Boehnlein J (2006) Religion and spirituality in psychiatric care: Looking back, looking ahead. *Transcultural Psychiatry* 43(4):634–651.

Brodman K, Erdman AJ, Wolf HG (1956) *Cornell Medical Index Health Questionnaire Manual*. New York: Cornell University Medical College.

Colon H, Canino G, Robles R, Lopez C, Orraca O (1998) *Household Study: Needs Assessment Program for Substance Abuse Services*. Commonwealth of Puerto Rico: Mental Health and Anti-Addiction Services.

Csordas T, Lewton E (1998) Practice, performance, and experience in ritual healing. *Transcultural Psychiatry* 35(4):435–512.

Cushman LF, Wade C, Factor-Litvak P, Kronenberg F, Firester L (1999) Use of complementary and alternative medicine among African-American and Hispanic women in New York City: A pilot study. *Journal of the American Medical Women's Association* 54:193–199.

Ezeji PN, Sarvela PD (1992) Healthcare behavior of the Ibo tribe of Nigeria. *Health Values* 16(6):31–35.

Gaines AD (1992) *Ethnopsychiatry: The Cultural Construction of Professional and Folk Psychiatries*. Albany, NY: State University of New York Press.

Garrison V (1977) Doctor, espiritista or psychiatrist? Health-seeking behavior in a Puerto Rican neighborhood of New York City. *Medical Anthropology* 1:64–85.

Gonzalez M (2007) Ecosicologia. *El Dia.* 2 September San Juan, Puerto Rico.

Hansen H (2004) Faith-based treatment for addiction in Puerto Rico. *Journal of the American Medical Association* 291:2882.

Harwood A (1977) *Rx: Spiritist as Needed.* New York: John Wiley and Sons.

Hess D (1991) *Spirits and Scientists: Ideology, Spiritism and Brazilian Culture.* University Park, PA: Pennsylvania State University Press.

Kaboru BB et al. (2006) Communities' views on prerequisites for collaboration between modern and traditional health sectors in relation to STI/HIV/AIDS care in Zambia. *Health Policy* 78:330–339.

Kiesser M, McFadden J, Belliard JC (2006) An interdisciplinary view of medical pluralism among Mexican-Americans. *Journal of Interprofessional Care* 20(3):223–234.

Koenig HG, ed. (1998) *Handbook of Religion and Mental Health.* San Diego, CA: Academic Press.

Koenig HG (2007) *Spirituality in Patient Care: Why, How, When and What.* Philadelphia, PA: Templeton Foundation Press.

Koenig HG, McCullough M, Larson DB (2000) *Handbook of Religion and Health: A Century of Research Reviewed.* New York: Oxford University Press.

Koss JD (1975) Therapeutic aspects of Puerto Rican cult practices. *Psychiatry* 38:160–170.

Koss JD (1976) Religion and science divinely related: A case history of Spiritism in Puerto Rico. *Caribbean Studies* 16(1):22–43.

Koss JD (1977) Social process, healing and self-defeat among Puerto Rican spiritists. *American Ethnologist* 4(3):453–469.

Koss JD (1980) The Therapist-Spiritist Training Project in Puerto Rico: An experiment to relate the traditional healing system to the public health system. *Social Science and Medicine* 14(B):255–266.

Koss-Chioino JD (1992) *Women as Healers, Women as Patients: Mental Health Care and Traditional Healing in Puerto Rico.* Boulder, CO: Westview Press.

Koss-Chioino JD (2000) "Traditional and Folk Approaches among Ethnic Minorities." In: *Psychological Intervention and Treatment of Ethnic Minorities: Concepts, Issues, and Methods.* 2nd edition. JF Aponte, J Wohl, eds. Needham Heights, MA: Allyn and Bacon, pp. 145–163.

Lake JH (2007) "Omega-3 Fatty Acids." In: *Complementary and Alternative Treatments in Mental Health Care.* JH Lake, D Spiegel, eds. Washington, DC: American Psychiatric Publishing, Inc.

Lake JH, Spiegel D, eds. (2007) *Complementary and Alternative Treatments in Mental Health Care.* Washington, DC: American Psychiatric Publishing, Inc.

Lambo TA (1978) Psychotherapy in Africa. *Human Nature* 1:38–40.

Maclean U, Bannerman RH (1982) Introduction: Utilization of indigenous healers in national health delivery systems. *Social Science and Medicine* 16:1815–1816.

Miller WR, Thoresen CE (2003) Spirituality, religion and health: An emerging research field. *American Psychologist* 58(1):24–35.

Moodley R, West W (2005) *Integrating Traditional Healing Practices into Counseling and Psychotherapy.* Thousand Oaks, CA: Sage Publications.

Moreira-Almeida A, Lotufo N, Koenig HG (2006) Religiousness and mental health: A review. *Revista Brasileira de Psiquiatria* 28(3):242–250.

National Drug Intelligence Center (2003) Puerto Rico and the Virgin Islands Drug Treatment Assessment. July. Available at: http://www.usdoj.gov/ndic/pubs3/3950/

index.htm#Contents. Cited in Hansen, H. (2004) Faith-Based Treatment for Addiction in Puerto Rico. *Journal of the American Medical Association* 291:2882.

Pargament K (1997) *The Psychology of Religion and Coping: Theory, Research, Practice*. New York: Guilford Press.

Puchalski CM (2006) *A Time for Listening and Caring: Spirituality in the Care of the Chronically Ill and Dying*. New York: Oxford University Press.

Ramsey, S (2002) WHO launches first global strategy on traditional medicines. *Lancet* 359:1760.

Ravi Shankar B, Sarvanan B, Jacob KS (2006) Explanatory models of common mental disorders among traditional healers in rural south India. *International Journal of Social Psychiatry* 52(3):221–233.

Rogler LH, Hollingshead AB (1961) The Puerto Rican spiritualist as psychiatrist. *American Journal of Sociology* 67:17–21.

Rogler LH, Hollingshead AB (1965) *Trapped: Families and Schizophrenia*. New York: John Wiley and Sons.

Ruiz P, Langrod J (1976) Psychiatry and folk healing: A dichotomy? *American Journal of Psychiatry* 133:95–97.

Sifre Lajara R (1974) *La Aurora del Pueblo* No. 71 (Sept.-Oct.).

West W (2004) *Spiritual Issues in Therapy: Relating Experience to Practice*. New York: Palgrave Macmillan.

WHO-UNICEF (1978) *The Promotion and Development of Traditional Medicine*. WHO Technical Report Series 622. Geneva: World Health Organization.

World Health Organization (2002) *Traditional Medicine Strategy, 2002–2005*. Geneva: World Health Organization.

9

Indigenization of Illness Support Groups for Lymphatic Filariasis in Haiti

JEANNINE COREIL AND GLADYS MAYARD

Introduction

Social scientists describe indigenization as the process of transformation that often occurs when social institutions developed in one context are transplanted into a totally different social context (Atal 1981; Bar-on 1999; Ho, Peng, Lai, and Chan 2001). As globalization transforms the cultural landscape near and far, observers are paying increasing attention to the process of indigenization of social forms and institutions. Cultural borrowing has intensified in pace and degree, in many directions, taking both predictable and surprising paths. No longer do we think of culture change as homogenizing and unidirectional; the post-colonial paradigm recognizes multiple sources of influence as well as the emergence of unique, localized patterns of cultural expression (Appadurai 1996; Sahlins 1999).

This chapter examines the process of indigenization that occurred within support groups organized by the authors with a grant from the World Health Organization (WHO) to provide psychosocial support and health education for women living with lymphatic filariasis (LF) in Haiti. It describes the cultural transformation of the groups into distinctly Haitian forms, and addresses the evolution of the groups to meet basic subsistence needs of members. Implications of this trajectory are the focus of the discussion.

Attention to indigenization, intended or not, is widely viewed as an essential component of directed change programs, variously labeled "local adaptation," "cultural tailoring," "cultural sensitivity," "cultural competence" or similar notions. However, in the latter approaches, adaptations are usually made by planners before implementing a program, while the focus of indigenization is on how program recipients themselves modify and transform activities. Despite notable attention to designing culturally competent programs in recent years, the concept of indigenization per se has received only limited theoretical attention in the social science literature.

The concept of indigenization gained currency during the 1970s when scholars from developing countries reacted to neocolonialist domination of social science by Western disciplines, calling for the development of independent, locally meaningful theoretical frameworks and methodologies for guiding research and scientific discourse. Interest grew during the 1980s, with much attention to disciplinary adaptation, including the epistemologies and practices of psychology, social work, and sociology (Adair 1999; Nimmagadda and Cowger 1999; Park 1988). Medical anthropological studies of indigenization have tended to focus on the ways in which institutions of Western medicine have changed in response to their introduction into different cultural contexts (Cheung 1989; Kleinman 1980). Others have examined the indigenization of popular culture within health contexts, such as Mattingly's analysis of how some children with disabilities in the United States come to terms with their conditions partly through identification with Disney characters (Mattingly 2006).

Illness support groups began to flourish in the latter half of the twentieth century in Western industrial nations. Propelled by the confluence of the self-help movement, increasing medicalization of everyday life, and resistance to biomedical dominance, support groups proliferated to encompass every conceivable misfortune from addictions, bereavement and victimization by violence, to cancer, disability, and sexually transmitted diseases (Powell 1994; Riessman and Carroll 1995). Self-help through peer support dovetailed with the rise of health promotion as a public health strategy, with its emphasis on empowering individuals to take charge of their health, achieving high levels of wellness through continual self-improvement, and incorporating community-based participatory approaches as key elements of a "healthy citizen" ethic (Petersen and Lupton 1992). Research on support groups has emphasized key features such as democratic principles of organization, core values of self-reliance and empowerment, and an antiprofessional stance. Groups rely on the use of catharsis, confession, modeling, problem solving and consciousness raising to promote change in attitudes and behavior. Finally, many groups promote social change through advocacy and public awareness (Humphreys and Ribisl 1999; Kessler, Michelson, and Zhao 1997).

Considerable variation in goals and fundamental principles occurs across different types of support groups. For example, "Twelve Step" addiction support groups are modeled on the principles of Alcoholics Anonymous, which rely heavily on spiritually based notions of personal change through "working the steps," and helping others on an individual basis. Because of the tenet of member anonymity and an organizational avoidance of political or social agendas, Twelve Step groups do not engage in advocacy activities, nor do they attempt to influence policy, legislation, or regulation. In contrast, cancer and other chronic disease support groups are often sponsored by larger organizations whose mission includes research funding, political action, and social change.

Apart from mission and goals, support groups also vary in terms of organizational culture, group ethos, or "community narrative" (Lavoie, Borkman, and Gidron 1992; Rappaport 1994; Riessman 2001). Each type of group tends to develop its own ideology or model for dealing with the shared problem, and this ideology is often codified in "sacred writings" such as the "Big Book" of Alcoholics Anonymous (Levine 1988). The group's culture provides a template for how one should ideally relate to and live with the shared condition. It has been suggested, for example, that gender composition of groups may influence the degree of emotional sharing that is normative within a group. Whereas prostate cancer support groups tend to stress keeping abreast of the latest scientific developments in treatment for the disease (Coreil and Behal 1999), breast cancer support groups typically emphasize the importance of maintaining a positive outlook on one's situation as a means of promoting personal growth and enhanced quality of life (Coreil, Wilke, and Pintado 2004).

Lymphatic Filariasis

Lymphatic filariasis (LF) is a parasitic disease transmitted by mosquitoes that damages the lymphatic system, causing painful inflammation and swelling of the legs and feet, and sometimes leading to severe disfigurement and elephantiasis. The disease is endemic in 83 countries, including Haiti, where a history of colonial settlement, heavy importation of African slaves, continuous sugar production, dense population and deforestation, and conditions of poverty perpetuates sustained transmission (Coreil 2000). Disease patterns vary by world region, and in the Americas lymphedema and elephantiasis of the leg are more common in women than in men, whereas men are more frequently affected by hydrocele, or enlargement of the scrotum.

Lymphatic filariasis is caused by tiny thread-like nematode worms called filaria that migrate to and live in the host's lymphatic vessels. Eight different kinds of filaria cause diseases in humans: about 90% of LF is caused by

Wuchereria bancrofti, the parasite found in Haiti. The parasite is transmitted in the larval stage (called microfilaria) from an infected host to another person through a mosquito bite. Several species of mosquitoes are involved in transmission, with the *W. bancrofti* parasite being carried by *Anopheles*, *Culex quinquefasciatus*, and *Aedes*. The life cycle of the parasite begins with the mating of male and female worms within a host. The female worm produces microfilaria, which circulate at night in peripheral blood vessels of the human body. Female mosquitoes ingest microfilaria while taking a blood meal from an infected person. The microfilaria develop into larvae in the thoracic muscles of the mosquitoes, and enter another human body through the punctured skin of a mosquito bite. After an incubation period of 6 to 12 months, millions of microfilaria enter the circulatory system. Most infected persons do not show signs of disease and never experience troublesome symptoms. It is estimated that about 120 million people worldwide have asymptomatic conditions (WHO 2000). For reasons that are poorly understood, a minority of people develop complications related to damage in the lymphatic system and kidneys. Lymphatic damage increases the risk of periodic adenolymphangitis (ADL), acute inflammatory attacks that can cause fever, vomiting, and painful swelling of the skin, lymph nodes, and lymphatic vessels surrounding affected limbs (Figure 9.1). Other parts of the body, especially genitals and breasts, can

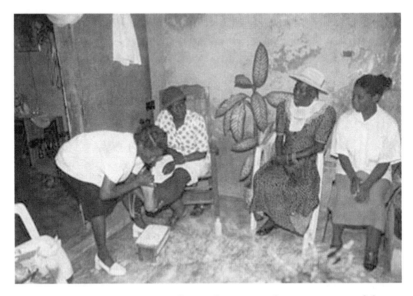

Figure 9.1. Support group members observe a demonstration of leg care practices for the management of lymphedema and prevention of acute attacks associated with lymphatic filariasis. http://www.who.int/tdr/tropical_diseases/databases/imagelib.pl

also be affected. Attacks occur several times a year and usually last 5 to 7 days. Lymphedema and fibrosis accompany acute attacks, and over time, repeated swelling of tissues leads to gradual enlargement of the limb or other affected area. The advanced stage of the condition called *elephantiasis* is characterized by enlargement, deep skin folds, dermatosclerosis, and papillomatous lesions. In Haitian women, lymphedema and elephantiasis of the lower leg and feet is the most common complication of LF. In men, as is the case worldwide, the most common impairment is hydrocele, or inflation of the sac surrounding the testes with fluid. Primary LF infection usually occurs in childhood, with the more advanced complications appearing in adulthood. The chronicity of the disease and its physical impairment make it one of the most serious disabilities associated with infectious disease (WHO 2006).

Global control of LF has experienced significant development over the past decade. In 1997 the WHO identified LF as one of 6 potentially eradicable infectious diseases, and in 2000 launched the Global Programme to Eliminate Lymphatic Filariasis (GPELF, WHO 2007). The program has 2 components, 1 focused on primary prevention through interruption of transmission of the infection, and another focused on morbidity control, through alleviation of suffering in affected individuals. Global health care companies and other private, public, and international organizations have partnered with the WHO to provide drugs free of charge to participating governments. The prevention strategy relies on mass distribution of the drug diethylcarbamazine (DEC) combined with albendazole or ivermectin, within endemic communities over several years. These drugs eliminate circulating microfilaria and prevent vector transmission. However, they do not destroy adult worms, and they have no impact on lymphedema, ADL, and other complications of LF. To alleviate suffering in affected persons, therapeutic programs focus on prevention of acute attacks through a regimen of careful skin hygiene and avoidance of skin punctures to prevent infections, antibiotic treatment of infections, and control of fever and pain. Morbidity control programs include patient and family education in disease management, professional training of health care providers in current treatment approaches, and community education to promote understanding and reduce social stigma attached to the condition.

Lymphatic Filariasis in Haiti: Background to the Support Group Study

Our study took place in the coastal town of Léogane (pop. 20,000), located about 30 km west of Port-au-Prince. In this community, the *W. bancrofti* antigen prevalence exceeds 50%, microfilaremia is present in about one-third of the population, 5% of women have chronic symptoms of lymphedema or elephantiasis, and about a third of men are affected by hydrocele (Eberhard, Walker, Addiss, and Lammie 1996; Lammie et al. 1998; Raccurt 1986). Sugarcane production and its related industries, including rum manufacturing, are important in the local economy. Most residents, especially the less wealthy ones, live in houses with limited protection from mosquitoes. An ethnographic study conducted in 1996 described the cultural context of LF in the Léogane community (Coreil, Mayard, Louis-Charles, and Addiss 1998). Lymphedema of the leg, locally known as *gwopye*, was traditionally considered to be a supernatural illness caused by spells and sorcery. Few natural explanations were offered, probably because of LF's incurable, lingering nature. The few natural causes identified included foot injury; exposure to cold, worms, or microbes; and stepping in foul water. Traditional treatments of lymphedema included bloodletting, cupping, and leeches to remove the "bad blood," and symptom-reducing herbal treatments.

Today, those with lymphedema and elephantiasis continue to suffer from community stigmatization and public ridicule. Further worsening the condition are the physical changes and disabilities inherent to lymphedema, which include limited mobility, walking, and standing, and the challenge of finding suitable footwear. These limitations further inhibit social and economic activities like family gatherings and marketplace selling, and are exaggerated by occurrences of bacterial ADL, or "acute attacks." They often cause the sufferer to be bedridden and completely dependent on others for basic needs such as eating (Dreyer et al. 2001).

Before the mid-1990s, global medical treatment for LF was limited to palliative care and in some areas, unnecessary surgery or amputation. Patients were advised that there was no cure for the disease and its debilitating sequelae, and they were counseled to learn to live as best as they could with its physical and social impairment. In the 1990s, Dr. Gerusa Dreyer of Brazil pioneered a simple regimen of skin hygiene and physical therapy that dramatically reduced secondary infections, acute attacks, swelling, and discomfort from LF (Dreyer, Addiss, Dreyer, and Noroes 2002). The regimen can be implemented at home using common household soap and water and elevation of affected limbs. Moreover, it does not require supervision by highly trained professionals and therefore requires minimal infrastructure and resources. The effectiveness of this low-cost regimen was demonstrated in populations around the world and has since become the standard of care for this disease (Dreyer et al. 2001). The basic LF regimen was first introduced to Haiti in 1994 at Sainte Croix Hospital in Léogane, an institution that has since been designated the National Referral Center for Filariasis.

Patients interviewed during our ethnographic study expressed profound gratitude to the hospital for offering them hope for a better life with this condition. For many patients, who were mostly women, it was the first time they had the opportunity to talk to others suffering from the same problem, and they were strongly motivated to sustain contact with other affected women. When asked about their preferences for learning more about LF and its management, and given a range of options including home visits by health workers, media communications, and support groups, respondents expressed a strong desire for women's support groups as a preferred strategy. Anticipated benefits of support groups reported by respondents included (1) sharing experiences of coping with common life situations affected by the disease; (2) reducing personal feelings of social isolation because one is "different"; (3) having the opportunity to observe reduction in symptoms among other patients, reinforcing confidence in treatment efficacy; and (4) exchanging practical advice about home care and adherence to the treatment regimen. Building on this perceived need, a support group program was designed to complement the clinical services of the hospital.

Funded through a grant by the World Health Organization/World Bank Program for Research and Training in Tropical Diseases, the Filariasis Support Group Program was initiated in 1998 by a project team consisting of the authors and outreach staff of the hospital filariasis treatment program. It was designed as a community trial of a low-cost intervention that offered many advantages for chronic disease management in resource-poor settings (Coreil, Mayard, and Addiss 2003). The objectives of the program were to assess the acceptability of support groups for LF in this setting, measure the educational and psychosocial benefits of participation in LF support groups, gain a better understanding of the process of indigenization of the support groups as they were adapted to fit the local cultural context, and evaluate the applicability of the support group model for community-based chronic disease management in other resource-poor settings. This chapter addresses the third objective of the study, by analyzing the theoretical and practical implications of the indigenization process that occurred in the Haitian context.

In Western societies, support groups attract a largely middle-class membership; rarely do socially disadvantaged populations like ethnic minorities or low-income groups participate in support groups (Kessler et al. 1997). Reaching these marginalized groups has been a challenge and has required specialized approaches. We expected to face this same problem when introducing the support group concept in Haiti, and in anticipation adapted a model used to develop ethnic minority support groups in the United States (Henderson, Gutierrez-Mayka, Garcia, and Boyd 1992). The model uses the concept of cultural competence within an ethnographic framework to foster the community's involvement in forming and growing support groups (Henderson et al. 1992). The model assumes that all populations, even those that are hard to reach, will engage in support group activities if these activities are introduced in a way that is congruous with the community's cultural values. The approach emphasizes participant recruitment using face-to-face personal contact and uses a 5-phase strategy: (1) targeted ethnographic survey; (2) indigenous support leader training; (3) participant recruitment; (4) support group implementation; and (5) feedback and evaluation. Since a focused ethnographic survey of

LF had already been completed in the study community, our project focused on phases 2 through 5.

The support group concept has affinity with a broader array of self-help groups such as contemporary "Mother's Clubs" and even deeper historical roots in Haiti, with some forms dating to the nineteenth century, such as the cooperative labor associations and grass-roots peasant societies that engage in mutual aid and civic projects (Smith 1999). Nevertheless, there existed no indigenous model for the peer support group focused on coping with illness. Only in recent years have illness-related support groups been organized in Port-au-Prince for chronic diseases such as diabetes and HIV/AIDS. In the global arena, Dr. Gerusa Dreyer has organized "Hope Clubs" for people with LF in Brazil, where large assemblies of affected individuals and their families gather to promote community awareness and understanding about the illness, as well as a more positive image of those living with the condition (Dreyer and Addiss 2000).

Implementation of the Support Group Program

Five support groups were organized in 1998 for women affected by LF in the study community. Groups were limited to women because of the low prevalence of leg disability among men in the study community and because informants expressed a strong preference for women-only support groups. The groups were recruited from the urban area of Léogane, and 3 groups were organized in rural areas surrounding the town and located at varying distances from the hospital (1, 3, and 8 km). By the end of the first year, there were 80 women enrolled in the groups. The groups began meeting once a week, and this schedule was maintained, by choice of the members, throughout the project. In the beginning, groups followed a common format; then over the course of the first year individual groups were given the flexibility to alter meeting format and content through processes of participatory planning and management.

Project personnel included the principal investigator (first author), the field director (second author), a support group coordinator, and 5 peer leaders recruited from the LF patient population of Léogane. The principal investigator was based in the United States and made quarterly trips to the study community for staff training, supervision of intervention activities, and planning of data collection. The field director lived in Port-au-Prince and commuted to Léogane most weekdays to manage all aspects of study activities. The project coordinator lived in the study community and had the responsibility for day-to-day operations, including planning and communication with group facilitators and purchase of supplies. The 5 group leaders were women from Léogane who had LF and showed the strongest potential to successfully carry out the role of a facilitator, as assessed by the field director through a process of training and evaluation of performance. During organizational meetings for the support group program, 10 candidates for the positions of facilitators were identified by the field director on the basis of evidence of leadership ability and communication skills. The field director then invited these candidates to participate in a week-long training workshop on development and management of illness support groups. Participants who showed the strongest potential for group facilitation were selected on the basis of ability to articulate the goals of support group meetings, organizational skills, and demonstrated ability to effectively moderate a group.

The American Cancer Society (Hermann, Cella, and Robinovitch 1995) describes 3 phases of support group development: phase 1, where members find commonalities, seek out information and explore alternative ways of alleviating problems; phase 2, where members provide mutual support, share experiences, offer help, redefine the illness experience, and uncover new ways of coping; and phase 3, in which the group may be brought to a close (if goals have been met) or become a long-term project (whether goals have been met or not). In later stages, it is also common for members to organize social action and advocacy. The focus of such advocacy and action initiatives is determined by how the members come to define the fundamental social conditions underlying the problem (Levine 1988). For example, the Women's Movement consciousness-raising groups of the 1970s produced a broad agenda for political action and societal change focused on achieving equal rights for women.

Our goal was to organize self-help groups for women with LF and achieve at least the first and second phases of support group development by the end of the second year. Achieving long-term sustainability of the program by the end of the project's duration, meaning that the groups would continue to meet after external funding ended, was a secondary goal. In the first year, facilitators were charged with establishing trust, formulating group norms and goals, encouraging the sharing of group members' experiences, and providing structure via planned agendas and organized activities. In the second year, facilitators were to develop a core participant group, recruit new members, and maintain group momentum.

We recruited support group participants through personal contact with patients during a clinic visit, expanding invitations through personal networks of program staff and patients, and through home visits by support group leaders. The urban groups met in a local school classroom, and the rural groups met on the verandas or in the yards of members or their relatives. The sociodemographic profile of the membership was fairly typical of the rural Haitian female population. About half were literate, with the typical participant having completed elementary school. About two-thirds of the women were Catholics;

most non-Catholics belonged to the Episcopal Church, which supports the local hospital. Approximately two-thirds of the women were married or partnered, and the group had an average of 4 living children. The majority of members made a living through small-scale farming, marketing of produce and other goods, and various small business enterprises. Most participants had been living with LF for 10 to 20 years.

The format and content of meetings initially was modeled along guidelines disseminated by the American Cancer Society for the development of peer-led self-help groups (American Cancer Society 1995). Peer leaders (women affected by the illness themselves) opened the meetings with an explanation of the purpose of support groups, generally described as a way to provide education and support for people living with a particular condition. Next, an educational segment provided information about home care practices for lymphedema and other symptoms of filariasis. Members were given an opportunity to share personal stories about living with LF. Sessions were concluded with the sharing of refreshments and socializing. We expected that in time this basic model would evolve, as it was adapted to the local cultural context.

The educational component of support group activities was adapted from the "listening group" method pioneered in Nigeria in which women listened to a series of audiotapes on the treatment and prevention of malaria. In Haiti, 10 tapes featuring culturally appropriate characters and stories were developed for a hospital LF patient education program. The tapes were broadcast on the Ste. Croix Hospital radio station to the entire Léogane community. These tapes and their accompanying take-home manual and illustrated booklets were the core educational tools used in the support groups. The stories on the tapes were dramatized vignettes with character dialogue that illustrated aspects of filariasis transmission and treatment. Each story's theme related to a verse from a song specifically composed for the program. Known as "the Filariasis Song," the tapes repeated the catchy song about a central character, Jesula, and each subsequent tape added new verses. Group members enthusiastically embraced the song as their theme song, making it popular in the community, especially among those with the illness and their families.

Project staff recorded the organizational activities that fostered program development and the indigenization process. This included making community contacts, distributing project information, making logistical arrangements, recruiting facilitators and participants, implementing the support groups, and troubleshooting problems. Special attention was given to documenting the decisions to modify program activities as circumstances dictated. The principal investigator kept separate notes on project development, relations with institutions such as hospitals and schools, staff training activities, and project management during supervisory visits and through telephone, fax, and written communications.

The support group coordinator kept a weekly log of coordinating responsibilities, including facilitator-planning meetings and meeting arrangements (e.g., purchase of refreshments and materials). Group leaders logged group activities, attendance, program format and content, and any problems encountered and their management. To facilitate monitoring the meeting process and quality a meeting assessment form was developed. Completed meeting assessment forms, weekly facilitator logs, and the group coordinator log were regularly collected by the field director; copies were mailed to the principal investigator.

At the end of the program's first and second years semi-structured questionnaires were given to all group members as well as to a comparison group of women with LF who did not participate in the support groups. The surveys elicited (1) demographic information; (2) illness history; (3) knowledge of and attitude toward *gwopye*; (4) quality-of-life measures; (5) home management practices; (6) daily living activities; and (7) assessment of support group participation. The first survey was administered in 1999 to 79 members and 77 controls; the second survey was administered during the summer of 2000 to 83 members and 101 controls. Members and controls did not differ in sociodemographic characteristics, with the exception of religion. More support group members were non-Catholic (41%) as compared to controls (25%). Items related to indigenization included perceived benefits of support group participation, ranking of preferred meeting activities, identification of problems in group functioning, and suggestions for improving the support group program. Univariate and bivariate analyses were conducted on indigenization-related variables using SAS software.

Indigenization of the Support Groups

During the support groups' first few months of meeting, a culturally meaningful, distinctly Haitian meeting format evolved that included several key features. Meetings began with a prayer recited by a selected member and made relevant to a particular time and place. The prayer was followed by a religious hymn, singing of the filariasis song, and then announcements and personal news. Some groups then did foot exercises or leg massages. Next came the educational portion of the meeting, which consisted of group discussion of health-related topics or discussion of the dramatized sketches from the tapes. Group members requested practical skills training in crafts, so lessons in paper floral art and sewing were incorporated into the meetings. Meetings were closed with another personalized prayer and hymn, and refreshments purchased with grant funds were usually served after the meetings. At first, light snacks of fruit juice and crackers or cookies were served, but when the women requested more substantial food, nutritious meal-like refreshments of chicken, vegetables, and rice were provided.

Key to maintaining group members' interest in the weekly meetings was to offer a variety of activities, practical skill instruction, nourishing refreshments, and ensuring that the meetings contained significant expressive and spiritual elements. Each group selected the skills they wished to be trained in; one group chose to learn sewing, another to assemble a collection of medicinal plants, a third focused on traditional handicrafts, and the large urban group chose paper floral art. Because group members expressed such strong interest in learning lucrative crafts, the budget for the second year was modified to provide more funding for handicraft instruction and materials. Educational topics at the meetings were also selected by the group members and included a comprehensive overview of filariasis and its management, male–female relationships, sexuality and contraception, family life, and other issues.

The Haitian women were less interested in sharing personal illness stories than is typical in North American and European support groups (Cain 1991; Cope 1995; Gray, Fitch, Davis, and Phillips 1997). In the Haitian groups, enthusiasm was fueled by opportunities to learn about and discuss a broad array of health topics beyond LF and family life issues, and to acquire income-generating skills. They wanted to learn "new" things at the meetings, not hear about the familiar problems of living with the disease, so leaders were challenged to develop a varied educational program. Spirituality and religion were clearly important to the meeting structure, and much of the meetings' style was influenced by church experiences. For almost all members, church groups (prayer, choir, sick visitation, missionary, church upkeep) were the only other type of small group meeting in which they had formally participated; it is not surprising that this experience shaped the support groups.

In Haiti, as in many places worldwide, many local organizations and groups hold large, end-of-the-year parties around Christmas. Likewise, the support groups had annual festival-like events during December in which all groups worked together to create a community-wide program. Occasions of much celebration, the parties displayed the women's crafts and were attended by community and hospital officials, providing an opportunity for increased program awareness. The 1999 party was particularly festive, with large pots of food, a special order cake, music, skits, a Master of Ceremonies, singing, speeches and a souvenir gift for members. Bright paper flowers crafted by the women themselves decorated the walls, and rows of handmade clothing and carved gourd bowls covered display tables. A large banner that was stretched across the street proudly announced the group's identity: *Groupe Support*.

Early in the first year, the 2 urban groups were combined into a single group because members of both groups preferred meeting on the same day, and as a means to conserve resources by paying a single craft instructor. We did not observe differences in process or outcomes of the program when the urban group was compared with the 3 rural groups.

Individual and Collective Outcomes

In the fall of 1999, stimulated by suggestions from project leaders, the groups began discussing the formation of an association that would represent all of the support groups. The motivations behind these discussions were to strengthen the organizational structure of the program, enhance long-term sustainability, and provide a mechanism for seeking local funding. Over several weeks, discussions with project management staff and hospital administrators took place in each support group. The idea was enthusiastically received at all levels, and by early 2000, a charter had been developed for FADES: *Femmes en Action Pour le Developpment et la Sante* (Women in Action for Development and Health). The project field director played a leadership role in facilitating the formation of the organization. The women wanted the association to be open to all women of the Léogane area. FADES was officially registered with the national Ministry of Social Affairs in August 2000. Soon after, the field director began work on a proposal for continuation of funding through FADES.

Possible association-sponsored projects were also discussed, with a focus on the prospect of a shoe-making operation. A consultant had developed a model shoe for large feet in 1997 with the idea of engaging patients in a microenterprise activity, and this idea was revisited as a potential FADES project. The principal investigator sought technical assistance from the shoe company Birkenstock USA and although the company could not respond to the request, they donated 80 pairs of sandals to the support groups. The idea of the shoe project resurfaced several times over the years, but never got off the ground.

Results from the annual surveys document both objective and perceived individual benefits of support group participation. Objective advantages of support group participation, as evidenced by comparing members with geographic controls, are summarized in Table 9.1 and reported in more detail in Coreil et al. (2003). Benefits of participation included better quality of life, greater understanding of the disease, more consistent home care practices, and fewer illness symptoms. Perceived benefits of support group participation identified by members are elaborated here because they relate more directly to the subject of indigenization. Overall, across the 2 years' surveys, the most commonly cited benefit of support group participation was learning new practical skills such as floral art and sewing. Other reported benefits included gifts, encouragement, refreshments, and new information.

Table 9.1. Summary of Benefits Found in Comparisons of Support Group Participants and Neighborhood Controls (Coreil, Mayard, and Addiss 2003)

COMPARISON GROUP	SIGNIFICANT FINDINGS	NONSIGNIFICANT FINDINGS
Support group members vs. controls	Greater knowledge of illness etiology (vector transmission)	No differences in illness history, leg size, and demographic variables
Support group members vs. controls	Higher proportion practice of daily foot hygiene and leg elevation	No differences in reported frequency of acute attacks
Core members vs. irregular attenders and controls[a]	Lower reported frequency of acute attacks	No differences in time spent thinking about the illness
Core members vs. irregular attenders and controls	Fewer reported difficulties living with the condition	No differences in reported shame or embarrassment
Core members, irregular attenders and controls	Dose response relationship with daily foot hygiene and leg elevation	Quality of life measures did not show clear dose-response relationship

[a]Core members are defined as having participated in both 1999 and 2000 surveys and having attended 65% or more of meetings across both years. Irregular attenders did not participate in both surveys or attended less than 65% of meetings. Controls did not participate in support groups.

Expressive Culture, Self-Help, and Entrepreneurialism

This project successfully demonstrated that the illness-focused support group model could be adapted to the Haitian context. Enthusiastic participation was sustained over 2 years, with consistent weekly meetings containing a high level of activity and an increasing demand for program expansion into new geographic areas and types of activity. Peer leaders and members alike showed great pride in their groups' accomplishments. Indigenization of the support groups occurred early in the development process. Unlike most support groups in developed country settings, the Haitian groups showed minimal interest in talking about illness-related problems; this kind of catharsis was viewed as a waste of time. Instead, members wanted to learn new things, master practical skills, and organize for economic ventures. They valued opportunities to develop and display their artistic talents. Strong religious and spiritual themes were expressed in meetings, with elements of the expressive Haitian culture incorporated into song, prayer, humor, role-playing and story telling.

Many of the elements featured in the support groups parallel themes discussed by Jennie Smith (1999) in her analysis of indigenous mutual aid groups in rural Haiti. Smith notes the important role of music and expressive culture in Haitian social life and Caribbean society generally. She writes that, "in rural Haiti, music is commonly employed as a tie that binds and defines collectivities of people" (p. 154). Songs, sayings, proverbs and story telling permeate everyday life and ritual activities. Joining together in cooperative labor groups and civic associations has deep roots in Haitian history, with some traditional forms dating to the colonial era. Collective labor efforts typically involve "drumming and singing, animated conversations, laughter, performance, disputes, and play" (p. 86). The ethic of sharing and helping one another (*yonn ede lot*) is deeply engrained in Haitian society, as reflected in myriad expressions and proverbs. Various indigenous aid groups contribute to the economic, material, social, health, and spiritual well-being of their members and communities, engaging in activities such as re-thatching houses, transporting heavy loads, or cultivating new gardens. It is common for such groups to direct their energy toward social change. Finally, the importance of religious expression in such institutions is noteworthy. In the Haitian context, "faith and social practice constantly presuppose and inform each other" (p. 190), a feature shared with Latin American social movements generally.

There were many reasons why the lymphedema support groups were interested in forming microenterprise endeavors. Of great influence was the strong entrepreneurial spirit that is an inherent part of Haitian culture. Born of the country's unstable history and economic necessity, this spirit of self-sufficiency motivates Haitians to take advantage of opportunity, and to find creative ways of "doing a little business" (*ti komès*) through side jobs to make ends meet. This clever business sense is particularly well developed among Haitian women, who are responsible for the marketing of produce and goods that supports their families. To expand their illness support group activities to include ways to generate income was a natural progression.

Another influence that caused an increased interest in microenterprise endeavors was the way in which the idea of microenterprise ventures was spread among the groups as they worked with community lymphedema programs. For example, a bednet-sewing cooperative, sponsored by the University of Notre Dame with funding from the Kellogg Foundation (KOLEMO 1999), began production in the program's second year, and some support group members were involved in various roles. A third influence on the rise in popularity of microenterprise endeavors was the discussion of creating profitable cooperatives in group meetings, which stimulated a great deal of interest and discussions on feasibility. The political and economic instability in Haiti was a final and significant cause of interest in forming microenterprises. Substantial increases in the cost of living were making it hard for Haitians to meet their basic needs and propelled people to explore every opportunity to earn more income.

Agency, Community Development, and Support Groups

Other studies of illness support groups in culturally diverse populations have documented a process of transformation to adapt group process to better fit the needs and expectations of members, analogous to what we describe as indigenization in this chapter. For example, Mathews (1999) studied African-American breast cancer survivors in eastern North Carolina, who broke away from a hospital-sponsored support group program to form their own peer support group modeled along traditional ethnic themes. The women rejected the dominant model of cancer survivorship espoused by the group that emphasized a positive outlook, a "fighting spirit," and used military and sports metaphors to idealize individual responsibility and decision making. The women's own culturally sensitive support group allowed members to express feelings of doubt and pessimism, and emphasized quality of life, spiritual values, and family relationships. In another study, Henderson et al. (1992) describe a process of cultural adaptation for support groups organized to help Hispanic caretakers of Alzheimer's patients in the United States cope with stress and role demands. Modifications to typical support group activities included use of local Spanish language media to recruit participants, finding a locale where members felt comfortable, serving ethnic foods for refreshments, and focusing discussions on topics salient to this cultural group.

The Haitian lymphedema support groups were transformed from a support group focused on education and coping with an affliction into a locally relevant self-help organization, with roots in indigenous Haitian mutual aid institutions, but clearly influenced by contemporary socioeconomic realities. The values of creative self-expression, spirituality, pragmatism, and entrepreneurialism emerged through the reinterpretation of support groups to meet context-specific circumstances. Groups evolved into utilitarian self-development associations focused on meeting material needs in a climate of political and economic insecurity. The shift in focus of the groups toward microenterprise activities can be viewed as a natural progression into social action and advocacy functions commonly found in many, though not all, support groups and interest groups in industrialized societies. Levine (1988) has suggested that what propels some groups into social and political action is the discovery that the fundamental conditions underlying their problem are *social* rather than *personal*. For example, he points out that what came out of the consciousness-raising groups of the women's movement in the 1970s was the realization that women's oppression was rooted in sexism and social discrimination.

What is noteworthy about the Haitian women's case is the focus of collective action on economic development rather than on social change or political advocacy. Although the local women recognized the social origins of their condition (e.g., poor housing, exposure to mosquitoes), the women's fundamental needs for income-generating skills took precedence over illness concerns and psychological well-being. In resource-rich countries, the standard of living is such that basic needs for food, housing, and education and the necessities of family life are readily satisfied for a majority of the population, thus enabling citizens to focus on higher-level needs such as quality of life and fulfillment through helping others. In affluent countries, a postmaterialist worldview gives priority to nonmaterial values such as self-expression, belonging, and intellectual or aesthetic satisfaction (Inglehart 1997). In contrast, people living in impoverished settings such as Haiti (as well as economically disadvantaged segments of rich countries) do not have the luxury of investing time and energy in activities focused *exclusively* on nonmaterial pursuits, although as we have seen, self-expression and creativity were indeed championed by the women's LF groups. Our results suggest that sustained participation in the support groups beyond the acquisition of illness management skills and expressive and spiritual engagement required the incorporation of economically beneficial activities in order to retain involvement of participants.

The Legacy

Our experience also points to the importance of community context from the standpoint of infrastructural support for self-help sustainability. The project described in this chapter was funded by an external grant that financed the support group operations for 2 years. Following this, the LF support group program was expanded and continued for 4 more years (2000–2004) in the Léogane area through a grant from the Presbyterian Church, USA. Excluding management salaries, the operational costs of the program were approximately $1.00 per participant per meeting. Sixteen groups continued the original program of education, support, and skills training, and closer ties were established between the local hospital treatment program for LF and the community-based support groups. However, the ending of the second grant coincided with the onset of political upheaval in Haiti following the military coup in 2004 that deposed President Jean Bertrand Aristide, as well as diminishing resources to sustain the hospital LF treatment program. The hospital has scaled down its clinical treatment program for LF dramatically, staffing has been reduced to a skeletal structure, and in the shuffle, support group activity has ceased altogether. In a resource-poor setting such as Haiti, without adequate infrastructural support it is extremely difficult to sustain a "luxury" program such as support groups. Interestingly, however, it appears that a long-term legacy of the support group program may be in the area of microenterprise activity. Group leaders learned in 2006 that a grant application submitted 2 years before to establish a "community store" managed by women with LF would be funded by a U.S. nonprofit foundation. The funding agency hopes that if the community store project is successful in Léogane, it can serve as a model for similar projects in other parts of Haiti. The viability of this opportunity is uncertain, however, given the precarious institutional and political–economic setting in which the model project would be implemented.

Conclusion: Indigenization and Beyond

In conceptualizing indigenization of self-help groups in resource-poor settings, local-level circumstances, and in particular material needs, have a strong influence on shaping the goals of the groups, particularly with regard to collective activity beyond the realm of individual coping with the common problem. In their review of women's movements in the Third World, Ray and Korteweg (1999) reached a similar conclusion, arguing for a shift of focus in comparative work from the macro level to the local level, to better understand how women's collective identities and interests are constructed, as well as the ideological and material conditions under which mobilization occurs (Ray and Korteweg 1999:66–67). Furthermore, our findings extend Levine's (1988) theory that self-help groups are mobilized to action when the group recognizes fundamental social causes of the problem. In poor settings, basic economic needs independent of the shared identity that brought the group together may take precedence over advocacy for the focal problem.

The findings also have relevance for contemporary discourse on cultural diversity and cultural competence in public health programs. Underlying this discourse is the assumption that best practice involves the tailoring of programs to fit the needs of ethnically and culturally diverse populations. Yet, the Haitian women took a "universalistic" approach (support groups) and, given free reign, "tailored" it themselves to meet their needs. The main difference here is that the identification of need remained in the hands of the program participants, whereas the design of most public health programs remains in the hands of experts, despite the infusion of "participatory" values in the planning process. The Haitian case also highlights the importance of planning for some degree of indigenization to occur during the implementation phase of a program. The concept of cultural tailoring must be broadened to include both program design and implementation, and should be redefined as an ongoing process of adaptation involving beneficiaries as active participants in shaping emergent outcomes.

Acknowledgments

Reproduced with modifications by permission of the Society for Applied Anthropology from Jeannine Coreil and Gladys Mayard, "Indigenization of

Illness Support Groups in Haiti", SfAA 2006, *Human Organization* 65(2): 128–139. Also, some content is taken from a report published in 2003 (Coreil, Mayard, and Addiss, 2003). The study was supported by Grant No. 970184, Social, Economic and Behavioral Branch, Tropical Diseases Research, World Health Organization, Geneva, Switzerland, 1998–2001.

References

Adair JG (1999) Indigenisation of psychology: The concept and its practical implementation. *Applied Psychology: An International Review* 48(4):403–418.

American Cancer Society (1995) *Guidelines on Support and Self-Help Groups*. Atlanta, GA: American Cancer Society.

Appadurai A (1996) *Modernity at Large: Cultural Dimensions of Globalization*. Minneapolis, MN: University of Minnesota Press.

Atal Y (1981) The call for indigenization. *International Social Science Journal* 33(1):189–197.

Bar-on A (1999) Social work and the "missionary zeal" to whip the heathen along the path of righteousness. *British Journal of Social Work* 29:5–26.

Cain C (1991) Personal stories: Identity acquisition and self-understanding in alcoholics anonymous. *Ethos* 19:210–253.

Cheung FM (1989) The indigenization of neurasthenia in Hong Kong. *Culture, Medicine and Psychiatry* 13(2):227–241.

Cope DG (1995) Functions of a breast cancer support group as perceived by the participants: An ethnographic study. *Cancer Nursing* 18:472–478.

Coreil J (2000) Local history and environment: Filariasis in Haiti. Paper presented at the Society for Applied Anthropology Annual Meeting. San Francisco, CA, March 21–25.

Coreil J, Behal R (1999) Man-to-man prostate cancer support groups. *Cancer Practice* 7(3):122–129.

Coreil J, Mayard G, Addiss D (2003) *Support Groups for Women with Lymphatic Filariasis in Haiti*. Geneva: World Health Organization.

Coreil J, Mayard G, Louis-Charles J, Addiss D (1998) Filarial elephantiasis among Haitian women: Social context and behavioral factors in treatment. *Tropical Medicine and International Health* 3(6):467–473.

Coreil J, Wilke J, Pintado I (2004) Cultural models of illness and recovery in breast cancer support groups. *Qualitative Health Research* 14(7):905–923.

Dreyer G, Addiss D (2000) Hope clubs: New strategy for lymphatic filariasis-endemic areas. *Bulletin of Tropical Medicine and International Health* 8(1):8.

Dreyer G, Addiss D, Bettinger J, Dreyer P, Noroes J, Rio F (2001) *Lymphoedema Staff Manual: Treatment and Prevention of Problems Associated with Lymphatic Filariasis*. Geneva: World Health Organization.

Dreyer G, Addiss D, Dreyer P, Noroes J (2002) *Basic Lymphoedema Management: Treatment and Prevention of Problems Associated with Lymphatic Filariasis*. Hollis, NH: Hollis Publishing.

Eberhard ML, Walker EM, Addiss DG, Lammie PJ (1996) A survey of knowledge, attitude, and perceptions (KAPs) of lymphatic filariasis, elephantiasis and hydrocele among residents in an endemic area of Haiti. *American Journal of Tropical Medicine and Hygiene* 54(3):299–303.

Erwin DO, Spatz TS, Stotts RC, Hollenberg JA, Deloney DE (1995) Increasing mammography and BSE in African American women using the Witness Project model. *Journal of Cancer Education* 11(4):210–215.

Fukui S, Kamiya M, Koike M, Kugaya A. (1996) Applicability of a Western-developed psychosocial group intervention for Japanese patients with primary breast cancer. *Psycho-Oncology* 9:169–177.

Gray R, Fitch M, Davis C, Phillips C (1996) Breast cancer and prostate cancer self-help groups: Reflections on differences. *Psycho-Oncology* 5:137–142.

Gray R, Fitch M, Davis C, Phillips C (1997) A qualitative study of breast cancer self-help groups. *Psycho-Oncology* 6:279–289.

Henderson JN, Gutierrez-Mayka M, Garcia J, Boyd S (1992) A model for Alzheimer's disease support group development in African-American and Hispanic populations. *Gerontologist* 33(3):409–414.

Hermann JF, Cella DF, Robinovitch A (1995) Guidelines for support group programs. *Cancer Practice* 3(2):111–113.

Ho DYF, Peng S, Lai AC, Chan SF (2001) Indigenization and beyond: Methodological relationalism in the study of personality across cultural traditions. *Journal of Personality* 69(6):925–953.

Humphreys K, Ribisl KM (1999) The case for a partnership with self-help groups. *Public Health Reports* 114:322–328.

Humphreys K, Woods MD (1994) "Researching Mutual-help Group Participation in a Segregated Society." In: *Understanding Self-Help Organizations: Frameworks and Findings*. TJ Powell, ed. Thousand Oaks, CA: Sage, pp. 62–87.

Inglehart R (1997) *Modernization and Postmodernization: Cultural, Economic and Political Change in 43 Societies*. Princeton, NJ: Princeton University Press.

Isaac DR (1989) A transcultural support group for Turkish women in poor health. *Community Health Studies* 13(1):49–58.

Kessler RC, Mickelson KD, Zhao S (1997) Patterns and correlates of self-help group membership in the United States. *Social Policy* 28:27–46.

Kleinman A (1980) *Patients and Healers in the Context of Culture: An Exploration of the Borderland between Anthropology, Medicine, and Psychiatry*. Berkeley, CA: University of California Press.

King G, Stewart D, King S, Law M (1999) Organizational characteristics and issues affecting the longevity of self-help groups for parents of children with special needs. *Qualitative Health Research* 10(2):225–241.

KOLEMO (1999) *Kolemo Annual Report*. South Bend, IN: Congregation of Holy Cross.

Lammie PJ, Reiss MD, Dimock KA, Streit TG, Roberts JM, Eberhard ML (1998) Longitudinal analysis of the development of filarial infection and antifilarial immunity in a cohort of Haitian children. *American Journal of Tropical Medicine and Hygiene* 59(2):217–221.

Lavoie F, Borkman T, Gidron B (1992) *Self-Help and Mutual Aid Groups: International and Multicultural Perspectives*. New York: Hawthorne Press.

Levine M (1988) An analysis of mutual assistance. *American Journal of Community Psychology* 16(2):167–188.

Lopez EDS, Eng E, Randall-David E, Robinson N (2004) Quality-of-life concerns of African American breast cancer survivors within rural North Carolina: Blending the techniques of Photovoice and grounded theory. *Qualitative Health Research* 15(1):99–115.

Luke DA, Roberts L, Rappaport J (1991) Individual, group context, and individual-group fit predictors of self-help group attendance. *Journal of Applied Behavioral Science* 29(2):216–238.

Maslow A, Lowery R (1998) Toward a Psychology of Being. 3rd ed. New York: Wiley & Sons.

Mathews HF (1999) Negotiating cultural consensus in a breast cancer self-help group. *Medical Anthropology Quarterly* 14:394–413.

Mattingly C (2006) Pocahontas goes to the clinic: Popular culture as lingua franca in a cultural borderland. *American Anthropologist* 108(3):494–501.

Moore RJ (1996) African American women and breast cancer: Notes from a study of narrative. *Cancer Nursing* 24(1):35–43.

Nimmagadda J, Cowger CD (1989) Cross-cultural practice: Social worker ingenuity in the indigenization of practice knowledge. *International Social Work* 42(3):261–276.

Park P (1988) Toward an emancipatory sociology: Abandoning universalism for true indigenization. *International Sociology* 3(2):161–170.

Petersen A, Lupton D (1992) *The New Public Health: Health and Self in the Age of Risk*. London: Sage.

Powell TJ, ed. (1994) *Understanding the Self-Help Organization: Frameworks and Findings*. Thousand Oaks, CA: Sage.

Raccurt CP (1986) La filariose lymphatique en Haïti: Sequelle historique ou problem d'avenir pour la santé publique a l'échelon régional? *Bulletin Société Pathologie Externe* 79:745–754.

Rappaport J (1994) "Narrative Studies, Personal Stories, and Identity Transformation in the Mutual-help Context." In: *Understanding the Self-help Organization: Frameworks and Findings*. TJ Powell, ed. Thousand Oaks, CA: Sage, pp. 115–135.

Ray R, Korteweg AC (1999) Women's movements in the Third World: Identity, mobilization, and autonomy. *Annual Review of Sociology* 25:47–71.

Riessman F (1992) Self-help is more than support groups: An interview with Frank Riessman. National Self-Help Clearinghouse. www.selfhelpweb.org/morethan.html. Accessed May 18, 2001.

Riessman F, Carroll D (1995) *Redefining Self-Help: Policy and Practice*. San Francisco: Jossey-Bass.

Sahlins M (1999) What is anthropological enlightenment? Some lessons of the twentieth century. *Annual Review of Anthropology* 28:i–xxiii.

Smith JM (1999) *When the Hands Are Many: Community Organization and Social Change in Rural Haiti*. Ithaca, NY: Cornell University Press.

Stewart GM, Gregory BC (1992) Themes of a long-term AIDS support group for gay men. *Counseling Psychologist* 24(2):285–303.

World Health Organization (2000) Lymphatic filariasis. Fact Sheet No. 102. www.who.int/mediacentre/factsheets/fs102/en. Accessed October 14, 2007.

World Health Organization (2006) Lymphatic filariasis: the disease and its treatment. www.searo.who.int/en/Section10/Section2096_10583.htm. Accessed October 14, 2007.

World Health Organization (2007) The Global Programme to Eliminate Lymphatic Filariasis (GPELF). www.who.int/lymphatic_filariasis/disease/en. Accessed October 14, 2007.

10

Using Formative Research to Explore and Address Elder Health and Care in Chiapas, Mexico

NAMINO GLANTZ

The Story of Doña Karina

My concern with elder well-being in Chiapas was initially inspired by my interaction with Chiapanecos during my extended residences (1990, 1991–1992, 1994–2000) there. The case of Doña Karina,[1] whom I met in 1995, helps to sketch the landscape that motivated me to delve into elder health and care.

I met Doña Karina, a 65-year-old woman, at the birthday party of a mutual friend. I arrived at the door just as she was struggling to knock with a plate of stuffed jalapeno peppers in one hand and a multicolored Jello castle in the other. Doña Karina lived around the corner, and ran a small convenience store out of her front room. It was stocked floor to ceiling with pasta, cereal, soap, candy, chips, soda, and trinkets. I became a loyal customer, and saw her a few times a week.

I worried whenever I saw Doña Karina's store closed, because it meant that she was not feeling well. This occurred more frequently as time went on. She had hypertension, but would take her medication only when she had enough money to buy it. She also said she was on a "forced diet," eating less "good food" because it was too expensive. Arthritis hit her during the dank rainy season. She used to crochet, but her sore joints and poor eyesight bothered her. These symptoms were punctuated by colds, coughs, and indigestion. But Doña Karina always worked.

Over the years, I learned a bit about her life. Among the youngest of 8 children, she was born on a farm, where her parents had toiled for the landowners. As a young girl, she moved to town and worked as a maid in an upper-class home. Around age 16, she married a mason's apprentice. They had 3 children, one right after the other. She hand washed and ironed clothes, charging by the dozen, sold snacks, and raised hens, but found it harder to make ends meet, as her children aged and her husband's drinking increased. When her children were in their early teens her husband left for good, which she described as a relief. Soon, her daughter married and moved to Mexico City. Her youngest son died in a car accident. Her oldest son helped her set up her front-room store and often dropped off her grandson when he and his wife needed a babysitter; but as she became weaker and the child grew bigger, he was a handful.

Doña Karina had very little income, and had lived without child support, pension, savings, or property. She lived in a house that her son "lent" her, a cement-block structure, with a few rooms, no frills, and a Coca Cola emblem painted on the front. As larger grocery stores sprung up around her, she began selling women's clothing, cilantro from her tiny garden, and *tostadas* in her doorway on weekend evenings. Every peso counted. Support from the government was meager. Doña Karina had no health insurance because neither she nor her husband or her children had formal employment. For health care, she waited in line at the Health Center, with varying results, or simply went to the nearby pharmacy. To her frustration, she was not old enough or poor enough to receive public assistance, although she did recount one instance of public investment. One year, when the governor was scheduled to tour the "quaint, colonial" streets of Comitán, all of the streets on the route between the Town Hall and the Mayor's mansion were paved. Doña Karina's dusty dirt road turned into a beautiful street, which increased car traffic and clientele.

Doña Karina had siblings, an ex-husband, children, nieces, nephews, grandchildren, neighbors, and acquaintances from the Catholic Church, but she could not really count on anyone for care. In the evenings, she would read the Bible or listen to the radio in the company of only her parrot.

Introduction

In many ways, Doña Karina is representative of the elder women in her city, all caught at the convergence of individual aging, shifts in household-level dynamics, societal health challenges, and nationwide limitations in infrastructure. My concern about whether the families, the state, and/or the community would care for them triggered research that continues to unfold (Figure 10.1).

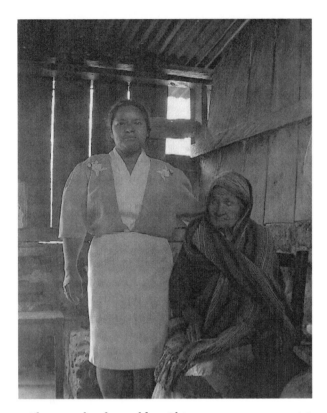

Figure 10.1. Photograph of an elder Chiapaneca survey participant in her home, and the granddaughter who cared for her. (Photo by Namino Glantz)

In this chapter, I detail how I used medical anthropological research to inspire engagement, critical reflection, and collaborative problem solving among key community members to facilitate primary health care for the elderly in Comitán, a small city in the Border Region of Chiapas, Mexico's southernmost state (see maps in Figure 10.2). I outline how broad sociohistoric circumstances have made elder well-being an urgent issue, and how I was propitiously located to study it, given my immersion in academic and in-the-field medical anthropology. After introducing the tenets of formative research, I describe the strategies I used to explore elder health care and to engage others in applying emerging insights. These methods include an interinstitutional forum, surveys, interviews, a strategic planning meeting, and a working group. For each, I illustrate the types of data obtained and the engagement it inspired in this nascent public health initiative. The cases of several study participants exemplify the challenges faced by the elders whom this research aims to help.

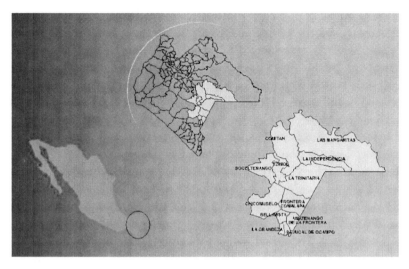

Figure 10.2. Maps of Mexico, the state of Chiapas, and the Border Region of Chiapas.

Context of Elder Care in Mexico

A brief description of the sociopolitical background shaping the nation's health services helps contextualize this research.[2] When the Mexican Revolution ended in 1918, the Constitution was drafted with high public health ideals. In the 1930s, however, depression hit. Recovery took the form of import-substitution industrial development[3] coupled with agrarian reform to assure production of cheap basic foods. The state's programs were managed by a one-party umbrella government under the PRI (*Partido Revolucionario Institucional*). Validated by managed elections from one presidential term to the next, the PRI fostered state-led petroleum and manufacturing industries, but the policy of holding down basic food prices ultimately brought about agricultural crisis and basic food shortfalls. Agrarian producers began to replace basic consumption products (such as corn and beans) with products destined for international commerce that were grown agroindustrially. Subsidies and agrarian reform, along with public education, social security, and health investment, helped keep unrest in check. In the post-OPEC years from 1973 to 1982, Mexico accepted loans for development of petroleum and other developmental infrastructure from the world banking system (Benjamin 1996; Collier 2005). Mexico seemed to have found a solution to its economic woes. But then, world oil prices plunged in 1982, leaving Mexico with ever-escalating external debt and a threat of default. To avert default, the World Bank, the International Monetary Fund, and the Inter-American Bank forced

Mexico to refinance the debt and restructure its budget. The public health budget froze, and the private health care sector grew. In 1994, the Zapatista rebellion, with its epicenter in Chiapas, drew international attention and resources to human rights (including health), and an influx of political refugees, civil society expansion, and entry of middle-class professionals into social and health services. It is in this context that Mexico faces demographic transition (increasing longevity due to decreasing fertility and mortality rates), and epidemiological transition (decreasing infectious and acute illness, with increasing disability and chronic degenerative illness).

Today, distinctive characteristics of Mexico's transitions call for a custom-designed health care response (Martínez and Leal 2003). These characteristics include unusually accelerated aging of the Mexican population (Frenk et al. 2004b; Reyes Fausto 2001), Mexico's growing noninfectious disease burden (García-Peña, Thorogood, Reyes Salmerón-Castro, and Durán 2001), and the perseverance of infectious diseases (Martínez and Leal 2003). Ill health and health care resources are inequitably distributed across the nation and throughout regions (Borges-Yáñez and Gómez-Dantés 1998; Phillips 1991; Salgado de Snyder, González-Vázquez, Jáuregui-Ortiz, and Bonilla-Fernández 2005). The current health system was designed to meet the needs of a younger, more homogenous population rather than those of the emerging group of older adults residing in very distinct contexts. The health-care system is inadequate in that it is characterized by fragmented design that divides people by employment and ability to pay; nonuniversal health insurance coverage; little attention to extra-clinical (household, self, alternative/complementary) care; and low prioritization of health care needs specific to the aged, especially elder women (Borges-Yáñez and Gómez-Dantés 1998; Frenk, Sepulveda, Gomez-Dantes, Knaul 2003; Frenk et al. 2004a, 2004b; Nichter 1995).

Compounding the problem, entitlement among Mexican elders to care and resources in the household may also be tentative and unpredictable. The government may derive some comfort from the pervasive notion that the family has traditionally been and will continue to be an important source of care in old age. Mexican elders are often represented as ensconced in extended family groups (Bonita 1998; CONAPO 2002). Further, demographic transition is supposed to usher in longer lives, a significant postponement of widowhood, a decrease in parents' experience of death among their children, and a greater potential for intergenerational family interaction (Tuirán 2000). These may be romanticized images inspiring a false sense of security, given that the country's "demographic revolution" has also resulted in cultural transformation; changes in household structure and family organization (CONAPO 2001), including a potential decrease in the number of family members physically present in Mexican elders' households (due to divorce, out-migration, urbanization, and falling fertility rates); and shifts in the values (such as familism, age hierarchy, gender roles, and reciprocity) presumed to underlie Mexican elders' entitlement to informal care, with unpredictable repercussions (Aguirre-Molina, Molina, and Zambrana 2001; Bonita 1998; CONAPO 2002; Salgado de Snyder et al. 2005; Soldo, Wong, and Palloni 2002; Tuirán 2000).

In Mexico, there is a sense that the government should be responsible for providing universal health care (Gobierno Federal 2001, 2002), and there is discourse on the moral obligation to provide family-based care. But there is also some recognition that family and state have not resolved the needs of certain subgroups. While not necessarily absolving these two institutions of their responsibilities, some segments of civil society have stepped in to address some of these issues, for instance, women and indigenous populations in Chiapas. Propitious engagement of Mexican civil society and interest on behalf of public policymakers has opened a window of opportunity in which to promote civic and state engagement and collaboration focused on the growing issue of elder well-being. The project I initiated in Comitán represents a step in this direction.

Formative Research through Medical Anthropology

I approached the exploration of elder Chiapaneco well-being from a privileged position—having been fully immersed in Chiapas academically, and then personally and professionally—because of my long-term residence there, during which time I worked at the Comitán Center for Health Research (*Centro de Investigaciones en Salud de Comitán*, CISC). Founded in 1990, CISC touts a deep involvement in health and care in Chiapas. The Center is attentive to vulnerable populations, such as people with HIV, women facing domestic violence, marginalized indigenous populations, and teens (who, in Mexico, generally have little legal control over their own health care). CISC is a trusted source of insight into health problems and interventions, and has honed its ability to facilitate multipartisan, interinstitutional participation. Although I was hired as a researcher, I envision my work as that of a translator—between Spanish and English, medicine and anthropology, quantitative and qualitative, men and women, North and South, rich funders and marginalized Chiapanecos, urban and rural, and theory and reality. My experience at CISC informed and was informed by my subsequent graduate training at the University of Arizona, in a department with a strong tradition of applied medical anthropology. So, concern initially inspired by people like Doña Karina, heightened by living in Chiapas and working at CISC, and shaped by graduate study, evolved into the guiding axes of my research: elders' health problems, their care resources, impact of sociodemographic change, ways to address elders' needs, and my role in the process.

To study these issues, I drew on formative research, defined by Nichter and colleagues (Nichter 1990; Nichter et al. 2002, 2004), as a multistage participatory process that is iterative and draws on multiple methods and participants to identify and define a problem, then develop, monitor, and assess locally congruent interventions. A fundamental tenet of formative research is that the process should be a partnership rather than a top-down study. This requires being sensitive to and working to level hierarchies of power and authority that traditionally frame researcher–subject relationships. All participants need to be self-reflective to promote mutual collaboration, reciprocal respect, and co-learning. The research ought to be sensitive to inequitable relations and tentative collaboration among the many stakeholders, all embedded in structures of power.

Further, each formative research project should become an iterative process, in which research informs subsequent research in an upward spiral of ever-improved methods and understanding. Growing insight and rapport among participants facilitate feedback so that strategies are evaluated and improved in real time. In this way, the research not only yields data, but is also intervention itself. The aim of formative research is to help meet local needs in a culturally congruent way requiring multiple methods, including qualitative research, to achieve a broad and deep understanding. Finally, formative research should be facilitated by ongoing participation of an invited social scientist.

To operationalize this model, Nichter lays out various iterative components:

- Becoming informed about what people do, say, and think about an issue
- Identifying problems and obstacles from perspectives of stakeholders in personal, household, community, and institutional contexts
- Generating intervention options via discussion with local participants invited to reflect on research findings
- Fostering critical assessment and problem solving among this inclusive group
- Investigating how best to implement interventions
- Introducing a process that monitors ongoing responses to interventions, enabling mid-course correction and stakeholder evaluation of the intervention process and outcome
- Evaluating process and outcome indicators of interventions. Evaluation entails being aware of how knowledge about issues and interventions is produced, distributed, and represented among public, institutional, and political audiences (for instance, via a review of popular media to see how health issues are framed, the way people view these issues, and their response in terms of implementing policies and changing behaviors) (Nichter 1990; Nichter et al. 2002, 2004).

The formative research stages help operationalize participatory partnerships to obtain crucial information on context, discourse, and actions that lends itself to meeting local needs in ways that make cultural sense. The iterative spiral of informing and becoming informed, planning, acting, evaluating, reflecting, and developing theory is its trademark. Participants constantly revisit the problem and, equipped with newly acquired insight, reframe it, and adjust responses. In this way, formative research allows for growing insight about people's needs and resources to continually enrich the cycle of research and intervention. Importantly, formative research spotlights often-ignored hierarchies of power and authority that influence health and care, as everyone involved is valued as an expert, and as stakeholders' roles, responsibilities, and relationships shift over the course of the project (Nichter et al. 2004).

In applying formative research to the nascent dilemma of elder well-being in Chiapas, my goal was as much to gather data and refine theories as to initiate and facilitate a process in which the local population was actively engaged. My trajectory through formative research took the form of conducting a number of activities in Comitán (population of 110,000), Chiapas, Mexico. First, I engaged the CISC in conversation and secured the Center's institutional backing. Then, I organized an elder health and care forum with relevant local institutions. Subsequently, I conducted an elder health and health care survey. At the same time, I interviewed elders, home-based caregivers, and formal care providers.[4] When I finished these data collection activities, I convened a strategic elder health and care planning meeting. In this context, I developed an independent elder health working group, and continued to facilitate this group's ongoing work. These steps are detailed subsequently, with examples of the kinds of data, insight, and engagement that each produced.

Interinstitutional Elder Health Forum

I drew on CISC's physical infrastructure (building, computers, library, etc.), accumulated research experience, and institutional stamp of approval to organize an elder health forum. The more than 30 forum participants included elders residing in Comitán, personnel from public and private health and social institutions, local researchers, and representatives from the region's radio and print media. At this forum, participants identified useful, urgent research issues, voiced initiatives for action, and committed to collaboration in research. Recommendations included creating a directory of the diverse individuals and institutions involved in elder health care, forming an elder health working group, and conducting an initial assessment of elder health and health care in Comitán. I later facilitated bringing all 3 of these initiatives to fruition.

In the days following the forum, I monitored media reports to see how issues were framed and the way people viewed and responded to these issues, in order to guide midcourse correction in the research. For instance, one report focused on elder women's health, associating the forum with International Women's Day, a link we had not featured. This spurred later emphasis on the needs of *all* elders (men and women), with the understanding that there are some gender-specific needs and resources. In 1 newspaper, the article on the forum was located next to a piece that stated that "health is a priority for the local government". This renewed my sensitivity to the need to reassert the state's good intentions in the face of emerging data that could be perceived as a critique. Two pieces highlighted the role of CISC in facilitating the forum far beyond contributions of other participating institutions. This prompted me to consider that future events might be hosted by other organizations while featuring CISC less prominently. Finally, to my horror, 2 newspapers featured photographs of me. One had also mistaken me as the director of CISC. I realized that my place in the project was portrayed much too obviously. I would have to transition from dominating the headlines to being a much less visible facilitator. The forum was a clear expression of research that is both intervention and data, and the merging of process and product.

The Elder Health and Care Survey and Interviews with Elders and Home-Based Caregivers

Forum participants designated the lack of baseline information on elders, their health, and health care in Comitán as problematic. Among providers' initial questions was, "Who are these elders and what are their lives like that they come to us so late and in such poor health?" Providers wanted a general description of the elder population in Comitán as well as a "diagnostic assessment" of their problems and care. Practitioners and clinical directors asserted that such an evaluation would provide trusted evidence of the types and distribution of problems and care. These data, they asserted, were required for legitimating the need for change and for negotiating the nature of such change with their superiors. For instance, a participating clinical director asserted, "research results should provide the evidence needed to strengthen and validate calls for funding." CISC, too, contended that such background information would strengthen proposals for funding more in-depth work on elder well-being. Participating elders fervently supported getting to know them and their cohort, asserting, "Yes! You don't know us! No one ever asks us!"

In response, in 2005, I coordinated the design and application of a 240-question survey among older adults in Comitán. Four CISC colleagues and I structured the survey, drawing on insight from previous research, bibliographic reviews, and long-term quotidian interaction with elders in Comitán. With this instrument, we gathered demographic, health, and care data from a purposive sample of 300 elders aged 50 and above, stratified by age, gender, and neighborhood. We sought basic information on the issues that forum participants had identified as relevant to their present challenges. We also included questions comparable to those posed in the nationally representative Mexican Health and Aging Study (MHAS 2003), so that the local state of affairs could be juxtaposed with that of the country, evidencing the urgent need for contextually appropriate action. Participation was voluntary. Recruitment was done largely via door-to-door canvassing. Surveys were often conducted while standing in the entranceway; some sitting inside homes, patios, yards, or businesses; others sitting on the sidewalk. Over 3 concentrated weeks, I conducted over half of the surveys, while my colleagues from CISC pooled their efforts to complete the other half.

This survey yielded quantifiable data, allowing me to generate a detailed description of elder health problems and health care strategies in Comitán. (Table 10.1 provides basic sociodemographic information on 300 elders.) I used the Pearson Chi-square two-tail test to determine the significance of the differences in statistics between men and women, and local and national statistics, reporting P-values for those differences that are statistically significant (at the standard minimal criterion of $P<0.05$). The value of these statistical differences is debatable. On one hand, as *no* subgroup of elders was doing well, the statistical significance of the difference between them is moot. On the other, I used these numbers to engage 2 groups of stakeholders. In the public health world, policymakers draw on statistics such as these to legitimate allocation of resources to populations at risk, in this case, elder women. Among health care practitioners, the hard survey data and numbers, even if not statistically significant, represented a warning sign that certain groups—especially Chiapanecan women—were underserved, striking a nerve in providers who did not need P-values to become engaged in the research.

The survey was posited as—and became—a means of contacting potential elders and caregivers for later interviews. Additionally, the survey elicited more open-ended, free-form information. Many were eager to discuss their experiences, problems, achievements, predicaments, and doubts. Seemingly straightforward survey questions prompted detailed responses. For instance, even the "simple" demographic question, "How many children do you have?" inspired detailed accounts of family and health.

Even before analyzing the data, researchers, elders, caregivers, and providers alike asserted that strategies we might consider as more "ethnographic" (e.g., "talking more with the elders," "asking people what they think, not just checking off boxes") would complement conventional measures, and allow elders more voice. The closed survey questions forced choices between a limited number of options and raised many issues. It was hard to keep elders "on track" in terms of getting through the survey without straying into less structured conversation about what they felt were key details. We decided to delve

Table 10.1. Basic Indicators for Survey Respondents

INDICATORS	% OF MEN SURVEYED	% OF WOMEN SURVEYED	% OF SURVEY SAMPLE
Women			54
Men			46
(Aged 50–105, mean = 64, median = 62)			
Born in Comitán	40	52	46
Speaking a Mayan language	8	9	8
Elementary school education or less	83	94	90
Illiterate	14	24	19
Catholic	79	86	83
No electricity at home	0	1	1
No indoor water faucet at home	21	16	18
No refrigerator at home	28	25	26
Cook with firewood/charcoal (vs. gas)	17	17	17
Television at home	93	91	92
Radio at home	90	87	88
Telephone at home	52	51	51
Ever married	97	98	97
Currently married	83	45	62
Widowed	6	36	22
Separated/divorced	9	17	13
Two or fewer living children	22	22	22
Living alone or with just one other person	28	30	29
Living in own home	78	71	74
Having small business or property (e.g., land)	41	30	35
Relying on public transportation	47	61	55
Owning a car (spouse or self)	20	6	12
Working at a steady job in the past year	63	41	51
Received pension in the past year	14	7	11
Received public assistance in the past year	22	26	24

deeper to access and record the experience behind the numbers, the details of elders' lives, work, and care in clinical settings and at home. This moved me to interview 20 elders and home-based caregivers (a spouse or close relative) in more depth. During survey visits, some informants and/or their caretakers requested that I return, and then agreed to be interviewed. I also made "follow-up" visits to those informants facing the most precarious situations. I oriented these semi-structured interviews with a loose guide consisting of questions designed to delve more deeply into their specific health problems, explore formal and informal health care utilization, broach the topics of male–female and local–national distinctions in health and health care, probe people's hopes and expectations in terms of satisfying their health care needs, and brainstorm about community elder health care needs and strategies. Mostly, however, my visits allowed people to share what they felt was important. This entailed listening and observing. Elders pulled prescriptions and pill bottles from cabinets and bags. Had I noticed the rash on their hands? Did I want to see their insurance card? This scar? They gestured to the material conditions of their home—the leaky roof, the muddy road, the empty water tank. They introduced me to their relatives, friends, and neighbors. Some joined the conversation; others made me promise to visit them again. Frequently, we were also accompanied by generations of relatives staring out from photographs on the walls. Elders offered me water, coffee, soda, a chair, shade. This hospitality came while they often continued their work, which I encouraged them to do. Women washed clothes, cooked, gardened, supervised children, tended their stores. Craftsmen continued sanding and sewing. Other men helped customers, shoveled dirt, arranged building materials. Others saw my visit as a time to rest. I attempted to be relaxed rather than rushed, to listen rather than talk and ask, and to pay attention to the most quiet, reserved people as well as to the dominating talkers. Some of the most quiet survey respondents became quite animated on subsequent visits. Some informants were familiar with earlier population censuses and epidemiological studies, and I wanted to offset biases based on these experiences as participants in—literally, objects of—research by treating them as my teachers, neighbors, fellow community members, and respected elders.

In moving from surveys to interviews, we attempted to shift from our knowledge, categories, and values to those of elders. Although it was convenient for statistical analysis, the survey essentially forced elders' realities to fit our frame of thought. In contrast, the semi-structured interviews were more open conversations. I had a mental checklist for reference, but not a preset sequence of questions. Our conversations were much more balanced or unbalanced in favor of the elders. Additionally, the interviews helped shift from measuring to understanding. For the survey, we wanted to know how many and how much, but the interview was about why and how. This type of question can be less threatening than measuring, especially for more private, sensitive topics, such as financial situation, marital relationships, fears, frustrations, and health problems. Elders truly enjoyed chatting about their family, past, livelihood, and health more than being subjected to a long survey. There was a shift in the nature of the interaction toward enjoyment, equity, and freedom of expression.

Partnering in research with multiple community members and using various methods facilitated triangulation of findings from the start. The forum, surveys, and interviews allowed for cross-checking and ongoing learning, as well as for comparing findings across methods, informants and groups of informants, disciplines, and researchers. We followed up on trends as well as exceptions, contradictions, and anomalies. Rather than pursuing rigor based on measurements, statistical tests, and replicability, we sought trustworthiness. While self-critical awareness was key, group activities (e.g., meetings and informal conversations) also helped, as individuals each added and amended details to develop a more complete and accurate account.

I wove insight from interviews with background data from the surveys to reconstruct real cases of individuals and couples who illustrate a range of scenarios lived by elders in this context. The case of Don Fernando and Doña Lolita is representative of the kinds of qualitative data I collected.

The Case of Don Fernando and Doña Lolita. Don Fernando, the veteran informant at 105 years, was quite wan and hunched over, and his 85-year-old wife, Doña Lolita, was just as slight. I found the two at, literally, the bottom of the town, on the edge of the eastern side of the city, living off a path so muddy and deeply rutted that surely no public transportation passed their door.

Don Fernando and Doña Lolita had grown up in the same Tojolabal farming community about an hour outside of Comitán. For many years before and after the marriage that their families had arranged, they farmed corn and beans. Neither had ever been to school. "There was no school," Don Fernando chuckled. Neither of them had learned to read or write. It was a hard life, they said, even dangerous. In a farming accident, Don Fernando's head had been slashed with a machete. Doña Lolita's glance was downcast as Don Fernando said that they had 7 children, but only 6 still lived. When his wife mentioned that he had been an alcoholic, Don Fernando was equally silent until she recounted convincing him to join an Evangelical church, upon which he stopped drinking. In the early 1970s, their sons became disillusioned with agriculture and decided to try their luck as manual laborers in Comitán. Without help on the farm, the couple followed their children to "the city." In Comitán, they could no longer support themselves without land, literacy, or even Spanish language skills (they spoke only Tojolabal, one of many Mayan languages spoken in Chiapas). Instead, they came to depend on their adult children in exchange for help around the house and with the grandchildren.

The couple lived in a 1-room clapboard structure with dirt floors and a hearth in 1 corner. Doña Lolita still cooked all of their simple meals over wood on her knee-high hearth. She boiled corn before grinding it up to make tortillas by hand. Her husband admitted that she had often burned herself, and that the smoke from the fire had taken its toll on her vision. The combination of her failing eyesight, a widespread symptom of aging, and the poverty that deprived her of both eye care and a gas stove put Doña Lolita at a heightened risk for burns and vision problems. The couple used a toilet in an outhouse next to their house that they had to flush out with a bucket of water from the water tank, next to the wash basin, where Doña Lolita still washed their threadbare clothing. In their house, an extension cord powered a single light bulb dangling from the rafters. The cord ran from next door, where their grandson and his family occupied a larger brick home with a cement floor, gas stove, and television. Occasionally, their son (the grandson's father) and his family would stop by to watch a soccer game and share a meal, but for the most part, their children and grandchildren were now absorbed by life elsewhere.

In much the same way that age and economy combined to expose his wife to health risks, Don Fernando's daily trips to the market illustrated the same problem. With little money, no refrigerator, and no means other than by foot to carry groceries, Don Fernando had to make frequent, energy-demanding trips to the market, where he would have to pay high prices for small quantities of perishable food. To do their shopping, he told me, he had to walk a mile and a half uphill to the market, which I did not believe until I saw him striding back home one day. He held a walking stick in one hand, and had a woven Tojolabal satchel over his shoulder, his two mutts on his heels.

It was clear that Don Fernando was very much in love with his wife, dedicating himself to caring for her and keeping her company. He thought it was unfair that she was so much younger but so much worse off physically, and he described to me how hard and fast she used to work on their farm and praised her for continuing to do their housework. He spoke of his wife in an animated and endearing way and worried aloud about her deteriorating health, functional difficulties, and failing vision. Doña Lolita nodded with a barely perceptible smile on her lips.

The couple's scant diet was made challenging by their nearly toothless mouths, which prevented them from chewing much more than soft tortillas and boiled beans. In addition to her vision problems, Doña Lolita also had itchy feet, headaches, and pain in her neck and extremities. When walking, she needed a broomstick to support her and to avoid tripping. Because of her eyesight, though, she rarely left home, even to go to church. Don Fernando, too, suffered from chronic pain in his waist, neck, and knees. He had grudgingly gone to the Health Center a few times over the past year, but "only when I feel like my blood pressure is high." On the other hand, both elders had self-medicated for pain with pills from a nearby pharmacy (where people often buy medication without a prescription, obtain medication not in stock in health services, and consult employees for advice). Don Fernando confessed, "I've taken more [pills] than I can count." Neither of these elders had been hospitalized recently. Neither had any health insurance, and would only consider going to the hospital in a major health emergency. Their grandson who lived nearby had the most sway over their health-related decisions, as he held the purse strings.

Until 4 or 5 months before I met them, the couple had received minimal financial support and free medication from the Municipal Integral Family Development center (*Desarrollo Integral Familiar,* DIF), a government support program. They were baffled at their last visit when they were told that they were no longer eligible for the cash. They expressed gratitude to their children and grandchildren for the help they provided. Despite this patchwork of assistance, they were visibly needy and openly lamented lack of money and food. Don Fernando said that they never had enough food, "2 or 3 tortillas, that's all." When I asked about wanting to gain weight, he said, "Sure, but what am I going to eat?!"

Elder Women's Health Problems. Surveys and interviews with elders and caregivers yielded an overview of elders and their lives in Comitán and baseline data about problems as experienced by elders. Rather than providing an exhaustive description of elders' demographics, problems, and care strategies, 20 assumptions about elder well-being and care that are commonly held by policymakers and the reality evidenced via formative research are outlined in Table 10.2. Correction of these misconceptions then informed subsequent stages of formative research, in which stakeholders generated and critically assessed intervention options.

In general, surveys and interviews revealed higher reported rates of certain health conditions among elders in Comitán than among their national counterparts. In many cases, however, the maladies plaguing elders in Comitán did not differ greatly from those faced by elders elsewhere; the distinguishing factor was that elders in Comitán confronted ill health with very limited social, economic, and structural resources. This made it difficult to avoid and address problems, and exacerbated them. Despite variation between the scenarios, 3 fundamental threads run through all: (1) economic vulnerability, (2) the inadequacy of local elder health care services, and (3) the differences in elder health and care by gender.

The surveys and interviews illuminated the nuances of these overarching trends as well (see Bonita 1998). Elaborating on the gender variations of elder health and care, I found a variety of problems more pronounced in women than in men (and often than in women nationally): noncommunicable diseases, such as hypertension and diabetes; chronic symptoms, such as swelling, dizziness, fatigue, and urinary problems; chronic pain, especially moderate and severe pain limiting daily activities; dental problems, which affected eating, nutrition, breathing, and self-esteem; poor vision; functional difficulties including climbing stairs, walking, and carrying bags; reproductive health problems, including menopausal symptoms; poor mental health, such as depression, overexertion, sleep deprivation, and memory loss; and nonhealth problems that

Table 10.2. Assumptions about Elder Well-Being and Reality Evidenced via Formative Research

ASSUMPTIONS	REALITY EVIDENCED VIA FORMATIVE RESEARCH
Elders had their basic survival needs covered	Not the case; even water supply was inconsistent, and housing was often substandard. Some suffered from meager diets and malnutrition
Having worked all their lives, elders were financially prepared for their later years and no longer needed to work	The majority was still trying to make ends meet, the men in farming, construction, and carpentry; the women doing domestic and caring work. Many operated small shops out of their homes. Scarcity was a defining facet of life, and many had seen a decline in prosperity over time. Most lived in a modest cement block, often belonging to their children. Many cooked with firewood or charcoal, had no indoor water faucet, refrigerator, or washing machine. Few had property to draw on for emergencies, long-term care, or even to pass on to their children
Poor elders could count on government assistance	Only one quarter had received public assistance in the past year. The gap between elders' needs and institutional responses widened with poverty
Elders were ensconced in large, caring households	Over a quarter lived alone or with just one other person. Over a third were widowed, divorced, or single. Nearly a quarter had 2 or fewer living children. Many were lonely; a few were outright abused and even abandoned
Elders could count on extensive extradomestic support networks	While many had relatives, friends, neighbors who might provide occasional light help, few believed that they could count on these acquaintances for significant support
Support for psychological and physical health needs was provided in clinic by physicians	The little support elders got was predominantly provided at home by close relatives. Beyond home and clinics, a few elders mentioned other institutions that had truly influenced their health for the better: religious (especially Protestant) groups and Alcoholics Anonymous
Elders could count on health insurance to cover their health expenses	Over a third were uninsured. Even those with insurance found coverage confusing and insufficient, with medication not covered, too expensive, or out of stock. Even when insured, tenuous resources meant that elders might be fine until a catastrophic event—a fall, a stroke, a bad stomach bug—forced them to scrape up resources for treatment, while preventing them from working. Chronic health problems—mental and physical—dried up resources, too, especially when drawn out over adulthood

(continued)

Table 10.2. Continued

ASSUMPTIONS	REALITY EVIDENCED VIA FORMATIVE RESEARCH
Health services targeted and addressed elders' most common and limiting health problems	Services targeted diabetes and hypertension, yet the most common problems were dental troubles, mental health issues, and chronic symptoms, such as pain, cough, stomachache, and fatigue. Diabetes and hypertension, too, often went uncontrolled and unsupervised by a physician, even when they limited elders' daily activities
Infectious disease was no longer a concern for the elderly	Elders faced conditions spanning acute and chronic conditions, both infectious and noninfectious in nature. Infectious diseases—especially those affecting the respiratory and digestive systems— plagued elders, predisposed them to later chronic disease, and exacerbated chronic disease
Elders relied on alternative health care	Elders rarely sought alternative care (herbalists, bone-setters, and healers) outside the home
Because there were clinics available in the city, access to and quality of care was not a problem	Elders were unhappy with health-care services because of low quality of care, excessive bureaucracy, long waiting times, poor rapport with providers, lack of medication, staff shortages, and differences in perspective regarding treatment. In the past year, over a third had not seen a physician at all and one fifth had suspected a serious health problem but did *not* consult a doctor, citing lack of money as the primary reason. Over a third had stopped taking necessary medication because of its high cost
Elders were noncompliant as they avoided consults and instead self-prescribed and self-medicated	Elders pieced together a mélange of care, generally ordered in a clear strategic sequence from home remedies and self-medication, through pharmacies, and then to doctors as a last resort. Given limited resources and poor-quality health services, elders used self-care, self-medication, and pharmacy consults as both a first course of action for an illness or injury episode, and as an ongoing strategy for managing chronic health problems. Over a third self-medicated at least once a week, including one-tenth who did so 4 or more times a week. Self-medication was abetted by visits to pharmacies. Nearly one-tenth consulted a pharmacy employee (rarely a trained pharmacist) more than 10 times in the past year. There was no home–pharmacy– physician communication or coordination. So, rather than elders being noncompliant, they were self-regulating in a context of scarcity. The health system was noncompliant by not being reality-based, e.g., by not offering quality care and by prescribing medication that elders cannot afford

(*continued*)

Table 10.2. Continued

ASSUMPTIONS	REALITY EVIDENCED VIA FORMATIVE RESEARCH
Health care satisfied preventive needs	Most elder health consults were aimed at curative and palliative care, rather than preventive care. This meant that elders' conditions were often discovered at a very advanced stage, making treatment more difficult
Elders were free from occupational health problems because they no longer worked	Elders still worked and suffered from past and present occupational health problems, especially common in men, but also in women, related to what is supposed to be a "safe" activity: housework. The burden on poorer elders was higher, as they did more hard manual labor and ate less
Reproductive health was no longer an issue among elders	While participants were beyond their childbearing years, women did complain of lingering reproductive health problems and many spoke of menopausal symptoms and medication
Age was the primary factor in elders' health problems	Elders suffered from a variety of nonmedical, age-independent problems that impacted their health, e.g., marital, occupational, and financial stresses
Elders had healthy lifestyles	Smoking and drinking, very common among men, impacted both men and women greatly. A fifth of men drank or had once drunk alcohol 5 to 7 days a week. A quarter of men had once smoked or currently smoked a pack or more of cigarettes a day
Elders were independent, economically and in terms of making decisions about their own health care	Elders endured economic dependence, looking to grown-up children, spouses, and siblings to cover expenses. Two-fifths were subject to others' decisions about their own health and care. For medical expenses in the previous year, less than half covered all of their own costs
Elders only received assistance	Many elders provided support to others. Some even wished to cut down on the support they provided
The health and care of elder men and women did not differ radically	Elderly women were at a disadvantage in terms of health status, health care, and life conditions

impact health, especially family and marital problems. Further, women in Comitán—more than local men and their national female cohort—had spent more days bedridden and nights hospitalized and had more negative perceptions of their health status.

In terms of health care, women visited doctors more often than did men; however, women, more than men, resisted seeking doctor's care when they suspected a serious health problem, for apparently gender-related reasons (such as shame, gossip, apprehension, and uncertain gains). Women also had less access to insurance-based services than did men. The women in this sample had sought less preventive care and diagnostic screening than did their male counterparts. Women also experienced more problems not prioritized by local services, including chronic pain, menopausal symptoms, and mental health problems. Further, women had less influence over decisions related to their own health than did men. Generally, women depended more on others to cover their health care expenses. In the end, women were more likely than men to simply put up with their health problems.

Research revealed at least 4 gender-specific life conditions that may challenge women's health and care compared to men. First, elder women in Comitán faced a trade-off—that men did not—in terms of marital status and well-being. On the one hand, marriage may allow women satisfying relationships as well as access to health-promoting economic and insurance benefits. On the other, living as single, separated, divorced, or widowed women may afford them more independence and tranquility, as marriage in this context often entailed enduring men's alcoholism and violence. Second, elder women tended to be more dependent than men on grown-up children for support, health-care expenses, and decision making; yet, these relationships were threatened by the dwindling numbers of adult children, and strained by the expectation that elder women would reciprocate with housework and childcare, an expectation not generally imposed on men. Third, elder women's work tended to be more life-long and day-long than men's. In Comitán, most elder women dedicated their lives to domestic work and/or food preparation and sales, patched together with unpaid housework and caregiving. If the "sandwich generation" refers to women who care for their parents and their children, then much of this cohort of women might be referred to as the "club sandwich generation," as they cared for their elderly parents, husbands, children, and grandchildren. Domestic, food, and caring work placed women at a disadvantage, offering them little pay, unsteady salary, and no health insurance or retirement benefits, and physical and mental health problems. Fourth, deficiencies in city infrastructure and household amenities had a greater impact on elder women than on men because prominent women's activities—housework, food preparation, and caregiving—were constrained by inadequate supply of water and cooking fuel and nonavailability of a refrigerator and washing machine. Elder women were also more limited than men by transportation obstacles.

Elder women's disproportionate health problems may be rooted in and exacerbated by the fact that they may not receive the health care that they needed and desired. It was also a function of gender-specific life conditions, primarily the accumulated effects of marriage, children, work, and infrastructure. In addition to noting key contrasts between elder men and women, these same factors permit contrasting among women. Elder women were not a homogenous group, and the "differences that make a difference" between women included whether they were in supportive marriages (with a husband who did not drink, was not abusive, was employed, insured, etc.); the nature of their relationship with their children; their working conditions; and whether they had access to household amenities and quality infrastructure. Women's cumulative gender-specific experiences throughout their lives meant that they frequently confronted illness in old age with less social, emotional, and economic capital than did men.[5]

The following narrative, pieced together from surveys and interviews with Doña Paty and Don Ruben, details how Doña Paty's health was failing; yet, she had not gotten the care she needed, and her life had been one long bout of suffering due to a marriage turned sour by alcoholism and violence, bittersweet interdependence with her children, unprofitable work in domestic service and food sales, and life with few amenities.

The Case of Doña Paty. Doña Paty, a 56 year-old woman, showed me into her front room, containing just a wooden table covered by a Christmas print tablecloth and a few wooden chairs, and nothing more. Perhaps noting my curious glance around the room, Doña Paty explained that the house was so stark because they had to sell most of their few belongings because of their poverty and her husband's alcoholism. "My parents were very poor, so I never went to school, not even one day. I helped my mother at home, and as a teenager began working as a servant, cleaning, washing, ironing. I've done that ever since." She also made *chalupas* (*tostadas* with beans, pork, cheese, and pickled vegetables) and sold them in her doorway on weekend evenings. Her street was not heavily traveled though, and she wondered whether she came out ahead. She had the same doubt about housecleaning.

Doña Paty had 4 children. She cared for her daughters-in-law following the births of her grandchildren, for whom she babysat quite a bit, while her children contributed what they could to keep Doña Paty's household (Doña Paty, her husband, and their youngest [15-year-old] daughter) afloat. Despite having the family around, Doña Paty maintained, "I have felt alone all my life." She was almost always depressed; only her children raised her spirits, but they also filled her with sadness and guilt. Most recently, she lamented that her youngest daughter had been forced to follow her footsteps, leaving school to work as a maid.

"My husband began drinking about 20 years ago. He drinks a lot, he yells at me, and he's very aggressive. I used to drink, too. I think I was even an alcoholic, because I sort of kept my husband company. I drank a lot, maybe half a liter of that liquor they make in Tzimol, almost every day. It all started when my mom passed away. It was just too much for me." Tears ran down her face, "I still walk up to the cemetery to visit her grave."

Doña Paty now seldom drank, but her husband continued to drink and smoke a lot. He had also stopped working. He had been a mason, and she was proud that he built their house. Now he never gave her a cent and he ran up debts, which they had covered at times by selling their possessions. Their only appliance was a television, and her husband dictated when it was on, who watched it, and what they would watch. He controlled many other aspects of their home life. He turned out the lights early. He broke the radio so that they would not listen to music. He no longer ate his meals with the family. He did not let his daughter go out and was always "hovering" over her. He did not let Doña Paty make her own decisions, and did not value her work. He had, in effect, extinguished life and happiness at home. She stopped sleeping with him 2 years ago, and wanted to kick him out of the house, but had been unable to figure out how. Since the onset of her husband's drinking, she had suffered from high blood pressure and severe headaches, "But I don't have any money to go see a doctor or pay for medicine, so I just try to get out of the house or shower to cool off." Don Ruben had also limited Doña Paty's opportunities to socialize with relatives, friends, and neighbors. None liked to be around when he was around, and he discouraged Doña Paty from going out to visit, and even from chatting with neighbors in her own doorway.

Doña Paty asked that I return to visit again, and I did. As I neared the house, I heard her husband, Don Ruben, yelling at their dogs. I knocked hesitantly. Doña Paty ushered me in and quietly explained, "He hasn't drunk for a week, but his character is just as ugly. It's almost worse than when he's drunk because when he's sober he doesn't sleep and he bothers me and my daughter all the time." Nevertheless, Don Ruben did sit and talk with us. He described that after working for 40 years as a mason, carpenter, and electrician, he "retired" 8 years ago. He admitted he often drank bottles of hard alcohol in a day, but asserted that he cut his 1-pack-a-day smoking habit down to 2 cigarettes a day since he began feeling ill. "My health is as low as the ground," asserted Don Ruben. He suffered from hypertension, heart and breathing problems, diabetes, knee pain, stomach discomfort, weight loss, insomnia, hallucinations, and memory loss. Everyday, he took over-the-counter pills from the pharmacy, in addition to prescribed medication. Don Ruben described the government as a scam and the clinics as good for nothing. Doña Paty scolded him for not working and worse. "He has no problem managing his money; he doesn't have any!" his wife quipped with an edge in her voice. Yet, she and their older children paid for Don Ruben's food and medical expenses, and he most likely diverted some of their resources to cover his alcohol and cigarettes.

The interviews and surveys together yielded detailed ethnographic description of elders' environments and challenges, such as that of Doña Paty and Don

Ruben and Don Fernando and Doña Lolita. The surveys and interviews only provided half the story; local health care providers' perspectives were needed to round out the characterization of elder health and care in this context.

Interviews with Health Care Providers

At the forum, mere mention of elder well-being seemed to hit a nerve, and practitioners were poised to share their experiences; however, I was wary of asking them to do so in a group setting, and wanted to avoid putting them on the defensive. In this culture in which "dirty laundry is washed at home," merely suggesting that practitioners and institutions were not doing an adequate job was risky. Beyond endangering their legitimacy and thus their employment, clinical directors might be provoked to put up barriers to future research in their institutions, and individual practitioners might hide shortcomings. I approached this delicate situation with interviews. The 10 practitioners I interviewed spanned the clinical echelons to include social workers, nurses, psychologists, physicians, administrators, and clinical directors. Over about an hour, I conversed with each person in the place of their choice: their office, a café, or a sitting room at home. With prior informed consent, I tape-recorded each interview, and later transcribed these. Some service providers also offered brochures and even CDs detailing programs and services.

I used a three-pronged interview strategy. First, to break the ice, I referenced general topics mentioned in the forum as well as preliminary findings from the surveys and interviews with elders and caregivers. Second, I asked practitioners to describe the official services provided by their institution or practice. This elicited flowery descriptions of what would seem to be an adequate array of support for elders in Comitán. Third, I asked them to share with me the challenges they faced in attempting to provide these services and their dreams for the future of elder care in Comitán. At this point, their official rhetoric rapidly shifted to an unofficial characterization in which they admitted that elder care did indeed fall short of expectations and needs. This exercise allowed me to generate an image of various local elder health care services, idealized as if they functioned as intended, and an illusion of a well-thought-out, well-functioning, comprehensive elder care system. I contrast this view with practitioners' assessment of the problems, shortcomings, and gaps. Their testimony evidences that the rights, programs, and facilities championed by the state may be little more than an empty shell. Large buildings, colorful brochures, and National Elder Health Cards create an illusion that contrasts with providers' critiques of the system. Prominent critiques were that access to services was insufficient and that the range of problems addressed was circumscribed. Another complaint was that providers had an immense task and very limited resources, which were poorly allocated, and aimed at state priorities (e.g., family planning) rather than local needs. Further, services were provided in clinic only, excluding elders with transport and mobility obstacles. Practitioners pointed out that there was no articulation among the individuals and institutions serving elders, making it easy for elders to fall through cracks and hard for providers to collaborate. Providers had not yet been made accountable for elder health care. Pressure from civil society, the state, and the international community to address elder health paled in comparison to pressure to control infectious diseases and safeguard maternal and infant health. Finally, practitioners observed that disconnects between providers and higher-ups were often rooted in centralized health planning.

In addition, providers blamed elders and their families for elders' poor health, while elders blamed the state and its employees. Practitioners argued that elders neither took care of themselves at home, nor took advantage of available health services. Instead, providers felt that elders self-prescribed and overmedicated themselves. Practitioners also contended that elders' families did not take care of their elders, while providers lacked the resources and institutional support to offer quality elder care.

The interviews illuminated that the schism between providers and elders was due to the fact that health practitioners and institutional directors were from the old elite families and the new professional class; elders, in contrast, tended to be of the marginalized social echelons. This situation persisted because providers spent their days in clinics, and did no home visiting. Given this lack of interaction, and despite their concern and good intentions, providers had a distorted view of elders' situations. On the other hand, practitioners were ideally positioned to identify interinstitutional challenges, underlying misallocation of state resources, and misguided priorities among policymakers. My next task was to create a space in which to discuss these contrasting perspectives and then engage stakeholders in using this insight.

Strategic Planning Meeting and Creation of Independent Working Group

The most widely embraced proposal at the forum and in interviews with providers was to hold a meeting in which interested individuals might strategize together. In response, I organized, this time independently of CISC, a strategic planning meeting. I created a CD of the forum's PowerPoint® presentations, proceedings, and a participant directory. I then visited stakeholders (providers, clinical directors, researchers), giving them a forum CD and newspaper clippings, and inviting them to the meeting.

This "strategic meeting" began with reflection on forum content. We then discussed progress of the survey and preliminary results, with the participants' insight directly applicable to subsequent research. Infused with both concern and hope, the conversation then turned to the formation of an independent (from government and nongovernment institutions) working group. Participants carefully created its title (Committee for Integral & Multidisciplinary Care for Older Adults, CAIMAM), crafted a mission statement, discussed guidelines for membership and decision making, and appointed a coordinator. In the past, providers in Comitán have gathered forces around other issues, from curbing infectious diseases to safeguarding maternal health. In forming CAIMAM, this group took a first step in developing a community of practice around elder well-being. My role was to facilitate dialogue and the social formation of the group while helping them develop future initiatives.

While CAIMAM was a group of motivated, well-intentioned individuals, research revealed that they were largely unaware of elders' lifestyles and constraints. Because they did not move in these elders' spaces, providers did not realize that many of the strategies they envisioned were problematic. Providers' "blame the victim" tone underlined the class and power differences between the educated providers who were mostly salaried professionals, and the more marginalized elders of the popular class whom they were to serve. The ethnographic data, however, provided a basis for identifying elder–provider power differentials and the real circumstances of elders in Comitán. For instance, practitioners argued for the importance of getting elders to work. One clinical director contended, for instance, that elders "can earn their money, they can support themselves rather than living off bones the government throws them." Elders, however, rarely received state handouts, and were indeed working hard. Providers seemed unaware of the extent of some elders' poverty, and of the fact that many elders were already doing salaried work, housework, grandchild sitting, and store tending. Further, given a general shortage of employment in Comitán, teaching elders other moneymaking skills might be useless. Providers also posited elders as upper-class retirees who should pass their time in leisure activities. In reality, many elders worked a lot and could not retire to a life of sitting in the park, doing crafts, and playing dominos, nor could they be expected to do much volunteer work when their next meal depended on paid work and tasks done in exchange for resources from relatives. Similarly, in suggesting that elders maintain better hygiene by bathing and washing clothing daily, providers presumed that elders had water (or could buy it), and that they could lift it, carry it, heat it, and afford the fuel to do so. This was not always the case. For example, many elder women had to haul water from a faucet outside their home, and few had a washing machine. Elders' diet, another target point, was often restricted by cash flow, cost of food, difficulty of preparation, and dental health. Likewise, what providers perceived as noncompliance with treatment, overmedication, and self-medication, was in fact elders self-regulation within the context of restricted resources. Finally, many recommendations, such as nutrition and diet, were not gerontological, but general public health issues, related to the economic infrastructure of Comitán and the surrounding region. It fell to me to draw on the data to inform this group and move them past their assumptions and class prejudice toward a more realistic understanding of elders' needs and resources.

At the strategic meeting, I aimed not only to inform and engage local people but also to hand over the reigns. I consciously worked to reverse roles so that rather than being an expert researcher and project organizer, I became a mere facilitator while local people took over as a group (rather than as disparate individuals). It was during the appointment of CAIMAM's coordinating team that I publicly withdrew as the project's point person and announced my return to the United States to finish my graduate studies. While many did ask me to stay, they eventually assumed responsibility. Indeed, the CAIMAM working group has gone on to initiate and carry out activities, including forging collaboration with the state through ongoing CAIMAM meetings, conducting interinstitutional elder care events, reviving previous proposals for changes in local government, and generating a new research proposal on quality of life among older adults.

Ongoing Facilitation

I now strive from afar to collect data, and facilitate and catalyze ongoing local engagement among stakeholders in Comitán. To illustrate, I recently attempted 2 strategies to engage stakeholders in reflection on survey results. I first tried sending to Comitán's providers and administrators the mass of survey data in a CD containing hundreds of tables of percentages (see Table 10.3).

I soon realized that these tables, and even the summary documents I produced from them, were too quantitative and inspired neither individual engagement nor group interaction. The format left a chasm between numbers and local environment. Seeking other ways to situate findings in context and inspire collective problem solving, I teamed with a fellow graduate student, Ben McMahan. We used Geographic Information Systems (GIS) to generate various sets of maps from the survey database, addressing a variety of health- and care-related issues and using an array of GIS visualization tools. For instance, the map in Figure 10.3 displays data from the table in Table 10.3—circles for women with hypertension and squares for men, plotted over the city of Comitán. (This map was originally generated with hypertensive men represented by blue dots and hypertensive women by red dots. The gender-specific distribution is much more evident with the color presentation.)

McMahan then went to Chiapas and shared the maps, individually and in groups with the elder health working group, CISC personnel (including those who helped design and conduct the survey), and local researchers. On one

Table 10.3. Standard Hypertension Survey Data Display, as Included in CDs Sent to Providers

Survey question: Have you ever been told by a doctor or other practitioner that you have hypertension or high blood pressure?

RESPONSE	COMITÁN MEN		COMITÁN WOMEN		COMITÁN ALL	
	FREQUENCY	%	FREQUENCY	%	FREQUENCY	%
Yes-dr.[a]	35	25.4	74	45.7	109	36.3
Yes-other	1	0.7	3	1.9	1	0.3
No	102	73.9	84	51.9	186	62.0
Don't know	0	0.0	1	0.6	1	0.3
Total	138	100.0	162	100.0	300	100.0

Source: Salud 3E: Encuesta para el diagnóstico de salud & bienestar, cuidados & atención en personas de la tercera edad en Comitán, 2005, SB_9_HIPER:Q8a

[a] "Yes-dr," the person is informed by a doctor that he or she has hypertension; "yes-other," the person is informed by some other practitioner (e.g., healer) that he or she has hypertension.

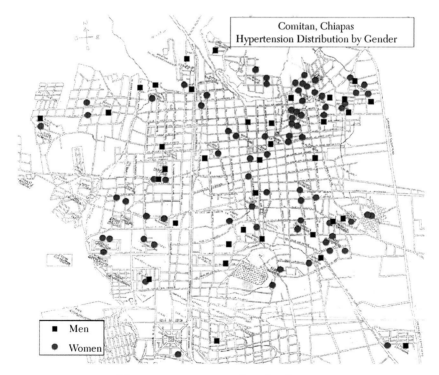

Figure 10.3. Map of hypertension survey data display using GIS.

Note: This map was originally generated with hypertensive men represented by blue dots and hypertensive women by red dots. The gendered distribution is much more evident with the color presentation.

level, the maps were prolific ethnographic elicitors, evoking direct reflection on and evaluation of the data. At a deeper level, the maps encouraged appropriation of the research and data, and inspired reflection on the power relations between researchers and local people. (See Glantz and McMahan 2007 for a more detailed account of this participatory GIS experience.)

To illustrate, the map in Figure 10.4 prompted looking at issues from a city-wide perspective, a new orientation to participants, most of whom were trained as physicians and were more accustomed to looking at individual-level data, such as a patient's chart. In this exercise, individual medical troubles became community problems. In response to this map, showing elders without an indoor water faucet, they discussed how scarce water supply and the need to carry water made life difficult, especially for elder women. They also pointed out that the question of indoor versus outdoor faucets is moot because Comitán's water supply is always limited, often nonexistent, and that this is probably due more to politics than to the water table. They indicated other variables on the map: if you live along the PanAmerican highway or downhill from the mayor's house, you almost always have water. In the more recently settled outskirts of town, you rarely have water. The hospital, perched on top of a hill, never has water and must rely on tanker trucks, an expensive solution. In this way, the maps triggered reflection on factors beyond the scope of the data presented.

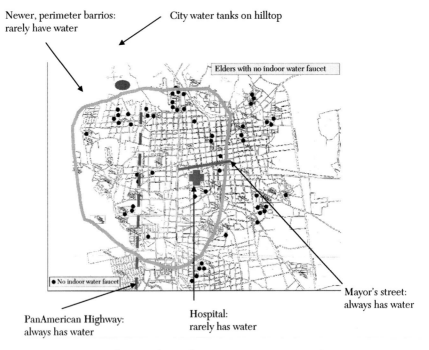

Figure 10.4. Map and notes from discussion on water supply.

The maps also spurred appropriation of research process and products. Rather than being a vertical dumping of results, presenting the maps was a horizontal exchange, sometimes even vertical, when participants oriented McMahan. The maps encouraged people to share their knowledge and expertise, often aimed at increasing the accuracy and breadth of map content. Maps also inspired thought about what is good for each subgroup (e.g., women) and location (e.g., city's perimeter). Participants saw social structural factors as causes of—and solutions to—biomedical problems. This data display—very scientific in their eyes—captured providers' attention. They realized that maps could be used from the research planning stage through interventions, and they considered learning GIS analysis themselves. They also wanted the maps to be shared—even when potentially compromising their institution's reputation—with local leaders and the public. For CISC personnel, seeing maps of the data they collected spurred satisfaction of a job well done.

The forum, interviews, strategic meeting, working group, and follow-up meetings allowed for setting up this space for nonconfrontational and honest dialogue among health care professionals. The map meeting helped sensitize providers about the lives of elders and about what elders wanted in terms of health and well-being (e.g., water, transportation, income, pain control versus vaccination, and diabetes checkups). Providers accepted this in a nonconfrontational way, and rather than contesting the maps, engaged with the maps and their colleagues to look at the distribution of problems—some of which they had not anticipated. In doing so, providers added to their capital as concerned practitioners in the capital of the science. Practitioners then began to discuss more in-depth problem solving regarding the practical details of operationalizing different interventions, such as a mobile clinic, community health workers, and a community center. They were able to think both upstream regarding matters of prevention and downstream about distribution of patients, resources, and needs. Rather than getting bogged down in the politics of critique and planning, the data, presented in a nonthreatening way, became a springboard to address realities. This entailed first accepting that their assumptions regarding elders' needs and resources differed from the life experiences of most elders in this context, and that this knowledge is needed for realistic planning. Again, the interaction with the data was as important as the data itself in generating questions, underscoring inequities, spurring local involvement in research, and leading to solutions.

Conclusion: My Role as Engaged Medical Anthropologist in Public Health Intervention

My long-term immersion in Chiapas and the region's unique elder health care context placed me in the ideal position, with appropriate skills, at a propitious time to address elder well-being. As a medical anthropologist, my role in the formative research process is as a catalyst, an invited facilitator, and stakeholder. Figure 10.5 illustrates the iterative process, in which I have been an engaged participant observer. Specifically, I have dedicated myself to

- identifying stakeholders,
- identifying the kinds of data stakeholders see as credible and respond to,
- obtaining these data, and then
- using them as the hook to inspire critical reflection with the goals of
- educating, linking, and motivating stakeholders, so that they can then engage in
- creative problem solving regarding interventions, while
- boosting their capital, which in turn gives rise to further opportunities of
- obtaining even better data and deeper understanding, and
- repeating the process.

In this dynamic, rather than provide answers, I outline the circumstances and ask and elicit questions that invite critical problem solving. I aim to engage

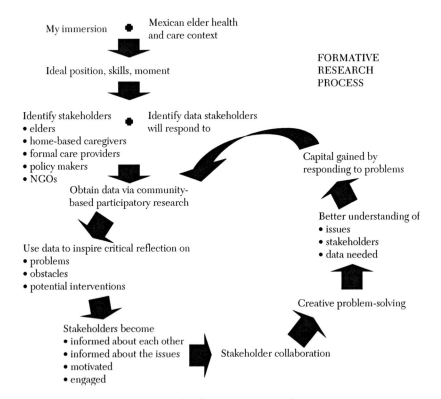

Figure 10.5. Iterative steps in the formative research process.

and mobilize stakeholders around what they feel they have a moral imperative to do (the politics of responsibility) and what they can do, and do well (the politics of possibility). I use the convertible capital inherent in practical lessons from qualitative research to support local people in on-the-ground community-based problem solving, while gleaning strengths of social science theory to critically examine and critique health practice, policy, and research itself. This anthropology *of* elder health and anthropology *in* elder health (see Nichter 2008) is a nascent effort, but with the potential of sparking a sustained movement. As a reporter said to me on his way out of the elder health forum, "If you had opened the doors to the public—anyone who is concerned about elder health—the city soccer stadium would not have been big enough to hold everyone!" Indeed, we are in the very first stages of what I anticipate will be a long-term formative research process with life-changing implications for elders and all those with a stake in elder health and care, in other words, each and every one of us.

Acknowledgments

I extend my utmost respect and gratitude to elders, home-based caregivers, and health and social service providers in Chiapas, Mexico. The Comitán Center for Health Research (CISC) provided generous institutional backing that enabled exploration of well-being in Chiapas. I am indebted to Imelda Martínez, Rolando Tinoco, Ben McMahan, and Julian Esparza for insight and support in the field. I am grateful for Mark Nichter's superior guidance and appreciate the University of Arizona Anthropology Department. The American Association of University Women, the Wenner-Gren Foundation, the Woodrow Wilson Johnson & Johnson Foundation, and the University of Arizona funded this study. This research is detailed in the Ph.D. dissertation entitled, "Formative Research on Elder Health and Care in Comitán, Chiapas, Mexico" (2007).

Notes

1. While narratives reflect real—not hypothetical—cases, all names are pseudonyms.

2. This history is described in detail by Collier (2005), Ocampo Guzmán (1999), and Benjamin (1996).

3. Import-substitution industrial development is a strategy for economic development based on encouraging industrial growth within a country to replace imports with locally produced substitutes, save foreign exchange, provide jobs, and reduce dependency.

4. They are hereafter referred to as "providers" or "practitioners" to distinguish them from people who care for elders outside the clinical setting, who are referred to as "home-based caregivers" or "caregivers."

5. This section coincides with Finkler's (1994) exploration of the relationship between culture, gender relations, and well-being in Mexico.

References

Aguirre-Molina M, Molina CW, Zambrana RE (2001) *Health Issues in the Hispanic Community*. San Francisco, CA: Jossey-Bass.

Benjamin T (1996) *A Rich Land, A Poor People: Politics and Society in Modern Chiapas*. Albuquerque, NM: University of New Mexico Press.

Bonita R (1998) *Mujeres, Envejecimiento y Salud. Comisión Mundial sobre la Salud de la Mujer*. Geneva: World Health Organization.

Borges-Yáñez SA, Gómez-Dantés H (1998) Uso de los servicios de salud por la población de 60 años y más en México. *Salud Pública de México* 40(1):13–23.

Collier GA (2005) *Basta! Land and the Zapatista Rebellion in Chiapas*. With Lowery Quaratiello E. 3rd ed. Oakland, CA: Food First.

Consejo Nacional de Población (CONAPO) (2001) Programa Nacional de Población 2001–2006: Hacia la Construcción de Nuestro Futuro Demográfico con Libertad, Equidad y Responsabilidad. www.conapo.gob.mx/pnp/pnp_pdf/044.pdf. Accessed April 26, 2006.

Consejo Nacional de Población (2002) Proyecciones de la Población de México, 2000–2005. www.salud.gob.mx/apps/htdocs/estadisticas/mortalidad/tabs/. Accessed January 17, 2007.

Finkler K (1994) *Women in Pain: Gender and Morbidity in Mexico*. Philadelphia, PA: University of Pennsylvania Press.

Frenk J, Sepulveda J, Gomez-Dantes O, Knaul F (2003) Evidence-based health policy: Three generations of reform in Mexico. *Lancet* 362:1667–1671.

Frenk J, Sepulveda J, Gomez-Dantes O (2004a) Mexican health system moves to an evidence-based model. *Reproductive Health Matters* 12(24):211.

Frenk J, Knaul F, Gómez-Dantés O, González-Pier E, Hernández-Llamas H, Lezana M, et al. (2004b) *Financiamiento Justo y Protección Social Universal: La Reforma Estructural del Sistema de Salud en México*. México, DF: Secretaría de Salud.

García-Peña C, Thorogood M, Reyes S, Salmerón-Castro J, Durán C (2001) The prevalence and treatment of hypertension in the elderly population of the Mexican Institute of Social Security. *Salud Pública de México* 43(5):415–420.

Gobierno Federal de los Estados Unidos Mexicanos, Cámera de Diputados (2001) *National Plan for Development 2001–2006*.

Gobierno Federal de los Estados Unidos Mexicanos (2002) Ley de los Derechos de las Personas Adultas Mayores.

Glantz N, McMahan B (2007) Merging formative research with participatory GIS mapping to address elder health in Chiapas, Mexico. *Practicing Anthropology* 29(4):6–14.

Martínez CS, Leal FG (2003) Epidemiological transition: Model or illusion? A look at the problem of health in Mexico. *Social Science and Medicine* 57:539–550.

Mexican Health and Aging Study (MHAS). www.ssc.upenn.edu/mhas/. Accessed September 30, 2003.

Nichter M (1990) Eight stages of formative research. www.medanthro.net/academic/tools/nichter_formative_research.pdf. Accessed March 8, 2003.

Nichter M (1995) Rethinking the household and community in the context of international health. Presented at American Anthropological Association Meeting, November 1995.

Nichter M (2008) *Global Health: Why Cultural Perceptions, Social Representations and Biopolitics Matter.* Tucson, AZ: University of Arizona Press.

Nichter M, Nichter M, Thompson PJ (2002) Using qualitative research to inform survey development on nicotine dependence among adolescents. *Drug and Alcohol Dependency* 68:S41–S56.

Nichter M, Quintero G, Nichter M, Mock J, Shakib S (2004) Qualitative research: Contributions to the study of drug use, drug abuse, and drug-related Interventions. *Substance Use and Misuse* 39:1907–1969.

Ocampo Guzmán A (1999) *La Economía Chiapaneca ante el Tratado de Libre Comercio.* San Cristóbal de Las Casas, Chiapas, Mexico: Centro de información y Análisis de Chiapas.

Phillips DR (1991) Problems and potential of researching epidemiological transition: Examples for Southeast Asia. *Social Science and Medicine* 33(4):395–404.

Reyes Fausto S (2001) *Population Ageing in the Mexican Institute of Social Security: Health Policy and Economic Implications.* Mexico City: Fundación Mexicana para la Salud, A.C.

Salgado de Snyder VN, González-Vázquez TT, Jáuregui-Ortiz B, Bonilla-Fernández P (2005) "No hacen viejos los años, sino los daños": Envejecimiento y salud en varones rurales. *Salud Pública de México* 47(4):294–302.

Soldo B, Wong R, Palloni A (2002) "Migrant health selection: Evidence from Mexico and the U.S." Paper presented at the Population Association of America Conference. Atlanta, Georgia. May 2002.

Tuirán R (2000) "Los desafíos demográficos en el nuevo milenio." CONAPO press release. www.conapo.gob.mx/prensa/reto2000.htm. Accessed April 26, 2006.

11

Anthropological Contributions to the Development of Culturally Appropriate Tobacco Cessation Programs: A Global Health Priority

MARK NICHTER, MIMI NICHTER, SIWI PADMAWTI,
C.U. THRESIA, AND PROJECT QUIT TOBACCO
INTERNATIONAL GROUP

Introduction

The impact of tobacco use on global health is quite simply staggering. One in 3 adults worldwide (>1.1 billion people) is a smoker and 80% live in low- and middle-income countries (Davies et al. 2006). At present, tobacco use is responsible for approximately 5 million premature deaths each year and if current patterns of tobacco use continue, the number is estimated to reach 10 million per year by 2030 (Peto and Lopez 2002). At least 70% of these deaths will occur in low to low middle income countries, the majority occurring in India, China, and Indonesia (TFI 2004). In India alone, mortality attributable to tobacco has been estimated to be 1 million at present and is projected to be 1.5 million by 2020 (Murray and Lopez 1996). In China 800,000 individuals were conservatively estimated to die of tobacco-related illness in 2000 and at current smoking uptake rates, tobacco use will kill about 100 million of the 300 million Chinese men under 29 years of age (Peto et al. 2000). Stated differently, tobacco use will cause one-third of all deaths in the next 20 years (Ezzati and Lopez 2003), and over 1 billion deaths this century (Stillman and Wipfli 2005). It has been estimated that between one-half and two-thirds of all long-term smokers will die because of tobacco use (Jamison et al. 2006). To place the public health impact of tobacco in a comparative perspective, tobacco smoking currently kills more people worldwide than malaria, maternal and major childhood conditions, and tuberculosis combined. On the other hand, if significant tobacco control efforts could be adopted and adult smoking levels reduced to 20%, over 100 million premature deaths could be averted by 2020 (Frieden and Bloomberg 2007).

However, it is not just body counts and mortality data that should be taken into account. Equally important, if not more, is the impact of tobacco-related morbidity on the households of the afflicted. The majority of those who become ill because of smoking, or who have an illness exacerbated by tobacco use, are men in the productive years of their life (Peto et al. 2000). Their wives, children, and elderly members of their households depend on their carrying capacity—that is, their ability to work and provide for others. The medical expenses of the afflicted present a major opportunity cost for families. Exposure to secondhand smoke in the household negatively impacts the household production of health. The suffering of the afflicted is also shared by all those around them and this takes a psychological toll.

The appropriate denominator for calculating the impact of tobacco is, therefore, not just those who die, but those whose lives are affected by tobacco-related disease and tobacco-related expenditures—expenditures covering both the cost of tobacco products and the burden of tobacco-related medical bills. Yet, it is not enough to consider the impact of tobacco on households. Many of the chronically ill are treated at government health facilities. The high cost of treating tobacco-related chronic illness taxes the capacity of national health systems to provide primary health care to its citizens. Also, despite misinformation offered by the tobacco industry (Jha and Chaloupka 1999), the costs of treating tobacco-related illness far exceed revenues that governments receive from tobacco taxes.

Given this alarming scenario, what can be done? Prevention of tobacco use and cessation of tobacco use, the two arms of tobacco control, obviously need to be promoted vigorously and supported by research that is sensitive to both the social and cultural dimensions of tobacco use and the marketing strategies of the tobacco industry. Tobacco control must be proactive on three fronts: tobacco policy (broadly conceived), community activism that makes tobacco control a community issue that includes women and children (not just an individual choice issue), and the mainstreaming of tobacco control in health care and medical education. To date, global prevention efforts, especially those related to policy, have far outpaced cessation efforts. This is one reason the percentage of current smokers who have expressed a desire to quit is far less in developing than developed countries (Abdullah and Husten 2004).

The prevention arm of tobacco control has focused on raising public consciousness about the dangers of tobacco use,[1] protecting vulnerable populations targeted by the tobacco industry to maintain and expand market share, and promoting tobacco-free environments. At the same time, the tobacco industry has worked to make tobacco use appear normative and appealing through aggressive marketing campaigns. In conjunction with the provisions of the Framework Convention for Tobacco Control (FCTC nd) tobacco prevention advocates have worked to introduce and enforce restrictions on tobacco sales to minors, limit the marketing of tobacco in ways that appear attractive to minors, restrict smoking in public places and work sites where others are exposed to secondhand smoke, and control tobacco smuggling. The FCTC has also called for the raising of prices of tobacco products as a proven deterrent to uptake and graphic product labeling to highlight the dangers of smoking on cigarette packs.

Millions of lives can be saved now—not just in the future—through tobacco cessation initiatives. The damage caused by smoking can be reversed substantially on an individual-by-individual basis by quitting tobacco use (Edwards 2004; US Department of Health and Human Services 1990, 2004). On a population basis, it has been estimated that by the year 2020, if adult consumption of tobacco were to decrease by 50%, approximately 180 million tobacco-related deaths could be avoided (Jha and Chaloupka 1999; Mackay and Eriksen 2002). Moreover, cessation is an important part of tobacco prevention (Abdullah and Husten 2004). In countries where tobacco use appears normative, exposing young people to adults engaging in cessation attempts serves as a counterbalance to images glamorizing tobacco use (Slama 2004).

How does one go about implementing tobacco cessation programs in other cultures and what role can anthropology play in developing this arm of tobacco control? In this chapter, we will describe formative research undertaken in Kerala, South India, and Central Java, Indonesia, over the last 5 years (2002–2007) as a first step toward developing tobacco cessation programs. The research was and continues to be funded by the Fogarty International Center of the National Institutes of Health and has involved 4 anthropologists (the coauthors) working in concert with multidisciplinary teams of addiction specialists, doctors, psychologists, and public health practitioners dedicated to establishing tobacco control centers in each country. A recent paper describes Project Quit Tobacco International (Project QTI) (Nichter 2006), and a project website (http://www.quittobaccointernational.net) provides additional information on project activities as well as those methods and instruments used in each stage of research to date. Highlighted here, after a brief introduction to Project QTI and formative research, are 6 areas of ethnographic research that can contribute to the development of culturally sensitive smoking cessation programs. They are (1) patterns of tobacco use and exchange; (2) perceptions of tobacco risk (to self and others) among currently healthy tobacco users, special patient populations, and health care providers; (3) tobacco harm reduction practices, reasons people quit or suspend tobacco use, and concern about withdrawal symptoms; (4) cognitive, visual, and evocative approaches to raising consciousness about tobacco harm in support of cessation; (5) cultural themes used to popularize tobacco use by advertisers that need to be confronted and reframed; and (6) current tobacco advice practices and willingness to be involved in cessation by physicians as a routine part of their medical practice.

Project QTI: Research Setting

Project QTI is an ongoing international research initiative having 4 main objectives: (1) to promote tobacco cessation as routine medical practice in developing countries such that all patients are asked about their tobacco use and then advised and assisted to quit; (2) to introduce tobacco education into medical and nursing school curriculum as well as continuing education and outreach programs; (3) to develop culturally sensitive clinic- and community-based tobacco education and cessation programs through a combination of formative and translational research (conceptual translation from science to lay understanding); and (4) to foster research collaborations that contribute to the formation of a community of practice (Wenger 1996, 1998) promoting tobacco cessation. By facilitating community-based cessation research as well as tobacco education in medical schools, Project QTI is endeavoring to build a critical mass of in-country experts and community activists that can make the dangers of tobacco use more visible to the general public, to the medical community at large, to patients, to the media, and to influential policy and decision makers.

For the first 5 years, Project QTI has been carried out in Thiruvananthapuram District, Kerala State, India and Jogjakarta Province, Indonesia. India and Indonesia were chosen initially for QTI research because they have high prevalence rates of tobacco use across all social classes, indigenous as well as imported tobacco products are popular, cessation is not currently a national public health priority or part of established medical school curriculum, and pharmaceutical aids for cessation are not readily available in the market. In India, almost 50% of men over 15 years of age either smoke or use smokeless tobacco (Rani, Bonu, Jha, Nguyen, and Jamjoum 2003; Reddy and Gupta 2004). In Kerala, between 30% and 50% of men and 1% to 2% of women are smokers and 10% to 23% of both men and women chew tobacco (International Institute for Population Sciences 2001; Sankaranarayanan et al. 2000). Notably, Kerala has the highest literacy rate and best health indicators of any state in India (Thankappan and Valiathan 1998) as well as a high rate of health service utilization (Kannan, Thankappan, Raman Kutty, and Aravindan 1991; Panikar 1998) giving health care practitioners ample opportunity to promote cessation. In Indonesia, fewer data are available on the prevalence of smoking, but it has been estimated that 60% of men and 5% of women are smokers (Achadi, Soerojo, and Barber 2005; World Health Organization 2005). An estimated 97 million Indonesians are regularly exposed to environmental tobacco smoke (ETS) in their own homes, 43 million of whom are children (Pradono 2002).

India and Indonesia are 2 of only 3 nations (China being the third) where tobacco consumption is rising. Moreover, although tobacco products have become more costly in many developing countries, tobacco products in both India and Indonesia have become 50% more affordable in the last 20 years. In both countries, tobacco is a highly influential industry. India is one of the largest producers of tobacco in the world and employs millions of workers at various points in the commodity chain. The tobacco industry in Indonesia is the second largest employer after the government. In India, major advances in tobacco control have been made in the policy arena, whereas in Indonesia tobacco control legislation is in its early stages. The sites chosen as tobacco cessation research centers in the 2 countries (Sree Chitra Tirunal Institute for Medical Sciences and Technology, Thiruvananthapuram, India, and Gadjah Mada University, Jogjakarta, Indonesia) are well established and highly prestigious public health and medical training centers supportive of multidisciplinary research.

Methods: Formative Research Process

Formative Research: an Overview

Formative research is a multistage iterative research process that employs a variety of qualitative methods to examine public health problems in context as well as to develop, critically assess, monitor, and evaluate public health interventions and the way they are represented (Nichter, Quintero, Nichter, Mock, and Shakib 2004; Ulin, Robinson, and Tolley 2004). Formative research considers multiple agents and environments associated with a public health problem as well as interactive—syndemic (Singer and Clair 2003)—relations between public health problems, and those factors that place particular populations at risk or are protective.

Figure 11.1 presents a biopolitical model of the epidemiology of tobacco dependency developed at the University of Arizona as a tool for medical anthropology training and research. The model draws attention to linkages between macro and micro environments of tobacco production, marketing, and consumption and applies lessons learned from the study of vector-borne disease, consumer behavior, and political economy. In this case the vector is the tobacco industry, which (1) actively (re)produces a favorable environment for expanding sales by socially engineering breeding sites through marketing

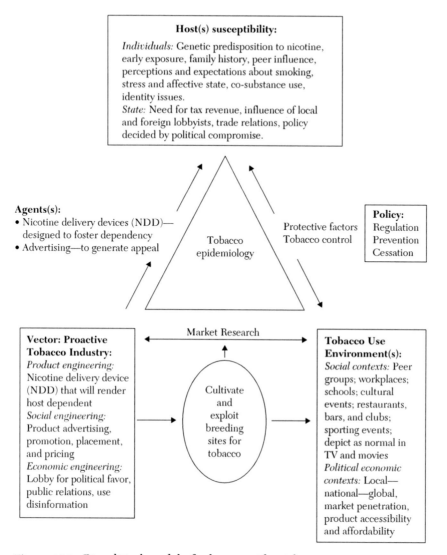

Host(s) susceptibility:

Individuals: Genetic predisposition to nicotine, early exposure, family history, peer influence, perceptions and expectations about smoking, stress and affective state, co-substance use, identity issues.
State: Need for tax revenue, influence of local and foreign lobbyists, trade relations, policy decided by political compromise.

Agents(s):
• Nicotine delivery devices (NDD)—designed to foster dependency
• Advertising—to generate appeal

Tobacco epidemiology

Protective factors
Tobacco control

Policy:
Regulation
Prevention
Cessation

Market Research

Vector: Proactive Tobacco Industry:
Product engineering: Nicotine delivery device (NDD) that will render host dependent
Social engineering: Product advertising, promotion, placement, and pricing
Economic engineering: Lobby for political favor, public relations, use disinformation

Cultivate and exploit breeding sites for tobacco

Tobacco Use Environment(s):
Social contexts: Peer groups; workplaces; schools; cultural events; restaurants, bars, and clubs; sporting events; depict as normal in TV and movies
Political economic contexts: Local—national—global, market penetration, product accessibility and affordability

Figure 11.1. Biopolitical model of tobacco epidemiology

(contexts where smoking is deemed normative) and identifying susceptible populations (cultivating market segments), and (2) pharmacologically engineers nicotine delivery devices (NDD) to more effectively render the host (user) dependent on tobacco. It is not just the individual as host who is rendered dependent (Nichter 2003). The land is rendered dependent on fertilizer and insecticide subsidies (Nichter and Cartwright 1991), the local population on tobacco-related jobs, the state on tobacco-related tax revenues (Wright and Katz 2007), and politicians on tobacco-related donations and lobbyist activities.[2]

Community- and clinic-based formative research conducted during Project QTI was primarily focused on tobacco use environments and factors encouraging tobacco use toward the end of developing culturally sensitive cessation interventions. We were interested in what led Javanese and Keralite men to adopt particular tobacco use patterns and trajectories as well as in what led them to quit or cut down tobacco use temporarily or permanently (See Figure 11.2).[3] Five areas of research were of central importance: (1) social and cultural factors that encouraged sustained smoking; (2) representations of cigarettes in advertising that fostered the perception that smoking was normative, culturally valued, and socially desirable in different groups; (3) perceptions of risk associated with different levels of tobacco use; (4) reasons for quitting or suspending tobacco use; and (5) factors that lead to relapse after someone has quit smoking for some time.

Research Methods

Several ethnographic methods were employed during Project QTI formative research. We engaged in participant observation in social contexts where

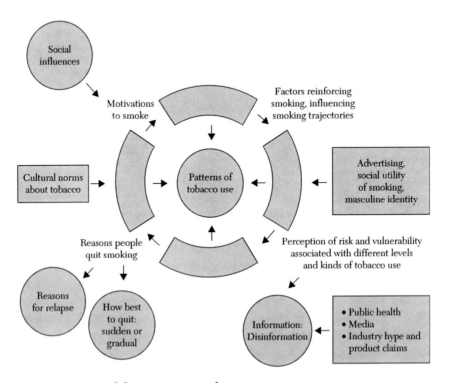

Figure 11.2. Initial formative research.

smoking was seen as normative and examined smoking-related behavior in both household and public spaces. We also observed ways in which cigarettes were offered, accepted, and refused in social settings. We conducted in-depth interviews with purposive samples of smokers hailing from different age cohorts and class backgrounds to gain insights into reasons for smoking, ideas about tobacco dependency, and perceptions of risk to health associated with different types of cigarettes smoked at different levels. We also interviewed people afflicted with diseases who continued to smoke or who quit tobacco. From these interviews we developed survey instruments that we administered to different groups of smokers to get quantitative measures of tobacco-related perceptions and behaviors to serve as a baseline against which to measure interventions.

We also created an archive of current tobacco advertisements, performed content (thematic) analysis of advertisements, and held focus groups to explore how advertisements were viewed by different groups of men. Focus groups were also used in translational research to explore how best to translate science into easy-to-understand ideas and images for lay populations and to develop tobacco cessation question-and-answer educational guides. Focus groups were used to select pictures of tobacco-related diseases for posters and educational materials and to develop counter-advertisements that challenged the positive imagery of smoking in advertisements. Narratives were collected from smokers who suffered an illness related to their tobacco habit and the economic and emotional impact of their disease on their families. We also interviewed and surveyed practitioners and medical students to find out about their tobacco use, perceptions of the risk of smoking at different levels, and how often and in what contexts they talked to patients about smoking. We present a few of our findings to illustrate why this information is of vital importance to tobacco cessation.

Research Findings

Why Do People Smoke? A Consideration of Utility

Motivations for smoking in India and Indonesia included several factors widely reported in the smoking literature as well as factors that are culturally specific. Cigarettes have 4 general forms of utility: (1) symbolic utility—they are employed in identity projects enabling one to appear more mature, masculine, modern, carefree, sophisticated, successful, in control, and so on, according to the "sign value" accorded a cigarette or brand of cigarette in a particular place (Nichter, Nichter, and Van Sickle 2004); (2) social utility—they facilitate social interaction, mark transitions between work and leisure, provide a break from routine or personal time, and so on; (3) affect regulation utility—smoking is at once associated with pleasure and perceived to be a means of reducing stress (beyond the pharmacological properties of nicotine contained in cigarettes, the physical act of handling cigarettes and the ritual of smoking cigarettes has a calming effect for some); and (4) physical regulation utility—smoking is used to regulate body rhythms from defecation to sleep–wake states and hunger cycles.

Each of these 4 types of utility has to be addressed in tobacco cessation. Studying how tobacco advertising manipulates cultural symbols to promote smoking as a socially valued behavior is important when trying to establish a positive nonsmoking identity. It is important to know one's adversary and learn what cultural values can be used to counter positive smoking images. Researching the social utility functions of smoking is also crucial. Quitting tobacco entails quitting established patterns of social interaction. Smokers in both India and Indonesia told us time and again that one of the biggest barriers to quitting would be learning how to handle invitations to smoke, especially in contexts where smoking facilitated particular types of social interaction. We were presented with the task of finding culturally acceptable means of turning down cigarette offers that would be comfortable for different types of people in different social settings.

Informants in both countries told us that saying that one's doctor had advised them not to smoke was an acceptable reason not to smoke, but this message came with a negative set of associations. For example, in Indonesia this signaled that a person was ill and literally not "healthy enough to smoke." Our challenge was clear: How could we turn doctors' advice to quit smoking from a marker of ill health to a marker of promotive health having a positive set of social associations?

Social Relations and Quitting

Research on the social utility of smoking also led us to consider social relations as a challenge to tobacco cessation. Smoking is one of the few forms of consumption that the average man can routinely afford to engage in with peers in both countries. The exchanging of cigarettes facilitates social solidarity, bonding, and affiliation, and the sharing of expensive cigarettes can mark a special occasion. An issue that immediately arose was whether quitting would compromise social relationships and reduce peoples' opportunities for socializing. Would quit attempts place individuals at social risk to loose valued social relations?

In both countries informants reported that friends encouraged them to smoke, even when they did not feel like doing so. However, if one did not smoke this did not exclude them from the group. Informants reported that it was difficult to establish a nonsmoking identity after having been known as a smoker. Smokers in both countries reported that their peers question their ability to give up smoking, rather than supporting their quit attempts. How to respond to being teased, and present oneself as strong and not weak in such situations, became an important research topic, a topic that demanded a consideration of cultural communication styles as well as cultural notions of strength and masculinity.

Culture and Communication Styles

Keralites and the Javanese have quite different communication and interactional styles. Keralites engage in far more direct communication, whereas indirect communication is a hallmark of Javanese culture. In Kerala, it is commonplace to challenge someone openly—and respond to a challenge directly, whereas in Java communication takes on a more subtle flavor. This requires that different strategies be developed for how one could respond to teasing by others in response to not smoking. In both cultures, the use of proverbs and analogies was valued as a display of wit, and QTI teams in India and Indonesia came to appreciate each others' use of folk wisdom to meet challenges to smoke.

Culture and Notions of Strength, Control, and Addiction

An examination of cultural perceptions of strength also proved insightful. Spiritual strength in each culture is important to men (but much less so for youth). Spiritual strength is perceived somewhat differently in each culture, but in both it is associated with control and the ability to withstand temptation (including the temptation to consume in excess), master and challenge desires, overcome fear, and maintain one's self composure. In both cultures, this ideal is articulated through practices such as fasting (among both Hindus and Muslims).

The extent to which smoking is associated with a state of uncontrol and addiction arose as a core research question. Although tobacco use was considered a minor vice capable of leading to addiction in Kerala, we rarely encountered terms for addiction being used to describe tobacco in Java. Terms such as *ketagihan* and *kecanduan* in Bahasa Indonesian were reserved for the use of alcohol and illegal drugs. One would have to smoke very heavily before being referred to as one who was addicted to tobacco. Instead, people would speak of someone finding smoking too pleasurable or enjoyable to stop—terms prominently used in many cigarette advertisements. The challenge for the QTI research teams in both countries was how to introduce the idea that routine smoking—even at low levels—was an addiction, a state in which the smoker was under the influence of tobacco and thus weak. In an advertising environment where smoking was graphically associated with strong men (sports figures, successful businessmen, etc.) we needed to reframe smoking as a weakness and not smoking as a sign of strength. We will have more to say about this shortly.

A further consideration of smoking as affect regulation led to a deeper understanding of the cultural association between smoking and control. The populations of both India and Indonesia have been inundated by images of actors in films smoking when stressed or distressed, and when relaxing or enjoying a moment of success. Marketing strategies have effectively bundled smoking with affective states and established expectancies for how people should feel when they smoke in different circumstances. But there is more to the association of smoking and affect regulation than this. Affect regulation is also cultural work, and smoking has become an important coping resource. This is clearly the case in Java.

In Java, emotional control is a cultural value, especially for men. Uncontrolled emotions are socially embarrassing and deemed dangerous. Men are socialized to keep displays of strong emotion in check. Cigarette smoking is utilized as a means of subduing, if not masking, strong emotions, and cigarettes are marketed as a coping device to use when upset or angry or when confronted by someone, such as a parent, wife, or girlfriend, displaying negative affect (Nichter 2005). Cultural concerns about affect regulation extend to times when unconscious desires emerge in daydreams, a time of "empty thoughts" (Ferzacca 2001), as well as times when one cannot stop "thinking–thinking" (stuck in an endless feedback loop). Smoking is "enjoyed" as a means of preventing these emotional states because when one smokes they return to an expected steady state of being.

Two challenges to cessation were presented by cigarettes being used as a means of affect regulation. Given that many people have come to rely on smoking as a device for coping with negative affect, we needed to identify other means of coping that could be offered as part of brief interventions. Second, we had to be prepared for encounters with people suffering from states of depression and anxiety, know how to recognize such states as they manifest culturally, and make provisions for referral (Wilhelm, Wedgwood, Niven, and Kay-Lambkin 2006).

Perceptions of Tobacco Risk to Self and Others

What is the perceived risk of smoking in Kerala and Java? To investigate this issue, we began by conducting research on what level of smoking was perceived to be relatively safe by the general population, health care providers, and groups having illnesses caused or exacerbated by smoking. In Kerala, it was widely believed that 5 to 10 cigarettes a day was relatively harmless to smoke, an impression shared by one-fourth of engineering students (n = 1000) and one-third of medical students (n = 1100). Among community- and hospital-based doctors (n = 300), 86% believed that smoking fewer than 10 cigarettes a day was within safe limits; 14% stated that smoking 4 to 5 cigarettes a day was relatively safe (Mohan et al. 2006). In Java, the mean number of cigarettes thought to be relatively safe to smoke a day was 12 among engineering students (n = 1200) and 9 among medical students (n = 1222). Eighty percent of physicians (n = 400) believed that smoking up to 10 cigarettes a day was not harmful for health (Ng et al. 2007). Research conducted in both countries revealed that although lung cancer was associated with smoking, the vast majority of people interviewed did not associate smoking with coronary heart disease, peripheral vascular disease, stroke, tuberculosis (TB).

We next surveyed patients afflicted with diseases strongly associated with tobacco use. We primarily focused on 2 patient populations: those having diabetes—as an exemplar of a chronic noncommunicable disease that affects rich and poor alike, and those treated for TB—as an exemplar of a curable communicable disease that primarily affects the poor. Let us briefly consider the seriousness of smoking in each case.

QTI Findings on Diabetes and Smoking. Diabetes mellitus has become a global epidemic (King, Aubert, and Herman 1998; Wild, Roglic, Green, Sicree, and King 2004). Between 1985 and 1995, the estimated number of people with diabetes *more than quadrupled*—from an estimated 30 million to 135 million. In 2000, there were an estimated 177 million diabetics, and that number is predicted to *soar* to 366 million by 2030. Forty million of those afflicted with diabetes currently live in India and Indonesia, and in 2020 the number will rise to a projected 100 million. Diabetes is a costly disease because of its chronic nature, the severity of complications, and the medical treatments necessary to control diabetes and treat its complications. Studies in India have estimated that a low-income family with an adult diabetic may devote as much as 25% of household income to diabetes care (Bjork, Kapur, King, Nair, and Ramachandran 2003).

Studies have shown that smoking is an independent, modifiable risk factor for the development of diabetes (WHO 2002), and there is a well-established link between smoking and complications of diabetes (Manson, Ajani, Liu, Nathan, and Hennekens 2000; Orth, Ritz, and Schrier 1997; Orth, Ogata, and Ritz 2000; Regalado, Yang, and Wesson 2000; Will, Galuska, Ford, Mokdad, and Calle 2001). Diabetic smokers have twice the risk of premature death compared to nonsmoking diabetics, and the combined cardiovascular disease risks from smoking and diabetes are nearly 14 times higher than the risk of either smoking or diabetes alone (Foy, Bell, Farmer, Goff, and Wagenknecht 2005).

Smoking impairs metabolic control and increases the risk of both macrovascular and microvascular complications including coronary artery disease, stroke, peripheral artery disease, proteinuria, renal failure, and neuropathy (Eliasson 2003). Secondhand smoke also increases the risk of having diabetes and its complications (Houston et al. 2006).

The data generated by QTI surveys were sobering. In both India and Indonesia, many men with diabetes smoke. Interviews with diabetes patients (n = 613) attending clinics in Kerala revealed that 30% (n = 182) had used tobacco in the last 6 months and of these smokers, 86% had smoked in the last 30 days. In Indonesia, interviews with patients with diabetes (n = 778) revealed that 21% (n = 160) had smoked in the last 6 months, and of these smokers, 81% had smoked in the last 30 days. We found that few diabetic patients suspected that tobacco use had anything to do with their disease. Notably, over one-half of the diabetic smokers interviewed in India reported that they did not think smoking or chewing tobacco affected their diabetes at all. Fifteen percent thought smoking or chewing might cause a mild aggravation of their symptoms, 21% reported that smoking or chewing might significantly aggravate their diabetes, and 9% had no idea. In Indonesia, 34% reported that smoking did not affect diabetes, 17% thought that it might cause mild aggravation, 24% that it might aggravate the disease a lot, and 25% had no idea.

We asked diabetic informants in both countries how many cigarettes they thought that a diabetic could smoke without it being very harmful for health. The number of cigarettes deemed relatively harmless to smoke was between 6 and 10. In India, there was a wide range of opinion: 43% thought 1 to 5 cigarettes were relatively harmless, 31% thought 6 to 10 cigarettes were harmless, and 26% thought more than 10 cigarettes was harmless. Only 5% of respondents stated that even 1 cigarette was harmful.

Another issue we investigated in each country was whether diabetics consumed tobacco as a way of keeping their weight down, and/or as a substitute for sweet or fried snacks in social settings. Only a few people consciously reported doing so, but some family members suspected that this might be the case, leading us to follow up on this possibility further.

QTI Findings on TB. Tuberculosis is the world's leading cause of death from a curable infectious disease and a major cause of both mortality and morbidity in the developing world. In 2004, TB was responsible for an estimated 1.7 million deaths, with 45% of all new cases occurring in Asia's 5 most populous countries (Dye 2006; Dye, Scheele, Dolin, Pathania, and Raviglione et al. 1999). India has over 2 million new TB cases every year, of which nearly 1 million are infectious smear-positive pulmonary cases (Gajalakshmi, Peto, Kanaka, and Jha P 2003). In India, 450,000 people die from tuberculosis every year (Khatri and

Freiden 2000). In Indonesia, TB is the second most common cause of death after cardiovascular disease. Notably, the incidence of TB in both countries is highest among the 20 to 49 age-group, which carries serious implications for social and economic development. This is also an age-group most likely to smoke (Pai 2007).

Smokers are at once at greater risk of developing TB (odds ratio [OR]: 1.8 light smokers, OR: 3.7 heavy smokers; Kolappan and Gopi 2002) and of dying from TB (OR: 4.5, Gajalakshmi et al. 2003).[4] Ex-patients are more than 3 times more likely to relapse if they smoke following short course TB treatment (Thomas, Gopi, Santha, Chandrasekaran, Subramani 2005). Those exposed to secondhand smoke (including children) are also significantly more likely to develop TB (Altet et al. 1996; Lin, Ezzati, and Murray 2007).

QTI has been examining TB patients' smoking behavior before diagnosis, during short course TB treatment, and following the completion of treatment. Six months before they were diagnosed with TB, more than 70% of a sample of current and recently treated TB patients in Kerala (n = 215) were smokers. Ninety percent of these people stopped smoking at the time they were diagnosed with TB largely because the disease rendered them too sick to smoke and because there is a general perception (in both countries) that one should not smoke or drink alcohol when taking medicine for an acute disease. For this reason, in India most TB patients (82%) did not resume smoking during their treatment. At the completion of treatment, 27% of these male patients began smoking and by 6 months post treatment, 31% had resumed their smoking.

In Java, the pattern was somewhat similar. Of a sample of ex-TB patients (n = 239), 91% (n = 218) were ever smokers. Almost two-thirds of ever smokers were daily smokers 6 months before their illness. When diagnosed with TB, the majority of daily smokers quit smoking, but 11% remained a daily smoker while under TB treatment. At the end of 6 months of TB treatment, only 7% of those who had quit smoking during TB treatment relapsed to become daily smokers. However, 6 months after treatment, 30% of the sample had resumed smoking daily and another 10% smoked occasionally. Only 59% of those who had quit during treatment remained nonsmoking 6 months after completing treatment.

QTI researchers are examining whether TB patients perceive smoking to be a possible cause of their illness, a factor rendering them vulnerable to TB, or a factor possibly leading to TB relapse. In India, of the TB/ex-TB patients surveyed (n = 215), only 13% thought that smoking *might* be a cause of TB. In Indonesia, however, 97% of TB patients (n = 202) and 51% of ex-patients (n = 209) thought that excessive smoking might be a cause of TB, and 74% of ex-TB patients believed that excessive smoking could increase the chance of TB relapse. A question begging further investigation was what did "excessive smoking" mean? In Indonesia, among current TB patients (n = 107) who had smoked before diagnosis, the mean number of cigarettes thought to be relatively safe to smoke a day for healthy people was 10, whereas among ex-TB patients (n = 178), 55% thought that smoking 5 to 6 cigarettes a day was safe. "Excessive smoking" generally meant 2 times the perceived safe limit.

On the basis of preliminary findings, QTI researchers began developing interventions in both countries focused on TB and diabetes patient populations. This has included training health care providers to ask about tobacco use behavior and offer specific cessation advice and developing patient-friendly question-and-answer booklets for patients and for use in community outreach programs. We will discuss these subsequently.

In sum, an awareness of the adverse health effects of tobacco use on health was largely limited to cancers, and quite low among both diabetics and those with TB. Cessation requires raising the consciousness of patient populations that tobacco not only increases your chances of becoming ill and dying prematurely from cancer, but also of suffering from complications as is the case with diabetes, or relapsing as in the case of TB.

Perceptions of the Harm of Secondhand Smoke and Household Smoking Bans

In both Java and Kerala, children's health is a focus of considerable attention, yet smoking in the home is very common. We discovered that smoking was not widely associated with children's illness, although some people did think smoking could exacerbate asthma. In Java, some informants believed that it was good to expose children to tobacco smoke to get them used to it. In this way, they would not be troubled when spending time in the many places where tobacco smoke was pervasive. It became clear that educating the public about the dangers of secondhand smoke was a necessary first step in promoting home-smoking restrictions and smoking at social gatherings attended by women and children. It was also clear that we needed to appeal to men's family responsibility and develop interventions that made home-based smoking restrictions into an issue of women's and children's health. We are currently exploring types of health data that may serve to mobilize women's groups that are already prominent in both Java and Kerala.

Encouraging a quit-smoking policy in homes requires research into several cultural issues. We are currently investigating what kind of messages women can give to men about not smoking in the home that are culturally acceptable and sensitive to gender roles. We are also investigating what role daughters and sons (of different ages) can play in giving nonsmoking messages to their fathers that address both their smoking in general and their smoking at home. What emotional appeal might family members use to make their point? We also need to examine what constitutes public and personal spaces within the home. Smoking appears far easier to restrict in private spaces of homes, and more difficult in public spaces. How could one ask visitors not to smoke in areas of the home or veranda traditionally set aside for social exchange? Our challenge is to find ways of changing existing home-based smoking norms so that it becomes culturally inappropriate to smoke both in one's own home and in the homes of others.

Harm Reduction and Quitting

In both countries, we discovered a number of practices intended to reduce harm related to smoking (Nichter 2006). In India, particular foods were thought to clean the lungs and remove heat from the body caused by smoking (Nichter, Nichter, and Van Sickle 2004). In both India and Indonesia, drinking copious amounts of water was likewise supposed to reduce toxins found in cigarettes and *beedi* (hand-rolled unfiltered cigarettes rolled in tendu leaves—*Diosyros melanoxylon*) by flushing them out of the body. And in Indonesia, it is widely believed that if a person smokes a brand of cigarettes that is "suitable" (*cocok*) for his body, no harm will come from smoking. These misperceptions have been addressed in the tobacco education material we developed in each country.

What leads people to quit smoking in Kerala and Java? As noted by researchers in the West, many more quit attempts appear to be unplanned and motivated by something that comes up in life than those planned after a period of contemplation and deliberation (Larabie 2005; West and Sohal 2006). In India and Indonesia, the most common reason for quitting smoking was illness, and the most common type of quitting was sudden, at a time of illness when medicine is taken. Quitting smoking signaled to others that they were ill, taking medication, and adopting a sick role. Resuming smoking signaled that they were once again well or at least that their condition was now manageable. We identified illness as an important opportunity to discuss quitting, especially if people were given a message by a health care worker not to smoke. Our challenge became turning cessation from being part of a sick role into an important part of a proactive health role.

We also queried people's impressions of quitting smoking suddenly rather than doing it gradually when not ill, given widespread concern about shocking the body and mind in both Indonesia and India. We were further interested in considering people's attitudes toward planning quit attempts in line with a stages-of-change model of cessation (Prochaska and Goldstein 1991; Prochaska and Velicer 1997; Prochaska, DiClemente, Velicer, Ginpil, and Norcross 1985). In both countries, we discovered a range of opinions about the best way to quit smoking as well as differences in opinion about quitting smoking suddenly. Some men argued that it was best to quit suddenly if one had the willpower to do so, or if an illness demanded this action. Many were interested in knowing if medicines could help one cope with withdrawal symptoms. Other men in both countries argued that it was better to quit smoking by gradually tapering down the amount one smoked. Some men in this group spoke of withdrawal symptoms as symptoms directly resulting from shocking the body by sudden change. A few stated that shocking the body in this way could prove more harmful than continuing to smoke. They believed that shocking the body caused latent illness to manifest—making quitters especially vulnerable to sickness.

Informants in both countries were of the opinion that different methods of quitting were likely to be better for different kinds of people. But overall, we found that people were less inclined to favor planning a quit in the future with an established quit date, than to endorse quitting at a moment when motivations to quit ran high for one reason or another (Larabie 2005; West 2005; West and Sohal 2006). Our charge became twofold. First, we needed to identify opportunities when motivations for quitting were likely to run high and ways we might tip the balance toward quitting at those times by offering cessation support. Below, we discuss attempts to create evocative quit messages to prime quit attempts. Second, we needed to encourage health practitioners to look at all illness experiences as opportunities to motivate patients to quit smoking. Training health care practitioners to ask patients about tobacco use as a routine part of their practice and to offer culturally appropriate cessation advice at teachable moments became 1 of our primary intervention goals.

Withdrawal Symptoms

A next consideration was the cultural significance attributed to specific withdrawal symptoms and culturally appropriate ways of coping with these symptoms. We faced 2 challenges: how to respond to questions about why such symptoms persist for some time after one quits and how to deal with withdrawal symptoms of greatest concern. We learned from experience that the best way to address the persistence of withdrawal symptoms question was to remind people that smoking was typically not initially pleasurable and that it took time to adjust to tobacco. After smoking for some years, it would take time for the body to re-adjust to its previous state of nonsmoking. In intervention settings, we have pointed out that withdrawal symptoms gradually lessen over time, and that people feel much stronger and healthier for the rest of their lives when they quit—a statement we backed up by testimonials of quitters as well as with facts about increased longevity.

Body and blood purification practices are part of popular health culture in both India and Indonesia. We are currently investigating whether cultural concerns related to purification might be used to reframe withdrawal symptoms as positive signs of toxins clearing the body. Could complementary medicine focused on purification (such as taking herbal medicine) be used to reinforce quitting?

A central focus of medical anthropology is how members of different cultures interpret bodily symptoms, and which symptoms they consider relatively serious and minor. To date, there has been little biosocial investigation of nicotine withdrawal symptoms in different cultures. The QTI teams found differences in what sensations people complained about most in India and Indonesia. In India, digestive complaints, gaseousness, constipation, dullness, throbbing in the head, and dizziness were common complaints. In Indonesia, the inability to think and concentrate, difficulty controlling anger, experiencing headache and dizziness, feeling too lazy to work, and bitterness in the mouth were commonly reported. Each team has searched for local methods and resources to deal with these symptoms, and continues to do so.

Developing Culturally Appropriate Cessation Interventions

Raising Consciousness and Priming Quit Attempts

In contexts where the association between smoking and health problems is not recognized, raising public consciousness is a primary step on the road to cessation. It sets the stage for quit attempts. However, reason is not the only path that leads people to be motivated to quit. Larabie (2005) and West and Sohal (2006) have emphasized that smokers must *want* to quit, and not just *think* that they should quit. What is critical here is adopting an image of being a nonsmoker that is attractive and that "feels" right to the individual. Figure 11.3

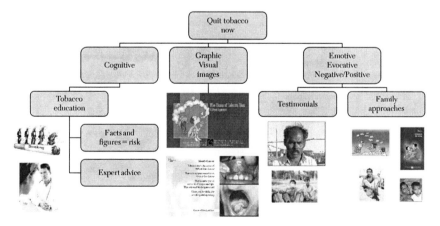

Figure 11.3. Approaches to promoting tobacco cessation.

highlights cognitive, visual, and evocative approaches to raising consciousness and making quitting an emotional as well as a reasonable course of action. We briefly describe our work on each of these three approaches.

The Cognitive Domain

As part of translational research, QTI teams have been developing question-and-answer guides to tobacco education that address misconceptions that people have about tobacco, as well as questions people have about smoking, health, and cessation. Here are just a few examples of the issues we have faced:

Common misconceptions

- Some cigarettes are relatively safe to smoke, including cigarettes that are expensive—filter tip, menthol, light cigarettes (Nichter, Nichter, and Van Sickle 2004).
- If one finds a brand of cigarette that is suitable for his body (Indonesia), then there is no harm. If one smokes a type that is incompatible, then there is illness.
- Low-level smoking is not harmful.
- Many old people who smoke are healthy, so smoking is okay if you are healthy otherwise.
- Smoking is okay for healthy people; only those who are sick already become very ill if they smoke.
- There are ways to reduce the harm of smoking including diet, drinking a lot of water to flush away toxins, herbal medicine, vitamins, and exercise.
- Since the environment is polluted anyway by smoke from vehicles and industry, it does little good to stop smoking.
- Being exposed to smoke is good because your body gets used to it and smoking by others will not bother you.
- It is dangerous to quit smoking suddenly because the body is used to tobacco and quitting will shock the body and make you vulnerable to ill health and becoming upset.

Questions raised by community members

- Does smoking decrease or increase blood pressure and why?
- What is the relationship between smoking and diabetes? (Diabetes is not a disease of the lung.)
- Is it true that people who do not smoke tend to be overweight or obese?

- Isn't it better for a diabetic to smoke and curb his appetite than to eat more?
- Are there any cigarettes that are safer for health; if so, which ones?
- How dangerous is secondhand smoke as compared to smoking?
- How can a person refuse a cigarette in a social context without losing face and feeling embarrassed?

For each issue, the QTI team has explored different ways of answering the question, responding to a doubt, or addressing a misconception. In each case, we have pretested candidate messages in focus groups composed of different types of people (by gender, age, education) to gauge people's responses. To identify the most effective responses, we have assessed both how popular the response is and how unlikely it is to be misinterpreted. This method has been used effectively in other health education initiatives (e.g., for nutrition, TB, and sexually transmitted diseases) (Datta and Nichter 2005).

Let us highlight two lessons we learned during the course of our research: details matter and folk wisdom is appreciated. In both field sites, local populations wanted more *specific* information on *how* tobacco caused specific health problems beyond general information about harm. They were not content with simply being told that tobacco was particularly harmful for people with diabetes; they wanted to know *how* tobacco consumption affected blood flow and how poor blood circulation was related to symptoms such as foot ulcers. In this case, a hydraulic model of flow and blockage was easily understood by diabetics.

Identifying appropriate responses to questions is often challenging. In the case of TB, former patients' questions about why smoking was particularly bad for them brought up the issue of the health of their lungs. We were faced with two possible messages. The first informs ex-TB patients that their lungs have been rendered weak for life and that smoking is especially dangerous for those with weak lungs. The second message conveys an image of the lungs of a TB patient as in a long-term process of healing and regaining strength. Healing is best accomplished if the person does not smoke. The question of which will prove most effective in each country requires further study.

A demand for specifics explained in simple terms and easy-to-grasp analogies and images influenced the development of our tobacco education materials (Nichter and Nichter 2001). It compelled QTI team members to engage in translational research that is attentive to practical logic and folk wisdom. In addition to analogies, proverbs also proved effective in making a point culturally salient. For example, in Kerala, some people with diabetes expressed a concern that if they quit smoking they would eat more and gain weight. A proverb was used to challenge their justification for continuing to smoke: "Smoking to reduce weight is like burning down the house to kill a rat" (local proverb). Another proverb was used in India to respond to TB patents who questioned whether it was appropriate to resume smoking at a low level if they consumed milk and ate healthy food. As a response, the QTI team stated that eating good food but continuing to smoke when you have TB was like "pouring water over a pot which is kept upside down" (local proverb).

We learned a different type of lesson during the course of presenting statistics to groups to enhance risk perception. Project teams first set out to determine through structured interviews and focus groups what types of global, national, and regional level tobacco facts were of most interest to local populations. Beyond identifying facts, we needed to pay attention to how risk was understood and best conveyed (Daley, James, Barnoskie, Segraves, Schupbach, and Choi et al. 2006; Gigerenzer and Edwards 2003; Weinstein 1999). Did the low- to middle-class populations in urban and periurban India and Indonesia respond well to statistics, and if so, what were the most relevant points of reference and frames of comparison? We found that lay people responded poorly to global statistics, were mildly interested in national statistics, and were far more interested in state and especially local level statistics and extrapolations. Some statistics that proved evocative in the West did not prove evocative in Asia. For example, statistics such as "lifetime economic expenditure on tobacco use" was poorly responded to and so was omitted from educational materials where space was at a premium. Another lesson we learned was that the person who presents statistics, such as a respected doctor, media person, or celebrity, is as important as the numbers themselves. This has led us to research whom people trust and respect to use as spokespersons.

Selecting Visual Images

A second way of raising consciousness that we have been developing is the use of graphic images. Our research has focused on how local populations would respond to graphic pictorial presentations of symptoms related to smoking (blackened lungs, mouth cancer, gangrenous feet, mouth ulcers, aging skin, and the like). The method we followed was similar to the one we used when developing question-and-answer frames. People were presented different pictures in focus groups and asked to chose ones they could relate to both cognitively (knowing what something was) and emotionally (horror and pity, but not so much horror one would look away). We found to our surprise that pictures selected for public use were quite graphic. Informants from both Kerala and Java also liked pictures of healthy and unhealthy body organs before and after smoking, respectively.

Evocative Appeals and Testimonials

A third approach we have been exploring is motivating smokers to quit through evocative appeals by loved ones. This has required 3 types of research.

First, we needed to investigate who could most effectively make such appeals. Exploring kinship relations in terms of power, status, and respect led us to the conclusion that the most evocative appeals to quit in both Kerala and Java would come from children younger than 10 and teenaged daughters, and not from wives or sons over the age of 10, as this would be seen as culturally disrespectful. To create emotional appeals to fathers to quit smoking, we are experimenting with invoking 2 types of images: images of children becoming ill and looking miserable after being exposed to smoke, and special times in a man's adult life (such as a child's marriage and the birth of grandchildren). Although responsibility is a subtext, the evocative images play on such things as a daughter's love for her father and her wanting him to be around to be a grandfather.

Another type of research we are involved in is the collection of illness narratives that might be used as evocative testimonials in print and short video formats. Stories that pull at the heartstrings of the listener may motivate them to quit or begin to think differently about smoking. We are in the process of developing different types of testimonials and testing them in focus groups, particularly testimonials that speak to the suffering of the smoker (e.g., a diabetic who smokes and becomes blind, or has a limb removed), the suffering of family members from secondhand smoke (e.g., a child who suffers from asthma), and family members who suffer as a result of a smoker's illness or death.

A third type of evocative image research QTI researchers are working on involves presenting juxtapositions that lead the public to think and feel in particular ways. For example, a popular image that won a poster contest in Indonesia juxtaposed a dead body wrapped in a white sheet before burial, and a cigarette drawn to look the same way (see Figure 11.4). Other images were appealing to the QTI team, but did not prove to be popular in some segments of the population, demonstrating the need for focus group research. For example, an image generated by a graphic artist that the team thought was very provocative pictured a cartoon character defending himself against cigarettes depicted as arrows. The figure held a shield and a *kris*, a ceremonial dagger associated with magical power and protection in Javanese culture. In focus groups, some teens to middle-aged men did not relate well to the cartoon character and deemed the imagery old fashioned. Others stated that the image might be useful for tobacco prevention among young children, but less useful for those who already smoke. We had hoped adults would also read the message as stating that one should resist temptation in the forms of cigarette promotions and tobacco industry advertising. We are currently investigating the appeal of the image for different age-groups, especially youth under 10 years of age familiar with cartoon heroes, and for those who are older and may immediately catch the cultural associations on a deeper level.

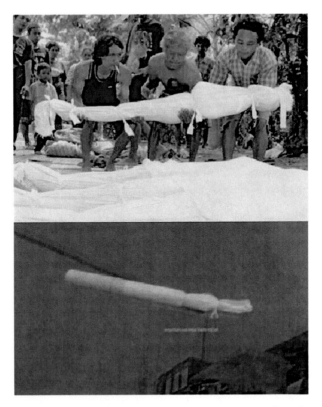

Figure 11.4. Counter-advertisement from Indonesia created to depict a body wrapped in a cloth for burial and a cigarette, the major behavioral risk factor responsible for premature death among men. (Photo by Mark Nichter)

Reframing Themes Used in Advertising

Advertising uses both cultural values and affiliation with the modern and global to position various brands of cigarettes. The QTI team in Indonesia was particularly keen to work on the reframing of advertising messages as part of our overall cessation strategy. We recognized the critical need to popularize and normalize a nonsmoking identity. Indonesia has some of the most sophisticated and aggressive tobacco advertising in the world and Java is awash in cigarette billboards, banners, and store signs. QTI Indonesia created a repository of cigarette advertisements, and analyzed them for thematic content (Nichter 2005). Focus groups were conducted to explore the types of people most likely to smoke different brands of cigarettes and what they liked about particular advertisements. Germane to this chapter, 2 popular themes used in advertisements were chosen for reframing following focus group research: masculinity and family values.

Rather than trying to confront global images of masculinity linked to images of sporting events and so forth directly, the QTI team has begun experimenting with a "challenge theme" and a "responsibility theme" that taps into Javanese images of strength related to willpower, having strength and confidence that draws others to follow your lead, and showing responsibility through one's actions. In focus groups among adults, this type of strength was thought to eclipse a macho image. Men are being asked in counter-messages if they are strong enough to quit smoking and if they have the strength to remain quit. Data from surveys of women are also being used to inform men that most women do not find smoking sexually appealing or attractive as advertisements would have them believe. The team is proceeding cautiously in light of observations made by Kohrman (2004) in China. In a country concerned about "quality citizens" and global image, mixed messages about the social and political appropriateness of smoking have led men to respond with considerable angst to tobacco control messages playing up a "strength to quit" theme. Kohrman notes that many men have begun to see themselves as too weak to engage in quitting as a form of self-management and desire regulation.

Family values are another theme commonly used in cigarette advertisements aimed at adults in Indonesia. Smoking is presented as a way to relax and enjoy social functions associated with cultural events, ranging from marriages and funerals to family gatherings. The QTI team is attempting to *take back culture* from the tobacco industry. Counter-images are being developed that present responsible men as never smoking anywhere near women and children. The tobacco industry is selling itself both as a bastion of authentic Indonesian culture through images of tradition and support of cultural events, and as a socially conscious industry through donations to schools and so forth.[5] It is important that such associations be broken.

Tobacco Cessation and Health Care Providers

In order for a downward shift in tobacco use to occur, health care providers must be at the forefront of tobacco cessation efforts (Davis 1993). To do so, they need to both quit using tobacco themselves and ask patients about tobacco use as a routine part of medical assessment (Fiore et al. 2000) and treat illness as a teachable moment (McBride, Emmons, and Lipkus 2003). A recent meta-analysis of the importance of health provider advice to quit tobacco concluded that provider advice delivered in routine care settings had greater impact on smoking cessation than all other major tobacco control strategies (Bao, Duan, and Fox 2006).

Surveys of doctors and medical students undertaken by QTI teams in India and Indonesia (Mohan et al. 2006; Ng et al. 2007) echo the findings of recent surveys by colleagues in India (*Indian Express* 2007) and China (Bezlova 2005; Li, Fish, and Zhou 1999; Smith, Wei, Zhang, and Wang 2006; Zhu, Feng, Wong, Choi, and Zhu 2004). Significant percentages of medical students and doctors currently smoke, and little time is allocated to tobacco-related health issues other than cancer in medical school (Richmond 2004; Tessier, Fréour, Belougne, and Crofton 1992). One of the major intervention goals of Project QTI in the next 5 years will be to introduce tobacco cessation training into all years of preclinical and clinical training in medical schools, and to mainstream tobacco education in all subject areas as distinct from being a stand-alone subject that appears to be peripheral. Our most basic goal is to train every medical student to ask patients routinely about their tobacco use and to convey to patients the message that quitting is one of the most important things that they can do for their own health and that of their family.

Of relevance to this chapter is a second set of research findings made by QTI teams related to messages doctors are currently giving to patients and how patients understand the messages delivered. Exit interviews with patients found that far fewer patients are asked about their tobacco habits than doctors report on surveys (Mohan et al. 2006; Ng et al. 2007). Qualitative interviews further revealed that advice given is often a one-liner offered in passing, not the type of brief intervention organized around the 5 As and 5 Rs (ask, advise, assess, assist, arrange; relevance of quitting to person, risk of smoking, reward of quitting, roadblock to quit, repetition) that has been recommended by cessation experts (Slama et al. 2007)—and which QTI has been trying to adapt for use in clinical and community settings in India and Indonesia. QTI interviews found that TB and diabetes patients often interpret the one-liners they receive (when they receive them) as general health advice—not advice specifically related to their illness, or advice not to smoke while sick or taking medication. QTI research also revealed that nurses, pharmacists, and TB treatment supporters (DOTS providers) rarely inquire about tobacco use or give advice to quit smoking. It is clear that QTI will not only need to promote the first two As of brief intervention in health care settings, but also to train health staff on how to answer common questions and provide them with culturally sensitive materials to assist them to participate in the process of cessation.

Project QTI has been recently funded for another 5 years to set up a tobacco cessation research network between medical schools and community groups in each country after introducing tobacco education into the schools of health professionals.[6] It is our intent to create a community of practice around tobacco cessation and cessation research (Wenger 1996, 1998). This will require additional formative research on the part of the medical anthropologists attached to the project. Introducing tobacco cessation in a packed medical school curriculum and knowing when and how to introduce brief tobacco interventions during a busy medical practice will be challenging. It will require culturally sensitive health service research attentive to the reality of medical practice in developing countries. We recognize that the devil is in the details—the when, how, and who issues that make or break an intervention. We also recognize that research will also need to be conducted on how to sustain the interest of health professionals in cessation in the face of failed quit attempts, given that cessation is a process typically characterized by multiple quit attempts. We also know that the efforts of health care providers will never be enough. Tobacco must become a primary health priority picked up by community groups and made into a women and children's—not just a men's—health issue.

Conclusion

Tobacco cessation is a high-priority public health intervention that can save millions of lives—in the short, not just the long term. We know little about how to introduce tobacco cessation in a culturally sensitive manner in developing countries. Project QTI is a pioneering attempt to find out what we need to know to encourage and successfully carry out smoking cessation. Transdisciplinary research has become a buzz word in the tobacco control field and anthropologists have an opportunity to participate in this emerging field of research (Abrams 2006; Nichter, Quintero, Nichter, Mock, and Shakib 2004; Sussman, Stacy, Johnson, Pentz, and Robertson 2004; Unger et al. 2003). To date, few medical anthropologists have actively participated in global tobacco control and even fewer have participated in tobacco cessation research. We have high hopes that this will change and have tried to illustrate some of the many areas of research in which anthropologists can contribute to tobacco cessation.

In this chapter, we have noted the importance of studying the social utility functions of smoking (and other forms of tobacco use) in different cultures, the social relations of accepting and turning down offers to smoke, the perceived risk of smoking at different levels by the general population, groups afflicted with illness, and by health care practitioners. We have called for ethnographies attentive to the sensorial aspects of smoking and quitting, cultural differences in how nicotine withdrawal is experienced and interpreted, and how sudden and gradual quit attempts are perceived. We have also noted the importance of translational research—research that finds the most culturally appropriate way of explaining to local populations (and patient populations such as those living with diabetes) how tobacco affects their bodies and leads to complications. Translational research is needed to identify appropriate analogies, pictures, ways to represent risk statistics, and so on. We have advocated the development of question–answer guides that address common misconceptions about tobacco use and health, and that address specific questions and concerns the local population has about smoking and quitting.

We have further called for the involvement of anthropologists in the analysis of tobacco advertisements and proactive attempts to reframe powerful symbolic associations cultivated by the tobacco industry tying smoking to masculinity, independence and strength, core cultural and family values, and so on. We have argued that tobacco cessation needs to be promoted as a family and women's health issue and not just a smoker's health issue. Smoking and smoking-related illness have a huge impact on the household in terms of second-hand smoke, the economic burden of morbidity, and shared suffering. And we have also suggested that cessation needs to be thought about in relation to space and place (e.g., household and public smoking bans) and not just person (individual smokers).

Thinking even more broadly, and in line with the biopolitical model of tobacco epidemiology presented in Figure 11.1, we see a role for engaged anthropologists in the study of tobacco policy as well as health service research related to smoking cessation (Abdulla and Husten 2004). How effective is existing tobacco policy and how can doctors and nurses be mobilized to better inform the public about the need for more stringent tobacco control measures—especially in spaces where nonsmokers are exposed to secondhand smoke? How can cessation services be best introduced in public and private clinics as well as in workplace environments? Also, how may tobacco cessation be best integrated into medical and nursing training programs as well as promoted in different urban and rural contexts through community outreach programs?[7]

Anthropologists will also have a role to play in monitoring the "vector" related activities of the tobacco industry and the industry's response to cessation efforts—efforts to both undermine and appropriate cessation toward its own ends. On a similar note, anthropologists will also need to monitor the marketing activities of the pharmaceutical industry as it enters the nicotine replacement market in developing countries, the response of local populations to the presence of cessation aids in the market, and the introduction of cessation aids by alternative medical systems.

Tobacco cessation is an urgent public health agenda that demands a keen assessment of people's motivations for smoking, how best to raise their consciousness about the health consequences of their actions for themselves and others, and how best to help them quit. It also requires an ongoing assessment of the promotion of a highly addictive product by a powerful industry that has proven to be unscrupulous on many well-documented occasions (Glantz, Barnes, Bero, Hanauer, and Slade 1996). Anthropologists working in the area of tobacco control are studying a moving target. They need to be ever vigilant and prepared to conduct research on not just changes in smoking behavior and response to national and international tobacco policy, but to do "ethnographies of spin." Moreover, anthropologists need to bear in mind that tobacco-related research—no matter how local—also demands a global perspective (Yach and Bettcher 2000). Tobacco control is the epitome of a global health problem demanding systemic ethnographic investigation.

Acknowledgments

The authors gratefully acknowledge support from the Fogarty International Center of the National Institutes of Health for research in India and Indonesia (RO1 TW005969). Project Quit Tobacco International is composed of three teams (India, Indonesia, and the US). The Indian team members are K.R. Thankappan, A.S. Pradeep Kumar, Sailesh Mohan, and C.U. Thresia from the Sree Chitra Tirunal Institute for Medical Sciences and Technology, Thiruvananthapuram, India. The Indonesian team members are Yayi Suryo Prabandari, R. Siwi Padmawati, and Nawi Ng, from the Department of Public Health, School of Medicine, Gadjah Mada University, Jogjakarta, Indonesia and the Centre for Bioethics and Medical Humanities, School of Medicine, Gadjah Mada University, Jogjakarta, Indonesia. The US team members are Mark Nichter, Mimi Nichter, Myra Muramoto (Department of Anthropology and Department of Family and Community Medicine, University of Arizona, Tucson, AZ), C. Keith Haddock, W. Carlos Poston, Felix Okah, and Kevin Hoffman, from the Department of Psychology, College of Arts & Sciences, University of Missouri–Kansas City, Kansas City, Missouri and Harry Lando, Division of Epidemiology, School of Public Health, University of Minnesota, Minneapolis, MN.

Notes

1. Raising consciousness involves getting across the message that tobacco is (a) the only legal product that, when used as intended by its manufacturers, eventually kills half its users (Beaglehole and Yach 2003); (b) a significant risk factor for over 25 major diseases; and (c) harmful and addictive even when consumed at low levels on a regular basis.

2. On the political economics of tobacco and the role of transnational corporations in promoting dependency through influencing state policy as well as involvement in contraband, see case studies by Stebbins (1991, 2001).

3. To date, Project QTI has focused on smoking. Many smokeless tobacco products are consumed in India, causing huge health problems such as oral cancer (Gupta and Ray 2003). These will be the focus of future QTI research and cessation interventions.

4. For an overview of the relationship between TB and smoking, see Chiang et al. (2007).

5. In Indonesia, religious organizations (like the *Nahdlatul Ulama*), members of Javanese royal families, and political parties have been tied to the tobacco

industry and particular brands of cigarettes. The tobacco industry has a history of giving scholarships to medical students and has been very active on college campuses.

6. Members of a tobacco cessation research network (TCRN) agree to be involved in the systematic study of various aspects of tobacco dependence and cessation including the evaluation of cessation interventions. The concept of a TCRN draws from the experience of practice-based research networks in medicine (Lindbloom et al. 2004; Nutting, Beasley, Werner 1999) and is attentive to the call for community participation in epidemiological studies (Leung, Yen, and Minkler 2004; Macaulay and Nutting 2006; Westfall, VanVorst, Main, and Herbert 2006).

7. An example of a community cessation outreach program that incorporates a formative research model and involves anthropologists is Project Reach, an Arizona-based program that trains laypersons on how to conduct brief tobacco cessation interventions (Campbell, Mays, Yuan, and Muramoto 2007; Castañeda, Nichter, Nichter, and Muramoto 2008).

References

Abdullah ASM, Husten CG (2004) Promotion of smoking cessation in developing countries: A framework for urgent public health interventions. *Thorax* 59:623–630.

Abrams DB (2006) Applying transdisciplinary research strategies to understanding and eliminating health disparities. *Health Education and Behavior* 33(4):515–531.

Achadi A, Soerojo W, Barber S (2005) The relevance and prospect of advancing tobacco control in Indonesia. *Health Policy* 72:333–349.

Altet MN, Alcaide J, Plans P, Taberner JL, Saltó E, Folguera LI et al. (1996) Passive smoking and risk of pulmonary tuberculosis in children immediately following infection. A case-control study. *Tubercle and Lung Disease* 77:537–544.

Bao Y, Duan N, Fox SA (2006) Is some provider advice on smoking cessation better than no advice? An instrumental variable analysis of the 2001 National Health Interview Survey. *Health Services Research* 41(6):2114–2135.

Beaglehole R, Yach D (2003) Globalization and the prevention and control of non-communicable disease: The neglected chronic diseases of adults. *Lancet* 362:903–908.

Bezlova A (2005) Curing the doctor in China. *Asian Times*, June 1. http://www.atimes.com

Bjork S, Kapur A, King H, Nair J, Ramachandran A (2003) Global policy: Aspects of diabetes in India. *Health Policy* 66(1):61–72.

Campbell J, Mays MZ, Yuan NP, Muramoto ML (2007) Who are health influencers? Characterizing a sample of tobacco cessation interveners. *American Journal of Health Behavior* 31(2):181–192.

Castañeda H, Nichter Mark, Nichter Mimi, Muramoto M (2008) Enabling and sustaining the activities of lay health influencers: Lessons from a community-based tobacco cessation intervention study. *Health Promotion Practice*, in press.

Chiang, CY, Slama K, Enarson DA (2007) Associations between tobacco and tuberculosis. *International Journal of Tuberculosis and Lung Disease* 11(3):258–262.

Daley CM, James AS, Barnoskie RS, Segraves M, Schupbach R, Choi WS (2006) Tobacco has a purpose, not just a past: Feasibility of developing a culturally appropriate smoking cessation program for a pan-tribal native population. *Medical Anthropology Quarterly* 20(4):421–440.

Datta M, Nichter Mark, for the IndiaCLEN Tuberculosis Study Group (2005) Towards ... introducing culturally sensitive tuberculosis education and context specific patient screening. http://www.inclentrust.org/downloads/pdf/ed_pack_mark_final.pdf and http://www.tnmmu.ac.in/edu.pdf

Davies PD, Yew WW, Ganguly D, Davidow AL, Reichman LB, Dheda K et al. (2006) Smoking and tuberculosis: The epidemiological association and immunopathogenesis. *Transactions of the Royal Society of Tropical Medicine and Hygiene* 100:291–298.

Davis R (1993) When doctors smoke. *Tobacco Control* 2:187–188.

Dye C (2006) Global epidemiology of TB. *Lancet* 367:938–940.

Dye C, Scheele S, Dolin P, Pathania V, Raviglione MC for the WHO Global Surveillance and Monitoring Project (1999) Global burden of tuberculosis: Estimated incidence, prevalence, and mortality by country. *Journal of the American Medical Association* 282:677–686.

Edwards R (2004) The problem of tobacco smoking. *British Medical Journal* 328: 217–219.

Eliasson B (2003) Cigarette smoking and diabetes. *Progress in Cardiovascular Diseases* 45(5):405–413.

Ezzati M, Lopez A (2003) Estimates of global mortality attributable to smoking in 2000. *Lancet* 362(9387):847–852.

Framework Convention Alliance for Tobacco Control (nd) www.fctc.org. Accessed 17 December, 2007.

Ferzacca S (2001) *Healing the Modern in a Central Javanese City*. Durham, NC: Carolina Academic Press.

Fiore M, Bailey WC, Cohen SJ, Dorfman SF, Goldstein MG, Gritz ER et al. (2000) *Treating Tobacco Use and Dependence: Clinical Practice Guideline*. Rockville, MD: U.S. Department of Health and Human Services, Public Health Service.

Foy CG, Bell RA, Farmer DF, Goff DC, Wagenknecht LE (2005) Smoking and incidence of diabetes among U.S. adults: Findings from the Insulin Resistance Atherosclerosis Study. *Diabetes Care* 28:2501–2507.

Frieden TR, Bloomberg MR (2007) How to prevent 100 million deaths from tobacco. *Lancet* 369(9574):1758–1761.

Gajalakshmi V, Peto R, Kanaka P, Jha P (2003) Smoking and mortality from tuberculosis and other causes in India: Retrospective study of 43,000 male deaths and 35,000 controls. *Lancet* 362:507–515.

Gigerenzer G, Edwards A (2003) Simple tools for understanding risks: From innumeracy to insight. *British Medical Journal* 327:741–744.

Glantz SA, Barnes DE, Bero L, Hanauer P, Slade J (1996) *The Cigarette Papers*. Berkeley, CA: University of California Press.

Gupta P, Ray C (2003) Smokeless tobacco and health in India and South Asia. *Respirology* 8(4):419–431.

Houston TK, Sharina DP, Mark JP, Kiang Liu, Carlos I, Catarina IK (2006) Active and passive smoking and development of glucose intolerance among young adults in a prospective cohort: CARDIA study. *British Medical Journal* 332:1064–1069.

Indian Express (2007) Most would-be docs smoke to bust stress, finds AIIMS. Monday, May 14, 2007.

International Institute for Population Sciences (IIPS) (2001) National Family Health Survey (NFHS-2) India, 1998–99, Kerala. Mumbai, IIPS, 28–30.

Jamison DT, Breman JG, Measham AR et al., eds. (2006) *Priorities in Health*. Washington, DC: World Bank.

Jha P, Chaloupka FJ, eds. (1999) *Curbing the Epidemic: Governments and the Economics of Tobacco Control*. Washington, DC: World Bank.

Kannan KP, Thankappan KR, Raman Kutty V, Aravindan KP (1991) Health and Development in Rural Kerala. Thiruvananthapuram, India: Kerala Sastra Sahitya Parishad.

Khatri GR, Frieden TR (2000) The status and prospects of tuberculosis control in India. *International Journal of Tuberculosis Lung Disease* 4:193–200.

King H, Aubert RE, Herman WH (1998) Global burden of diabetes, 1995–2025. *Diabetes Care* 21:1414–1431.

Kohrman M (2004) Should I quit? Tobacco, fraught identity, and the risks of governmentality in urban China. *Urban Anthropology* 33(2–4):211–245.

Kolappan C, Gopi PG (2002) Tobacco smoking and pulmonary tuberculosis. *Thorax* 57:964–966.

Larabie LC (2005) To what extent do smokers plan quit attempts? *Tobacco Control* 14:425–428.

Leung MW, Yen IH, Minkler M (2004) Community based participatory research: A promising approach for increasing epidemiology's relevance in the 21st century. *International Journal of Epidemiology* 33(3):499–506.

Li HZ, Fish D, Zhou X (1999) Increase in cigarette smoking and decline of anti-smoking counselling among Chinese physicians: 1987–1996. *Health Promotion International* 14(2):123–131.

Lin H-H, Ezzati M, Murray M (2007) Tobacco smoke, indoor air pollution and tuberculosis: A systematic review and meta-analysis. *PLoS Medicine* 4(1):e20.

Lindbloom EJ, Ewigman BG, Hickner JM (Year) Practice-based research networks: The laboratories of primary health care research. *Medical Care* 42:45–49.

Macaulay A, Nutting P (2006) Moving the frontiers forward: Incorporating community-based participatory research into practice-based research networks. *Annals of Family Medicine* 4:4–7.

Mackay J, Eriksen M (2002) *The Tobacco Atlas*. Geneva: World Health Organization.

Manson JE, Ajani UA, Liu S, Nathan DM, Hennekens CH (2000) A prospective study of cigarette smoking and the incidence of diabetes mellitus among US male physicians. *American Journal of Medicine* 109(7):538–542.

McBride CM, Emmons KM, Lipkus IM (2003) Understanding the potential of teachable moments: The case of smoking cessation. *Health Education Research* 18(2):156–170.

Mohan S, Pradeepkumar AS, Thresia CU, Thankappan KR, Poston WSC, Haddock CK et al. (2006) Tobacco use among medical professionals in Kerala, India: The need for enhanced tobacco cessation and control efforts. *Addictive Behaviors* 31(12):2313–2318.

Murray CJ, Lopez AD, eds. (1996) *The Global Burden of Disease: A Comprehensive Assessment of Mortality and Disability From Diseases, Injuries and Risk Factors in 1990 and Projected to 2020*. Cambridge, MA: Harvard School of Public Health.

Ng N, Prabandari YS, Padmawati RS, Okah F, Haddock CK, Nichter M et al. (2007) Physician assessment of patient smoking in Indonesia: A public health priority. *Tobacco Control* 16(3):190–196.

Nichter Mark (2003) Smoking: What does culture have to do with it? *Addiction* 98(1):139–145.

Nichter Mark, for the Project Quit Tobacco International Group (2006) Introducing tobacco cessation in developing countries: An overview of Project Quit Tobacco International. *Tobacco Control* 15(1):12–17.

Nichter Mark, Cartwright E (1991) Saving the children for the tobacco industry. *Medical Anthropology Quarterly* 5(3): 236–256.

Nichter Mark, Nichter Mimi (2001) "Education by Appropriate Analogy." In: *Anthropology and International Health: Asian Case Studies.* M Nichter, M Nichter, eds. New York: Routledge, pp. 401–426.

Nichter Mark, Gilbert Quintero, Mimi Nichter, Jeremiah Mock, Sohaila Shakib (2004) Qualitative research: Contributions to the study of drug use, drug abuse, and drug use(r)-related interventions. *Substance Use and Misuse* 39(10–12):1907–69.

Nichter Mimi (2005) Developing tobacco cessation in Indonesia: Reframing advertising messages. Paper presented at the Society for Applied Anthropology Meetings, Vancouver, BC, April 2005.

Nichter Mimi, Mark Nichter, David Van Sickle (2004) Popular perceptions of tobacco products and patterns of use among male college students in India. *Social Science and Medicine* 59:415–431.

Nutting PA, Beasley JW, Werner JJ (1999) Practice-based research networks answer primary care questions. *Journal of the American Medical Association* 281:686–688.

Orth SR, Ritz E, Schrier RW (1997) The renal risks of smoking. *Kidney International* 51:1669–1677.

Orth SR, Ogata H, Ritz E (2000) Smoking and the kidney. *Nephrology Dialysis Transplantation* 15:1509–1511.

Pai M (2007) Lethal interaction: The colliding epidemics of tobacco and tuberculosis. *Expert Review of Anti-infective Therapy* 5(3):385–391.

Panikar PGK (1998) Health Transition in Kerala. Discussion Paper No. 10. Kerala Research Programme on Local Level Development. Thiruvananthapuram: India Centre for Development Studies.

Peto R, Lopez A (2002) "Future worldwide health effects of current smoking patterns." In: *Critical Issues in Global Health.* C Koop, C Pearson, MR Schwarz, eds. San Francisco: Jossey-Bass, pp. 154–161.

Peto R, Darby S, Deo H, Silcocks P, Whitley E, Doll R (2000) Smoking, smoking cessation, and lung cancer in the UK since 1950: Combination of national statistics with two case-control studies. *British Medical Journal* 321:323–329.

Pradono JK (2002) *Passive Smokers, the Forgotten Disaster.* Jakarta: National Institute of Health Research and Development, Ministry of Health.

Prochaska JO, Goldstein MG (1991) Process of smoking cessation: Implications for clinicians. *Clinical Chest Medicine* 12:727–735.

Prochaska JO, Velicer WF (1997) The transtheoretical model of health behavior change. *American Journal of Health Promotion* 12:38–48.

Prochaska JO, DiClemente CC, Velicer WF, Ginpil SE, Norcross JC (1985) Predicting change in smoking status for self-changers. *Addictive Behaviors* 10:395–406.

Rani M, Bonu S, Jha P, Nguyen SN, Jamjoum L (2003) Tobacco use in India: Prevalence and predictors of smoking and chewing in a national cross sectional household survey. *Tobacco Control* 12(4):e4.

Reddy KS, Gupta P, eds. (2004) *Report on Tobacco Control in India.* New Delhi, India, Ministry of Health & Family Welfare.

Regalado M, Yang S, Wesson DE (2000) Cigarette smoking is associated with augmented progression of renal insufficiency in severe essential hypertension. *American Journal of Kidney Diseases* 35:687–694.

Richmond R (2004) The process of introducing a tobacco curriculum in medical school. *Respirology* 9:165–172.

Sankaranarayanan R, Mathew B, Binu JJ, Thomas G, Somanathan T, Pisani P et al. (2000) Early findings from a community-based, cluster randomized controlled oral cancer screening trial in Kerala, India. *Cancer* 88:664–673.

Singer M, Clair S (2003) Syndemics and public health: Reconceptualizing disease in bio-social context. *Medical Anthropology Quarterly* 17:423–441.

Slama K (2004) Current challenges in tobacco control. *International Journal of Tuberculosis and Lung Disease* 8(10):1160–1172.

Slama K, Chiang CY, Enarson DA, Hassmiller K, Fanning A, Gupta P et al. (2007) Tobacco and tuberculosis: A qualitative systematic review and meta-analysis. *International Journal of Tuberculosis and Lung Disease* 11(10):1049–1061.

Smith DR, Wei N, Zhang YJ, Wang RS (2006) Tobacco smoking habits among a cross-section of rural physicians in China. *Australian Journal of Rural Health* 14(2):66–71.

Stebbins KR (1991) Tobacco, politics and economics: Implications for global health. *Social Science and Medicine* 33(2):1317–1326.

Stebbins KR (2001) Going like gangbusters: Transnational tobacco companies "making a killing" in South America. *Medical Anthropology Quarterly* 15(2):147–170.

Stillman FA, Wipfli H (2005) New century: Same challenges. *British Journal of Cancer* 92:1179–1181.

Sussman S, Stacy AW, Johnson CA, Pentz MA, Robertson E (2004) A transdisciplinary focus on drug abuse prevention: An introduction. *Substance Use and Misuse* 39(10–12):1441–1456.

Tessier JF, Fréour P, Belougne D, Crofton J (1992) Smoking habits and attitudes of medical students towards smoking and antismoking campaigns in nine Asian countries. *International Journal of Epidemiology* 21:298–304.

Thankappan KR, Valiathan MS (1998) Health at low cost—the Kerala model. *Lancet* 351:1274–1275.

Thomas A, Gopi PG, Santha T, Chandrasekaran V, Subramani R (2005) Predictors of relapse among tuberculosis patients treated in a DOTS programme in South India. *International Journal of Tuberculosis and Lung Disease* 9:556–561.

Tobacco Free Initiative (TFI) (2004) Why is tobacco a public health priority? World Health Organization, December 12, 2004.

Ulin PE, Robinson T, Tolley EE (2004) *Qualitative Methods in Public Health.* San Francisco, CA: Jossey-Bass.

Unger JB, Cruz T, Shakib S, Mock J, Shields A, Baezconde-Garbanati L et al. (2003) Exploring the cultural context of tobacco use: A transdisciplinary framework. *Nicotine and Tobacco Research* 5(1):S101–S117.

US Department of Health and Human Services (1990) The health benefits of smoking cessation. A report of the Surgeon General, Washington, DC. DHHS Publication No. (CDC) 90–8416.

US Department of Health and Human Services (2004) "Introduction and Approach to Causal Inference." In: *The Health Consequences of Smoking: A Report of the Surgeon General.* Atlanta: US Department of Health and Human Services, Centers for Disease Control and Prevention, National Center for Chronic Disease Prevention and Health Promotion, Office on Smoking and Health, pp. 1–33.

Weinstein ND (1999) What does it mean to understand a risk? Evaluating risk comprehension. *Journal of the National Cancer Institute, Monographs* 25:15–20.

Wenger E (1996) Communities of practice: The social fabric of a learning organization. *Healthcare Forum Journal* 39(4):22–26.

Wenger E (1998) *Communities of practice—learning, meaning, and identity.* New York: Cambridge University Press.

West R (2005) Time for change: Putting the Transtheoretical (Stages of Change) Model to rest. *Addiction* 100:1036–1039.

West R, Sohal T (2006) Catastrophic pathways to smoking cessation: Findings from national survey. *British Medical Journal* 332:458–460.

Westfall JM, VanVorst RF, Main DS, Herbert C (2006) Community-based participatory research in practice-based research networks. *Annals of Family Medicine* 4:8–14.

Wild S, Roglic G, Green A, Sicree R, King H (2004) Global prevalence of diabetes: Estimates for the year 2000 and projections for 2030. *Diabetes Care* 27:1047–1053.

Wilhelm K, Wedgwood L, Niven H, Kay-Lambkin F (2006) Smoking cessation and depression: Current knowledge and future. *Drug and Alcohol Review* 25(1):97–107.

Will JC, Galuska DA, Ford ES, Mokdad A, Calle EE (2001) Cigarette smoking and diabetes mellitus: Evidence of a positive association from a large prospective cohort study. *International Journal of Epidemiology* 30:540–546.

World Bank (1999) Curbing the Epidemic: Governments and the Economics of Tobacco Control. Washington, DC: World Bank

World Health Organization (2002) The cost of diabetes. Fact Sheet Number 236. Geneva, Switzerland: WHO.

World Health Organization Global InfoBase Team (2005) The SuRF Report 2. Surveillance of Chronic Disease Risk Factors: Country-Level Data and Comparable Estimates. Geneva: World Health Organization.

Wright AA, Katz IT (2007) Tobacco tightrope—balancing disease prevention and economic development in China. *New England Journal of Medicine* 356(15):1493–1495.

Yach D, Bettcher D (2000) Globalisation of tobacco industry influence and new global responses. *Tobacco Control* 9:206–216.

Zhu T, Feng B, Wong S, Choi W, Zhu SH (2004) A comparison of smoking behaviors among medical and other college students in China. *Health Promotion International* 19(2):189–196.

12

From Street Research to Public Health Intervention: The Hartford Drug Monitoring Project

MERRILL SINGER, GREG MIRHEJ, CLAUDIA SANTELICES, AND HASSAN SALEHEEN

Introduction

It is estimated that over 200 million people worldwide consume illicit drugs (Kavan 2003). In the United States in the year 2004, over 19 million Americans, or about 8% of the population over the age of 12, reported using illicit drugs—including marijuana/hashish, cocaine, heroin, hallucinogens, inhalants, and diverted pharmaceutical drugs (i.e., medicine with psychopharmacological properties that are diverted from the legal to the illegal drug market)—during the 30-day period before being interviewed in the National Survey on Drug Use and Health (2005). The annual economic cost of drug abuse in the United States is estimated to be over $180 billion (Lewin Group 2004). The human cost, in terms of disease and social suffering, is also enormous (Farmer and Kleinman 1989). More than one-third of all HIV/AIDS adult cases in the United States are directly or indirectly linked to injection drug use, through either high-risk sexual contact under the influence of drugs or the sharing and reuse of nonsterile syringes and other drug paraphernalia (CDC 2004).

A significant dimension of drug-related health problems arises from the interaction of 2 or more present diseases simultaneously and noxious social conditions, a phenomenon known as a *syndemic* (Singer and Clair 2003; Singer et al. 2006). Research among almost 1,000 not-in-treatment injection drug users (IDUs) in Connecticut and Massachusetts (Singer 2006b), for example, found high rates of a range of major diseases, including HIV/AIDS (26%), hepatitis B (24%), hepatitis C (33%), other sexually transmitted diseases (23%), and tuberculosis (TB) (8%). While 24% of the individuals in the sample reported none of these diseases and an additional 23% reported only 1 of the diseases, the remaining 53% reported 2 or more of these diseases. Bodily interactions among these diseases and other health conditions have been shown to magnify the damage done to the health status of drug users beyond the sum of their individual contributions to user morbidity (CDC 2002).

Importantly, drug use is an ever-changing behavior. While the concept of addiction suggests inflexible adherence to the use of specific drugs (e.g., "heroin addiction") and routinized ways of using them (e.g., "drug injection"), the shadowy domain of illegal drug use is in a continuous and consequential transformation, much like the complex social world that drives it—a place of quickly shifting technologies, transportable ideas, mobile populations, and changing market-driven commodities. While in local settings consumption may remain stable for varying periods, viewed globally and over longer periods of time, the lesson that has been learned by drug researchers is "that 'drug problems' are an ever-shifting and changing phenomena. There are fads and fashions, rages and crazes, and alternative trends in drugs of choice and patterns of use" (Inciardi, Lockwood, and Pottieger 1993:1). The types of changes that occur include the appearance of new drugs and novel drug combinations, innovations in ways of using older drugs and adoption of new kinds of drug use equipment, and the development of new populations of users and contexts of drug use (Singer 2006a). Moreover, as evidenced by the HIV/AIDS pandemic, as well as the rapid diffusion of viral hepatitis among drug users, the emergence of TB as a drug-related disease, the increasingly global spread of injection drug use, the ever wider distribution of methamphetamine consumption, rising rates of drug overdose, and the increasing dominance of polydrug use patterns, change in drug use dynamics can have significant effects on public health.

Despite the magnitude of the drug abuse problem, most communities have limited programming in place to either monitor changing drug use patterns or assess the public health implications of changes that occur. As a result, new patterns of use can emerge and become widespread before they are identified and their potential public health implications assessed. This occurred, for example, both in the case of the appearance of crack cocaine in the mid- to late-1980s and the first detection of injection drug-related spread of HIV around the same time.

As these examples suggest, as drug use practices are modified, society is confronted with new diseases or disease expressions, renewed diseases (i.e., new epidemics of older diseases), and other health and social consequences (e.g., overdose cases, injury-causing drug-related violence, and other drug-related crimes) that it is unprepared to handle. Existing programs, including both drug treatment and prevention, may not have the means of monitoring behavioral change. Moreover, as drug treatment programs age, their defining missions become less flexible and their procedures routinized. One consequence is that programs can become resistant to change even in the face of significant shifts in drug use patterns among local populations (Singer et al. 2005b, 2005c).

As a result of these factors, periodic drug use assessment has been identified as an important and needed public health initiative. Ouellet, Wiebel, and Jimenz (1995:182) observe: "Given the potential impact of substance abuse on matters as grave as health, education, and crime, intelligent policy formation often requires that accurate information be produced quickly." Some researchers and policy makers have begun to point to the need for ongoing monitoring that is capable of rapidly spotting new behaviors or new health and social consequences of older behaviors performed under changed conditions. While traditional public health surveillance analyzed trends in mortality and, to a somewhat lesser extent, morbidity, such an approach is inadequate when there is a major time lag between preventable exposure and the clinical manifestations of disease, as is the case with AIDS, for example, in which the gap can be 10 years or longer. As Morabia (1996:625) emphasizes, under these circumstances, "monitoring distributions of risk factors in populations [based on actual monitoring of behavior] provides short-term indicators to identify prevention strategies, assess their effectiveness, and predict emerging epidemics."

In this light, this chapter reports on the Community Responses to Risks of Emergent Drug Use Project, also called the Drug Monitoring Study, an anthropologically initiated CDC-funded project in Hartford, CT, that was designed to (1) use ethnographic and epidemiological methods to identify and track emergent drug use trends; (2) analyze these trends across key socio-demographic traits, including age, gender, ethnicity, and neighborhood of residence; (3) assess the potential impact of changes in drug use on public health; and (4) use a Participatory Action Research (PAR) model to implement community-based public health responses to research findings in collaboration with a Community Response Team (CRT) composed of representatives of local health-care provider institutions (e.g., emergency room physicians), community-based organizations, HIV prevention initiatives, drug treatment services, local high schools, and related programs and institutions. The chapter demonstrates the utility of field-based anthropological methods in the rapid identification of emergent drug-related cultural conceptions (e.g., new understandings of old drugs, as occurred with the development of crack cocaine); new behaviors (e.g., new drug combinations such as the mixing of phencyclidine [PCP], embalming fluid, and marijuana); changing social relationships (e.g., the array of local drug distributors and their supply sources exemplified by the replacement of so-called "mom and pop" small scale methamphetamine producers in the mid-west and south by large laboratories in Mexico); and cultural artifacts (e.g., drugs and drug paraphernalia, such as the crafting of crack pipes from available glass tubes of various sorts) that can have significant public health effects.

The chapter specifically focuses on several drug use trends that were examined in the study, including the spread of methamphetamine among hard-core drug users, PCP among emergent adult users, and sweetened cigars among youth, as well as the anthropological methods (field immersion, participant observation, casual interviewing, in-depth interviewing, and ethnographically informed surveys). Moreover, the chapter shows the value of ethnographic and related methods in tracking the diffusion of new drug use patterns across urban neighborhoods and subgroups (Page 1990). Finally, the chapter affirms the capacity of anthropologists to take the lead in local public health efforts in collaboration with colleagues from other disciplines by describing applied initiatives designed to address the public health implications of identified drug use trends.

Monitoring Risk Among Drug Users: An Overview of Initiatives in the United States

Traditional methods for monitoring drug-related mortality and morbidity emphasized the use of surveys and various statistical mechanisms (e.g., emergency room mentions of drug use, tracking of the causes of death using death certificates). The shift to field-based public health surveillance of drug-related risk, including actual observations of drug use combined with assessment of the social relationships, cultural understandings, and life contexts that shape risk behaviors, requires a change in the focus of research from outcome to onset, from ultimate consequences to on-the-ground behaviors, and development of rapid approaches for the identification of contextual sources of risk. This methodological transition creates the opportunity for "ethno-epidemiology" or "cultural epidemiology" (Trostle 2004), the productive collaboration between traditional ethnographic and epidemiological approaches to the definition of research questions and the collection, analysis, and interpretation of findings. As a result, field investigation in natural settings takes on a dramatic new importance in public health research, as does "technique triangulation" (Fielding and Fielding 1986), that is, the collection of diverse data using various strategies in a multimethod research design involving the analytic integration of heterogeneous types of data.

While movement toward public health monitoring of risk began in the 1970s, the effort especially gained momentum with the AIDS epidemic and recognition of the link between behaviors involving drug use and HIV transmission. In 1994, the Committee on Substance Abuse and Mental Health Issues in

AIDS Research of the Institute of Medicine, in response to a Congressional directive to the Alcohol, Drug Abuse, and Mental Health Administration, initiated a study of AIDS that concluded that among IDUs it is "critical to develop effective epidemiological surveillance mechanisms for identifying new drug injectors within populations, to be able to track trends in drug injection over time" (Auerbach, Wypijewska, and Brodie 1994:71). The Committee recommended that the National Public Health Service coordinate new interagency efforts "to monitor and respond to concurrent epidemics (such as drug use, violence, and infectious diseases) that will alter the course of the HIV epidemic" (Auerbach et al. 1994:6). The Committee explicitly emphasized the value of expanding the role of behavioral and social science research, including cultural and ethnographic studies, as part of these efforts. The National Research Council reached a similar conclusion:

> Monitoring changes in risk-associated behaviors that can lead to subsequent acquisition and spread of infection is ... critically important. During the first decade of the [AIDS] epidemic, investigators who considered the risks associated with drug use focused primarily on injection practices. As the epidemic has matured, however, greater appreciation of the role of other drugs, such as crack, has emerged ... (Miller, Turner and Lincoln 1990:69).

This recognition further supported the development of new surveillance strategies capable of drawing "attention to the appearance of new drugs whose use may pose additional risk to [the drug using] population" (Miller, Turner, and Lincoln 1990:71).

Monitoring Efforts at the National Institute on Drug Abuse

In the field of drug studies, an important influence on the growing awareness of the benefits of perpetual monitoring is the Community Epidemiology Work Group (CEWG) of the National Institute on Drug Abuse. The CEWG is a loosely affiliated network of field researchers from major urban areas across the United States but also includes affiliated researchers in other countries. The network meets semiannually,

> with the primary objective of providing ongoing community-level public health surveillance of drug use and abuse, principally through collection and analysis of epidemiologic and ethnographic research data. Through this program, the CEWG provides current descriptive and analytical information regarding the nature and patterns of drug abuse, emerging trends, and characteristics of vulnerable populations (Kozel 1997:iii).

Implied in the accounts above is the primary public health objective of systematic behavioral monitoring, namely to "get out ahead" of shifting trends in drug use and their health consequences through the expeditious implementation of research-driven educational, behavior change, treatment, or other efforts designed to minimize the health effects of drug use shifts. Exemplary are several national efforts by the National Institute on Drug Abuse (NIDA), including the 29-site National AIDS Demonstration Projects (NADR), and the 23-site Cooperative Agreement for AIDS Community-based Outreach Intervention Research (CA), in which our research team participated (Coyle, Needle, and Norman 1998). Through these projects, ethnographer/indigenous outreach worker field teams (in varying configurations) were deployed in local communities to identify, recruit, and (in some cases) provide intervention to active, not-in-treatment drug users. These teams, which link ethnographic researchers with trained outreach and recruitment specialists, often drawn from the target community, were in a position to rapidly identify new or emergent drug use trends and related health risks, and to monitor the changing drug scene locally (Carlson, Jichuan, Siegal, and Falck 1994; Koester 1994a, 19994b, 1996; Koester and Hoffer 1994:1990).

Through NADR and the CA, our research team was able to develop a profile of street drug use in Hartford, CT, including, among other findings, a pattern of high frequency drug injection as compared with IDUs in other cities, important (African American vs. Puerto Rican) ethnic differences in drugs of consumption and injection frequencies, an absence of methamphetamine injection, notable levels of injection equipment sharing, and high rates of HIV and hepatitis infection as compared to IDUs elsewhere in the country (Dushay, Singer, Weeks, Rohena, and Gruber 2001; Singer 1999a; Singer, Himmelgreen, Singer, Richmond, and Romero-Daza 1998; Weeks, 1998; Weeks, Singer, Grier, Hunte-Marrow, and Haughton 1993; Weeks, Williams, Schensul, Singer, and Grier 1995; Weeks, Singer, Grier, and Schensul 1996). Currently, the CEWG and the Monitoring the Future study (MTF) constitute NIDA's two main national-level epidemiological tracking studies. NIDA has used findings from both of these to implement public information campaigns targeted to both drug users and the broader community concerning dangerous new trends in drug use, such as a sharp rise in the use of anabolic–androgenic steroids, significant increases in the use of so-called club drugs like ecstasy, the spread of methamphetamine use across many parts of the United States, and the diversion of pharmaceutical drugs to illicit use (Leshner 2000).

Monitoring Efforts at the Centers for Disease Control and Prevention

Also important is the Centers for Disease Control and Prevention (CDC) effort to build multicity collaborative programs in response to AIDS, beginning in 1984, with its funding of a U.S. Conference of Mayors effort to enhance information exchange on AIDS prevention activities. In 1985, the CDC began funding community-based HIV prevention demonstration projects, but initially only government public health programs could apply for funding. Two years later, the CDC began to enter into cooperative agreements with nongovernment organizations focused on AIDS prevention and soon launched its AIDS Community Demonstration Projects initiative (O'Reilly and Higgins 1991). By 1994, over 500 organizations were directly or indirectly funded by the CDC. That same year, the CDC's HIV prevention strategies were assessed through an external review by health professionals, social scientists, and prevention experts organized by the CDC Advisory Committee on the Prevention of HIV Infection. One recommendation of this review was that the CDC's AIDS/HIV surveillance be expanded from "counting cases" of disease or infection to include the monitoring of behaviors like drug use that facilitate acquisition and transmission of HIV. In the language of the review committee, "[m]oving the focus of surveillance to the 'front end' of the epidemic is a critical prerequisite to the identification, development and evaluation of prevention interventions" (CDC 1994:34).

An exemplary movement in this direction was CDC support of an 8-city community assessment process (CAP) involving (in the first year) a series of qualitative interviews with IDUs and youth in high-risk situations (e.g., homeless youth who support themselves through the illicit street economy), followed (in the second year) by a survey with representative samples of these 2 target populations. The CAP was designed to learn (1) the distribution of prevention materials and messages; (2) the locations of intervention delivery by street outreach workers; and (3) the delivery of other services to the target populations. In the CDC-supported AIDS Community Demonstration Projects (Corby and Wolitski 1997; Wolitski, Corby, Fishbein, and Galavotti 1996a; Wolitski, Fishbein, Johnson, Higgins, and Esacove 1996b), formative research to identify sources of HIV information, such as community experts knowledgeable about local risk patterns in targeted populations (such as IDUs), was a prerequisite for the development of community-level HIV prevention efforts.

Project RARE and the Office of HIV/AIDS Policy

In the late 1990s, in response to the rise of a significantly disproportionate rate of AIDS cases in African American and other ethnic minority communities, the U.S. Surgeon General's Office of HIV/AIDS Policy (OHAP) adopted a rapid ethnographic assessment model called RARE (Rapid Assessment, Response, and Evaluation) for use by U.S. cities in identifying, targeting, and implementing effective local interventions. The RARE model was based on the development of local field teams charged with building on existing knowledge of at-risk communities and settings through focused research. The core set of methods utilized by RARE field teams include focus group interviews, key informant interviews, direct observations, mapping and geocoding, and rapid assessment interviews containing both qualitative and quantitative questions (Bowser, Quimbey, and Singer 2007). The multimethods mixture found in RARE parallels that utilized in other rapid assessment and response programs (see Rhodes, Stimson, Fitch, Ball, and Renton 1999; Stimson, Fitch, Rhodes, and Ball 1999). Rapid assessment provides information for spotting emerging conditions that are not yet apparent in other data sets and allows for the development of interventions successfully configured for local contexts, especially where local cultural conditions and values are different from the dominant cultural system.

Additionally, critical to the RARE model is the rapid research-based development of specific recommendations for public health action (Trotter and Singer 2005, 2007). These recommendations, and the RARE model overall, are designed to bridge the gap between science and public health practice and policy (Shriver, de Burger, Brown, Simpson, and Meyerson 1998). As designed, the RARE model has been shown to lead to the successful development of targeted, community-appropriate prevention/intervention recommendations; however, operationalization and implementation of recommendations is left to local public health and political officials (Singer, Bowser, and Quimbey 2007). Consequently, there has been an uneven response to recommended changes in public health practices/policies, in part reflecting local political issues as well as traditional tensions between research and practice. Moreover, even when attempted, the successful transfer of research findings to community-based and public health service organizations to help guide intervention efforts remains a significant challenge. Various translation barriers have been identified, including those found in community organizations (e.g., lack of appropriate personnel, lack of needed resources, lack of adequate staff training, and lack of required information) or in the original intervention model (e.g., too costly to implement by a community organization, too time consuming, and culturally inappropriate for local target populations) (Hitt et al. 2006; Singer et al. 2005a). Another issue is community participation in the formation of prevention research to ensure the relevance and applicability of tested models. As Auerbach and Coates (2000:1031) emphasize, "how best to do this translation, transferal, and collaborative research is an undeveloped scientific question that requires further investigation."

The National HIV Behavioral Surveillance

Continued high levels of HIV infection among men who have sex with men, heterosexuals who engage in high-risk sexual practices, and IDUs led the CDC to develop a model—called the National HIV Behavioral Surveillance

(NHBS)—for ongoing AIDS behavioral tracking in municipal areas with the largest number of AIDS cases (Gallagher, Denning, Allen, Nakashima, Sullivan 2007a; Gallagher, Sullivan, Lansky, and Onorato 2007b; Lansky et al. 2007). The method was implemented in 25 metropolitan areas across the United States beginning in 2005, with plans to continue surveillance at least through 2010. The sampling method used for the recruitment of IDUs in this program—which is implemented every 3 years (in rotation with the other 2 target groups)—is Respondent-Driven Sampling (RDS) (Broadhead et al. 1998). RDS is a controlled form of chain-referral sampling that involves using the social networks of drug users as recruitment pathways to contact new participants as embedded recruiting agents. The method has been proved to allow the development of statistically valid samples from hidden and hard-to-reach populations (and those for which no clear sampling frames exist) (Salganik and Heckathorn 2004). As Heckathorn, and colleagues (1999) note, just as drug user social networks serve as the route of transmission for the virus, they also have great potential to be used as the route of transmission for HIV prevention information and services.

On the basis of a formative data collection phase using observational and other qualitative methods, RDS researchers identify various locations in the target area from which to recruit a small sample (e.g., 10 to 15) of first-level "seeds" (i.e., individuals from the target group who are capable of using their social networks to recruit additional individuals who meet project inclusion criteria). Recruitment of first-level seeds is critical because those selected as seeds must have adequate social networks to allow the recruitment of new participants.

In implementing this approach, it has been found necessary to ensure through recruitment ethnic, gender, age, and other diversities among the initial seeds, as individuals tend to recruit others who share their sociodemographic characteristics (e.g., recruiting only Hispanic seeds would bias the overall sample in favor of Hispanics). Seeds are provided with numbered recruitment coupons that they give to drug-injecting members of their social network. These second-level participants are instructed by the seeds to bring the coupon to the local project site to enlist. The staff record all coupon numbers to allow identification of the originating seed and to track the numbers and characteristics of participants recruited by each seed. Second-level participants, in turn, are trained to recruit members of their respective networks and so forth. RDS-based research indicates that recruitment to the sixth level ensures representative sampling from the target population despite the use of a nonrandom recruitment method (Heckathorn 2002). The NHBS structured interview asks participants about drug use and sexual behavior, HIV testing history, and access to and use of HIV prevention services. Findings are available to local communities for use in the development of targeted prevention efforts.

The Drug Monitoring Study

Context

The Drug Monitoring Study was implemented in Hartford, the capitol of Connecticut and one of the 14 poorest cities in the United States. Hartford was 1 of only 4 U.S. cities that saw an increase in the rate of poverty between 1990 and 2000, with the percentage of people living below the federal poverty line in the city increasing from 3.1% to 9.2% of the city's total population during this period (Trinity College 2001). The average per capita income in Hartford is $13,428, the lowest of any city in the state (Annie E. Casey Foundation 2003). With such a high concentration of poverty, social conditions in Hartford are tenuous: 58% of families with children are headed by a single woman; 39% of adults lack a high school degree; and unemployment is 3 times that of the state. Moreover, 22% of all births in Hartford in 2000 were to teenage mothers (compared to 14% across the 50 U.S. cities with the highest teen birth rates). In Hartford, more teenage girls give birth than graduate from high school (Trinity Collect 2001). During 1999, the rate of the STI (sexually transmitted infection), Chlamydia, in Hartford was more than double the national rate and 4 times the rate in the state of Connecticut (Singer et al. 2006). Across the indicators used by the Annie E. Casey Foundation (2003) as an interlocked set of factors that effectively measure child well-being (i.e., rates of low birth weight, infant mortality, child deaths, teen deaths, teen births, school dropout, parental unemployment, teens not working or going to school, child poverty, single parent households, and lack of employment opportunities), Hartford compares poorly to other cities in the nation.

Finally, there is the issue of ethnic disparities. Of the children born in Hartford in 2000, 48% were Latino and 42% were African Americans. These statistics roughly reflect the ethnic composition of the city, which is 38% African American and 40% Latino (U.S. Census Bureau 2000), with the majority of the former being concentrated in the north end of the city, and the majority of the latter living in the south end of city (in the neighborhoods immediately surrounding the Hispanic Health Council). In addition to poverty, Hartford residents suffer de facto ethnic/racial discrimination, as other, wealthier cities in Connecticut, which are populated by mostly Whites, resist efforts to use state dollars to solve the capital's socio-economic woes. All of these factors put Hartford at high risk for poor health indicators given existing national patterns of ethnic differences in health status (Smedley, Brian, Stith, and Nelson 2003). In reference to the AIDS epidemic, Hartford forms part of the hinterland of the New York/New Jersey megalopolis, an epicenter of the national and international AIDS epidemic. Consequently, Connecticut ranks ninth in its rate of AIDS cases per 100,000 population nationally, and within the state of Connecticut, the city with the most reported cases of AIDS is Hartford (Connecticut Department of Public Health 2003). Notably, 63% of people living with AIDS (PLWAs) in Hartford were infected through drug injection behaviors. Forty-eight percent of PLWAs in Hartford are Latino, while 38% are Black. Twenty-nine percent of all PLWAs in Hartford are women. The high percentage of AIDS cases tied to drug use reflects a broader pattern, namely a city with a high rate of drug users and comparatively risky drug use patterns. These features underline the importance of a project designed to identify, assess, and respond to the risks of drug use in a city like Hartford.

Background

The Drug Monitoring Study developed as a result of efforts by Hartford-based applied anthropologists to respond to the explosive growth in HIV infection among drug users during the first decade of the AIDS epidemic. Within a few years of the identification of AIDS, almost 50% of IDUs in the city, as in some other Northeast cities (Hahn, Onorato, Jones, and Dougherty 1989), were testing positive for HIV infection (Singer, Jai, Schensul, Weeks, and Page 1992). Initial response by our research team included the testing of several alternative approaches for lowering AIDS risk among IDUs and other street drug users. Our tested interventions showed considerable promise (Dushay et al. 2001; Weeks et al. 1995, 1996). Along with research-supported changes in state law that allowed the implementation of syringe exchange and over-the-counter pharmacy access to sterile syringes, these interventions contributed to a decline in the HIV epidemic among local street drug users (Singer et al. 1997). Nonetheless, findings from a series of studies among drug users showed continued high morbidity and mortality rates from an array of causes beyond HIV/AIDS. As a result, the public health value of continuous behavioral monitoring, with a special focus on emergent and changing risk factors, became increasingly evident (Singer 2006a, 2006b) and served as impetus for the development of the Drug Monitoring Study.

Specific identification of the local need for drug use surveillance emerged during a set of CDC-sponsored regional meetings intended to help organize local consortia to enhance the coordination of prevention and intervention efforts. At the Northeast regional meeting, which was held in Princeton, New Jersey, in the mid-1990s, the invited organizations from Hartford, which included researchers, representatives of community-based agencies, drug treatment providers, and officials from city and state health departments, identified the monitoring of drug use behavior as a pressing need in local AIDS prevention. Following lengthy discussions with state public health officials, in 1997 the Connecticut Department of Public Health funded the Hispanic Health Council and the Institute for Community Research, 2 organizations with a long history of collaboration in AIDS and other work, to initiate a citywide surveillance project designed to closely monitor drug use practices and populations in the city, and to identify, describe, and assess the public health implications of emergent and changing patterns in the local drug use scene (Singer, Juvalis, and Weeks 2000). Findings from this 1-year pilot project included the identification of several emergent drug use practices as well as the realization that local drug treatment, HIV prevention, and other health and social service providers welcomed the flow of local research findings on changing drug use behaviors and user populations.

Based on this experience, the decision was made to seek longer-term federal funding for a citywide surveillance study, leading to submission of a grant application for this purpose to the CDC, which was funded in 2002. Design of this 4-year Drug Monitoring Study was guided by an experience-based conceptual framework—known as the drug use and health risk trends model (Singer and Mirhej 2004)—comprised of the following principles. First, drug use, like other market-driven consumption behaviors, is in constant flux, with new products and use patterns introduced regularly over time with the intention of retaining older markets and attracting new ones. Second, street drug users are driven by addiction, limited resources, and (because of police action and other factors) market fluctuations in availability and price to explore alternative strategies to get high. Third, the illegal nature of drug consumption accelerates the pace of behavior change, as distributors and users must find means of averting and adapting to the threats of law enforcement and the criminal justice system. Fourth, the public health consequences of changes in drug use are not of immediate concern, at least initially, to illicit drug distributors and users, and hence unexpected and usually unintended health consequences of drug use often emerge with the initiation of new behaviors. Fifth, the intersection of certain spatial, temporal, and population segments (e.g., weekend nights at certain parks when urban and suburban populations meet to buy and use drugs and engage in commercial sex) create zones of hyper-risk that lead to the rapid spread of HIV and other drug-related diseases. Finally, close monitoring of emergent drug use practices over time and the timely sharing of research findings can contribute to rapid public health responses to changing risk configurations in a volatile climate.

Project Goals and Models

In light of these understandings, the goals of the Drug Monitoring Study were as follows:

1. To combine ethnographic and epidemiological methods to identify and track the diffusion of new and changing drug use patterns and contexts, including the local adoption of new drugs and drug combinations, the development or diffusion of new drug consumption methods, the

appearance of new drug-using populations, and the surfacing of new drug use contexts, and to determine associated HIV and other health risks of these emergent patterns

2. To identify and assess the epidemiological importance of particular time/place/drug-using population intersections (Trotter et al. 2001), sometimes called "hot spots" of health risk, such as a park, city block, alleyway, abandoned building, or dance club at particular times of the day/week, characterized by concentrated patterns of risk, including sites that involve the mixing of population groups (e.g., stroll areas where urban commercial sex workers and suburban customers meet, dance clubs where inner city and suburban youth mingle, injection sites near large copping areas that attract drug users from a wide area, and the areas around late night bars, rapid check cashing businesses, and stores that sell X-rated commodities)

3. To track and analyze emergent drug use and risk trends across key socio-demographic characteristics including age, gender, ethnicity, and location in the city

4. To implement a research/health planning and policy community partnership to allow for the timely flow of research findings on drug use trends and emergent health risks to local and regional public health officials and providers concerned with implementing policies and programs related to drug abuse issues, including immediate public health responses by a researcher/provider team

The last of these components was guided by a Participatory Action Research (PAR) model. PAR has its roots in the seminal effort of Paulo Freire (1970) to break down the barriers between teachers and students in the process of education. The distinctive features of the PAR approach to problem solving are its emphasis on scientific study, its insistence on theoretically informed intervention, and its commitment to democratic community involvement (Fals-Borda 1987). According to Gilmore, Krantz, and Ramirez (1986:161),

> Action research ... aims to contribute both to the practical concerns of people in an immediate problematic situation and to further the goals of social science simultaneously. Thus, there is a dual commitment in action research to study a system and concurrently to collaborate with members of the system in changing it in what is together regarded as a desirable direction. Accomplishing this twin goal requires the active collaboration of researcher and client, and thus it stresses the importance of co-learning as a primary aspect of the research process.

As applied to the domain of public health, the concern is with uniting research and action, researchers and health and service providers, and professionals and communities in a participatory effort to address pressing health problems. Participatory research methodologies, which developed during the

1960s, have been used to investigate and build responses to a range of public health issues and related social concerns. Whatever the health issues of concern, in this approach to research, "Much of the researcher's time is spent on refining the methodological tools to suit the exigencies of the situation, and on collecting, analyzing, and presenting data on an ongoing, cyclical basis" to community collaborators (O'Brien 2001:3). This feature of action research is especially suited to the monitoring of behaviors like drug use in that such research requires repeated measures to spot and track changes over time as well as the fine-tuning of existing methods and the addition of new research elements attuned to the study of behaviors not anticipated at the beginning of the project.

Data collection in the Drug Monitoring Study was organized around annual cycles of ethnographic discovery and exploration of new behaviors and trends, and the implementation every 9 to 12 months of a survey among street drug users and service providers to assess the range and distribution of newly identified drugs and drug combinations, emergent and changing drug use behaviors, and the social contexts in which the behaviors of concern were found. Findings were presented at the end of each cycle to the CRT, which participated in decision making about appropriate public health responses. Each of these components, discussed subsequently, presented specific challenges to the effective conduct of cultural epidemiology.

Monitoring National Trends

To ensure awareness of possible new drug use trends, coincident with the ethnographic phase, we implemented a broad literature and computer-based search for information about emergent drug use patterns nationally. This search included government (e.g., NIDA, DEA), police, public health, medical, social science, and drug treatment reports about various drug-related trends spotted in one or more locations over the last several years. For example, the Connecticut Clearinghouse reported that it had several fact sheets on a street drug called "dust" that had been useful in alerting our pilot project to the use of this drug locally. Similarly, the director of the Bridgeport, CT Needle Exchange Program provided the project with a transcript of a focus group he had conducted with a group of drug users on the emergent behavior of converting crack cocaine back into an injectable solution. Additionally, we found the weekly FAX (called "Cesar FAX") on new drug use trends and research findings distributed by the Center for Substance Abuse Research at the University of Maryland quite useful. For example, one Cesar FAX received by the project included a glossary of new local drug user language terms from the drug scene (e.g., "lace" is used in Miami to refer to a marijuana and cocaine cigarette, "primo" is used in the Southwest to refer to a marijuana and crack cocaine cigarette, and "ozone" is used in Chicago to refer to a cigarette that contains marijuana, PCP, and crack cocaine, distinctly different terms from those among study participants in Hartford). Newspaper and magazine articles provided another source of information about emergent trends around the country, such as the spread of methamphetamine from the West Coast to the Midwest and South. Computer-assisted searchs also allowed project staff to spot reports on new drugs and growing trends in drug use behaviors. Monitoring of national trends was used to alert the project ethnographer to possible emergent behaviors that might be encountered in the field.

Ethnography

The target group for the Drug Monitoring Study comprises a "hidden population" (Griffiths, Gossop, Powis, and Strang 1993; Singer 1999b). Hidden populations are social groupings that reside outside of institutional and clinical settings, and whose "activities are clandestine and therefore concealed from the view of mainstream society and agencies of social control" (Watters and Biernacki 1989:417) as well as from local community-based organizations. It is well known that such groups are at special risk for infection and for transmitting infection to other populations. Lack of knowledge about daily activities and emergent behaviors in these groups, however, hampers intervention strategies, while intentional or inadvertent concealment makes it difficult to reach them with general services. Ethnography has proven to be an effective approach for overcoming this dilemma (Carlson et al. 1994) because it has an inherent capacity for the discovery of unknown social beliefs and behaviors; it emphasizes "experience-near," on-the-ground data collection; and it directs attention to understanding the insider's perspective. Within this framework, there are 4 specific methodological features of ethnography that make it optimal for studying hidden populations:

1. observation of behavior in natural contexts, including the noticing of rare events (e.g., initial instances of new behaviors) and detailed recording of witnessed activities, interactions, material objects in use (e.g., drug paraphernalia), and physical locations
2. in-context informal interviewing during behavioral observation to clarify insider understandings, experience, meanings, and emotional reactions
3. key informant interviewing with active drug users and frontline drug treatment staff on issues of emergent concern (e.g., specific behaviors or social actors of concern, new trends in drug use)
4. the need for focused attention on rapport building and maintenance (useful both during ethnographic data collection and during the subsequent recruitment of survey participants)

Ethnography, as used in the Drug Monitoring Study, involved the project ethnographer (Claudia Santilices) spending large blocks of time with target group members in their natural settings as they went about daily life, including closely observing their drug use behaviors, drug-related and other risky behaviors, and social interactions; listening to their conversations; noting the places they visit and the activities they undertake; and engaging them during the course of daily activities in casual conversations about established and emergent drug use and drug-related behaviors. Settings for this work included abandoned buildings, street corners, drug treatment organizations, soup kitchens, homeless shelters, and participant apartments. As a result of prolonged presence in the field, over time, the ethnographer became well versed in common behaviors in the target population, and was in a position to rapidly spot heretofore unobserved behaviors. This discovery was enhanced by constantly inquiring about particular behaviors, investigating the popularity of identified behaviors, and letting it be known on the street that the ethnographer was keenly interested to learn about new drugs and drug combinations, new ways of preparing and consuming drugs, and health problems that are being faced by street drug users. Attention to rapport building allowed the ethnographer to gain access to hard-to-reach places, events, and information. The ethnographer was able to move about the local drug scene, visiting and mapping the social locations of target group life, thereby allowing a more comprehensive picture of the target group to emerge, including insight into how group members might respond to public health prevention/intervention initiatives that grow out of the research effort. During this process, the ethnographer treated existing and potential study participants with sensitivity and respect, assisting as appropriate in facilitating access to medical or other services, distributing prevention materials, and providing prevention information as appropriate. Given the many years of drug-related street ethnography that have occurred in Hartford by Singer and others, dating back to early in the AIDS epidemic, participants recognize the role of the researcher as part of the wider social service system and, while sometimes initially cautious, are generally ultimately willing to openly share information on risky behavior, including participation in illegal activities. Most participants have been arrested for drug-related charges, and hence know that their involvement in illicit behavior is known to the police.

Interviews with key informants were used to solicit insider understandings of the potential effectiveness of possible intervention strategies. Key informants were selected on the basis of their demonstrated knowledge about and involvement in the local drug scene, ability to articulate an insider's perspective, and willingness and interest in working with the ethnographer to produce an accurate picture of the world of the target population. Studies have shown that contrary to what might be expected with individuals who are often under the influence of mind-altering drugs and engaged in illegal behaviors, drug users tend to provide accurate answers to research questions (Weatherby, Needle, and Cesari 1995). Although immersed in the target group, its life style, culture, and social settings, the best key informants were found to be individuals who were capable of pulling back from their day-to-day cultural immersion and offering objective accounts of group behavior, beliefs, experiences, and related matters, including recognizing and describing emergent drug-related behaviors. Some not only answered the ethnographer's questions, but, as they developed in the role of key informant, also anticipated questions. In other words, they grasped the ethnographer's objective and helped in the acquisition of needed information (e.g., location where particular drugs were sold). In addition to active drug users, the project also relied on frontline health care, drug treatment, AIDS prevention, and social service providers (some of whom were in recovery from drug addiction) who regularly interacted with the target population and were likely to be aware of new behaviors related to drug consumption and drug use lifestyles. Together, these 2 sets of key informants constituted a drug monitoring network that could alert the project to the appearance of new drug-related behaviors. Interviews with key informants, when possible, were tape-recorded, transcribed, and entered into the project data base for content analysis.

Atlas-TI, a flexible and powerful qualitative data analysis program (Lewins and Silver 2007), allowed us to sort text segments based on assigned codes, index our database by topic, and use multiple readings of grouped text segments to identify patterns, trends, and relationships across all the cases represented in our data, such as drug use patterns/preferences, chronology and history of drug initiation, knowledge about drug composition, and perceptions of drug-related risk. For example, given that one of our primary interests was "new drug use practices," all project narrative data (which had been loaded into a computer file), including interviews and records of observations, were carefully read, and all references in the text to new behaviors related to drug use were coded with the "new drug use practices" code (including sufficient surrounding text to clarify the actual behaviors involved, the contexts in which they were found, participants involved in the behavior, and related conceptions and ideas of participants about the activity). Subcodes were used to label specific kinds of new behaviors (e.g., use of methamphetamine). This enabled a focused reading of all references in our data to specific behaviors of interest to identify patterns and trends (e.g., who was involved in this behavior, where did it tend to occur, when did it begin locally, what factors appeared to be influencing its spread, how widespread was it in the city).

During the first year of the project, ethnography was used to investigate (1) baseline drug use behaviors; (2) local drug use/acquisition sites that might be critical "geotemporal centers" of disease transmission; and (3) emergent or previously unknown drug use patterns (including the local presence of behaviors identified through the literature and online search component of the study). In subsequent years of the project, specific issues were selected for further investigation based on project findings. Thus in the last year of data collection, the project focused, among other topics, on the smoking of flavored cigars among underage youth (i.e., illegal use of tobacco), a topic that had not been on the agenda at the beginning of the project.

The biggest challenge faced by the ethnographic component of the study was the difficulty in always getting a clear picture of the frequency and distribution of new behaviors. While an informant might mention a new behavior, it was not always possible to either witness it or find others who affirmed its local presence or the characteristics of the initial adopters of the behavior. Additionally, the ethnographic segment of the project was challenged at any point in time by project interest in several different behaviors that were found among different subgroups of drug users (e.g., as differentiated by age). As a result, the ethnographer's time was divided and the extent of information gathered about some topics was limited. Despite these problems, ethnography helped the project to include important observational and contextual information about emergent and changing behaviors. Information gathered during the ethnographic phase in each cycle was used to update the project's survey instrument as well as to interpret findings from the project surveys, which helped address the issues of frequency and distribution of specific behaviors.

Surveys

Structured survey interviews were administered to approximately 250 drug users in each cycle for 3 years. The purpose of the survey was to assess the range, frequency, distribution, and correlations of drug-related risks of concern. With each cycle, questions about new behaviors were added on the basis of the prior wave of qualitative and quantitative data collection. Consequently, the project survey instrument included a set of core sociodemographic, drug use, and risk-related questions, as well as new questions that were added each time (while others were eliminated) to reflect the changing research focus. Participants for the survey were recruited through street outreach by experienced community outreach/interviewers.

To recruit survey samples that reasonably reflected the street drug–using population of primary concern to the proposed project, recruitment was based on a neighborhood sampling design supplemented by advertising in community newspapers and other community media, strategies that we have found effective in recruiting the target population. This design allowed contact with a heterogeneous group of active drug users from the 6 target neighborhoods known from prior research, AIDS surveillance data, and police reports to have the highest densities of street drug users in the city. Inclusion criteria included being at least 18 years of age, active consumption of illicit drugs (beyond marijuana) during the last 30 days, and not being involved in drug treatment for the last 30 days. Participants were paid $20 for an interview that lasted approximately 1 hour. Data collection for each wave of the survey required approximately 6 months. In the second and third waves of the survey, no attempt was made to re-recruit or to exclude participants from earlier waves of data collection. Data from the survey were entered by the interviewer onto Teleform data sheets, which allowed respondent responses to be scanned directly into the project's computer database. Quantitative data were analyzed using SPSS.

The core component of the survey instrument was based on the AIDS Risk Assessment (ARA). This research tool, originally developed for use with drug users in Houston, is a shortened (more rapid) version of the Risk Behavior Assessment developed and widely used and validated by NIDA. The instrument has been found to have acceptable reliability test–retest scores of between 0.69 and 0.78 and internal consistency between 0.87 and 0.89 (Dowling-Guyer et al. 1994; Needle et al. 1995; Weatherby, Needle, and Cesari 1995). The ARA systematically collects information on drug use, syringe-related and sex-related AIDS risk behaviors, health status, and related health information. Our research team modified the instrument (subsequently called ARA-M) to add missing key items on specific drug use and sexual practices, the locations of potential geotemporal epicenters of risk, and emergent drug use patterns (e.g., relatively recent—within 1 year—drug-related behaviors that a participant had heard about, seen, or participated in). The completed instrument for each cycle was pilot tested with a small sample of drug users for (1) length of administration (no more than 1 hour); (2) clarity for interviewers; (3) clarity for participants; and (4) consistency of answers across sections of the interview. On the basis of this testing, the instrument was finalized and translated for participants who preferred to be interviewed in Spanish.

The survey component of the study faced some of the same kinds of challenges as the ethnographic component. Because the use of many drugs differs across social segments, and each survey wave included several issues of special concern, it was not always easy to recruit a sample that could be informative about some topics (especially very new or narrowly distributed behaviors). For this reason we began going beyond neighborhood recruitment (e.g., by advertising in community newspapers) to recruit individuals who would be more likely to report involvement in particular behaviors. Additionally, because various issues of interest to the project emerged with each new cycle of data collection, it was a challenge to keep the interview time within the 1-hour limit that was known from past research with drug users to be acceptable. As it was, and as is common in drug use studies, more data were collected than were analyzed, and a number of analyses were not completed by the end of the project (and now must compete with analyses done on newer data sets collected in subsequent projects).

Presentation of Findings

Following the PAR model, findings from each wave of qualitative and quantitative data collection were reported as they became available to the CRT. The purposes of this presentation were to inform community collaborators about the research, to solicit input on the health implications of the newly identified behaviors, and to discuss approaches for public health interventions needed. Some of the findings triggered spirited discussion about public health implications or the best public health responses, such as presentation of participant interview data showing that use of the drug called "dust" or "wet" on the street was very widespread among drug-using youth and young adults in Hartford. Many CRT members were unfamiliar with this drug and what its risks to health might be. Collaborators in the medical laboratory at Hartford Hospital suggested testing the urine of dust users to confirm the actual chemical contents of the drug. As a result, a substudy was developed. Forty-one individuals were recruited who reported to project outreach workers that they had used dust during the previous 48-hour period. These individuals provided urine samples, which were toxicologically analyzed by our laboratory collaborators, and 31% of the samples tested positive for the presence of PCP, an anesthetic developed during the 1950s that was discontinued for human use because it was found to induce postoperative psychosis and dysphoria (although it has continued since then to be available in veterinary medicine and as an illicit drug). Additionally, the project collected 12 of the small plastic bags in which dust is commonly sold on the street from litter debris on the ground at known drug use sites. All of these bags tested positive for PCP. Given the fact that PCP is a dissociative drug that produces both hallucinogenic and neurotoxic effects and leads to risky or even violent behavior in some users, the findings were seen by the CRT as raising an important public health concern (Singer et al. 2005b).

Inclusion of the CRT in the project produced several challenges, including inconsistency in the ability of CRT members to attend project meetings given their other responsibilities at their home institutions and difficulty in reaching decisions about appropriate courses of action. While members of the CRT generally showed enthusiasm about the project and its ability to generate important public health findings, it was not always easy for them to stay actively involved. As a result, meetings were often difficult to arrange. Moreover, given the extent of drug problems in Hartford, it was not always clear to CRT members what the right course of action should be for the identification of new drug-related threats to public health. Many advocated strongly for issues that most impacted their own agencies or client population, and competing philosophies of drug use and treatment at times derailed conversations. While some CRT members argued that it might be possible to successfully warn people about the dangers of one drug, this would only lead them to switch to other drugs, a common enough pattern among regular drug users. Some members were also concerned that social marketing for education and prevention of a new drug could also attract new users who had not heard of it. Despite these concerns and differences, the project was able to launch several efforts to respond to the health implications of its research findings. Examples of two of these initiatives are described here.

Public Health Responses

Youth Drug Use

As noted, the prevalence of dust use in Hartford among youth and young adults, as well as the seriousness of potential long- and short-term health consequences associated with the use of PCP, were cause for alarm within the project (Moriarty 1996). The Drug Monitoring Study research team determined that although an intervention was necessary, there was at that time little local community awareness of the drug beyond users. Possible interventions identified by the team included (1) a primary prevention educational campaign targeting parents, teachers, and students through public schools; (2) a program to improve diagnostic awareness by informing hospital and walk-in clinic providers about the symptoms and treatment of dust-related illnesses; (3) a program to educate current dust users through outreach, peer educators, and flip cards; and (4) integration of findings into the Hispanic Health Council's ongoing community drug education and counseling. The team chose an inclusive approach in which teenagers in the Hispanic Health Council's youth program would be invited to design dust prevention posters as part of a drug awareness educational contest. A presentation about the contents and effects of dust was made by team members to the after-school program at the Hispanic Health Council's Center for Youth and Families. In response, student participants created a group of prevention posters in Spanish and English. The goal was to expand the peer education model used in the program by allowing youth to develop their own drug prevention images and messages and reach peers using their own "language." A professor in graphic arts at a local college was contacted and agreed to make a digital duplication of the winning poster (as part of a class project)—entitled "*DUST: Doing Uncontrollable Stupid Things*" by its creators—so that it could be sent to schools and modified for classroom use. Meetings were arranged with the director of health and education programs for the Hartford City School System to develop strategies to bring dust prevention educational materials and messages into the schools and to use them in in-service training with teachers.

Additionally, a PowerPoint presentation on dust was developed and shown to a wide audience at a citywide community drug conference that included representatives from local drug treatment, education, church, law enforcement, health care, community, government, and public health institutions and organizations. A representative of the project also presented findings about dust to a community meeting organized as a follow-up to the citywide drug conference. Through these strategies, information about dust and its associated health risks was disseminated in the local community. Funding limitations, however, did not allow a pre-/posttest assessment of the impact of these activities in raising community awareness about this drug.

The Spreading Methamphetamine Epidemic

In identifying and tracking emergent drug use trends, the project assessed the spread of methamphetamine in Hartford between 2003 and 2005. Before the initiation of the project, drug use patterns in Hartford had been monitored in a series of studies involving several thousand participants (Singer 2006b; Weeks et al. 1998). Comprehensive surveys administered to them and ethnographic information revealed that although amphetamine-type substances had been sporadically used in Hartford over a long period, methamphetamine use specifically had been fairly limited. To the degree that methamphetamine use was reported in these studies, it was primarily reported as something participants had done while living in other parts of the country. Within the Drug Monitoring Study, in 2003, only 4.4% of the surveyed participants ($N = 300$) reported having ever used methamphetamine, with only one individual reporting current use (in the last 30 days). The following year, 19 individuals, or 7.9% of the sample, reported having ever used the drug, with one individual reporting current use. In 2005, by contrast, of the participants surveyed ($N = 241$), the number of individuals reporting having ever used methamphetamine rose to 15.8%, with 26% of this group indicating that they had used the drug during the previous 30 days. While the number of participants reporting current methamphetamine use was still numerically small (9 of the 241 participants interviewed), statistically this represented a significant increase (600%) (Singer et al. 2006). Without a doubt, reported levels of methamphetamine use in Hartford did not match those being reported at the time for places like Sioux City, Iowa, a well-recognized regional center for methamphetamine trafficking, or other places in the United States where the use of this drug had already had a major impact on drug use and public health patterns (Singer and Mirhej 2004). However, growing evidence suggested that an equally devastating epidemic could be approaching the Northeast. For example, in the last project, conducted between January and July 2005, a set of questions was added to evaluate the availability of methamphetamine. We found that 60% of participants ($N = 25$) answered "yes" to having acquired the drug in Hartford, with 56% of these participants citing "raves" (all-night dance parties characterized by high-energy electronic music) as the acquisition site and 33% reporting "dance club/bars" and "streets." Findings from in-depth interviews with current methamphetamine users and other key informants made it clear that, even though it was not as widely available as crack cocaine, heroin, marijuana, or "dust," methamphetamine was available from various dealers in and around Hartford, and that the drug was no longer used by just one group (e.g., gay men). Rather, methamphetamine users in our study revealed that the range of use included people from various cultural, ethnic, and economic backgrounds—from street syringe sellers, who at times traded syringes for drugs, to college students who reported acquiring the drug on the street and bringing it back to campus for parties. This information, coupled with the police raids of two methamphetamine labs in Connecticut during 2005, suggested a potentially significant rise in local use. A project account submitted to CDC in January 2006 reported:

> It is possible that geographic location has granted Hartford a short reprieve from the devastating [methamphetamine] wave that has leveled other parts of the country. However, by looking at the most recent local research and drug arrest findings, as well as a national map of how the methamphetamine epidemic is moving across the country, the period of reprieve may be short-lived. And, although it is in some ways the nature of government and people to address problems only after they occur, we believe that Hartford has a rare and vital opportunity to create a task force and plan of prevention that could possibly save innumerable lives and the relentless drain of resources from which other cities have yet to recover.

These findings gave rise to the Methamphetamine Primary Prevention Campaign, which was intended as a concerted and integrated response from the public health community, health-care institutions, policymakers, community-based service and treatment providers, the Hartford school system, night/dance club owners, and community members. Components of this effort included

- *coordination* of prevention efforts through a citywide coalition to effectively reach diverse populations at risk for use of methamphetamine
- *saturation* through multiple methods, mediums, and target locations/populations with a single redundant message pointing at the detrimental impact of methamphetamine use on people's health, social relationships, and users' quality of life

- *education* through the use of culturally tailored models for prevention to target populations at risk
- *representation* through the use of methamphetamine addicts in recovery of diverse ages, ethnicities and sexual identities as knowledgeable spokespersons
- *access* through advocacy for high quality treatment programs of sufficient duration to effectively treat methamphetamine addicts
- *support of policy changes* that monitor the purchase or theft of chemicals used in the production of methamphetamine, and the emergence of methamphetamine use

Specific activities that were initiated included:

- An editorial on the dangers of rising rates and risks of methamphetamine published in the Hartford Courant in September 2004
- Presentation of findings to the Hartford Health Department (HHD) and at a citywide meeting of providers organized by the HHD
- A methamphetamine community forum held in December 2004. Approximately 50 people were invited to the event, including health care and drug treatment providers, AIDS outreach workers, people in drug recovery, and the press. Attendees received a packet with a description of the project and a compilation of methamphetamine-related materials, including a copy of a newspaper article showing a former methamphetamine user's before and after picture, which demonstrates the toll of the drug on the user's health, and a fact sheet prepared by project staff with national and statewide findings
- Presentation of findings at AIDS Science Day in April 2005 hosted by the Center for Interdisciplinary AIDS Research at Yale University
- Participation in a symposium at the Connecticut State Legislature with representatives from the legislature, the state public health department, law enforcement, drug treatment providers, and the media, including distribution of a report on project findings
- Presentation of findings and recommendations at the Hartford Drug Summit, a policy and providers' conference organized by a member of the Hartford city council, including distribution of the project's report on methamphetamine
- Development and citywide distribution (to community organizations, stores, health institutions, local colleges, bars and night clubs, and libraries) and display of a Methamphetamine Makeover Poster (revealing the rapid toll of use on user health and appearance)
- A year-long distribution of a fact sheet (in English and Spanish) on the risks of methamphetamine use at community health fairs, community organizations, community events, the media, and drug treatment providers, as well as the state Deputy Commission of Public Health and to city schools

As a result of these efforts, a series of articles appeared in the Hartford Courant newspaper detailing project findings and recommendations. Additionally, the largest drug treatment program in Connecticut began testing new patients for methamphetamine use. Subsequently, pharmacies in the state withdrew precursor over-the-counter medicines used in the making of methamphetamine from store shelves and buyers were required to show identification when purchasing these items. Our research team has continued to monitor evidence of the diffusion of methamphetamine in the city, and while the drug continues to be present and have a set of regular users, the feared epidemic of use seen in other parts of the country has not, as yet, occurred.

Conclusion

The Drug Monitoring Study represents a successful initiative launched with significant anthropological leadership and participation that used a participatory action and culturally sensitive approach to addressing urgent public health issues. Working through a well-established community-based organization and in collaboration with local providers, educators, and community representatives, the project combined multimethod behavioral surveillance and translation of research findings into community education initiatives in addressing the significant health risks associated with changing patterns of illicit street drug use.

Research initiated by the project identified and tracked several trends in drug use, including the spread of methamphetamine among street drug users, PCP among youth and young adult users, and sweetened cigars among youth. Using anthropological methods, including immersion in local drug use scenes, observation of drug user behavior, casual interviewing with active drug users as they went about their daily routines of acquiring and using drugs, in-depth interviewing with both drug users and drug treatment staff, and the implementation of 3 ethnographically informed surveys, the project collected data on current drug use practices by neighborhood as well as by age and ethnic subgroup that were assembled and presented to a team of public health officials, health-care providers, and community organization staff. This team assessed the public health implications of project findings, discussed appropriate and achievable public health interventions, and implemented several culturally sensitive intervention programs designed to improve community awareness of the risks of specific drugs or to improve public health and drug treatment responses to health risks associated with drug use. Although funded only for 4 years, the project was able to continue afterward through various innovative strategies, including working with the anthropology department of a local college in the development of a student honor's thesis project designed to monitor the emergence and consequences of a popular new drug known as salvia (*Saliva divinorum*) among college students.

The Drug Monitoring Study illustrates the capacity of anthropologists to take the lead in local public health efforts in collaboration with colleagues from other disciplines and the utility of anthropological research in the public health surveillance of changing behavioral risks in vulnerable populations. Further, the project offers a model for applied public health research that promotes collaboration between anthropologists, public health officials, community organizations, and health-care providers. Given the extent of drug-related health problems in the United States and globally, there is a critical need for research-based assessment of changing drug use patterns, contexts, and populations in the development of effective intervention strategies. Given its field-based approach to data collection, demonstrated capacity for studying hard-to-reach populations, and capacity for informing intervention with local data on target groups, anthropology has a significant role to play in this effort.

Acknowledgments

This project was supported by grant R01/CCR 121652 awarded by the CDC (Merrill Singer, PI), with additional support for the lead author in the preparation of this paper by grant 1 PO1 CD 000237 awarded by the CDC (Leslie Snyder, PI).

References

Annie E. Casey Foundation (2003) *The Right Start for America's Newborns: A Decade of City and State Trends* (1990–2000). Baltimore, MD: Annie E. Casey Foundation.

Auerbach J, Coates T (2000) HIV prevention research: Accomplishments and challenges for the third decade of AIDS. *American Journal of Public Health* 90(7):1029–1032.

Auerbach J, Wypijewska C, Brodie HK, eds. (1994) *AIDS and Behavior: An Integrated Approach*. Washington, DC: National Academy Press.

Bowser B, Quimby E, Singer M, eds. (2007) *Communities Assessing Their AIDS Epidemics: Results of the Rapid Assessment of HIV/AIDS in Eleven U.S. Cities*. Lanham, MD: Lexington Books.

Broadhead R, Heckathorn D, Weakliem D, Anthony D, Madray H, Mills R, et al. (1998) Harnessing peer networks as an instrument for AIDS prevention: Results from a peer-driven intervention. *Public Health Reports* 113(Suppl 1):42–57.

Carlson R, Jichuan W, Siegal HA, Falck RS (1994) An ethnographic approach to targeted sampling: Problems and solutions in AIDS prevention research among injection drug and crack cocaine users. *Human Organization* 53(3):279–295.

Centers for Disease Control and Prevention (1994) *External Review of CDC's HIV Prevention Strategies by the CDC Advisory Committee on the Prevention of HIV*

Infection. Atlanta, GA: US Department of Health and Human Services, Public Health Service.

Centers for Disease Control and Prevention (2002) *Hepatitis C Virus and HIV Connection*. Atlanta, GA: CDC.

Centers for Disease Control and Prevention (2004) Fact sheet: Drug-associated HIV transmission continues in the United States. www.cdc.gov/hiv/resources/factsheets/idu.htm. Accessed January 26, 2007.

Connecticut Department of Public Health (2003) *Epidemiologic Profile of HIV and AIDS in Connecticut–2003*. Hartford, CT: Connecticut Department of Public Health.

Corby N, Wolitsk R (1997) *Community HIV Prevention*. Long Beach, CA: Statewide Technical Books.

Coyle S, Needle R, Normand J (1998) Outreach-based HIV prevention for injecting drug users: A review of published outcome data. *Public Health Reports* 113(Suppl 1):19–30.

Dowling-Guyer S, Johnson M, Fisher D, Booth R, Needle R, Rhodes F, et al. (1993) Reliability of drug users' self-reported HIV risk behaviors and validity of self-reported recent drug use. *Assessment* 1:383–392.

Dushay R, Singer M, Weeks M, Rohena L, Gruber R (2001) Lowering HIV risk among ethnic minority drug users: Comparing culturally targeted intervention to standard intervention. *American Journal of Alcohol and Drug Abuse* 8:17–25.

Fals-Borda O (1987) The application of participatory-action research in Latin America. *International Sociology* 2:329–347.

Farmer P, Kleinman A (1989) AIDS as human suffering. *Daedalus* 118(2):135–162.

Fielding N, Fielding J (1986) *Linking Data*. Beverly Hills, CA: Sage Publications.

Freire P (1970) *Pedagogy of the Oppressed*. New York: Continuum.

Gallagher K, Denning P, Allen D, Nakashima A, Sullivan P (2007a) Use of rapid behavioral assessments to determine the prevalence of HIV risk behaviors in high-risk populations. *Public Health Reports* 122(Suppl 1):56–62.

Gallagher K, Sullivan P, Lansky A, Onorato I (2007b) Behavioral surveillance among people at risk for HIV infection in the U.S.: The national HIV behavioral surveillance system. *Public Health Reports* 122(Suppl 1):32–38.

Gilmore T, Krantz J, Ramirez R (1986) Action based modes of inquiry: Research as praxis. *Harvard Educational Review* 56(3):257–277.

Griffiths P, Gossop M, Powis B, Strang J (1993) Reaching hidden populations of drug users by privileged access interviewers: Methodological and practical issues. *Addiction* 88(12):1617–1626.

Hahn R, Onorato I, Jones T, Dougherty J (1989) Prevalence of HIV infection among intravenous drug users in the United States. *Journal of the American Medical Association* 261(18):2677–2684.

Heckathorn D (2002) Respondent-driven sampling II: Deriving valid population estimates from chain-referral samples of hidden populations. *Social Problems* 49(1):11–34.

Heckathorn D, Broadhead R, Anthony D, Weakliem D (1999) AIDS and social networks: HIV prevention through network mobilization. *Sociological Focus* 32:159–179.

Hitt J, Robbins A, Galbraith J, Todd J, Patel-Larson A, McFarlane J, et al. (2006) Adaptation and implementation of an evidence-based prevention counseling intervention in Texas. *AIDS Education and Prevention* 19(SA):108–118.

Inciardi J, Lockwood D, Pottieger A (1993) *Women and Crack-Cocaine*. New York: Macmillan Publishing Co.

Kavan J (2003) U.N. Information Service. www.unis.unvienna.org/unis/pressrels/2003/gasm322.html. Accessed July 16, 2006.

Koester S (1994a) Copping, running, and paraphernalia laws: Contextual variables and needle risk behavior among injection drug users in Denver. *Human Organization* 53:287–295.

Koester S (1994b) "Applying Ethnography to AIDS Prevention among IV Drug Users and Social Policy Implications." In: *AIDS Prevention and Services: Community Based Research.* J. Van Vugt, ed. Westport, CT: Bergin and Garvey, pp. 35–58.

Koester S (1996) "The Process of Drug Injection: Applying Ethnography to the Study of HIV Risk among IDUs." In: *AIDS, Drugs and Prevention: Perspectives on Individual and Community Action.* T Rhodes, R Hartell, eds. London: Routledge Press, pp. 133–148.

Koester S, Hoffer L (1994) "Indirect sharing": Additional HIV risks associated with drug injection. *AIDS and Public Policy Journal* 2:100–104.

Kozel N (1997) *Foreword. Epidemiologic Trends in Drug Abuse, Volume II, Proceedings. Community Epidemiology Work Group.* Rockville, MD: National Institute on Drug Abuse.

Lansky A, Abdul-Quader A, Cribbi, M, Hall T, Finlayson T, Garfein R, et al. (2007) Developing an HIV behavioral surveillance system for injecting drug users: The National HIV Behavioral Surveillance System. *Public Health Reports* 122(Suppl. 1):48–55.

Leshner A (2000) NIDA's epidemiological compasses. *NIDA Notes* 15(3):3–4.

Lewin Group (2004) Bush and Kerry health care proposals: Cost and coverage compared. www.lewin.com/NR/rdonlyres/F46F96C3–0562-44DF-BA21–969EAD747052/0/LewinPresidentialComparison.pdf. Accessed January 27, 2007.

Lewins A, Silver C (2007) *Using Software in Qualitative Research.* London: Sage.

Miller H, Turner C, Lincoln M (1990) *AIDS: The Second Decade.* Washington, DC: National Academy Press.

Morabia A (1996) From disease surveillance to the surveillance of risk factors. *American Journal of Public Health* 86(5):625–627.

Moriarty A (1996) What's "new" in street drugs: "Illy." *Journal of Pediatric Health Care* 10:41–43.

National Survey on Drug Use and Health (2005) Substance abuse or dependence in metropolitan and non-metropolitan areas, 2004 update. http://oas.samhsa.gov/2k5/metro/metro.cfm. Accessed January 8, 2007.

Needle R, Fisher DS, Weatherby N, Chitwood D, Brown B, Cesari H, et al. (1995) The reliability of self-reported HIV risk behaviors of drug users. *Social Science and Medicine* 9:242–250.

O'Brien R (2001) Theory and practice of action research. www.web.ca/~robrien/papers/arfinal.html. Accessed on January 3, 2007.

O'Reilly K, Higgins D (1991) AIDS community demonstration projects for HIV prevention among hard-to-reach groups. *Public Health Reports* 106:714–720.

Ouellet L, Wiebel W, Jimenez A (1995) "Team Research Methods for Studying Intranasal Heroin Use and its HIV Risks." In: *Qualitative Methods in Drug Abuse and HIV Research.* E Lambert, R Ashery, eds. NIDA Research Monograph 157. Rockville, MD: National Institute on Drug Abuse, pp. 182–211.

Page JB (1990) Shooting scenarios and risk of HIV infection. *American Behavioral Scientist* 33(4):478–490.

Rhodes T, Stimson GE, Fitch C, Ball A, Renton A (1999) Rapid assessment, injecting drug use, and public health. *Lancet* 354:65–68.

Salganik M, Heckathorn D (2004) Sampling and estimation in hidden populations: Using respondent-driven sampling. *Sociological Methodology* 34(1):193–240.

Shriver M, de Burger R, Brown C, Simpson H, Meyerson B (1998) Bridging the gap between science and practice: Insight to researchers from practitioners. *Public Health Reports* 113(Suppl 1):189–193.

Singer M (1999a) Why do Puerto Rican injection drug users inject so often? *Anthropology and Medicine* 6(1):31–58.

Singer M (1999b) "Studying Hidden Populations." In: *Mapping Networks, Spatial Data and Hidden Populations, Book 4, The Ethnographer's Toolkit*. S Schensul, M LeCompte, R Trotter, E Cromley, and M Singer, eds. Walnut Creek, CA: Altamira Press, pp. 125–191.

Singer M (2006a) *Something Dangerous: Emergent and Changing Illicit Drug Use and Community Health*. Prospect Heights, IL: Waveland Press.

Singer M (2006b) *The Face of Social Suffering: Life History of a Street Drug Addict*. Prospect Heights, IL: Waveland Press.

Singer M, Bowser B, Quimby E (2007) "Assessing Primary, Secondary and Future Benefits of Project RARE." In: *Communities Assessing Their AIDS Epidemics: Results of the Rapid Assessment of HIV/AIDS in Eleven U.S. Cities*. B Bowser, E Quimby, and M Singer, eds. Lanham, MD: Lexington Books, pp. 231–248.

Singer M, Clair S (2003) Syndemics and public health: reconceptualizing disease in bio-social context. *Medical Anthropology Quarterly* 17(4):423–441.

Singer M, Clair S, Schensul J, Huebner C, Eiserman J, Pino R, et al. (2005c) Dust in the wind: The growing use of embalming fluid among youth in Hartford, CT. *Substance Use and Misuse* 40:1035–1050.

Singer M, Erickson P, Badiane L, Diaz R, Ortiz D, Abraham T, et al. (2006) Syndemics, sex and the city: Understanding sexually transmitted disease in social and cultural context. *Social Science and Medicine* 63(8):2010–2021.

Singer M, Himmelgreen D, Dushay R, Weeks M (1998) Variation in drug injection frequency among out-of-treatment drug users: A national study. *American Journal of Drug and Alcohol Abuse* 24(2):321–341.

Singer M, Himmelgreen D, Weeks M, Radda K, Martinez R (1997) Changing the environment of AIDS risk: Findings on syringe exchange and pharmacy sale of syringes in Hartford, CT. *Medical Anthropology* 18(1):107–130.

Singer M, Jia Z, Schensul J, Weeks M, Page JB (1992) AIDS and the IV drug user: The local context in prevention efforts. *Medical Anthropology* 14:285–306.

Singer M, Juvalis JA, Weeks M (2000) High on illy: Studying an emergent drug problem in Hartford, CT. *Medical Anthropology* 18:365–388.

Singer M, Mirhej G (2004) The understudied supply side: Public policy implications of the illicit drug trade in Hartford, CT. *Harvard Health Policy Review* 5(2):36–47.

Singer M, Mirhej G, Santelices C, Hastings E, Navarro J, Vivian J (2006) Tomorrow is already here, or is it? Steps in preventing a local methamphetamine outbreak. *Human Organization* 65(2):203–217.

Singer M, Mirhej G, Shaw S, Saleheen H, Vivian J, Hastings E, et al. (2005b) When the drug of choice is a drug of confusion: Embalming fluid use in inner city Hartford, CT. *Journal of Ethnicity and Substance Abuse* 4(2):71–96.

Singer M, Stopka T, Susan S, Santelices C, Buchanan D, Teng W, et al. (2005a) Lessons from the field: From research to application in the fight against AIDS among injection drug users in three New England cities. *Human Organization* 64(2):179–191.

Smedley B, Brian, Stith A, Nelson A (2003) *Unequal Treatment: Confronting Racial and Ethnic Disparities in Healthcare*. Washington, DC: The National Academic Press.

Stimson G, Fitch C, Rhodes T, Ball A (1999) Rapid assessment and response: Methods for developing public health responses to drug problems. *Drug and Alcohol Review* 18:317–325.

Trinity College (2001) *Hartford Primer and Field Guide*. Hartford, CT: Cities Data Center, Trinity College.

Trostle J (2004) *Epidemiology and Culture*. New York: Cambridge University Press.

Trotter R, Richard H, Needle R, Goosby E, Bates C, Singer M (2001) A methodological model for rapid assessment, response, and evaluation: The RARE program in public health. *Field Methods* 13(2):137–159.

Trotter R, Singer M (2005) "Rapid Assessment Strategies for Public Health: Promise and Problems." In: *Community Interventions and AIDS*. E Trickett, W Pequegnat, eds. Oxford, UK: Oxford University Press, pp. 130–152.

Trotter R, Singer M (2007) "Rapid Assessment: A Method in Community-based Research." In: *Communities Assessing Their AIDS Epidemics: Results of the Rapid Assessment of HIV/AIDS in Eleven U.S. Cities*. B Bowser, E Quimby, M Singer, eds. Lanham, MD: Lexington Books, pp. 9–28.

U.S. Census Bureau (2000) Census 2000: Summary File 4: CT Hispanic or Latino (of any race) Median Family Income in 1999 (Dollars) by Family Size. Washington, DC: U.S. Census Bureau.

Watters J, Biernacki P (1989) Targeted sampling: Options for the study of hidden populations. *Social Problems* 36(4):416–430.

Weatherby N, Needle R, Cesari H (1995) *Validity of Self-Reported Drug Use*. Washington, DC: National Institute on Drug Use.

Weeks M, Himmelgreen D, Singer M, Richmond P, Romero-Daza N (1998) Drug use patterns of substance abusing women: Implications for treatment providers. *Drugs and Society* 13(1/2):35–61.

Weeks M, Singer M, Grier M, Hunte-Marrow J, Haughton C (1993) AIDS prevention and the African American injection drug user. *Transforming Anthropology* 4(1–2):39–51.

Weeks M, Singer M, Grier M, Schensul J (1996) "Gender Relations, Sexuality, and AIDS Risk among African American and Puerto Rican Women." In: *Gender and Health: An International Perspective*. CF Sargent, B Brettell, eds. Upper Saddle River, NJ: Prentice-Hall, pp. 338–370.

Weeks M, Williams S, Schensul J, Singer M, Grier M (1995) AIDS prevention for African American and Latina women: Building cultural and gender appropriate intervention. *AIDS Prevention and Education* 7:251–264.

Wolitski R, Corby N, Fishbein M, Galavotti C (1996a) Sources of AIDS information among low and high-risk populations in five U.S. cities. *Journal of Community Health* 21:293–310.

Wolitski R, Fishbein M, Johnson D, Higgins D, Esacove A (1996b) AIDS community demonstration projects: Sources of HIV information among injecting drug users in three U.S. cities. *AIDS Care* 8:591–555.

13

Sexual Risk Reduction among Married Women and Men in Urban India: An Anthropological Intervention

STEPHEN L. SCHENSUL, RAVI K. VERMA, BONNIE K. NASTASI, NIRANJAN SAGGURTI, AND ABDELWAHED MEKKI-BERRADA

Introduction

Worldwide, the number of people living with HIV/AIDS is currently estimated at 33.2 million (UNAIDS 2007). In the early stages of the epidemic, the disease primarily affected men (Mann, Tarantola, and Netter 1992), but this proportion quickly changed, so that women manifested the most rapid increase in global infection rates (Vuylsteke, Sunkutu, and Laga 1996). In sub-Saharan Africa, there has been a dramatic shift in gender ratios over the past decade, with HIV-positive women now outnumbering men (1.3 to 1; UNAIDS 2004a).

The global epidemiological picture is being replicated in India. As the epidemic accelerated in India in the early 1990s, gender distribution estimates for 1994 indicated a male-to-female ratio of 5:1, with female cases mostly among sex workers (Pais 1996). By the end of the decade, the epidemic had crossed over to the general population and gender ratios had reduced to a 3:1 ratio. Currently it is estimated that the ratio is between 1.7:1 (UNAIDS 2004b) and 1.2:1 (Hawkes and Santhya 2002), with infection rates increasing most rapidly among women (NACO 2004), who now represent an estimated 40% of people aged 15 to 49 living with HIV/AIDS in India (NACO 2004; UNAIDS 2004b). Much of this rapid increase in prevalence among women in India is a result of male-to-female transmission within marriage (Gangakhedkar et al. 1997; Newmann et al. 2000).

The prevention challenge in India, as elsewhere in the world, is to identify effective approaches to reduction of risk behavior that will serve to lower
transmission rates. The approaches to this problem need to move beyond the
standard interventions to risk and harm reduction that have characterized the
mainstream approaches to HIV prevention and to work with men and women
within the context of their own culture and worldview to reduce the risk of
HIV transmission. In the case presented in this chapter, the focus is on married women and men living in urban poor communities (referred to locally as
"slums") in Mumbai, the largest city and economic center of India. Our first
step in these communities was to understand the broader issues of men's and
women's sexual and reproductive health beliefs and behaviors.

Sexual Health Concepts in India

Men's Culturally Based Sexual Health Concepts

The work of Verma, Rangaiyan, Singh, Sharma, and Pelto (2001) at the
International Institute for Population Sciences (IIPS) in Mumbai on men's
sexual concepts, conducted in the late 1990s, provided the "opportunity" to
address HIV/STI (sexually transmitted infection) risk from a cultural perspective. Male sexual dysfunctions, such as a lack of sexual interest, premature
ejaculation, impotence (erectile dysfunction), and infertility and the anxieties
they produce are widely distributed across societies and cultures. Male sexual
performance is seen in most cultures as the benchmark of masculinity, virility, personal adequacy, and fulfillment (Kulhara and Avasthi 1995). Verma and
colleagues, research showed that men living in both urban and rural areas of
India have widespread anxieties associated with sexual matters (Pelto, Joshi,
and Verma 1999; Verma et al. 2001; Verma and Schensul 2004). South Asian
and Indian culture amplifies these concerns with a focus on the dangers associated with "semen loss" through nocturnal emission and masturbation (Kulhara
and Avasthi 1995). According to Indian tradition (writings in *Upanishads*),
semen is known as *virya*, derived from a Sanskrit word that means bravery,
power, or greatness (Verma, Khaitan, and Singh 1998) and is considered the
source of physical and spiritual strength. The loss of *virya* through sexual
acts or imagery (including masturbation and nocturnal emission) is considered harmful both physically and spiritually. The focus on semen loss makes
premature ejaculation, nocturnal emission, and masturbation special concerns
among Indian men (Verma et al. 1998). Although nocturnal emissions and
masturbation are the main sources of "sexual release" in the years before marriage among the majority of males, they are also major causes of anxieties
among unmarried young men in South Asia.

Men are more concerned about performance issues related to semen loss than they are about STIs (Pelto et al. 1999). Strongly held cultural beliefs cause the vulnerable individual to develop concerns about sexual performance, thereby leading to anxiety, which may then act as a mediator for the genesis and perpetuation of problems (Verma et al. 1998). The term *gupt rog* ("secret illnesses" in Hindi) refers to the range of symptoms that are caused by semen loss and other factors that range from eating meat to having sex with "wrong" women. It became clear that *gupt rog* would provide a cultural route to addressing HIV/STI risk reduction among men in the study communities.

Women's Culturally Based Sexual Health

Many Indian women living in poor rural and urban communities are faced with numerous life challenges that include a difficult work schedule, limited financial resources to support the household, and male domination that limits mobility, empowerment, and control over their own sexuality. One way that the difficulties in life situation are manifested in some Indian women is in part through sexual and reproductive health symptoms, particularly *safed pani* (vaginal white discharge) and *kamjori* (general state of weakness) (Patel and Oomman 1999; Prasad, Abraham, Akila, Joseph, and Jacob 2003). Research studies on women's health in India indicate that women express the psychological, social, and economic difficulties in their lives in the form of culturally defined gynecological problems, including *safed pani*, as "idioms of distress" (Nichter 1981) or as "metaphors for psychological distress" (Patel and Ooman 1999).

As a consequence, community-based studies in India have reported a high level of gynecological morbidity. Of the 90,303 ever-married women sampled nationwide in the 1999 National Family Health Survey (IIPS 2000), 39% reported at least one gynecological and related symptom within the past two months that included vaginal discharge (31%) and urinary tract problems (17%). A number of community-level studies in India have also shown that from 55% to 100% of ever-married women respondents self-reported one or more current symptoms (Bang et al. 1989; Bhatia and Cleland 1995; Garg et al. 2002; Kambo, Dhillon, Singh, Saxena 2004; Koenig, Jejeebhoy, Singh, Sridhar 1998; Oomman 2000; Prasad et al. 2003).

The most prevalent problem mentioned by women in India is *safed pani* (Bang and Bang 1991, 1994), a nonspecific vaginal discharge related to a number of causes, most of which reflect normal physiology and micro-organisms in the reproductive tract. *Safed pani* is deeply embedded in cultural beliefs about causation of *kamjori*, menstrual complications, and symptoms related to their husbands having sex with other women; *safed pani* is considered by women to be a serious health problem (Bang and Bang 1994; Bhatia and Cleland 1995; Kambo et al. 2004; Patel 1994; Patel, Barge, Kolhe, and Sadhwani 1994).

Another condition, *kamjori* includes a wide range of general bodily complaints such as pain related to menses, pain in joints (hands and legs), dizziness, loss of appetite, and chronic fatigue. *Kamjori* as a health concern is pervasive throughout South Asia (Nichter 1989). In South Asia, women associate *kamjori* with *safed pani* (Bhatti and Fikree 2002; Gittelsohn et al. 1994). Another culturally defined health problem linked by many Indian women to gynecological and related symptoms is *tenshun*, an English-derived term used by Urdu- and Hindi-speaking women to define psychological distress that is expressed in terms of anxiety and sadness or depression. *Tenshun* has also been viewed as associated with high levels of poverty, low education, excessive household chores, husband's alcoholism, low empowerment, domestic violence, and marital difficulties (Oomman 1996; Patel and Oomman 1999; Prasad et al. 2003; Ramasubban and Rishyasringa 2001). *Tenshun*, as well as *safed pani* and *kamjori*, are associated with women's heavy social burden, low self-esteem, and gender-based inequalities that in turn prevent women from seeking proper health care (Jejeebhoy and Koenig 2003; Patel and Oomman 1999; Weiss and Gupta 1998).

Sexual Health Concepts and HIV Risk

How can we use these folk concepts of illness to develop a responsive HIV preventive intervention? From the perspectives of the authors, there were several "hooks" on which to hang an approach to HIV prevention. The first of these hooks is that the domains of *gupt rog* and *stree rog* (women's illness) can provide a cultural base for raising issues related to the sexual and reproductive risks of HIV and other sexually transmitted diseases (STDs). Second, *gupt rog* and *stree rog* are seen as problems that need to be treated, and therefore men and women can be engaged in intervention at the "point of service." Third, *gupt rog* and *stree rog* symptoms may be markers of sexual risk or the behaviors that contribute to sexual risk. Finally, the concepts of *gupt rog* and *stree rog* are highly salient among men and women in the study communities and create a pathway to addressing sexual risk.

The NIH Projects

The Male Grant

Utilizing these concepts, the first author, an anthropologist and the principal investigator, Verma, an Indian-based psychologist, and Nastasi, a US-based psychologist, developed a 5-year (2002–2007) grant entitled, "Sexual Health Concerns and Prevention of HIV/STD in India" (the Male Grant) that was funded by the National Institute of Mental Health (RO1-MH64875). The same collaborators developed a supplement funded by the Office of AIDS Research (2002–2006) entitled "Assessing Women's Risk of HIV/STD in Marriage in India." These grants were the product of collaboration between the University of Connecticut School of Medicine and the Institute for Community Research in the United States and the IIPS in Mumbai, India. They led to the formation of the IIPS-based program, Research and Intervention in Sexual Health: Theory to Action (RISHTA, an acronym meaning "relationship" in Hindi and Urdu). (For a more detailed discussion of grant development and basic design, see Schensul, Verma, Nastasi [2004] and Schensul et al. [2006a]).

The Male Grant focused on married men between the ages of 21 and 40. Married men in this age range were selected because (1) risky sex primarily occurs close to and after marriage for young Indian men; and (2) we were interested in the role of marriage and spouse in the dynamics of sexual risk. The grant involved a quasi-experimental design that was implemented in 3 stages. The first stage consisted of "formative research," a mix of qualitative and quantitative data collection methods in which the objectives were to (1) understand the cultural and community context; (2) provide the empirical base for intervention design; and (3) develop culturally appropriate instruments for measurement of change. Formative research methodology included a community ethnography, 52 male in-depth interviews, a rapid assessment of all 245 private allopathic and nonallopathic providers in the 3 communities (Schensul et al. 2006b), in-depth interviews with 37 nonallopathic providers, and a baseline survey of a random sample of 2,408 married men, aged 21 to 40, in the 3 slum communities in Mumbai. A randomly selected subset of 642 men was tested for STI, including acute and lifetime syphilis and herpes simplex virus-2 using 5 ml of blood, and gonorrhea and Chlamydia through polymerase chain reaction (PCR) testing of urine.

The intervention stage involved the implementation of a multilevel intervention involving community education, provider training, and patient counseling. The third stage involved a follow-up instrument that was consistent with the baseline survey to provide a final evaluation of the impact of the intervention, built on a comparison with the baseline survey. The follow-up survey was administered to a systematic random sample of 2,710 men (a new sample from that of the baseline), and a subset of 910 men were administered STI testing to assess the impact of the program on the community and a patient sample of 537 married men who utilized allopathic and nonallopathic providers in the communities to address *gupt rog* problems.

The Women's Supplement

The Women's Supplement represented a pilot effort and involved the collection of both qualitative and quantitative data. Field staff conducted in-depth qualitative interviews among married Hindu and Muslim women (n = 66) in the 3 study communities. In addition, 260 married women were administered a survey instrument that was comparable to the men's baseline survey. The women's project sample was generated from the men's project sample. A random sub-sample of men (n = 311) was asked for their verbal consent to have their wives interviewed for the women's project. When these men agreed, their wives were recruited into the sample after the women's project was explained to them and they gave their written consent. Of the 311 women who were contacted, 9.3% refused to be interviewed and an additional 7.1% had family members (principally husbands) who refused to allow them to be interviewed. Therefore, the women's project survey instrument was administered to a final sample of 260 married women whose husbands had also participated in the study. A subset of 193 women consented to be involved in a gynecological exam and STI testing for Chlamydia, gonorrhea, HSV-2 and syphilis.

The Study Communities

The 3 study communities, with an estimated total population of 700,000, are located in a fringe area of Mumbai. They are large settlements of people relocated from the central part of Mumbai in the late 1970s. Over a period of about 2 decades the slum population has grown rapidly, with a large number of illegal and unauthorized structures added by migrants coming from various parts of the country. The population in the baseline sample is mixed: Hindu (42%), Muslim (54%), and Christian (4%), with migrants coming from Uttar Pradesh (51.2%), rural Maharashtra (22.2%), and Tamil Nadu (9.1%) among other states. The majority (66%) of the population are migrants, with almost half of the migrants coming with their natal families, while the rest came as older male youth or adults on their own (28%) or with friends (21%). For those coming as older youth or adults, the typical pattern (68.8%) is to live with family (frequently a brother) or in a rented room with other migrants from the same location or from the same workplace (25.2%). After migrant men have established work and residence, they frequently return to their native village to marry or bring wives left in the village to Mumbai on a permanent basis. Close to 16% of married men are living without their wives for a mean of 8.6 months.

Most (90.7%) marriages in the study communities are arranged, with most wives and husbands coming together on their wedding day as virtual strangers. This emotional distance can be exacerbated by the fact that men who migrate to Mumbai from rural areas for jobs, leave wives in the husbands' parental homes until they finally settle in Mumbai, seeing them only during periodic visits to the rural village. Once women join their husbands, the opportunities for increased intimacy with their husbands are limited by the presence of husband's parents, children, and other family members in extremely limited residential space. Households consist primarily of one (81.3%) or two (17.5%) rooms with an average of 6.4 people per household. Nuclear households are most common (47.0%), followed by joint and extended households (37.1%), with 15.8% of households consisting of men only that may include same-age relatives, friends, and coworkers sharing a single residence.

Men in the study communities are daily wage workers (39.8%), petty traders and business owners (27.5%), salaried factory and private workers (13.2%), drivers (8.3%), government employees (5.3%), and construction workers (4.4%), with only 1.5% reporting being unemployed. The mean income for men is Rs. 3272 per month (approximately US$72) with only 4% of wives working for cash income, either inside the home (40.6%) or outside the home (59.4%) for a mean income of Rs. 1353 ($31) per month. Of the total households, 22% have another wage earner (other than wife), frequently a younger brother, who brings in an additional mean income.

Sexual behavior was explored with married men responding to the baseline survey instrument. Close to 40% (37.8%, $N = 910$) of married men in the baseline survey reported that they had had sex before marriage. Age at first sex was relatively late in adolescence/young adulthood at 18.5 years. For those men reporting premarital sex, only 12.3% of men reported that their first sex was with a sex worker, with 87.7% reporting that their first sex partners were friends, neighbors, and relatives. For those men who had premarital sex, they reported a mean of 2.6 partners before marriage. The relatively high age at marriage corresponds to reports of men masturbating before marriage (62.7%) and experiencing nocturnal emission (93.5%). Only 1.4% of men reported sex with a male before marriage.

In terms of extramarital sex, 22.5% reported ever having sex with women other than their wives and 12.4% reported sex with women other than their wives in the past 12 months. Of those who had extramarital sex in the last year, 30.7% reported sex with a sex worker and 73.7% with women who were not sex workers. Five percent of married men reported having sex with men after marriage, both sex workers and non–sex workers.

On the baseline survey men were asked about marital sex. Since almost all of the households consist of a single room, frequently occupied by children and extended family members, marital sexuality presents its own unique problems. Those men whose wives lived with them reported having sex with their wives a mean of 10.9 times per month, with a mean number of sexual acts of 11.1 including penetrative sex, despite the environmental constraints.

Condom use in the baseline survey with sex workers at last sex was 81.9%; with non–sex workers, 43.6%; and with wives at last marital sex, 11.7%. Of the

13 men who did not use a condom with a sex worker, none used a condom with their wives in last intercourse. Of 102 men who had sex with a woman who was not a sex worker, 92 did not use a condom with their wives.

Formative Research Results

Men's *Gupt Rog*

Analysis of the baseline results of the 2,407 married men between the ages of 21 and 40 showed that 53% reported at least one symptom of *gupt rog* in the last 3 months. Men's interviews, further confirmed by provider interviews, identified three primary symptom clusters through principal components analysis and consensus modeling (Weller and Romney 1988): men's *kamjori*, which can be defined as "sexual weakness" (distinguished subsequently from women's *kamjori*, which relates more to general weakness/tiredness); *dhat*, which indicates a problem with the quality and quantity of semen and the loss of semen; and *garmi*, which primarily relates to external and internal genital symptoms. Table 13.1 presents the symptoms reported by men in the baseline survey in these 3 clusters.

More than half the men sampled in the study communities reported that they had a *gupt rog* problem in the last 3 months. Further, the more likely men were involved in extramarital sex without a condom, the greater the number of *gupt rog* problems (Schensul et al. 2007). It is unclear whether men who have *gupt rog* problems compensate for those problems through extramarital sexual activity or whether the *gupt rog* problems are a result of risky sex. In any case, these problems serve as markers for those men involved in risky sex outside of marriage.

In India and elsewhere in the world, occupational migrants are seen as a population at greater risk for engaging in high-risk sexual behavior. The data from these study communities, however, show that it is the nonmigrant sector, including those individuals who have migrated as children with their natal families, who are involved to a significantly greater degree in premarital and extramarital sex. In addition to the nonmigrant status, it is occupational mobility as defined by being away from home overnight as a part of work, which shows a significant relationship to sexual risk behavior. Individuals who show greater occupational mobility are more likely to be involved in risky extramarital sex.

A significant number of men seek treatment for *gupt rog* problems, primarily from the many nonallopathic providers (225) who practice Indian systems of medicine and have small "cabinets" in the 3 study communities (Schensul et al. 2006b). For those men who have at least 1 symptom in any of the clusters,

Table 13.1. Men's *gupt rog* symptoms

CLUSTER AND SYMPTOMS	FREQUENCY	PERCENTAGE (N = 2407)
Kamjori	630	26.0
• Early ejaculation	388	16.1
• Loss of sexual desire	185	7.7
• Loss of erection	47	2.0
• Penis shape and size	52	2.2
Dhat	348	14.0
• Quantity of semen	64	2.7
• Thinning of semen	104	4.3
• Color of semen	17	0.7
• Nocturnal emission	178	7.4
• Masturbation	37	1.5
• Infertility	36	1.5
Garmi	877	36.0
• White Discharge	78	3.2
• Hot urine	221	9.2
• Burning urine	276	11.5
• Itching on the genitals	335	13.9
• Pain in the penis	39	1.6
• Pimples on the penis	55	2.3
• Sores on penis	28	1.2
• Pain in the abdomen	125	5.2

the frequency of treatment is 58% for *garmi* with a mean number of treatments of 1.5; 23% for *kamjori* with a mean number of treatments of 1.7; and 18% for *dhat* with a mean number of treatments of 2.3. Men are the most frequent users of the nonallopathic providers both for general health problems and for *gupt rog* specifically. The results of the formative research demonstrate the significance of *gupt rog* in terms of frequency, saliency, and a stimulus for seeking treatment with nonallopathic providers.

Gupt Rog and Sexual Risk

The baseline survey data show a statistically significant relationship between men's reports of *gupt rog* symptoms and extramarital sex (see Schensul et al. 2007). The qualitative interview data (Schensul et al. 2004) illustrate men's perceptions of the complex relationships of their sexual behavior to *gupt rog* symptoms. Many men associate their sexual performance problems with their wives to semen loss through masturbation and early ejaculation. This view is frequently supported by the nonallopathic practitioners. Other causal behaviors include watching pornographic films and ideating about sex resulting in nocturnal emission, having sex with an older woman (e.g., a neighbor whose husband is away or a sister-in-law), sex with a sex worker and being involved in an occupation where heat is generated from machinery (e.g., driving or factory work), and wives' lack of satisfaction with their husband's sexual performance. Thus a variety of etiological factors that include risky sexual behavior can contribute to *gupt rog*.

At the same time, *gupt rog* symptoms, particularly those involving men's sexual performance, are related to men's conceptions of their masculinity and status as a husband and household leader. Early ejaculation and lack of interest in marital sex leads some men to seek more willing and compliant women with whom to have extramarital sex or on-going affairs. Men see these affairs as validation of both their sexual potency and their masculinity. In addition, *gupt rog* symptoms are significantly related to intimate partner violence with spouse as a further indication of the need, in their view, to find alternative approaches to male domination.

Women's Culturally Based Symptoms

Results from the female baseline survey (designed to be comparable to the male baseline survey) provided data from 260 women about whether they had experienced any of 32 sexual and reproductive health and related symptoms in the previous 3 months (these symptoms had been identified through in-depth interviewing). Utilizing principal components analysis (Tabachnick and Fidell 1996), 5 clusters were identified: (1) *kamjori;* (2) *safed pani;* (3) *tenshun;* (4) sexual dysfunction; and (5) vaginal symptoms. *Kamjori* (80.8%) was the most frequently reported cluster, with *safed pani* (31.2%) being the second, and *tenshun* (28.1%) being the third, followed by sexual dysfunction (9.6%) and vaginal symptoms (6.9%; Table 13.2). The average number of reported symptoms was 4.1 per woman. There are a variety of terms for these overall symptoms within the community; we have chosen to call them *stree rog* (women's illnesses in Hindi, see Table 13.2).

Once again, we see that the culturally based symptoms of *stree rog* take on greater importance when examining their relationships to factors in a woman's life and her risk of HIV/STI. Path analysis (Wright 1921) of these survey data shows that a greater number of women's *stree rog* symptoms are significantly associated with more negative women's life situations, as defined by less empowerment, increased domestic violence, poorer self-assessment as a wife and sex partner, and lower self-esteem. Further, there is a significant association between men's extramarital risky sex and women's *stree rog* symptoms indicating that they can be a marker for greater risk of transmission of HIV/STI for women (Schensul et al. 2007).

Table 13.2. Women's reported gynaecological and related symptoms

SYMPTOMS AND CLUSTERS	FREQUENCY	PERCENTAGE (N = 260)
Cluster 1: Kamjori	210	80.8
Lower backache	126	48.5
Headache	116	44.6
Pain in body	94	36.2
Giddiness (Dizziness)	67	25.8
Pain/cramps during menses	57	21.9
Pain in lower abdomen	53	20.4
Loss of appetite	42	16.2
Palpitations	40	15.4
Chest pain	38	14.6
Irregular menses	34	13.1
Cluster 2: Safed Pani	81	31.2
Cluster 3: Tenshun	73	28.1
Anxiety	73	28.1
Depression	56	21.5
Cluster 4: Sexual Dysfunction	25	9.6
Loss of sexual desire	13	5.0
Pain in vagina	9	3.5
Sexual dissatisfaction	9	3.5
Cluster 5: Vaginal and urinary tract symptoms	18	6.9
Burning urination	18	6.9
Itching in and around vagina	15	5.8
Pain while urinating	13	5.0
Obstructed urine flow	9	3.5

In terms of available health facilities, women can choose to travel to a public hospital involving high costs and time commitment, or to services in the community, which include the public urban health centers and private allopathic and nonallopathic providers. Treatment patterns for women in the survey sample showed considerable variation based on symptoms. The predominant pattern is for women with *safed pani* and those with *kamjori* to seek treatment most often (34% and 33% respectively), compared to a lesser proportion of women seeking treatment for vaginal and urinary tract problems (20%), with only a limited number of women seeking treatment for psychological distress (5%) and none for sexual dysfunction (0%). Those women who are not able to access treatment must live with the problem. The high rates of treatment for the most frequent symptoms indicate that it is important to engage women for risk reduction intervention where they seek health care, since for many women in the study communities mobility on a regular basis is restricted to proximity to home.

Culturally Based Symptoms as a Marker of Sexual Risk

The formative research showed a significant correlation between *gupt rog* symptoms and men's sexually risky behavior (Schensul et al. 2007). The formative research also showed that there was a significant relationship between greater *stree rog* symptoms, women's negative life situation, and HIV/STI risk. Therefore, men's and women's culturally based symptoms can be markers for sexual risk. In addition, these symptoms are a motivator for men and women to seek care, primarily from the practitioners of Indian systems of medicine in their communities. These and other results developed in the formative stage of the research led to a multilevel intervention involving community education, provider training, and altered provider treatment procedures for current patients.

Focal Intervention Concepts

The preliminary research of Verma et al. and the RISHTA formative research led to a series of core foci on which the intervention plan was developed. These concepts centered on the high degree of utilization on the part of community residents of nonallopathic private practitioners drawn from a holistic tradition of medicine, the development of a model of individual treatment and community education drawn from that holistic tradition, and from an understanding of community social and political organization.

Indian Systems of Medicine

The syndromes of *gupt rog* and *stree rog* represented the starting positions for the development of culturally based interventions. The next step was to identify approaches to these syndromes that would make cultural sense and thus be in accord with the local understanding of disease prevention efforts. We found that the holistic understanding in traditional Indian systems of medicine (Schensul et al. 2006b) provided just such an approach. There are several medical traditions in India including those derived from within the Indian civilization(s) and those that find their origins in other cultures. The most popular of the traditional medical traditions are *Ayurveda* and *Siddha*, although there are many other practices including yoga, magico-religious practices and supernatural healing, bone setting, and midwifery. Several "imported" medical traditions are *Unani*, homeopathy, naturopathy, and allopathy. *Ayurvedic*, *Unani*, homeopathic, and allopathic providers are the dominant treatment resources available to residents in the Mumbai study communities.

Ayurveda (the "science of life" in Sanskrit) stems from ancient Indian culture through the *veda* tradition. According to *Ayurveda*, the human body is a microcosmic replica of the universe, containing elements, humors, and substances, one of which called *sukra*, enters into the formation and cycle of sperm and ovum. When *sukra* is disturbed, it results in reproductive and sexual health problems; in the same way, any disturbance in the equilibrium of the elements, humors, and substances results in disease. *Ayurvedic* medicine is considered holistic in its focus on a balanced state of the body, mind, and emotions, as well as environmental, social, moral, and spiritual welfare (Basham 1976; Dash 1999; Lad 1990; Ministry of Health and Family Welfare 2004; Obeyesekere 1976). The main principle of treatment is thus to maintain or restore equilibrium. Ayurvedic medicine promotes a preventive and positive health approach, and when treatment is needed, it is aimed at avoiding causative factors such as risky behaviors and unbalanced diet.

Unani (meaning "Greek" in Arabic) is derived mainly from the Greco-Hellenic and Islamic civilizations. According to *Unani* medicine, all beings are made up of basic elements, temperaments, qualities, humors, and forces. In this healing system, health is a state of the body in which there is equilibrium of these components, and when this equilibrium is disturbed, disease occurs. The main goal of *Unani* medicine is to achieve an optimal balance (*eukrasia*) for each person. *Unani* treatment is based on the *contraria contraris* principle, "to treat a disease by its opposite" (e.g., a "hot" disease is cured with a "cold" medicine). *Unani* medicine is also considered holistic in its consideration of physical and mental activity, environment, and diet, which contribute to the preservation of health (Dols 1984; Leslie 1976; Ministry of Health and Family Welfare 2004).

Homeopathy (derived from the Greek *homois*, "similar," and *pathos,* disease/suffering) was developed in Germany and first appeared in the midst of the medical experimentation in India in the nineteenth century. According to homeopathy, "miasm" (from the Greek, to pollute), is the main cause of all diseases. The human body contains an innate vital force that is weakened during illness. Treatment is based on *similia similibus* principle (Latin, "like are cured by like"); a remedy, which by its "nature" is most similar to the symptom, is prescribed and administered to the patient in a minimum dose. This remedy stimulates the "vital force" or existing defense mechanism of the body, which fails when disease occurs. Homeopathy is also considered holistic in its concern with environmental, social, and emotional determinants on which action is taken for better treatment (Gala 2000; Jacobs and Moscowitz 1996; Leslie 1976; Ministry of Health and Family Welfare 2004).

While a greater number of Muslim patients seek care with *Unani* providers, there is considerable use by members of the various ethno-religious groups of the providers from each of the medical disciplines. Selection of a private provider is primarily based on location and relationship rather than on discipline. In fact, analysis of reported use of providers on the baseline survey instrument indicated that close to three quarters of men and women misidentified the discipline of their private provider. In addition, there is considerable evidence (Schensul et al. 2006b) that the treatment methodologies of over 80% of the nonallopathic providers are primarily focused on allopathic medicines (particularly antibiotics) resulting in a symptom–prescription orientation that undermines the holistic traditions of these disciplines.

There are a small number (less than 10%) of private providers in the 3 study communities who are allopaths with MBBS or MD degrees. The majority of allopathic services is provided by 2 urban health centers and 3 smaller health posts run by the Mumbai Municipal Corporation with faculty, residents, and students from a Mumbai-based Medical College. These governmental primary care services are primarily geared to the needs of new and expectant mothers and young children. This orientation leaves little room for women's *stree rog* symptoms and as a result, women prefer presenting these problems to the non-allopathic private practitioners. The allopathic health service system has had little respect for *gupt rog* symptoms and their perceived etiology. As a result, men are the highest utilizers of private, nonallopathic services and very low users of public allopathic services.

The Narrative Intervention Model

At the core of the projects is the Narrative Intervention Model (NIM), a theory-driven, ecological approach that addresses men's and women's sexual health symptoms and their link to cultural, relational, and psychological factors that increase the risk for HIV/STI. The NIM builds on the saliency of the holistic approach embodied in several Indian systems of medicine. We developed the NIM as a model for culture-specific intervention for HIV/STI risk reduction and prevention, which integrates principles and strategies from narrative therapy (Eron and Lund 1996), cognitive therapy (Beck 1976), multicultural or culturally sensitive approaches to counseling and therapy (Ivey and Ivey 2003), and cognitive-behavioral approaches to sexual risk prevention and risk reduction (Azjen and Fishbein 1980; Fisher and Fisher 1993). The theoretical underpinnings of NIM reflect the social and cultural origins of people's systems of belief and behavior (Nastasi et al. 2000), bioecology (Bronfenbrenner 1999), and anthropology (Good 1994; Kleinman 1986; Pelto and Pelto 1997; Wallace 1961).

The NIM posits that behavior, specifically behavior related to sexual health, is influenced by the interaction of biological, psychological, and cultural factors, and that through repeated experiences, individuals and communities develop narratives or scripts that guide their behavior. These assumptions have implications for behavior change efforts, in this case, the development of health-promoting and risk-reducing behaviors related to HIV/STI prevention. First, understanding a person's cognition and behavior requires knowledge of the individual's social–cultural history, which can be represented as their personal story, their individual as well as community narrative. Through the use of focused interpersonal interactions, trained practitioners can help individuals to (a) identify the story related to the presenting problem, (b) critically examine the psychological and social–cultural factors that influence or maintain the problem, and (c) create a revised narrative that leads to solving the problem. This process leads to the development of a revised personal narrative that supports health-promoting and risk-reducing behaviors related to HIV/STI prevention and treatment. The narrative approach requires that interventionists make use of a process of conceptual revision in which ideas and beliefs linked to risky sexual behavior are challenged through the introduction of alternative culturally rooted views, and risk reduction narratives are constructed through dialogue. These principles are applied in interventions directed both at doctor–patient relationships and at community education.

Community Dynamics

We found that the 3 study communities had a wide range of communal, collective advocacy organizations that represent potential partners in the intervention process. These include governmental functionaries (the lowest level of government officials in Mumbai) and their community offices; political parties, including local and national parties; nongovernmental organizations (NGOs) providing health, literacy, and other services; *mandals* (community-based organizations) that include those for youth, women (*mahila*), and men (*purush*); and Hindu temples, Islamic mosques, and associated religious organizations and schools, both public and private. The 3 communities included 2 government-run allopathic urban health centers and smaller health worker–staffed health posts conducted by the Mumbai Municipal Corporation (local Mumbai government) and police stations in each of the communities. Each of the communities is divided into sections and lanes providing reference points for community coverage. This high degree of organization provided many opportunities for RISHTA to gain permission for the project with community gatekeepers that included political, organizational, government, and religious leaders; describe the goals and nature of the projects to community groups; enlist aid for conducting formative research (including providing sites for the collection of blood and urine for STI testing); and generate the active involvement of community members in the community education component of the intervention. In addition, RISHTA worked closely with organizers of festivals (e.g., *Ganpati, Diwali, Eid*) and other community-wide celebrations to include RISHTA presentations and materials. The early involvement of these community collaborators provided both a venue for dissemination of research, evaluation of results, and recruitment of community groups and individuals who could provide sustainability of the RISHTA interventions.

Intervention for Men

A year and a half (2001–2002) of formative research led to the development of a multilevel intervention at the community, provider, and patient levels. Implementation at each level was based on the holistic approach, drawn from Indian systems of medicine and cognitive learning theory, and embodied in the NIM.

Community Level

Community-level intervention has involved a series of community-familiar mechanisms to deliver messages concerning the factors that contribute to men's sexual risk. These mechanisms have included street dramas and follow-up meetings, community meetings, opinion leader meetings, individual consultation and referral, informal group discussions, poster competitions and exhibitions, involvement in festivals, and the development of written materials on topics related to sexual risk.

1. In collaboration with a local NGO with experience in developing and performing street dramas, RISHTA presented over 200 performances with 3 scripts in each of the lanes (roadways for travel in the community that serve to designate neighborhoods) in the 3 communities. Street dramas have become a significant part of rural and urban community life in India. The scripts depicted the linkages of *gupt rog* to alcohol use, hypermasculinity, poor marital relationships, intimate partner violence, and behavior risky for *gupt rog*. The street dramas were presented in each section of the 3 communities on a rotating basis; when all sections were covered, additional scripts were generated, and continued to rotate through the communities.

2. Follow-up meetings were held on the day after a street drama to collect reactions from men who attended the street plays and to identify their questions related to sexual health. The answers to questions and further discussion were provided in a second community meeting that took place within the following week.

3. Community meetings were held on a regular basis with informal community-based organizations (*purush mandals*) and more formal community-based NGOs to provide information on sexual risk reduction and to recruit members of these organizations into participation in community-level education.

4. Opinion leader meetings were held with a panel of official and informal leaders in each of the three study communities to gauge community reaction to RISHTA programs and to receive feedback on new program initiatives.

5. Individual consultation and referral were provided by RISHTA field staff to community men with sexual health questions or problems. It is estimated that over 3000 men have contacted the RISHTA staff for these problems and have received informal advice concerning the nature of the problem and referral.

6. Informal group discussions have been utilized by RISHTA field staff to provide education, referral, and marketing of project activities to clusters of men as they form in tea shops, bars, and other community gathering locations.

7. Special community projects have included a poster competition, conducted with over 60 local secondary school students, emphasizing HIV/STI prevention measures and factors involved in sexual risk and exhibitions of the posters in community gatherings, which have attracted over 7,500 people. The poster competition generated pictorial materials for communication on sexuality and sexual health. The posters are displayed once a month in the 3 communities.

8. RISHTA has also participated in all festival events in the 3 communities involving education and risk reduction, referral, and marketing of the interventions.

9. Our qualitative data indicated that men in the study communities have many questions about masturbation, nocturnal emission, and STDs and

RISHTA (I. I. P. S.)

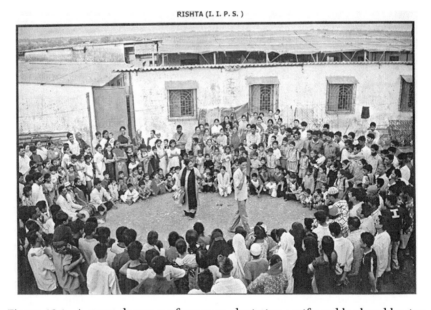

Figure 13.1. A street drama performance, depicting a wife and husband having a fight as a result of his coming home after drinking with his friends.

their treatment. As a result, a 40-page book was developed and printed by the RISHTA team that addressed sexual health problems and their solutions. This book provides insights in a lay language that best meets the informational needs of the men in the study communities. Copies were distributed to men who were contacted during meetings, poster exhibition sessions, or street plays. Men have found the book useful in clarifying many apprehensions with regard to sexual health. Finally, there have been a series of brochures developed on the project domains of lifestyles, masculinity, STDs and their treatment; these have been distributed to men in the communities.

Provider Intervention

The formative research identified the treatment seeking behavior of men with *gupt rog* problems and found that the greatest majority sought care from *Ayurvedic, Unani,* and homeopathic providers in their communities. There were several reasons for focusing on the local practitioners of Indian systems of medicine. *Gupt rog* symptoms were a centerpiece of their practice and the various healing disciplines provided herbal and other remedies for these problems. In contrast, the public allopathic system (present in urban health centers and health posts) had little respect for *gupt rog* problems; their focus was maternal and child health.

As a result, it was decided that the provider level intervention would consist of two alternatives: in one community all the practitioners of Indian systems of medicine would be trained in the NIM approach to *gupt rog* problems and the reduction of sexual risk, while in a second community, a "male health clinic" (MHC) would be organized at the urban health center and allopathic staff trained in the NIM approach to gupt rog and management of STDs (WHO 1997).

The Nonallopathic Providers

The RISHTA program convened a meeting of all of the *Ayurvedic, Unani,* and homeopathic providers in the community to discuss the training program and its objectives. There was almost unanimous support for the training and an appreciation for the opportunity to learn more about HIV and other STDs.

While the practitioners were well-versed in *gupt rog* problems, the nature of their "practiced medicine" (Schensul et al. 2006b) had moved away from the holistic approach that characterized their training. The NIM approach was viewed as a return to their holistic tenets that had been left behind in the rapid integration of allopathic medications in their practice. In October 2003, a 4-day training program was organized for the practitioners of the Indian systems of medicine. The curriculum was based on the results of the formative research and covered an introduction to the RISHTA project; a review of men's sexual health problems (*gupt rog*) with data from the baseline survey; an examination of the factors that contribute to, co-occur, and result from *gupt rog*; treatment of *gupt rog* through the use of NIM, to include attention to biological, psychological, and sociocultural factors; etiology, treatment seeking, treatment, and prevention of *gupt rog*; education and counseling for prevention of sexual risks; appropriate testing and treatment of STIs through syndromic management; referrals for medical, psychological, and social services as needed; and creation of a support system for providers in implementing the NIM, consisting of RISHTA intervention staff.

Results from evaluations, conducted before and after the training, indicate that the training was positively received and that the holistic perspective drew providers back to their disciplinary roots. RISHTA conducted refresher training, which was held in each quarter from 2004 to 2006, on syndromic management of STDs, and the processes of counseling and education. In the interim between refresher sessions, RISHTA field staff stayed in regular contact with the trained providers, assisting in referrals and responding to questions concerning the NIM process.

Male Health Clinic

In December 2003, the "male health clinic" (MHC) opened in another of the study communities. The MHC is based in the urban health center run by the Mumbai Municipal Corporation and staffed by a local medical college in Mumbai. The head of the Department of Social and Preventive Medicine and her faculty were very positive about a new approach to men and sexual risk. With a relatively small amount of financial support from the RISHTA project (<$5,000), a special clinic, the Male Health Clinic (MHC), was organized for men in the hours after work during the weekdays and on the weekend. The MHC is open 3 days per week (Monday, Friday, and Sunday) from 5 PM to 8 PM, times that were convenient for working men. The clinic was announced to the community through street dramas and meetings held in the community. The MHC was available to men of any age and with any presenting problem. The data from the patient records show that since the opening of the MHC, there has been a steady flow of male patients into what has been an almost exclusive female health clinic. From December 2003 to January 2006, the clinic saw close to 4,000 patient visits, an average of 14 patients for each clinic session, of whom 56.3% presented with sexual health problems and 12.9% were diagnosed with an STI. Of those with sexual health problems, 57.9% were in the 21 to 40 age-group and 74.2% (156) were married. The results indicated that an MHC in a government urban health clinic, in a community where men tend to avoid the governmental facilities, is capable of attracting men, of whom a significant percentage will present with a sexual health problem.

Physician faculty and interns were trained in NIM jointly with providers of the Indian systems of medicine. While this joint training at first seemed problematic, considering the antipathy between allopaths and traditional providers, it turned out to be positive. The NIM was a model that was well accepted by the allopaths, who felt that their approach to patients was becoming too narrow, and by the nonallopaths, who also found the approach salient. Allopaths accepted the greater expertise of the nonallopaths in relation to *gupt rog*, while the nonallopaths accepted the greater expertise of the allopaths in the realm of STDs. Allopaths participated in all 4 days of the initial training and all the refresher sessions alongside the nonallopathic providers.

Evaluation Design for Men

The intervention used a quasi-experimental design (Campbell and Stanley 1966) in which all 3 study communities received community-level education, 2 of the communities were "experimental" (the community with the MHC and the community with trained traditional providers), and the third community was the control, not receiving either of the additional services. To assess multilevel differences between the 3 communities and between the patients of the different providers using and not using NIM, the following data collection methods were used:

- The baseline survey of a systematic random sample of 2,407 married men from 21 to 40, drawn evenly from the 3 communities has been compared with a separate random sample of 2,710 randomly selected men administered the follow-up survey to assess community-level trends and impact of the RISHTA project.
- A panel (cohort) sample of 403 men who responded to the baseline survey have also been administered a follow-up survey to assess individual change at the community level.
- A patient sample of 537 men from 21 to 40 years of age presenting to providers with *gupt rog* problems was drawn randomly from the practices of the allopathic and nonallopathic providers trained by RISHTA and the untrained private allopaths and nonallopaths in the control community. Each of the sampled men received a pre-treatment interview, a post-treatment interview (within 48 hours) and a 6-month follow-up interview.
- A random sub-sample of men responding to the baseline (641) and the follow-up survey (902) participated in blood draws and collection of urine

specimens to test for the presence of acute and lifetime HSV-2, acute and lifetime exposure to syphilis, and current gonorrhea and Chlamydia infection (HIV testing was not conducted; it was estimated that there would be a six times greater rate of STDs than HIV and as a result, STDs would be a better indicator of sexual risk behavior).

Intervention for Women

The Women's Supplement provided an opportunity to collect formative research on married women and their relative sexual risk of contracting HIV/STI from their husbands. It also provided the opportunity to develop a pilot women's health clinic to provide women with gynecological examinations, as well as drawing blood and collecting urine for STI testing. The pilot women's health clinic was conducted at the same urban health center where the MHC was established. The procedure for examination of married women involved female field staff conducting the survey interview and then establishing a day for the women to come to the clinic in the early afternoon (a period where women had some free time). Of the 260 women who were administered the survey, 193 participated in the gynecological examination and STI testing. Most of the women who did not participate did not do so because of the decisions made by husbands and mothers-in-law. Once at the clinic, we found that almost all women had never had an internal pelvic examination and had only come to the urban health center in the past for prenatal care and well-child care. The procedure at the clinic involved a medical history with a female intern, an internal examination with a gynecologist (not regularly available at the urban health center), examination of cervical specimens in the laboratory organized for the pilot clinic, and urine collection and blood draw by a trained phlebotomist. The positive reception to the women's health clinic both by the married women in the sample and by the faculty and staff of the clinic raised the possibility that a specialty clinic devoted to *stree rog* would make an important contribution to women's needs and be a "point of service" in which married women's sexual risk could be addressed.

Two additional formative research methods were utilized in assessing women's needs with regard to the potential for HIV/STI transmission in marriage; both of these methods recognized the need to involve husbands in women's health needs and risk reduction. The first method involved interviews with 51 couples. Each couple was provided a series of scenarios concerning the problems of "another couple" in the community (these scenarios were drawn from composites of problems related to sexuality, domestic violence, husband's alcohol use as identified in the women's and men's in-depth interviews). Field researchers took detailed notes on how the couple would resolve the problem as well as the interactive dynamics of the way couples dealt with each other in problem resolution. It became clear in these interviews that working independently with women would not fully address the issues of male dominance and risk taking and would present problems for women who sought risk reduction through unilateral action (El-Bassel et al. 2001; Becker and Robinson 1998; Padian, O'Brien, Chang, Glass, and Francis 1993).

A second approach was pilot testing of "couples' intervention." To assess feasibility and acceptability of a couples' intervention, we piloted a 7-session intervention with 21 married couples recruited from 1 of the study communities. Drawing on the results of men's, women's, and couples' interviews, we adapted the NIM to the objectives and format of the couples' intervention. The intervention targeted skills related to communication and negotiation, coping with tensions and conflicts, and sexual risk reduction within the marital relationship. Sessions of 60 to 90 minutes duration were conducted in small group format and held weekly in a centralized and easily accessible community location. The first 3 sessions were conducted with wives and husbands separately and the remaining 4 sessions were conducted jointly with husbands and wives. Sessions were facilitated by field staff (2 women, 2 men) who participated in development of the intervention program, with support from an experienced Mumbai-based social worker. Sessions with women were cofacilitated by female staff, male sessions by male staff, and joint (couples) sessions by female–male dyads. The initial 5 sessions addressed the following topics: (1) roles and responsibilities in marriage; (2) tensions in marriage; (3) sex in marriage; (4) negotiating roles and responsibilities in marriage (joint couple session); and (5) negotiating tensions in marriage (joint couple session). Participants requested and received 2 additional sessions focused on sexuality and sexual risk.

Evaluation addressed the capacity of field staff to implement and facilitate single- and mixed-gender group sessions, appropriateness of activities for married couples, response of couples to session content and activities (participation, acceptability), and perceived utility and relevance of the topics for their marital lives. Evaluation strategies included participant observation (by same-gender field staff member), structured group feedback activity at the conclusion of each session, and individual feedback from a sample of participants following each session. Evaluation data indicated a high level of feasibility. Sixteen of the 21 couples participated consistently across the 7 sessions. All the female and male participants reported a high level of interest and enthusiasm toward the program. They participated actively in session activities and were supportive and cooperative in group activities. They indicated a high level of agreement regarding the appropriateness of session topics and activities and relevance to their daily lives.

Outcomes

Each of the 3 study communities was provided community education over a period of 3 years. The quasi-experimental design at the community level called for a comparison of the baseline and follow-up surveys for the 2 experimental communities vs. the control community and for the allopathic (MHC) experimental community vs. the nonallopathic experimental community. At the patient level, the design called for a comparison of the patients seen by the trained providers vs. those seen by the untrained providers and a comparison of the patients seen by the trained allopathic providers at the MHC vs. those seen by the trained nonallopathic providers. Among 16 indicators, the primary outcome indicators included extramarital sex, biologically determined STD status, intimate partner violence, alcohol use, STI knowledge, satisfaction with marital sexual life, and a masculinity scale ranging from "hypermasculine" to gender equitable.

Preliminary outcome results comparing the baseline at 2003 to the follow-up at 2006 show that all 3 communities had a dramatic decline in extramarital sex (12.5% to 2.9%, $P < .001$) and a consequent reduction in gonorrhea and Chlamydia (4.2% to 1.7%, $P = .013$). There was no significant difference between the 2 experimental communities and the control community on these outcomes. Given the design, we cannot conclude that community education in all 3 communities produced these dramatic results; however, informal feedback from surveys in other Indian communities has noted a decline in STDs, but not as dramatic as those in our study communities.

Other results support the basic hypotheses of this study. First, intimate partner violence showed a greater decline in the experimental communities vs. the control community, with reduction in the MHC community greater than that in the nonallopathic community. Second, there was significantly greater gender equity among the experimental communities than in the control community, with the MHC community showing greater equity than the nonallopathic community. Finally, marital sexual satisfaction showed a greater increase in the experimental communities than in the control community and there was greater satisfaction in the nonallopathic community than in the MHC community.

At the individual level, those who reported direct exposure to community education showed a significantly lower rate of extramarital sex than those who had no exposure. Those individuals who utilized the trained providers showed a significantly lower rate of extramarital sex than those who saw either no provider or an untrained provider. Finally, those individuals who were exposed to both community education and trained providers showed the greatest decrease in extramarital sex.

From the individual patient level, the data indicate (1) a significant reduction in alcohol use by the patients of trained vs. untrained providers, with trained allopaths showing the greatest reduction; (2) a significant increase in STD knowledge among the patients seen by the trained vs. untrained providers, with the nonallopathic providers showing the greatest increase; and (3) a significant reduction in extramarital sex among the patients seen by the trained vs. the untrained providers, with Chlamydia and gonorrhea showing the greatest reductions in the nonallopathic community.

The results indicate that the experimental communities where provider training has taken place have shown better outcomes at the community level than the control community where there has been no provider training. The comparison of the 2 experimental communities has shown that each approach has specific strengths and that training of both types of providers will achieve complimentary outcomes. In terms of patients, those using trained providers have shown better outcomes than those using untrained providers. Similar to the community-level results, patients of both trained allopaths and trained nonallopaths show complementary outcomes that suggest the need to work with both types of providers. Finally, we saw the positive effects of both exposure to community education and to trained providers and the synergy that can result in greater sexual risk reduction.

Sustainability and Dissemination

A significant portion of the final year of the project (2006–2007) was devoted to finding mechanisms for sustaining educational activities focused on sexual risk reduction within the study communities and replicating the RISHTA approach in other communities in India. In the beginning of the final year we began a process that we have labeled "ethnographic dissemination," which utilized our knowledge of the communities to disseminate research and evaluation results to opinion leaders, community-based organizations, and residents. In total, 21 dissemination sessions were conducted in the 3 study communities, focusing on presentation of baseline vs. follow-up results and evaluation of the community and provider level interventions. These presentations stimulated the development of 5 "community action groups" that committed themselves to continuity of community education with special emphasis on street drama and community meetings with the support of community-based institutions and NGOs.

In terms of "replicability," the project has had the good fortune of being in the right place at the right time when the National AIDS Control Organization (NACO) of the Ministry of Health and Family Welfare announced an initiative to involve nonallopathic providers in the prevention of HIV/AIDS. The RISHTA model, with special emphasis on the training of nonallopathic providers in NIM and in diagnosis and referral of STIs has become center stage in the NACO effort. RISHTA principal investigators, including Ravi Verma and Niranjan Saggurti, are now providing leadership for a technical assistance group involved in the implementation of training, counseling, and referral for nonallopathic providers. In August 2007, RISHTA held a national dissemination in New Delhi, where project results were presented by all of the collaborators to an audience of key policy makers and the RISHTA manual, *Health Care Practitioners' Guide to Prevention of HIV/STIs: Narrative Prevention Counseling for AYUSH, Allopathic and Other Providers* (Population Council 2007) was officially released. The national dissemination and the manual were the stimulus for training programs to be conducted at the state level in various locations in India.

The Women's supplement demonstrated the centrality of *stree rog* symptoms as a marker for sexual risk and a way of reaching married women to prevent HIV/STI transmission within marriage. It also identified the importance of male involvement in risk reduction for married women and in the need to upgrade clinical services related to women's health. These developments provided the empirical base for a new NIH grant entitled, "Prevention of HIV/STI among married women in urban India" (RO1-MH75678). The components of the new grant include a focus on *stree rog* among married women, the development of an enhanced clinic in the urban health center for women with *stree rog* problems, and involvement of women and their husbands in couples' intervention. This project was funded in September 2007 for a 5-year period, which will provide continuous funding for HIV/STI risk for reduction for men and women in the same 3 communities for a period of 11 years.

Conclusion

While the U.S.-based anthropologist has the role of principal investigator in this work, the projects described in this chapter are a transdisciplinary collaboration that includes public health practitioners, epidemiologists, demographers, psychologists, physicians, and microbiologists based in India, the United States, Canada, and the United Kingdom. The term "transdisciplinary" (see Schensul et al. 2006a) is used because the collaboration is not simply a set of specific tasks for each discipline but a shared and unified conceptual model involving the role of culture and local community dynamics, linked to extant theory, in the conduct of the research and the design of the intervention.

Anthropological leadership of public health projects is not a requirement for cultural and community relevant models. A more significant requirement is the need to avoid the domination by any one discipline and to pursue the creation of a more egalitarian project environment in which a variety of disciplinary perspectives can be considered in the development of a unified model. This notion is embedded in the "NIH Roadmap" (NIH 2007), a call to move beyond artificial discipline boundaries to further science and empirical research.

At the same time, it is necessary for anthropologists and members of public health disciplines alike to understand what anthropology can bring to the scientific table and to the design of public health interventions. In the projects in this chapter, these contributions are as follows:

1. A cultural perspective: Anthropologists see culture as a coherent body of behavioral guidelines, with consistency and saliency across generations, but also a dynamic process responding to environmental change and producing significant intracultural variation. Anthropologists have a cultural focus, which allows them to identify salient cultural behavior and beliefs on which to base endogenously derived interventions. In the case of the men's component of the RISHTA project, these cultural elements were drawn from the "great traditions" of *Ayurvedic* and *Unani* medicine and belief systems about semen loss, *safed pani*, *kamjori*, and *gupt rog* that are widespread throughout South Asia. The development of an understanding of this medical culture and its salience for men and women made it a fundamental component of the intervention. HIV and other STDs are an increasingly important concern for Indian men and women, but *gupt rog* and *stree rog* problems were far more salient. At the same time *gupt rog* and *stree rog* provided a "doorway" to enter the realm of sexual risk and begin a dialogue with the study communities, the providers and the patients. The link with a cultural element(s) also means that Western theories (cognitive learning, social ecology) can be brought into an integrative model without imposing such theories on non-Western cultures.

2. A holistic perspective: Anthropologists use the concept of holism to signify their interest in a broad view of the problem under study and a view of that problem as a product of a number of interrelationships with different parts of the culture and community. This process of contextual understanding of public health problems and outcomes avoids reductionist thinking and seeks to identify both multilevel interventions and multivariate outcomes. The RISHTA project has viewed sexual risk in the context of community dynamics, the structure and nature of health care resources, the organization of the family, and the behavior of individual men and women. The interventions also take a holistic perspective in the process of providing community education, provider training, and impact on the patient–provider interaction. Finally, the holistic perspective calls for multiple outcomes that go beyond extramarital sex, STD status, and condom use to include behaviors such as alcohol use, risky activities with friends, access to pornographic materials and the nature of marital sex

and attitudes that include gender equity, assessment as a spouse and sex partner, self-esteem, and other variables that measure significant parts of individual lives in a community context.

3. A local perspective: Anthropologists are concerned about the perspectives and worldview of the communities and individuals with whom they are involved. Much of the data that anthropologists collect involves face-to-face discussions and interviews with key informants (cultural and community experts) and residents in an effort to understand the "inside looking out" perspective on key aspects of the community and individual lives. In the RISHTA project, understanding of the subset of men who have problems in sexual performance, their rationale for seeking sex workers and other "compliant women" who will not challenge their performance, the threats of their performance problems to their masculine role and the function of intimate partner violence as a means of reasserting their male domination over their wives is derived from these kinds of interviews.

4. An emphasis on the micro-level: Anthropologists have traditionally focused their attention on geographic communities of a size that allows them to develop rapport with both leaders and residents, participate in and observe daily life, and generate support and collaboration among residents for research and intervention efforts. This focus means that anthropologists bring a perspective derived from the ecological context rather than treating research subjects as independent individuals. Further, the relationship develops expectations on the part of community residents that become a required part of the design of projects. RISHTA is now well known in the 3 communities, recognized for its role in research, intervention, and the sustainability of interventions. Anthropologists can play a significant role in research-resident collaboration and institutionalizing projects in communities rather than the more typical "drive-by" intervention.

5. The qualitative contribution: "Mixed" qualitative and quantitative data collection procedures have now moved into the mainstream of public health research. Despite this shift, the participant observation and in-depth interviewing that anthropologists have used in their qualitative methods have frequently been short-circuited by other disciplines as a means of simply adapting Western-derived instruments or using rapid methods such as focus groups to locally modify externally derived instruments and interventions. The methods used by RISHTA have involved a heavy investment of time and effort in securing observational and interview data that provide an independent understanding of the community and its residents and a complement to statistical methods by providing explanatory evidence for quantitative results.

6. Culturally based interventions: The anthropological approach described in this chapter provides an argument for the continued development of culturally based interventions that are derived from a local setting and have an impact on that setting. While public health searches for global "magic bullets" in the realm of HIV and other prevention efforts, there is room and necessity for local interventions that use cultural elements that are salient to residents in addressing significant problems. At the same time, anthropologists need to become more involved and experienced in translating their work into intervention design. This orientation involves several steps: the application of both traditional and nontraditional anthropological methods to generate empirically validated results; the need to identify facilitating resources and collaborative organizations in the local community; the ability to disseminate research results to a variety of disciplinary representatives and community residents; participation in the translation of research results into intervention design that is locally relevant and innovative; modification of interventions to meet the realities of community needs and responses; participation in the evaluation of the intervention, both from the perspective of intervention improvement and assessing the validity of research results; and involvement in the sustainability of interventions for local communities and the replicability of interventions in other communities.

These projects have demonstrated the need for a cultural and community "hook" for intervention programs. The concepts of *gupt rog* and *stree rog* in the context of Indian systems of medicine have proved to be useful in our study communities. There are comparable cultural hooks upon which to hang intervention programs in all communities and groups and for all health issues. The identification of these hooks and their integration in intervention may be anthropology's greatest contribution to public health.

References

Azjen I, Fishbein M (1980) *Understanding Attitudes and Predicting Social Behavior.* Englewood Cliffs, NJ: Prentice-Hall.

Bang R, Bang A (1991) Why women hide them: Rural women viewpoint of reproductive health infections. *Manushi* 69:27–30.

Bang R, Bang A (1994) "Women's Perceptions of White Vaginal Discharge: Ethnographic Data from Rural Maharashtra." In: *Listening to Women Talk about Their Health: Issues and Evidence from India.* J Gittelsohn, ME Bentley, PJ Pelto, M Nag, S Pachauri, AD Harrison, et al. eds. New Delhi: Har-Anand Publications, pp. 79–94.

Bang RA, Bang M, Baitule M, Chaudhury Y, Sarmukaddam S, Tale O (1989) High prevalence of gynaecological diseases in rural Indian women. *Lancet* 8629:85–88.

Basham AL (1976) "The Practice of Medicine in Ancient and Medieval India." In: *Asian Medical Systems: A Comparative Study*. C Leslie, ed. Berkeley, CA: University of California Press, pp. 18–44.

Beck AT (1976) *Cognitive Therapy and Emotional Disorders*. New York: International Universities Press.

Becker S, Robinson JC (1998) Special communication—reproductive health care: Services oriented to couples. *International Journal of Gynecology and Obstetrics* 61:275–281.

Bhatia J, Cleland J (1995) Self-reported symptoms of gynecological morbidity and their treatment in south India. *Studies in Family Planning* 26(4):203–245.

Bhatti LI, Fikree FF (2002). Health-seeking behavior of Karachi women with reproductive tract infections. *Social Science and Medicine* 54:105–117.

Bronfenbrenner U (1999) "Environments in Developmental Perspective: Theoretical and Operational Models." In: *Measuring Environment across the Life Span: Emerging Methods and Concepts*. SL Friedman, TD Wachs, eds. Washington, DC: American Psychological Association, pp. 3–28.

Campbell DT, Stanley JC (1963) *Experimental and Quasi-experimental Designs for Research*. Chicago: McNally.

Dash V (1999) *Fundamentals of Ayurvedic Medicine*. Delhi: Konark Publishers.

Dols MW (1984) *Medieval Islamic Medicine: Ibn Ridwan's Treatise on the Prevention of Bodily Ills in Egypt*. Berkeley, CA: University of California Press.

El-Bassel N, Witte SS, Gilbert L, Sormanti M, Moreno C, Pereira L, et al. (2001) HIV prevention for intimate couples: a relationship-based model. *Families, Systems, and Health* 19(4):379–397.

Eron JB, Lund TW (1996) *Narrative Solutions in Brief Therapy*. New York: Lyle Stuart.

Fisher WA, Fisher JD (1993) "A General Social Psychological Model for Changing AIDS Risk Behavior." In: *The Social Psychology of HIV Infection*. JB Pryor, GD Reeder, eds. Hillsdale, NJ: Erlbaum, pp. 127–153.

Gala D (2000) *Homeopathy for Common Diseases*. Mumbai: Navneet Publishers.

Gangakhedkar RR, Bentley ME, Divekar AD, Gadkari, D, Mehendale SM, Shepherd ME, et al. (1997) Spread of HIV infection in married monogamous women in India. *Journal of the American Medical Association* 278:2090–2092.

Garg S, Sharma N, Bhalla P, Sahay R, Saha R, Raina U, et al. (2002) Reproductive morbidity in an Indian urban slum: Need for health action. *Sexually Transmitted Infections* 78(1):68–69.

Gittelsohn J, Bentley ME, Pelto PJ, Nag M, Pachauri S, Harrison AD, et al. (1994) *Listening to Women Talk about Their Health: Issues and Evidence from India*. New Delhi: Anand Publications.

Good BJ (1994) *Medicine, Rationality, and Experience: An Anthropological Perspective*. Cambridge, UK: Cambridge University Press.

Hawkes S, Santhya KG (2002) Diverse realities: sexually transmitted infections and HIV in India. *Sexually Transmitted Infections* 78:1–8.

International Institute for Population Sciences (IIPS) (2000) *National Family Health Survey: India (NFHS-2)*. Mumbai: IIPS, Measure DHS+, and ORC MACRO.

Ivey AE, Ivey MB (2003) *Intentional Interviewing and Counseling: Facilitating Client Development in a Multicultural Society*. 5th ed. Pacific Grove, CA: Brooks/Cole.

Jacobs J, Moskowitz R (1996) "Homeopathy." In: *Fundamentals of Complementary and Alternative Medicine*. MS Micozzi, ed. New York: Churchill Livingstone, pp. 87–99.

Jejeebhoy S, Koenig M (2003) "The Social Context of Gynaecological Morbidity: Correlates, Consequences and Health Seeking Behaviour." In: *Investigating Reproductive Tract Infections and Other Gynaecological Disorders*. S Jejeebhoy, M Koenig, C Elias, eds. Cambridge, UK: Cambridge University Press, pp. 30–81.

Kambo IP, Dhillon BS, Singh P, Saxena BN (2004) Self reported gynaecological problems from twenty three districts of India (ICMR task force study). *Indian Journal of Community Medicine* 29(1):8.

Kleinman A (1986) *Social Origins of Distress and Disease*. New Haven, CT: Yale University Press.

Koenig M, Jejeebhoy S, Singh S, Sridhar, S (1998) Investigating women's gynaecological morbidity in India: not just another KAP survey. *Reproductive Health Matters* 6(11):84–95.

Kulhara P, Avasthi A (1995) Sexual dysfunction on the Indian subcontinent. *International Review of Psychiatry* 7(2):231–240.

Lad V (1990) *Ayurveda: The Science of Self Healing*. Twin Lakes, WI: Lotus Press.

Leslie C (1992) "Interpretation of Illnesses: Syncretism in Modern Ayurveda." In: *Paths to Asian Medical Knowledge*. C Leslie, A Young, eds. Berkeley, CA: University of California Press, pp. 177–208.

Mann JM, Tarantola D, Netter TW (1992) *AIDS in the World: The Global AIDS Policy Coalition*. Cambridge, MA: Harvard University Press.

Ministry of Health and Family Welfare (2004) Department of Ayurveda, Yoga and Naturopathy, Unani, and Siddha. http://indianmedicine.nic.in/

NACO (2004) HIV estimates in India (based on HIV Sentinel surveillance). www.naco.nic.in/indianscene/esthiv.htm

Nastasi BK, Varjas K, Schensul SL, Silva KT, Schensul JJ, Ratnayake P (2000) The Participatory Intervention Model: a framework for conceptualizing and promoting intervention acceptability. *School Psychology Quarterly* 15:207–232.

National Institutes of Health (nd) NIH roadmap. http://nihroadmap.nih.gov/interdisciplinary. Accessed October 5, 2007.

Nichter M (1981) Idioms of distress: Alternatives in the expression of psychosocial distress. *Culture, Medicine and Psychiatry* 5:379–408.

Nichter M (1989) "Lay Perceptions of Medicine: A South Indian Case Study." In: *Anthropology and International Health: South Asian Case Studies*. M Nichter, ed. Dordrecht, Netherlands: Kluwer Publishers, 187–213.

Newmann S, Sarin P, Kumarasamy N, Amalraj E, Rogers M, Madhivanan P, et al. (2000) Marriage, monogamy and HIV: A profile of HIV-infected women in south India. *International Journal of STD and AIDS* 11:250–253.

Obeyesekere G (1976) "The Impact of Ayurvedic Ideas on the Culture and the Individual in Sri Lanka." In: *Asian Medical Systems: A Comparative Study*. C Leslie, ed. Berkeley, CA: University of California Press, pp. 201–226.

Oomman N (1996) *Poverty and Pathology: Comparing Rural Rajasthani Women's Ethnomedical Models with Biomedical Models of Reproductive Morbidity: Implications for Women's Health in India*. Ann Arbor, MI: UMI Dissertation Services.

Oomman N (2000) "A Decade of Research on Reproductive Tract Infections and Other Gynaecological Morbidity in India: What We Know and What We Don't

Know." In: *Women's Reproductive Health in India*. R Ramasubban, SJ Jejeebhoy, eds. New Delhi: Rawat Publications, pp. 236–271.

Padian NS, O'Brien TR, Chang YC, Glass S, Francis D (1993) Prevention of heterosexual transmission of human immunodeficiency virus through couple counseling. *Journal of Acquired Immune Deficiency Syndromes* 6:1043–1048.

Pais P (1996) HIV and India: looking into the abyss. *Tropical Medicine and International Health* 1(3):295–304.

Patel BC, Barge S, Kolhe R, Sadhwani H (1994) "Listening to Women Talk about Their Reproductive Health Problems in the Urban Slums and Rural Areas of Baroda." In: *Listening to Women Talk about Their Health Issues and Evidence from India*. J Gittelsohn, ME Bentley, PJ Pelto, M Nag, S Pachauri, AD Harrison, et al. eds. New Delhi: Har-Anand Publications, pp. 131–144.

Patel P (1994) "Illness Beliefs and Health-seeking Behavior of the Bhil Women of Panchamahal District, Gujarat State." In: *Listening to Women Talk about Their Health Issues and Evidence from India*. J. Gittelsohn, ME Bentley, PJ Pelto, M Nag, S Pachauri, AD Harrison, et al. eds. New Delhi: Har-Anand Publications, pp. 55–66.

Patel V, Oomman N (1999) Mental health matters too: Gynaecological symptoms and depression in South Asia. *Reproductive Health Matters* 7(14):30–38.

Pelto PJ, Joshi A, Verma R (1999) *The Development of Indian Male Sexuality*. Population Council: South and Southeast Asian Regional Office.

Pelto PJ, Pelto GH (1997) Studying knowledge, culture and behavior in applied medical anthropology. *Medical Anthropology Quarterly* 11(2):147–163.

Prasad J, Abraham S, Akila B, Joseph A, Jacob KS (2003) Symptoms related to the reproductive tract and mental health among women in rural southern India. *National Medical Journal of India* 16(6):303–308.

Ramasubban R, Rishyasringa B (2001) "Weakness (*ashaktapana*) and Reproductive Health among Women in a Slum Population in Mumbai." In: *Cultural Perspectives on Reproductive Health*. CM Obermeyer, ed. New York: Oxford University Press, pp. 13–37.

Schensul SL, Hawkes S, Saggurti N, Verma RK, Narvekar SS, Nastasi BK, et al. (2007) Sexually transmitted infections in men in Mumbai slum communities: The relationship of prevalence to risk behavior. *Sexually Transmitted Diseases* 34(7):444–450.

Schensul SL, Mekki-Berrada A, Nastasi BK, Saggurti N (2006b) Healing traditions and men's sexual health in Mumbai, India: The realities of practiced medicine in urban poor communities. *Social Science and Medicine* 62(11):2774–2785.

Schensul SL, Nastasi B, Verma, R (2006a) Community-based research in India: A case example of international and transdisciplinary research. *American Journal of Community Psychology* 38(1–2):95–111.

Schensul SL, Verma RK, Nastasi BK (2004) Responding to men's sexual concerns: research and intervention in slum communities in Mumbai, India. *International Journal of Men's Health* 3(3):197–220.

Tabachnick B, Fidell L (1996) *Using Multivariate Statistics*. New York: HarperCollins.

UNAIDS (2004) *India: Epidemiological Fact Sheets on HIV/AIDS and Sexually Transmitted Infections*. Geneva: UNAIDS/WHO.

UNAIDS (2007) *AIDS Epidemic Update, December 2007*. Geneva: UNAIDS/WHO.

Verma KK, Khaitan BK, Singh OP (1998) The frequency of sexual dysfunctions in patients attending a sex therapy clinic in North India. *Archives of Sexual Behavior* 27(3):309–313.

Verma RK, Rangaiyan G, Singh R, Sharma S, Pelto PJ (2001) A study of male sexual health problems in a Mumbai slum population. *Culture, Health and Sexuality* 3(3):339–352.

Verma RK, Schensul SL (2004) "Male Sexual Health Problems in Mumbai: Cultural Constructs that Present Opportunities for HIV/AIDS Risk Reduction." In: *Sexuality in the Time of AIDS: Contemporary Perspectives from Communities in India.* RK Verma, PJ Pelto, SL Schensul, A Joshi, eds. New Delhi: Sage Publications, pp. 243–261.

Vuylsteke B, Sunkutu R, Laga M (1996) "Epidemiology of HIV and Sexually Transmitted Infections in Women." In: *AIDS in the World II: The Global AIDS Policy Coalition.* JM Mann, DJM Tarantola, eds. New York: Oxford University Press, pp. 97–109.

Wallace AFC (1961) *Culture and Personality.* New York: Random House.

Weiss E, Gupta GR (1998) *Bridging the Gap: Addressing Gender and Sexuality in HIV Prevention.* Washington, DC: International Center for Research on Women.

Weller S, Romney A (1988) "Systematic Data Collection." Series #10 in: *Qualitative Research Methods.* J. Maaren, P. Manning, and M. Miller, eds. Thousand Oaks, CA: Sage Publications.

WHO (1997) *Management of Patients with Sexually Transmitted Diseases.* Geneva: Global Programme on AIDS.

Wright S (1921) Correlation and causation. *Journal of Agricultural Research* 20:557–585.

Part III

ANTHROPOLOGICAL EVALUATIONS OF
PUBLIC HEALTH INITIATIVES

14

Honorable Mutilation? Changing Responses to Female Genital Cutting in Sudan

ELLEN GRUENBAUM

Maryam's Story

"I'm not afraid anymore." Freshly bathed and dressed in a pretty, blue cotton dress with gingham collar and puffed sleeves, Maryam, 10, smiled sweetly as she told me her story. When she was 8 years old, all the other girls in her village in central Sudan were having their turns being circumcised, but she was too scared. Her mother and grandmother wanted to schedule the date, but even when her best friend was about to be "purified," Maryam refused. Her father had intervened to stop the pressure, assuring everyone that it was okay not to be circumcised.

But now, Maryam had changed her mind. She wanted to be grown up like the other girls. In addition, her father was away for some weeks, working at a distant factory.

Maryam's mother had sent word to the midwife the night before, and Besaina, the midwife whose career I have followed since the 1970s, invited me along. We met at Besaina's house early in the morning. She carried her equipment box and her professional uniform—the white veil that she would change into later—and we walked along the dusty paths between the adobe houses, past the mosque, to the other side of the village. We entered a large courtyard with a small vegetable garden, a rectangular two-room house with veranda, a separate kitchen, and outbuildings for latrine and shower. We heard the cold water splashing in the shower, probably Maryam getting ready.

Maryam's mother and an aunt greeted us and ushered us into the screened veranda. Honored by my surprise appearance—offering hospitality to visitors is a source of pride in Sudan—Maryam's mother hurried to the kitchen and shook the fire back to life and sent a child on an errand to buy bread, signs of hurried preparation of a meal to follow the operation.

How different from the 1970s, I thought! In those days, a circumcision was a big family event and a group of women would have been cooking for hours to prepare for the guests.

And, how different Besaina's procedures! Many things were the same—the family's sweeping and sprinkling of the dirt floor, Besaina's thorough washing of her hands with pink carbolic soap, the waterproof cloth on the wood-framed rope bed, open shutters for good light, the bowl of boiling water to sterilize the instruments, the Dettol disinfectant, the xylocaine injection. But this time there was no crowd of visitors, and the girl was much older than the little ones Besaina had cut in the 1970s. Most significantly, Besaina was no longer performing "pharaonic" circumcisions (Figure 14.1.).

I had a chance to talk to Maryam while the family finished cleaning the room. When everything was ready, Besaina asked the mother, "How much of the clitoris do you want me to take off? The whole thing or just half?"

Maryam's mother choked back tears. I wondered if she was regretting the decision to circumcise. But the aunt who sat nearby decorating Maryam's feet with henna, explained. "She is just sad because Maryam's grandmother died a few months ago—she would have been so happy to see this day!"

"Take the whole thing," the mother said.

To my surprise, Maryam sat up with great curiosity during the short operation, trying to watch as Besaina washed, injected, waited, and then snipped with her surgical scissors. Besaina made just two stitches to close the wound, but unlike the past, she left the vaginal and urethral openings untouched, open. No crying this time.

The aunt finished putting henna on Maryam's hands to stain them beautifully—something that would not happen again until her wedding—then tied the traditional protective strings with some beads around her wrist, fluffed up her cotton pillow, and brought her a glass of a sweet red drink. Besaina packed up her things while giving aftercare instructions—give her an aspirin if needed when the anesthesia wears off, keep her in bed for a while, be sure she urinates.

Maryam's circumcised girlfriend arrived and we left them chatting amiably as we were called to the veranda, where her mother had carried in the breakfast tray.

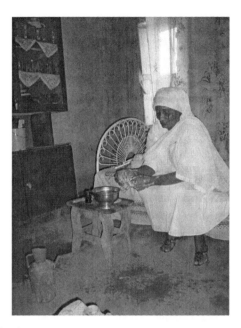

Figure 14.1. Midwife in a Gezira community preparing to perform a circumcision, wearing her white tobe as a uniform. She scrubs with carbolic soap, sterilizes instruments with disinfectant, and prepares local anesthetic for injection. The dirt floor has been sprinkled to reduce dust. Note the traditional facial scarification, no longer performed in this area. (Photo by Ellen Gruenbaum).

Female Genital Cutting and Public Health

More than 100 million women and girls worldwide have undergone some form of female genital cutting (FGC), many with far more traumatic experiences or damaging results than Maryam's.[1] The practices are usually referred to as female genital mutilation, or FGM, to emphasize its mutilation of the female genitalia. FGC/FGM practices are traditional cultural, nontherapeutic practices that often cause harm to health. Because the practices are so widespread and so shocking from international perspectives, FGC/FGM has taken a prominent place in international discourse on women's and girls' health. Variations of these practices are found in at least 28 countries of Africa, with additional cases in parts of southwest Asia and among immigrants in Europe, North America, and elsewhere. Current estimates are that about 3 million girls undergo some form of FGC each year, and additional numbers of adult women are affected by its long-term health or psychological consequences and/or recircumcision practices. Based on self-report data in Demographic and Health Surveys for several countries, prevalence appears to be declining slowly, at least in some countries (Yoder, Abderrahim, and Zhuzhuni 2004:ix–x), and incidence, severity, and attitudes are shifting, with younger generations of women being less supportive of the practices (Yoder et al. 2004:48–50). Nevertheless, rapid progress toward eradication has not occurred—with the possible exception of the areas impacted by Senegal's TOSTAN project (www.tostan.org)—despite the 3 decades of activity against FGC following the WHO's international conference on the subject in Khartoum in 1979.

Cultural Relativism or Universal Values?

As an anthropologist committed to utilizing cultural relativism—the idea that cultural practices need to be understood from within their own cultural contexts rather than examining a different culture's values only to disparage them—I can understand the importance of such rituals to the development of gender identity, as a rite of passage, as the underpinning of family honor, and even as an aesthetic preference. The exercise of cultural relativism helps us to see that it is not parents' intent to mutilate their daughters but rather to give them proper, socially expected treatment. Their intent is simply to "circumcise" or "purify."

And yet as humanists seeking to improve health and the human condition, to find ways to protect children from harm, and to participate with our fellow human beings in positive social development, anthropologists and public health advocates engage in critiques of behaviors, education against unsound beliefs, and encouragement of healthy lifestyles. Knowing the harm that can result from genital cutting and recognizing the growing international consensus that the practices need to end, anthropologists have embraced a process of strengthening human rights and improving human health while offering the cultural analyses that could make the process more culturally sensitive, effective, and less disruptive to culturally valued social institutions. Our goal is to prevent well-intentioned efforts from slipping into ethnocentric, paternalistic programs that impose a solution. Instead, we draw attention to the need for beneficiaries of programs to have the resources and opportunities they need to discuss and work on their futures.

In short, anthropologists engaged in this public health issue locate the resistance to ending the practices in their cultural embeddedness; medical anthropologists and other social scientists are then partners with grass-roots activists and policy makers, analyzing the issues to develop better strategies for change.

In this chapter, I provide an overview of this vexing public health problem and an analysis of the situation in Sudan based on my ethnographic research there over the past 30 years. My goal is to assess the effectiveness of current public health interventions by tracking some of the changes that are occurring. As I see it, both the practices themselves and their justifications are shifting. What accounts for these processes is neither a vague trend toward "modernization" nor success of public health measures. Indeed, the woefully underfunded, unevenly distributed, and sporadic public health measures— though not without some effect—cannot account for the limited progress that has occurred in the movement toward abandonment of FGC.

In essence, my research has become an ethnography of change, since the cultural rationales for continuing FGC in Sudan are not only variable in differing cultural contexts but are also in the process of evolution. Indigenous initiatives from change agents who have targeted this issue have been important, and these deserve greater attention. Also, individual midwives, religious leaders, communities, and families—responding to media, travel, education, and influential leaders—have been debating the issues, talking about FGC in new ways, and making choices about FGC, as individuals or with groups. Yet this indigenous evolution of practices and cultural rationales raises questions about the cultural and social consequences of preservation or abandonment of the practices, including unanticipated effects on social relationships and gender roles. If change is strongly pushed from the outside, it is well known that backlash can occur, and might the same thing happen with other change dynamics that are perceived to be locally inspired? Also, the question arises whether—from a public health perspective—the evolution to less harmful forms, falling short of complete abandonment of the practices, is beneficial or desirable as a positive step. In short, understanding the dynamics of change— whether it be the public health "stages of change" model that Shell-Duncan examines (2006), a loosely coordinated social movement, or some other process of social transformation—is key to improving policy and public health initiatives in the efforts against FGC.

Research Methods

My research in Sudan since the 1970s has been guided by my desire to understand the political and economic contexts of health and social phenomena, using comparative participant observation research in more than one community, supplemented by archival research and interviews with selected leaders of social movements. In the 1970s, during my 5 years of residence in Sudan as a teacher and researcher, and again during my return research visits in 1989 and 1992, I chose to focus on 2 communities with different ethnic compositions and differing situations with respect to FGC practices for short-term participant observation studies (here I will call them Wad Hassan and Garia Jadida, located in the Gezira irrigated project and the Rahad irrigated project, respectively) (Gruenbaum 1982, 1996, 2001). I stayed with families in each community, observed daily life and celebrations, participated in group discussions, and interviewed key members of each community. I attended whatever births or genital cutting rituals occurred during my visits to the villages and interviewed midwives, religious leaders, folk healers, government health care providers, and teachers. Although I sometimes used a research assistant for a few days, I relied on my own interactions in Arabic for collecting ethnographic data. In cases where Hausa and Zabarma ethnic minority women knew little Arabic, I was not able to obtain as much information directly. However, because of the long-term connections with them, I was fortunate to return more than once to visit women who had, in the intervening years, learned better Arabic, in the neighborhoods of their multiethnic village. This allowed me to fill in some of the gaps and observe changes.

The opportunity to return to Sudan for short research visits in 1989 and 1992 enabled me to make this a longitudinal ethnographic project focusing on change in FGC attitudes and practices. I stayed with the same families, interviewed a number of the same individuals, and followed the careers of the midwives I met (Gruenbaum 1996, 2001).

In 2004, I conducted additional participant observation and interviewing in both communities, and expanded the number of case study communities using short-term, intense observation and interviewing with the help of research assistants—what one might call rapid ethnography—in 5 additional rural communities. I also interviewed 20 Sudanese activists in the movement against FGC, mostly in urban settings, using open-ended interviews and participant observation in meetings and public events.

The additional 5 communities provided a broader view of the cultural contexts of Sudanese FGC. The communities were selected on the basis of the research needs of UNICEF Sudan and CARE Sudan, respectively, on the topic of FGC. Two of the 4 communities selected for the UNICEF study were in what was then Western Kordofan state and 2 were in Kassala state in the east. I worked with Sudanese research assistants to collect qualitative data through interviews, observations, conversations, and group discussions over a period of 1 week in each location. Four of the communities were chosen from among those where an on-going multi-year epidemiological research project on FGC prevalence was being conducted by Ahmed Bayoumi for UNICEF and the Sudanese government (Bayoumi 2003). Bayoumi's research design labeled approximately 10 communities as controls and 10 as intervention communities in each of the 3 states in Sudan in which UNICEF was conducting its Child Friendly Communities Initiative in cooperation with state government units. With UNICEF's FGC project director Dr. Samira Amin Ahmed, we chose 1 control—a community that had not been a target of programs to end FGC—and 1 community that had received program efforts in each state for ethnographic investigation of the community's knowledge about FGC and its complications, people's attitudes toward the practices and toward change in their cultural contexts, and their actual practices. A security crisis in South

Darfur prevented us from carrying out the planned studies there, so we completed just 4 sites.

In these 4 communities, I worked with 1 male interviewer and 1–3 female interviewers. We collected qualitative data—stories, opinions, explanations, and background information—on the topics and questions on the research outline. We used ethnographic participant observation—for example, taking notes on conversations and observation at social occasions, during visits to schools, at the market, while helping with chores, and other activities—as well as interviewing key community members and conducting group discussions. To strengthen the relevance of data for the epidemiological study, we interviewed as many of the adults as possible (usually mothers, fathers, or grandmothers) from the homes of the cohort of 5-year-old girls chosen in the Bayoumi epidemiology baseline study, focusing on their knowledge, attitudes, and practices with respect to FGC and their awareness of efforts toward change. We also interviewed key informants selected for their particular community roles.

CARE Sudan selected the seventh community I studied in Sudan in 2004. Located in North Kordofan, it had previously received intensive educational ("awareness raising") efforts in reproductive health and against FGC, including monthly programs at the school using various teaching aids (charts, anatomical models, a dramatized video) and the training of volunteers to carry out home educational visits. Working with a female Sudanese research assistant, I conducted participant observation using the earlier research outline. In addition, we investigated the events that led to a pledge by the men of the village some 2 years earlier to end FGC, as well as the aftermath of this decision.

The research in each community lasted about 1 week. All ethnographic interviews and discussions were conducted in Arabic, which was the first or second language of participants. My own notes were recorded in English, and all Arabic interview notes by assistants were verbally reported to me in English or Arabic and transcribed in English with some Arabic quotations. My study of anti-FGM movement leaders (Gruenbaum 2005) relied on interviews of feminist leaders, health personnel, NGO staff, and others, usually in urban areas. These were conducted in either Arabic or English.

Clitoridectomy, Excision, and Infibulation

The term "female genital mutilation," or FGM, has been widely used to describe various forms of what practitioners refer to in many different ways in many countries, using indigenous terms that suggest its ritual significance, such as "female circumcision" or "purification." "Mutilation" is technically accurate for most variants of the practices, since they entail damage to or removal of healthy tissues or organs, and the provocative term, as well as the realities it conveys, has stimulated great international concern and action. But since "mutilation" connotes harmful intent, some people, even those who favor stopping the practices, have been deeply offended by the term FGM.

The word commonly used for FGC in Arabic-speaking countries, *tahur* or *tahara*, means "purification," that is, the achievement of cleanliness through a ritual activity. "Female circumcision," however, echoes the term for the removal of the foreskin in the male, which has been considered nonmutilating (Toubia 1993:9)—at least until the recent movement to end that practice as well (see the work of the organization NOCIRC)—and is therefore rejected by many people, since it seems to trivialize the damage done and the huge scale of the practices. I prefer the term "Female Genital Cutting," or "FGC," which has also become well established in international discourse, particularly among social scientists. FGC avoids disparaging the practitioners, yet does not minimize the seriousness of the issue.

There are several types of cutting and removal of tissues of genitalia of young girls and women, done to conform to social expectations. The form varies not only from one sociocultural context to another but even within a single village, such as one Sudanese village of my research, where different ethnic groups do different types of cutting. Forms vary between families, too, with some preferring their ethnic group's traditional forms while other families seek less harmful forms. Also, trained midwives and other practitioners (including traditional birth attendants, other older women, barbers, and even medical doctors in varying country contexts) have their own individual techniques of doing the procedures, resulting in varying amounts of tissue taken and various levels of hygiene. (In most countries, medical doctors are now strongly discouraged or forbidden by their professional organizations and governments from doing any form of FGC, but the degree of enforcement is unclear.)

In some cultural contexts, it is very young children who are cut, including infants or toddlers (Toubia 1993, 1994). Anne Jennings reported southern Egyptian girls undergoing genital cutting at age 1 or 2 (1995:48), and I encountered some Hadendawa in eastern Sudan who claim to do it in the first weeks or months of a girl's life. In Sudan, it is most commonly done between the ages of 4 and 8, but in some cultural contexts (e.g., the Maasai of East Africa), cutting is delayed until a young woman is in her teens and is about to be married (14–15 years or even older).

The World Health Organization developed a comprehensive typology that technical experts use for the different types (for description and illustrations, see Toubia 1999:15–19). People who practice FGC have their own terms for different types in their many languages, of course, which may or may not fit well with the World Heath Organization's 4 types. Researchers can, however, place the range of the practices into the following categories (Figure 14.2).

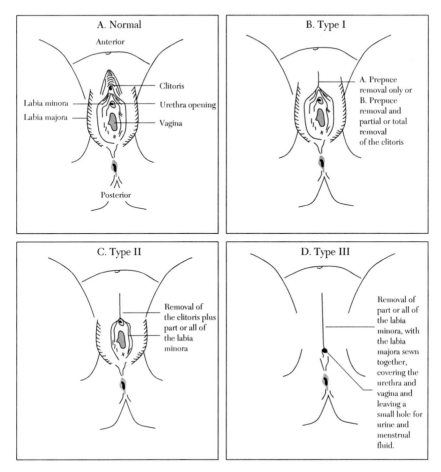

Figure 14.2. (A) Normal Vulva; (B) WHO Type I, Clitoridectomy; (C) WHO Type II, Excision; (D) WHO Type III, Infibulation.

Clitoridectomy

The World Health Organization's Type I includes both the least severe form of the operations, the cutting away of part or all of the clitoral prepuce, or hood, and also forms that cut away part or all of the external (protruding) portion of the clitoris, called clitoridectomy. The removal of the prepuce only is analogous to the foreskin removal of male circumcision, and it is evidently fairly rare, but the removal of a large part of the external clitoris is fairly common. Since erectile tissue of the clitoris normally extends well below the surface, it is inaccurate to say that the entire clitoris can be removed.

Clitoridectomy, whether partial or more radical, is often referred to by Muslims and others as *tahur as-sunna* (Arabic for "*sunna* circumcision" or "*sunna* purification"). *Sunna* means "in the tradition of the Prophet Mohamed," and it is a cognate of the word for the branch of Islam known as Sunni. "*Sunna* circumcision" is a controversial term in Sudan because of disputed associations with religion (discussed subsequently). But it is precisely because of the positive association between "*sunna*" and Muslim religious values that the term has been popularly applied to a wide variety of forms. Reformers seek to ban "*sunna* circumcision" as a descriptive term, and I use it here only as part of the folk terminology used by my interviewees.

Excision

The World Health Organization's Type II is called "excision." In this type, the cutting goes further than clitoridectomy to include removal of the prepuce, the entire external clitoris, and partial or total excision of the labia minora (the smaller inner lips of the vaginal opening). In Sudan this form is also usually labeled with the controversial term "*sunna*," even though it is more damaging than what some people mean by "*sunna*." In common parlance, there are just two basic folk terms—*sunna* and pharaonic circumcision—and they use the "*sunna*" terminology for both clitoridectomy and excision. (In fact, this controversial term, discussed subsequently, is often applied to any circumcisions that are not "pharaonic.") Imprecise terms (such as *nuss* for "half") are also used for some of the in-between forms that would be included in Type II.

Infibulation and Reinfibulation

The most severe cutting occurs with Type III, or infibulation. It is the main type in Sudan, where it is commonly called "pharaonic circumcision," a term reflecting its purported origins in the ancient Nile Valley at the time of the pharaohs. In Egypt, where infibulation is rare today, it is called "Sudanese circumcision." In this type, part or all of the external genitalia—prepuce, clitoris, labia minora, and all or part of the labia majora—are removed and the raw edges on opposite sides are infibulated, that is, held together by stitching, binding, or using thorns until the joined edges are sealed with scar tissue. When healed, infibulation leaves a perfectly smooth vulva of skin and scar tissue with only a single tiny opening for urination and menstrual flow, preserved during healing by the insertion of a small object such as a piece of straw. In a variation of infibulation that is slightly less severe, the trimmed labia minora are sewn shut but the labia majora are left alone. In either case, it is essential that a midwife be present for childbirth to make an incision in the tissue to allow the baby to be born. The new mother is then reinfibulated by the midwife, a practice that is repeated after each pregnancy. The new mother often asks the midwife to make the opening very small, "like a virgin," to enhance her husband's sexual pleasure. This is analogous to, although more severe than, what some North American obstetricians have done when they take an extra stitch, called "the husband's stitch," when closing an episiotomy, for the purpose of restoring tightness to the opening.

Other Variations of FGC

WHO labels any other nontherapeutic or cultural alterations to the female genitalia that do not include tissue removal as Type IV. This category includes practices such as pricking, piercing, incision, stretching of the clitoris or labia, cauterization, cuts or scrapes on the genitalia, or the use of harmful substances in the vagina. Labia stretching to pursue culturally preferred aesthetics of the body is not particularly harmful, but other variations can be painful or damaging. In some East African countries, to satisfy some men's preference for "dry sex," women or men introduce dangerous or painful astringents into the vagina to dry it out before intercourse, which is included in Type IV. In Europe and North America, the fad of labia or clitoris piercing among some young people, as well as cosmetic reduction of labia through plastic surgery, could be included as a Type IV practice.

FGC as It Is Practiced in Sudan

The most common Sudanese form of FGC is the World Health Organization's Type III, consisting of the removal of the prepuce, clitoris, labia minora, and most of the labia majora, followed by infibulation of the labia across the urethral and vaginal openings, leaving a single tiny opening for urination and future menstrual flow. Usually performed before girls reach the age of 7, the result, once healed, is a smooth surface of skin and scar tissue that later presents a barrier to intercourse, which many people hope will help prevent premarital sex and pregnancy. At the time of marriage and first intercourse, the opening must be stretched, torn, or surgically opened.

Although there are no accurate data on the types of cutting practiced (since self-report is inadequate and clinical examinations impractical), the consensus among activists and health care providers today is that a growing proportion of people in Sudan have begun to practice a less severe form of cutting, the World Health Organization's Type I or II, removing all or part of the prepuce and external clitoris but avoiding infibulation. Another proportion of families has abandoned the practices entirely, particularly among the urban, educated classes. The percentage of women 15 and older in the northern two-thirds of the country who had some type of FGC was reported at 89% in the period from 1989 to 1990 (Yoder et al. 2004:26). According to preliminary unpublished results of a survey for UNICEF Sudan, there appears to be a recent substantial drop in prevalence (Ahmed 2007); such information should be published on the Internet when completed, at www.unicef.org/infobycountry.

Harmful Effects

Predictably, such cutting practices, regardless of type, can be expected to have harmful health effects, particularly when performed in unhygienic circumstances. These effects include the immediate risks for girls at the time of cutting and later complications with first intercourse, birth, sexual function, physical sequelae, and psychological effects (see Toubia 1994, 1999).

The immediate complications documented include cases of excess bleeding (hemorrhage), infections, blood poisoning (septicemia), retention of urine, or shock. Such complications can be life threatening. Later on, the infibulated state sometimes results in retention of menses (if the vagina is blocked by scar tissue), difficulty in urination (if there is excess scar tissue around or over the urethra), and a high incidence of urinary tract and chronic pelvic infections. At first intercourse, the extremely small size of the opening created by infibulation presents a barrier, which can make first sexual intercourse difficult, painful, or impossible. Often the scar tissue around the opening must be painfully ruptured or is cut by the husband, a midwife, or a doctor.

Obstetrical complications have included problems with the inelastic scar tissue of infibulation, which of course must be cut by the birth attendant at the right time so labor will not be obstructed. Not only is obstructed labor dangerous to the baby but the mother's internal tissues can also be damaged, creating a fistula (opening in the tissue separating the vagina from the urinary bladder), which can result in an embarrassing condition with constantly leaking urine (Gruenbaum 2001; Shell-Duncan and Hernlund 2000; Toubia 1994). While early pregnancy may be the primary cause of the high rate of fistula problems in Africa, infibulation may be a contributing factor. Also, prolonged second stage of labor may be related to other adverse obstetric outcomes (WHO Study Group 2006).

While it seemed unlikely that the lesser forms of FGC would cause obstetrical complications, the WHO-sponsored prospective study of 28,393 women studied during singleton deliveries at 28 obstetric centers between November 2001 and March 2003 in 6 African countries (Burkina Faso, Ghana, Kenya, Nigeria, Senegal, and Sudan) determined that Types I, II, and III (based on clinical examination) all correlated with increased rates of adverse obstetric outcomes (WHO Study Group 2006). Predictably, Type III, infibulation, was associated with the greatest increased risks. As compared with women without FGC, 31% more women with FGC III required caesarean sections and there were 69% more cases of postpartum hemorrhage, 98% more cases requiring longer hospital stays than uncircumcised women, 66% more infant resuscitations, and 55% more stillbirths or early neonatal in-patient deaths. Researchers estimated that FGC leads to "an extra one or two perinatal deaths per 100 deliveries" (WHO Study Group 2006:1835), and they concluded that all forms of FGC create increased risk of adverse obstetric outcomes.

The psychological effects of FGC practices are less well understood, not systematically researched, and no doubt differ a great deal from one cultural context or individual situation to another. In some situations, girls are circumcised in groups in celebratory circumstances, allowing moral support for a shared experience. In other cases, girls may experience their FGC as a surprising and forced violation. Where it is performed on individual girls in a family context, there may be significant pride and celebration involved, leading to fond memories of the day. In other cases, a girl may have no memory of the act, as she was an infant. Nevertheless, there is anecdotal evidence of adverse psychological effects, which merits further research.

Sensitivity to the feelings of already circumcised women is important for medical practitioners, public health educators, and counselors. Professionals and activists should be sensitive to the feelings of circumcised women so that, in the course of changing social attitudes to view "mutilation" as no longer acceptable, they do not stigmatize circumcised women or add to their psychological difficulties. Similarly, those who have done circumcisions or allowed circumcisions to be done to their daughters under cultural imperatives that define it as good, can be expected to have complex feelings to deal with as the social convention shifts away from the practices.

Damage to sexual responsiveness is reported for many women, yet there are also data suggesting that the frequency and extent of problems vary greatly. Women do not necessarily lose sexual interest, and even those with extensive tissue removal, such as those who are infibulated, can retain the ability to achieve sexual satisfaction and orgasms (Gruenbaum 2001, 2005, 2006; Lightfoot-Klein 1989). Sexual responsiveness could be affected differently depending on the location and extent of tissue damage, whether the surrounding or underlying tissues retain sensitivity, whether there is severe infibulation, and of course whether the emotional attachment of the partners is strong and the relationship loving and supportive. Some midwives have been careful to avoid cutting too much of the sensitive tissue (clitoris and erectile tissue) hoping to preserve sensitivity, but still make the result look like an infibulation by joining the labia across the opening. In short, it is erroneous to assume that all women who have been cut lose their sexual responsiveness. Similarly, although many experience very harmful medical consequences, many do not.

But Why?

That loving parents can allow their daughters to be held down and cut, often causing fear, pain, and possible major immediate or long-term damage to health and physical functions, seems shocking, especially when it is very young girls who are surprised and frightened by their powerlessness against a violent act at the hands of those they trust. In the discourse of the West and North, it is often argued that the prevalence of these customs is intended to punish or suppress women by depriving them of their sexuality, that it is an outgrowth of patriarchal male dominance, or that the fault lies with one or more particular religions, patriarchy, or "blind tradition." But as I have argued more extensively elsewhere (Gruenbaum 2001), FGC defies reductionist explanations that neglect the tremendous cultural diversity of rationales and practices.

People believe FGC practices to be right, necessary, sexually appropriate, or spiritually and ritually purifying if their cultural traditions have given them these perspectives. Often, their beliefs and practices are reinforced by the idea (whether well-founded or not) that it is their religion (whatever it may be) which requires it, that their health will be improved, that a future husband will prefer it, or that their family's honor will be enhanced by assuring that their daughters are properly circumcised (and virgins) at marriage. Gender identity is often involved, making one a true woman or constituting a rite of passage to a marriageable status. One's ethnic identity, too, may be marked by a particular type of circumcision operation or ritual.

Although many cultures believe the girl's sexual impulses and other behavior will be better controlled following circumcision, I have found that people are not seeking to destroy sexuality, but to tame it. While it is painful, people say that creating pain is not the reason for it, but a consequence—are there not other painful experiences that women go through to be wives and mothers? Even in cultures where virginity is not strongly valued at marriage, propriety is, and circumcision is often part of its definition.

Religion

The practice of FGC is not commanded in the sacred texts or dominant interpretations of any of the major religions of the world (see Gruenbaum 2001 for a fuller discussion of the religious issues). Nevertheless, the practices are found in many countries and among people of widely different ethnic groups and religions, including Judaism, Christianity, Islam, and traditional African religions. Yet, people who follow circumcision traditions often do associate the practices with their own religious beliefs, whether their theologians would agree or not.

For example, although many learned Islamic teachers and scholars have declared that infibulation has no place in Islam, and some say that no form whatsoever should be permitted, other Islamic teachers consider female circumcision as an "ennobling" act that is very proper for Muslims, so long as they don't go beyond clitoridectomy, which (unfortunately) is commonly called "*sunna* circumcision" in the Sudanese folk taxonomy. It is unfortunate because it suggests a tie to Islam.

The lack of agreement about Islamic rules can be traced to the differing sources of authority in Islam. Muslims believe the Holy Qur'an to be God's direct revelation and the chief source of guidance for righteous living. The Qur'an is silent on the subject of female circumcision. But Muslims also respect the sayings and actions attributed to the Prophet Mohammed during his lifetime (570–622 C.E.) as a secondary source of guidance, handed down through oral tradition and the writings known as the *Hadith*. Which stories and quotations offer the most reliable versions of the Prophet's advice is a matter of disagreement among Muslims, as is the interpretation of them. Many Muslims have concluded that the Prophet Mohammed's oft-quoted but somewhat ambiguous and nonspecific pronouncement on the subject of female circumcision—"Reduce but do not destroy"—means that only the less severe cutting of the female genitalia is acceptable, though not required. Others believe the Prophet thereby advocated doing some form, making it either an obligation (a *sunna*, or tradition of the Prophet) or at least a blessing to do it. Or perhaps, some think, he was saying only that you can do it if it is your custom, but it is really unnecessary.

It appears that a growing consensus of Islamic leaders supports the idea that Muslims should avoid female circumcision completely, since it is not mentioned in the Qur'an as a duty of the faithful and the handed-down sayings may be inaccurate, "weak Hadith." Since using the term *sunna* seems to imply that it is expected of Muslims, some reformers are leery of it; while the term may help convince Muslims to give up infibulation, it may reinforce their continuing clitoridectomy. No doubt there will be many lively discussions among Muslim scholars about this in the coming years!

All 7 communities of my long-term and recent studies in Sudan are comprised of Muslims of varying sectarian affiliations. Their views on FGC have become increasingly diverse, yet all of them hope to find justification in their Islamic faith for their cultural practices. During the 1970s, despite a religious and medical proclamation facilitated by British colonial powers in the 1940s which led to the outlawing of the most severe "pharaonic circumcision" in Sudan in 1946, religious leaders in Wad Hassan and Garia Jadida, like their counterparts throughout the Muslim north, ignored the pamphlet, the *fatwa*, and the law, not viewing this as a matter for religious debate but rather a custom of Muslim women. In the 1970s, people told me they believed FGC (whether pharaonic or "*sunna*") was permitted and even encouraged by Islam as "ennobling" and protecting honor. However, at that time the ethnic minority groups in Wad Hassan and Garia Jadida (Hausa and Zabarma, respectively, both of West African origin) though pious practitioners of Islam, did not consider infibulation Islamic and either did not practice FGC or chose to do only the most minimal cutting possible.

Subsequently, as a result of influence from economic migration of a significant number of educated people from Wad Hassan to the oil-rich Arab countries, many of the younger generation began to realize that not all Muslims practiced FGC and that in fact the residents of the holy places of Saudi Arabia considered FGC a pre-Islamic African holdover that Sudanese ought not do. Following greater attention to these religious aspects, the discourse in Wad Hassan, particularly as articulated by some of the school teachers and the trained midwife, whose son had worked in Saudi Arabia and sponsored her to make the pilgrimage to Mecca, began to shift during my research trips in 1989 and 1992 to a position favoring only the lesser forms of Type I or II, what they called "*sunna.*" Although a few girls had escaped infibulation by 1992, as I have been able to reconstruct events from the 2004 interviews, there was a fairly clear shift in convention in about 1994, and all of the girls circumcised since then have (reportedly) not been infibulated. My interviews and discussions found both religious and health reasons as explanations for the change.

The same has not been the case in the other village of long-term study, Garia Jadida. In an area with fewer schools in the past and therefore less outward migration and less access to urban influences, television, etc., the ideas about FGC not being Islamic have only recently begun to be discussed. Unfortunately, the minority group that did not consider FGC to be Islamic (the Zabarma) and did either nothing or Type I in the past, have adopted FGC (Type I or II) under social pressure for a degree of conformity with the higher status ethnic group. So for them, change has gone in the wrong direction over the past decade. (A similar expansion of FGC to groups that did not formerly practice it has been reported for some of the ethnic groups of Southern Sudan who became internal refugees in the national capital Khartoum during the civil war that lasted until 2004.) The discussions about religious appropriateness do not seem to have gained much influence among either ethnic group in the community. Instead, some of those I interviewed are beginning to think about change based on the rumor of future legal sanctions on midwives who violate the new professional ban on all forms of FGC.

In the other 5 communities, people also have considered FGC to be permitted by Islam. In the 2 communities in West Kordofan (Tuwaifra and Wad Shaefoun), religious and secular leaders have now declared themselves against pharaonic circumcision (Type III), based on exposure to discussions with Sudanese activists. Tuwaifra has not completely shifted, and many of those we held discussions with were unconvinced, but articulate and active leaders are working to change that through women's literacy classes, youth theater, and local development committees. In the case of Wad Shaefoun, the religious leader and the midwife said that for the past decade they both had been opposed personally to all forms, for religious and health reasons, respectively, but that the people so strongly supported FGC for cultural reasons that they felt it was difficult to convince people—the religious *shaykh* said he felt he was "standing alone" in his religious view, based on his understanding of the teachings of the Qur'an, that no form of FGC should be done. The midwife and the religious *shaykh*, however, had managed to convince many people to move in the direction of modification to Type I or II (they called it "*sunna*") in the last decade. But in the past few years, they have received a group of student activists and a religious leader who influenced local discussions. The activist religious leader met with the senior religious council of the community and discussed passages of the Qur'an and several documents of religious interpretation. As the group studied and pondered these, they came to the conclusion that they should ban all forms of FGC. Gratified, the local *shaykh* announced the council's decision as a new policy in the name of Islam for the entire community. In our interviews and discussions there in 2004, we found that many families were still not fully convinced, adopting a wait-and-see attitude. Typical was one man's view, "I don't want to be alone. If others decide to stop, then we will, too." Still, despite the lack of a clear, firm resolve to end it, the midwife reported that no circumcision of girls had been performed in 2 years.

Another example of the role of religious leadership comes from the town of Wad Sharifae in Kassala State, a large community in eastern Sudan with a large number of Beni Amer and migrants from Eritrea as well as several minority ethnic groups. Several local men who had spent some years as labor migrants in Saudi Arabia became involved in the more conservative Wahhabist Islam of that region and affiliated with a sect called the *Ansar Sunna* that receives funds from wealthy Saudi patrons. When they returned to Sudan, followers of the movement promoted several extreme practices not found among most Sudanese Muslims, including the seclusion and chaperoning of women, face veils for women, and headscarves for even very young schoolgirls. They also ban music and pictorial representations on walls. While strongly supporting basic education for girls, the sect also discourages outside higher education for young women and limits women's participation in the work force except for teaching and local missionary work. Women I interviewed, who graduated from their schools, enthusiastically embrace these practices. Others seemed less enthusiastic, but accepting.

The Beni Amer ethnic group, from which many of the *Ansar Sunna* adherents are drawn, traditionally practiced pharaonic circumcision and considered it a prerequisite for marriage. The *Ansar Sunna* religious leaders, however, now argue that pharaonic circumcision is wrong and Muslims should do the Type I or Type II "*sunna*." At the same time, workshops being held in the village by nongovernmental and government-sponsored groups working to end FGC—the "interventions" being tested in the Bayoumi epidemiological study—have given a clear message that all forms of FGC should be stopped.

Parents of young girls are thus caught in the middle of a swirling ideological controversy—shall they do what the government (through these workshops) advocates, to prevent being criminals and avoid the possible harmful health consequences? Or will that leave their daughters unmarriageable in the ethnic group, with all the stigma and poverty that might entail? Should they infibulate their daughters and risk the religious sect's condemnation for not doing the *"sunna"* form? Or should they do the *"sunna"* and risk both governmental censure and unmarriageability?

As one Beni Amer, *Ansar Sunna* mother caught in this dilemma told me, "I want to do the right thing, but I don't know what that is. I wish I didn't have daughters, because I am worried about them."

Marriage, Morality, and Infibulation

Although ideological supports such as religion and ethnic identity promote continuation of these practices, the most fundamental and emotionally charged foundation for FGC in Sudan is morality, honor, and the marriageability of daughters.

Marriage is important not only because of its cultural value and religious aspects but also because it is vital to women's economic and social well-being. In a society where the family and one's offspring constitute the source of status and economic living as well as one's social security system during illness, misfortune and old age, marriage is essential. Without marriage, a young Muslim woman's life is considered wasted and pitiful, while marriage and children provide for economic security, social standing, and the fulfillment of religious expectations.

Where marriageability is tied to FGC—as is especially the case in infibulating cultures where the community knowledge of a girl's ritual "purification" along with the intact scar across the opening constitute proof of virginity—the cultural complex supporting the practices is often profoundly reinforced by emotional, moral, and aesthetic values that create major obstacles to change.

FGC protected virginity, it was believed, by reducing a girl's interest in sex with clitoridectomy and by creating a barrier to illicit penetration with the scar of infibulation. For Sudanese Muslims, protecting virginity is vital to maintaining family honor and a daughter's marriageability. Pharaonic circumcision created the smooth, tight opening that husbands expected for their sexual pleasure. As the norm, the smooth vulva was aesthetically pleasing and protruding parts were considered masculine or ugly, and people feared they could grow larger if not cut back. Also, FGC was believed to be good for health, keeping the area clean and preventing some specific folk illnesses.

Family honor is at stake in the preservation of virginity and the daughter's marriageability. When marriageability is defined by virginity, and virginity is defined by infibulation, then the alternative—no circumcision and no socially defined confidence in virginity—is profoundly shameful.

In my interviews in all 7 communities, people consistently referred to "shame" as a reason for their reluctance to change their FGC practices. For example, in the North Kordofan community of Kubur Abdal Hameed, where a large number of men and unmarried youths had pledged 2 years before to discontinue FGC in their community, I found that many local women could not countenance its total abandonment. The women, like their mothers and grandmothers before them, believed FGC to be moral, clean, Islamic, and aesthetically pleasing.

In 1 group discussion with women in Kubur Abdal Hameed, I asked how they felt about FGC and the men's earlier pledge to end circumcision. Several women acknowledged that FGC is painful and can cause complications, but they saw this as just one of the many challenges of being a woman. For them, no amount of suffering would be worse than the shame that would result from one's daughter's morality being questioned or her being tempted to have sex before marriage. If a groom were to find his wife not a virgin, he would be within his rights to divorce her on the spot, leaving her virtually unmarriageable. Thus, FGC continued to be valued by these women for its protection of honor and marriageability. In addition, they said, it plays a role in pleasing husbands sexually because of the narrowed vaginal opening (Gruenbaum 2006).

Many, if not most, of the women of the community still hold to these beliefs and values, but they are also aware of the movement for change, especially since it has been embraced by many of the male and some of the female community leaders. The result is a situation of contradictions, where even women who now voice their opposition to FGC also talk about why it is, or has been, good. In a single discussion, women might slip into talking about FGC in a comfortable way, explaining its benefits, extolling it as a good practice. Then, within the same conversation they might switch and say, "But that was in the past. Now we have stopped it."

In other cases, women mentioned their intentions to circumcise their daughters, even in the presence of others who were denying that circumcisions took place anymore. "We do the *sunna*," several women in a group discussion agreed. Since the term "*sunna*" has been used primarily for lesser types such as clitoridectomy or partial clitoridectomy, which do not occlude the vaginal or urethral opening, I sought clarification and asked what they meant by it. "We do it so she won't be open like that door." "We do it covered a little." "We don't want the girl to be dirty, open, with smelly underwear." They wanted to prevent the sound of urine passing and the little hole in the sand the stream produces, so they just "take the clitoris and close a little, over the urethra, and that's *sunna*." Clearly, this so-called "*sunna*" is closer to Type III than Type I or II!

While their current cutting may be less severe than the previous type of pharaonic circumcision, it is still infibulation, Type III, if they "close a little."

But by labeling it "*sunna*" they seem to believe they are avoiding the sinful or forbidden ("*haram*") form, pharaonic circumcision, and bringing the modified practice under the tent of the Prophet Mohamed's "traditions." This group, like most of the women I discussed this with in rural Sudan, continued to assume that "*sunna*" circumcision, variously done, was good and permitted in Islam.

It was clear from our participant observation in this community over the next few days that many of the women were resistant to the idea of change while others had been convinced that they should give it up. The convinced women were persuaded both by religious arguments and medical arguments, with their own painful memories to reinforce their changed attitudes. But those who were opposed to or reluctant about change feared the possible moral and sexual consequences of being uninfibulated and grounded these in powerful emotions and ideas about shame and ugliness. Their lifelong experience of the fear of sexual impropriety, risks to honor and marriageability, and derogatory regard for uncircumcised women continue to hold many of them back from embracing change.

Ethnography of Change

All but 1 of the 7 communities I studied seem to be in the process of change, although most have not been recipients of any extensive targeted programs of public health education. Change has occurred in a gradual and irreversible process for Wad Hassan, while, from a health and human rights perspective, change has moved in the wrong direction in Garia Jadida. Yet even in Garia Jadida, the tenor of discussions and the change in the senior midwife's intentions suggest that people are softening toward modification at least.

Understanding what creates cultural change is vital to future public health education interventions and requires further research (see also Abusharaf 2006). Where female circumcision rituals are an important rite of passage, there have been some successes with alternative rituals that do not involve cutting, such as the Maendeleo Ya Wanawake Organization's "Circumcision Without Cutting" in Kenya (Abusharaf 2006), but alternatives have also been opposed for fear they perpetuate the desire for FGC (see Catania and Hussen 2005). The experiences of the highly successful Senegalese organization known as TOSTAN (which means "breakthrough" in Wolof, see www.tostan.org) suggest that public declarations against FGC made by whole communities are the keys to successful abandonment, but these need to be done in the context of a commitment to broader community development efforts that the community selects—a new school, a literacy program, or other desired change. While not framed as a reward for FGC abandonment, there may be an element of that, as the agendas for change in most of rural Africa put peace, economic development, health (clean water supply, clinics), and schools at the top of their lists. The concerns of the community of the single case of an abandonment pledge in my Sudanese research suggests that other sorts of rewards were exactly what the community expected. Abandonment, clearly, was not its own reward.

Pledges are expected to be successful because they allow people to overcome their fears of shame or lack of marriageability for their daughters—if everyone promises to stop, then no one needs to take the risk of being the first or the only ones to make the change (Mackie 1996). And yet, before a community can be ready to make such a pledge, a process of persuasion needs to take place. Thus, interventions that emphasize health information, religious instruction, and human rights ideas must be accompanied by facilitation of community dialogue, where people can hear their leaders and neighbors voicing opinions. People need to know how others in their social worlds are reacting to the new messages. The message techniques being used in various countries of Africa include TV advertisements, music videos, radio and television programming, posters, roving theater groups, and programs of sponsored community meetings for education and discussion; ideally all should pose quandaries or questions that stimulate people to talk to each other in conversations, just as those who have television access love to talk about the dilemmas of the soap opera characters.

Not all communities or segments of communities are equally well placed to receive these social influences as can be seen from my assessment of the 7 communities I studied. But documenting the process of changing cultural values and practices could help in the successful design of interventions.

Harm Reduction or Human Rights?

In Sudan, many of those willing to begin to change their FGC practices do not want to go all the way to abandonment, but only to a modification to a less harmful form. There can be no doubt that stopping infibulation (Type III), even if partial clitoral removal or fuller excision (Type I or II) were to continue, would be beneficial from a harm reduction orientation (see Shell-Duncan 2001). Certainly, maternal mortality and morbidity as well as neonatal outcomes could be expected to decline for women protected from infibulation. Trends in the direction of less severe forms should be welcomed.

Yet as a matter of policy, public health advocates must consider the human rights impact of their approaches. Ending FGC is not only about improving health outcomes. It is also about protecting the human rights of girls and women: preserving their rights to bodily integrity and preventing harmful violence to them.

Human rights protections have commonly been conceived as protections against oppressive governments' use of torture or other forceful suppression of civil and political rights. But in the last 3 decades the human rights discourse has increasingly been addressed to the urgent concerns of women and children, even if it is not the state itself that is the agent of discriminatory and harmful treatment. Instead, several international agreements hold governments accountable if they fail to protect their female and minor residents from sociocultural conditions that are oppressive to them and deprive them of their rights; these agreements include the 1979 United Nations Convention on the Elimination of All Forms of Discrimination Against Women (known as CEDAW), the 1994 U.N. Declaration on the Elimination of Violence Against Women, and others. Adult women are able to exercise a greater degree of agency in determining what happens to their bodies than are children, so it is salutary that these international agreements are especially clear about the need to protect children and that cultural and religious arguments should not be permitted to interfere. Particularly noteworthy is the section on "the girl child" in the program of action from the 1994 United Nations International Conference on Population and Development (held in Cairo, Egypt): "Governments are urged to prohibit female genital mutilation wherever it exists and to give vigorous support to efforts among non-governmental and community organizations and religious institutions to eliminate such practices" (United Nations 1994: B.4.22:29).

Sudanese activists have discussed this issue extensively in recent years, concluding that despite the possibility that modification to a lesser form would have short-term benefits to public health, the abandonment of all forms is the only meaningful goal. They argue that even if there were only the most minor negative health effects associated with a mild form of genital cutting, anything short of complete abandonment of all forms would be to allow continued violation of the rights of girls. Having any sort of justification—religious, cultural, or social—for any form creates a slippery slope that might allow supporters of FGC to preserve, unsupervised, whatever form they choose, in the privacy of their homes. The only reasonable way to prevent this is to ban all forms.

The evidence from my interviews that terminologies for the mild and severe forms are inconsistently used supports this position, since there are some people willing to use the term *"sunna"* for even Type III operations. A policy that allowed for or encouraged "modification" only could result in just a change in nomenclature rather than substance. That would be a Pyrrhic victory indeed, serving neither human rights nor health.

Conclusion

My anthropological research on the cultural contexts of FGC in Sudan, conducted over a 30-year period and with additional comparisons in 7 rural communities in Sudan in 2004, points to the tenacity of this harmful traditional practice. Yet the long-term efforts of both indigenous and international activism, first for modification to a lesser form to reduce the harmful health effects, then later for complete abandonment of the practices to also protect human rights, have begun to show progress, with evidence of somewhat lower prevalence in UNICEF and other UN statistics.

My ethnographic findings suggest that FGC, though still deeply embedded in important cultural values like morality, identity, and aesthetics, is in the process of change as people seek to improve their health and their religious observances and as they become more aware of alternatives and more confident about the possibility of change. Strong countervailing social pressures are preserving the practices, including peer pressure among girls and the desire to conform to practices of higher status groups, and these contribute to the spread of FGC in some contexts. Deep cultural values associated with gender identity, honor, shame, and morality create visceral, emotional responses rejecting ideas of change. Thus, the ethnographic landscape includes a gamut of responses to the movement to end FGC: undesirable, negative directions of change; strong preservation of traditions and resistance to change; contemplation of change without action; gradual change; and rapid change.

In my assessment, it will take a multipronged approach—one that includes health education, religious leadership, cultural leaders, media, and the arts—to accelerate change. These efforts should be embedded in an awareness of the long agenda of needs of the rural poor. Improving girls' lives and well-being requires more than just the preservation of their intact genitals, of course.

Anthropologists and public health advocates have important roles to play in helping assure a culturally sensitive yet effective process of engaging people in change, one that acknowledges the breadth of their self-defined needs and that works to ameliorate their poverty along with protecting their health. In the time-scale of public health projects—with the need to evaluate outcomes and demonstrate results—there is often an urgency that precludes in-depth evaluation of the process of behavior change in favor of rapidly scaling up and replicating the solution, rather like a social "vaccination campaign." Yet long-term anthropological engagement that documents and tracks change efforts that emerge indigenously from the grass-roots level and in concert with larger social movements for health and human rights is also important, particularly for health-related behaviors that are deeply embedded and passionately defended.

Acknowledgments

My research in Sudan in 2004 was funded by California State University, Fresno, and I am grateful for research affiliation with the Institute of Women, Gender, and Development Studies at Ahfad University for Women, Omduran, Sudan. I am also grateful to UNICEF Sudan and CARE Sudan for allowing me to use information gained from my research consultancies with these organizations in 2004. All findings, interpretations, and opinions expressed are my own and do not represent those of any organization. Special thanks for their advice and facilitation go to Sudanese anthropological colleagues Samira Amin Ahmed, Samia El Nagar, and Balghis Badri. Thanks also to Nahid Toubia. I am grateful for research assistance from Lena El Sheikh, Mohamed Omer Abdal Magied, Asma Tiya, Samia Abdalla Mohamed, and Affaf Osman Mohamed. Portions of this chapter were presented at the Sudan Studies Association (August 2005) and the Society for Applied Anthropology (April 2004). Thanks to Rebecca Allen and Merrily McCarthy for assistance with drawings.

Note

1. For more on health consequences, cultural contexts, and efforts at change, see also Abusharaf 2006; Boddy 2007; El Dareer 1982; Gruenbaum 2001; Shell-Duncan and Hernlund 2000; Toubia 1994, 1999; WHO Study Group 2006.

References

Abusharaf RM, ed. (2006) *Female Circumcision: Multicultural Perspectives.* Philadelphia, PA: University of Pennsylvania Press.

Ahmed S (2007) Sudan Country Update, presented at UNICEF Task Force Global Meeting on the Research on the Social Dynamics of Abandonment of Harmful Practices, Addis Ababa and Afar, Ethiopia, March 19–23, 2007.

Bayoumi A (2003) *Baseline Survey on FGM Prevalence and Cohort Assembly in Child Friendly Community Initiative, Three Focus States.* Khartoum: UNICEF Sudan.

Boddy J (2007) *Civilizing Women: British Crusades in Colonial Sudan.* Princeton, NJ: Princeton University Press.

Catania L, Hussen AO (2005) *Ferite per Sempre (Damaged Forever).* Rome, Italy: DeriveApprodi.

El Dareer A (1982) *Woman, Why Do You Weep? Circumcision and Its Consequences.* London: Zed Press.

Gruenbaum E (1982) The movement against clitoridectomy and infibulation in Sudan. *Medical Anthropology Newsletter* 13(2):4–12.

Gruenbaum E (1996) The cultural debate over female circumcision: The Sudanese are arguing this one out for themselves. *Medical Anthropology Quarterly* 10(4):455–475.

Gruenbaum E (2001) *The Female Circumcision Controversy: An Anthropological Perspective.* Philadelphia, PA: University of Pennsylvania Press.

Gruenbaum E (2005) Feminist activism for the abolition of female genital cutting in Sudan. *Journal of Middle East Women's Studies* 1(2):89–111.

Gruenbaum E (2006) Sexuality issues in the movement to abolish female genital cutting in Sudan. *Medical Anthropology Quarterly* 20(1):121–138.

Jennings A (1995) *The Nubians of West Aswan: Village Women in the Midst of Change.* Boulder, CO: Lynne Rienner.

Lightfoot-Klein H (1989) *Prisoners of Ritual: An Odyssey into Female Genital Circumcision in Africa.* New York: Harrington Park Press.

Mackie G (1996) Ending footbinding and infibulation. *American Sociological Review* 61:991–1017.

Shell-Duncan B (2001) The medicalization of female "circumcision": Harm reduction or promotion of a dangerous practice? *Social Science and Medicine* 52:1013–1028.

Shell-Duncan B (2006) Are there "stages of change" in the practice of female genital cutting? Qualitative research findings from Senegal and the Gambia. *African Journal of Reproductive Health* 10(2):58–71.

Shell-Duncan B, Hernlund Y, eds. (2000) *Female "Circumcision" in Africa: Culture, Controversy, and Change.* Boulder, CO: Lynne Rienner.

Toubia N (1993) *Female Genital Mutilation: A Call for Global Action.* New York: Women, Ink.

Toubia N (1994) Female circumcision as a public health issue. *New England Journal of Medicine* 331(11):712–716.

Toubia N (1999) *Caring for Women with Circumcision: A Technical Manual for Health Care Providers.* New York: Rainbo.

United Nations (1994) *Programme of Action, Report of the International Conference on Population and Development.* Cairo, Egypt. 5–13 September.

WHO Study Group on Female Genital Mutilation and Obstetric Outcome (2006) Female genital mutilation and obstetric outcome: WHO collaborative prospective study in six African countries. *Lancet* 367:1835–1841.

Yoder S, Abderrahim N, Zhuzhuni A (2004) Female Genital Cutting in the Demographic and Health Surveys: Critical and Comparative Analysis, DHA Comparative Reports No. 7. Calverston, MD: ORC Macro. www.measuredhs.com/pubs/

15

Making Pregnancy Safer for Women around the World: The Example of Safe Motherhood and Maternal Death in Guatemala

NICOLE S. BERRY

Introduction

Maternal mortality, or the death of a woman due to pregnancy-related causes up to 42 days after being pregnant (United Nations Development Group 2003), constitutes one of the greatest challenges to global health today. Maternal mortality kills over half a million women per year, 99% of whom reside in developing countries (World Health Organization, United Nations Children's Fund, and United Nations Population Fund 2004). Pregnancy-related problems are one of the top causes of morbidity and mortality for women of reproductive age who live in the third world (World Health Organization 2006).

The challenge to make pregnancy and birth safe for women around the world has gained more importance since it was first introduced as a worldwide goal in 1987. That year marked the creation of the Safe Motherhood Initiative (SMI), which, for almost 20 years, has been the predominant authority on policies and interventions to decrease maternal mortality (AbouZahr 2003; Rosenfield 1997; Starrs 2006). Originally, the SMI outlined a broad agenda for decreasing maternal mortality by 50% by the year 2000 (AbouZahr 2003). As a decade of championing a wide array of programs failed to decrease international ratios of maternal mortality,[1] by the end of the millennium SMI policies had become more focused on the direct medical causes of maternal mortality (e.g., postpartum bleeding and infection or obstructed labor) (Maine 1999). Accordingly, a crux of the effort to decrease maternal mortality over the last decade has been decidedly focused on changing the quality of biomedical care accessible to women during pregnancy and birth (Bullough et al. 2005; Carlough and McCall 2005; Fauveau and de Bernis 2006; Hussein and Clapham 2005; Miller, Sloan, Winikoff, Langer, and Fikree 2003). While this approach, which mirrors the management of pregnancy in developed countries where maternal mortality is not a pressing issue, would appear to be promising, by itself it has done little to lower global ratios of maternal mortality (Ronsmans and Graham 2006).

The recent inclusion of improving maternal health as the fifth United Nations Millennium Development Goal has renewed the 1987 commitment to making pregnancy and birth safer for women around the world. The primary indicator of this goal, which was approved by 189 countries in 2000 as one of the most pressing current problems that developing countries must solve, is to decrease global maternal mortality ratios by three quarters (Rosenfield, Maine, and Freedman 2006). Inspired by this strengthened commitment to maternal health, the World Health Organization (WHO) has organized the Partnership for Maternal, Newborn, and Child Health (PMNCH) as the new focal point for safe motherhood.[2] While the PMNCH takes its lead from the SMI, it is committed to revisiting the problem of maternal mortality and reevaluating current approaches (Partnership for Maternal Newborn and Child Health 2007).

Given this striking array of powerful, international actors who have cooperated in the fight against maternal mortality for almost 20 years, it is even more surprising that global ratios of maternal mortality have not budged. The ethnographic research presented in this chapter explores some reasons why lowering maternal mortality has been so challenging. It explores how understandings of pregnancy-related problems in areas where maternal mortality is high can be antithetical to those assumed by SMI policies. In doing so, it provides an important example of how to reframe understandings of why women die, which, hopefully, can lead to new ways of addressing the problem.

Ethnographic Setting

If global maternal mortality represents one of the greatest health disparities between the developed and the developing world (Mahler 1987), Guatemala embodies this distinction on an internal level, where only the poorest women experience high rates of pregnancy-related death. Indeed, a woman who dies from pregnancy-related causes in Guatemala is most likely Indian, unemployed, and lacking a high school education (MSPAS 2003). For nonindigenous women, many of whom live in the capital city, rates of maternal mortality hover around 70 per 100,000 live births (MSPAS 2003). Yet in Sololá, a predominantly indigenous *departamento* (or province) with low rates of literacy and widespread poverty, the ratio continually exceeds 280—one of the highest ratios in the country (Medina-Giron 1989; MSPAS and JHPIEGO 2003; Schieber and Stanton 2000).

Because of these characteristics, over the last 18 years, Sololá has been the focus of an intense Safe Motherhood campaign waged by a partnership between the Ministry of Health and international organizations. In 1989, MotherCare began working with United States Agency for International Development (USAID) and the Ministry of Health on the problem of maternal mortality in Sololá and other departments in Guatemala with high maternal mortality (MotherCare, MSPAS, and USAID 1999; MotherCare and USAID 1994). MotherCare received 2 cycles of 5-year funding from John Snow, Inc. In 1999, that funding was transferred to JHPIEGO, a nonprofit organization affiliated with Johns Hopkins University, which coordinated the Safe Motherhood campaign for the duration of this research.

While MotherCare programs had emphasized working with midwives to lower maternal mortality, with JHPIEGO, policy shifted toward bolstering emergency obstetric care in the regional Sololá hospital (located in the same-named town of Sololá) as the center of the Safe Motherhood campaign (Maine and Rosenfield 1999). This particular approach was typical of the SMI's endorsement of policies that focused on reforming the quality of biomedical care available. While bolstering emergency obstetric care can mean many things, in Sololá the important components of this effort involved improving the ability of biomedical personnel in the hospital to respond to a pregnancy-related emergency. An obstetrician was hired part time. The general practitioners and the nurses who regularly staffed the hospital were given extra training to ensure that they were up-to-date on the latest treatment protocols for the most common obstetric emergencies. The hospital was also concerned with ensuring that basic drugs necessary for treating obstetric emergencies were continuously available.

In Sololá, however, the efficacy of the policy of investing in emergency obstetric care was challenged by the lack of access that biomedical providers had to birthing women (Hinojosa 2004a). Women and their families staunchly preferred homebirth with a traditional birth attendant over hospital birth. 2002 was a typical year, where, for example, only 6% of women in Sololá *departamento* had hospital deliveries (MSPAS 2002). Biomedical providers did not have access to women with obstetric problems either: *departamento* records from 1999 through 2003 also show that almost all maternal deaths still occurred outside of the hospital (MSPAS and JHPIEGO 1999, 2000, 2001, 2002, 2003). The reluctance to come to the hospital was regarded by local ministry personnel as fueled by a deep resistance among Mayan families to break with the cultural tradition of homebirth. As no social scientists staff the local Ministry of Health, they were very interested in me, a medical anthropologist and someone they regarded as specializing in cultural issues, to look into the problem.

Ministry officials recommended that I base myself in Santa Cruz la Laguna (population of 1200), the seat of a Kaqchikel Maya municipality that had recently experienced unusually high rates of maternal mortality. Women and men in Santa Cruz depend on a variety of local and extra-local resources for their health needs. Officially, Santa Cruz has a health post staffed by an auxiliary nurse.[3] Although this is an excellent resource, the health post has limited hours of operation. The auxiliary nurse gets paid only to work from 8:00 AM to 4:30 PM Monday through Friday, making it difficult for men to access the care there since these are the exact hours that they work. The nurse is required to attend an in-service meeting every Monday morning (a peak time of demand since the post has been closed all weekend), and thus the post is only open for half a day on Mondays. While she does attend emergencies in the middle of the night during the week, on the weekend, when she is not being paid, the nurse returns to her natal village and the health post remains closed. Participating in the internationally well-funded campaign to vaccinate all children (one of the main measures by which the nurse's performances is evaluated) occupies another 3 days of the nurse's time every month, and again, the health post is closed. Finally, Ministry policy dictates that nurses get 1 month off per year, normally taken around Christmas time, and, though theoretically a substitute worker is supposed to fill in during the nurse's vacation, the district is never allotted enough money to maintain the surplus worker, so the health post remains closed. Despites it restrictions, the health post is a health resource frequently used by both women and children.

The Ministry of Health in Guatemala is organized so that in addition to the nurse, villagers in every health district have access to more skilled biomedical practitioners. In the VII health district, to which Santa Cruz belongs, there is a health *center* (as opposed to health *post*) located a few villages away in San Pablo. A doctor and a *professional* nurse both staff the health center. Theoretically, this doctor is supposed to be at the disposal of all 15,469 people who live in the VII health district and should attend patients in each health post every week. Practically, as the doctor is responsible for attending patients in San Pablo every day, and is also responsible for the entire administration of the VII health district (which necessitates both a weekly meeting of district personnel and a weekly meeting at the Ministry headquarters in the town of Sololá), it is untenable to think that he actually could also travel to each of the other 3 health posts every week. While the health center in San Pablo is there for the Cruceños (residents of Santa Cruz), they practically never use it. Transportation between Santa Cruz and San Pablo is expensive and sporadic and the health center is not well equipped. Most Cruceños see that for the same effort, they can get better care elsewhere.

The hospital is another medical resource provided to all Guatemalans as part of their free medical care. The regional Sololá hospital, *San Juan de Rodas*, located in the town of Sololá, is the closest one to Santa Cruz. While any sick person with an acute condition can be treated in the emergency room, the hospital also offers *consulta externa* (outpatient care), which functions like a visit to the doctor. Patients arrive at the hospital from 7:00 AM onward and are given a number to see 1 of 4 medical specialists or the dentist. The consultation is free, but patients must purchase any prescriptions. Medicines are available at discount prices from the hospital's own pharmacy. People in Santa Cruz go to the hospital frequently, especially for getting stitches, pulling teeth, obtaining an ultrasound or an X-ray, or visiting a patient. Its popularity is probably due in part to the relative proximity of Sololá to Santa Cruz, its easy accessibility, and the fact that the Sololá market is the largest and cheapest market around.

Outside of the public biomedical providers, Cruceños frequently visit private doctors' offices to seek treatment for themselves and for their children. Many people use pharmacies as a biomedical alternative to a private doctor. While technically pharmacists in Guatemala are not supposed to prescribe medicines, in practice, many pharmacists function like, and are treated as, a doctor (Rosenthal 1987).

In addition to biomedical options, people in Santa Cruz also use "traditional" medical alternatives. While there is no one in the village who claims to be a shaman, many Cruceños rely on their own knowledge of herbs, that of an elder in their family, or a helpful neighbor to treat some health problems. For example, many people fought the common cold by making teas out of eucalyptus, cedar, and hibiscus. Other people boiled the leaves of a certain tree and applied them to swollen joints. There are also a number of traditional practitioners in the area who can be accessed for more severe problems. A trusted and popular herbalist lived in the village of Santa Clara, about two hours away. Like many doctors, the herbalist diagnosed for free and then sold the necessary medicine, but unlike the doctors, the herbalist's medicines were very inexpensive. She was also willing to accept less money from poorer people. The other popular herbalist was a man who lived near the hospital in Sololá, who was also reported to be a shaman. Finally, a few people sought help in the herb stalls in the market in Sololá.

Besides herbalists, one of the most important area resources are the traditional bone doctors of San Pedro (Hinojosa 2002, 2004b). Bone doctors treat anything from a fall to a fracture. Many of them have a special instrument that they use to push bones back into place, while others use their hands to manipulate. For example, one woman hit her elbow as she woke from bed.

A painful swelling developed and she could not move her arm without it hurting. She went to a bone doctor, who pushed her bone back into place. She immediately regained full motion without pain, she told me, and the swelling subsided shortly thereafter. Since there is really nothing similar to a bone doctor available in biomedicine, even people who normally depend on biomedical treatments still use bone doctors.

Nonbiomedical practitioners who deal in supernatural powers are also available. There are several Evangelical diviners who have received their gift from God. Diviners have a variety of different abilities, but in general, they are able to see some aspect of the future and are thus consulted the way an oracle might have been. Santa Cruz has one diviner and his power is to say whether a person is going to live or die, presumably when they encounter some sort of sickness. Shamans are another health resource who harness supernatural powers for their treatments, and one can visit a shaman in Sololá.

Finally, Santa Cruz boasts the help of several midwives or *iyoma*. Despite the fact that almost all babies are delivered at home by an *iyom*, midwives have no official role in the public health system in Guatemala. On the local level, *iyoma* are well identified in the community, and health posts keep track of who delivers each baby. Nevertheless, *iyoma* are not paid or employed by the Ministry of Health. Nor do they show up in the institutional diagrams mapping out the hierarchical relationships of health resources throughout the country.

When I first began my fieldwork, there were 6 practicing *iyoma* in the village. During the course of this research, 2 died,[4] one claimed that she had become too old to work, and another one stopped working because she could not get more clients after a maternal death. People worried that perhaps a curse on her had caused the parturient's death. The 2 remaining working midwives were busy indeed.

Research Methods

Over 24 months of fieldwork (2000–2001 and 2002–2003), I pursued 2 main activities to investigate indigenous women's reluctance to use the hospital for an obstetric emergency. My first aim was to compare women with obstetric emergencies who had sought care in the hospital to those with obstetric emergencies who had not sought care. I was interested in finding out if perhaps there was some background difference that predisposed some women to go to the hospital while others stayed home. I accomplished this first aim through a combination of 2 different methods. First, I interviewed women, their families, and midwives in the regional hospital when they came seeking help for an emergency. I used this same interview (described subsequently) in a randomly chosen sample of parous Kaqchikel women living in 3 different villages of the

VII Health District. During these interviews, I elicited a reproductive history, detailed information about birthing events and problems experienced, and information about the use of different traditional and biomedical health resources for different problems, and I asked open-ended questions concerning beliefs and feelings about birth and pregnancy and health care resources, such as the hospital and midwives. This allowed me to find women who had had obstetric emergencies and had not gone to the hospital.

Second, I carried out participant observation in one of the villages, Santa Cruz, over a 2-year period. This hallmark of anthropology has the researcher join in normal everyday life in the research setting. The experiences and observations made in the course of daily life are recorded and treated as data to be analyzed (I explain how this is done more thoroughly subsequently). Since I maintained an interest in villagers' use of health care resources as part of my participant observation activities, I offered to accompany women to a variety of different doctors' appointments and also participated in emergency evacuations from the village to the hospital of several women who experienced birthing-related problems.

My second aim was to investigate the Safe Motherhood effort itself to better understand the campaign's policy and how it was being carried out. On this topic, I also relied on participant observation and systematic observation as my primary methodologies. First, to familiarize myself with the policy initiative, I participated with other agency representatives in Safe Motherhood organizational efforts at the department level. I also attended all agency and public events related to Safe Motherhood in Sololá. To understand the attempt to bolster emergency obstetric resources in the hospital, I participated in all of the trainings of emergency room (ER) doctors to improve their own diagnosis of and response to obstetric emergencies, as well as to orient them to general improvements in the hospital aimed at strengthening obstetric care. I sat in on many weekly review sessions between hospital doctors and the directors, in which individual cases of obstetric emergencies were discussed and specifics of the Safe Motherhood policies were assessed. I spent 2 months observing in the ER to see how obstetric emergencies were handled. I also followed up on 33 women who came with an obstetric emergency, beginning at the entrance to the ER, through to the maternity ward (where I obtained their consent), and then to their discharge from the hospital. Finally, I participated in Safe Motherhood efforts to better orient midwives toward recognizing obstetric emergencies and refer their clients to the hospital. Toward this end, monthly meetings were held in the hospital with an ambassador group of midwives representing the entire department (Berry 2005), as well as individual meetings with midwives in every village. I attended both these department-wide meetings and the monthly meetings of midwives in each of the 3 villages where I worked.

What marks my project most significantly as "ethnographic" is its inductive design (Bernard 1994); rather than going to Sololá with 1 predetermined hypothesis to test, my research depended on finding out new information while in the field that would reshape the focus of my study. The core process that supported this inductive design involved participant observation, recording, and analyzing field notes daily. As I learned more about Sololá, the everyday lives of indigenous families, and the particulars of birth through this process, the questions that I asked and the particulars I paid attention to evolved. For example, while I had gone to Sololá expecting to understand why women were reluctant to go to the hospital with an emergency, the more I interviewed and talked to local participants in these events, the more I realized that I needed to focus on the specifics of referral: When were women referred to the hospital? Whose job was it to refer them? Whose decision was it for them to go? What was at stake when making a referral or deciding to go? Both my interview guide and informal conversations changed to accommodate this new line of inquiry. Ultimately, the goal of my ethnographic project was to ensure that the important themes and lines of inquiry were defined by the participants of this study, rather than by having my own categories of analysis take precedence.

My typical day when conducting interviews helps demonstrate the intertwining of methods and analysis that is the hallmark of inductive ethnography. When I conducted interviews in a village, I was accompanied by another woman, usually from the village itself.[5] Our interviewees ranged from 16 to more than 70 years old, and most were unaccustomed to the constant question-and-answer format of an interview. We took a number of steps to make the interview more comfortable and, by doing so, to ensure the quality of our data. First, we memorized the interview protocol and attempted to make the interview resemble a conversation as much as possible. One interviewer conversed with the participant, while the other filled in the surveys and took notes.[6] If a participant, for example, began discussing pregnancy complications while listing all of her gestations, we would make sure to cover both categories at once, instead of returning to complications after learning about gestations. We interspersed open-ended questions with closed-ended ones in an attempt to make speaking time between the interviewer and interviewee more equitable. We also made sure to leave pauses, as might occur in a normal conversation. All interviews were conducted in Kaqchikel by my assistant or infrequently, myself.[7] After each interview, my assistant and I would debrief by reviewing what had been written down during the interview and add missing information or make other notes.

At the end of the day, I would return home and "write up" the interviews. First, I would enter quantifiable information into a spread sheet. Then I would type up the responses to the open-ended questions into word processing documents. I would then write field notes about the conditions of each interview and my impressions concerning the day in general. In short, I would generate a corpus of written texts that composed my raw qualitative data. I analyzed these texts by first entering them into a software package for qualitative data analysis (Muhr 2004), and then "coding" them. To code them, I would reread the text and highlight sections—these could be groups of words or lines of text or paragraphs. The software would allow me to attach a label (or "code") to each highlighted section. I could then use the software to compare similar pieces of information from different sources side by side. This process helps the researcher see the patterns that are emerging in people's responses. For example, I knew that I was interested in obstetric complications and asked women to tell me about times that they had had problems. When I would read over interviewees' answers, I would highlight text that explained why they had not gone to seek biomedical care and label it. The more interviews I coded, the more I found I was using the label "religious reasons" to explain why a woman had not sought help. I then asked the software to pull up all instances of "religious reasons" to see if I could find new, important subcodes or themes within these pieces of text. Coding helped me interpret my data and to generate new hypotheses or lines of inquiry that I needed to follow up on. Thus, my day would end with notes concerning further research activities that I needed to carry out—for example, informal conversations that I could have or new questions that could be added to my next interview guide that might help me substantiate or nullify my interpretation of my data.

Adopting a "holistic" approach was important to understanding how the problem of maternal mortality related to my participants' lives. Instead of limiting my inquiry to maternal health, I participated in various facets of people's everyday lives and took and coded fieldnotes on all of it. This approach allowed me the freedom to pursue avenues that did not occur to me before I arrived in the field, permitting me to move beyond many of the ways that the problem had been approached (e.g., a focus on distance or cost). The comprehensive view that this approach provided helped me understand how, in this setting, pregnancy and birth are thought about very differently than they are among health workers in the Safe Motherhood campaign and the hospital. I now turn to describe more about these important differences and about how they were at the root of the problems that made the Safe Motherhood interventions in Sololá ineffective.

Using the Social to Understand the Physical: Connecting Religion and Birth

Local representatives of the Ministry of Health in Sololá did a good job of framing their concerns about the Safe Motherhood program for me: Namely, as long as Mayan women preferred the tradition of homebirth with a local midwife and eschewed modern medical resources available in the hospital, working with international counterparts to make the hospital better would not decrease maternal mortality. While I was suspicious of this depiction of indigenous Mayans as traditional and unwilling to join the modern world (Cosminsky 2001), the point that investing in emergency obstetric resources would never lower pregnancy-related deaths if women did not access them was well taken. I now want to focus on some of the reasons why a woman might not go to the hospital at the first sign of an obstetric problem.

From the perspective of health planners working on Safe Motherhood, "a problem" in pregnancy or birth was conceived of as a physiological dysfunction, revealing a normative assumption that birth is primarily a biological event. Since the late 1970s, however, anthropologists have recognized that the birthing process is *biosocial*—that it is composed of both biological and social processes (Jordan 1978). In many communities, the importance of pregnancy and birth in affirming or compromising social relationships, roles, and cosmologies is prioritized over biological facets of the birthing experience (Chapman 2003; Krause 2005; Paxson 2004; Uzendoski 2005). The intertwining of pregnancy, birth, and religion in Santa Cruz illustrates such a view.

In Santa Cruz, it is impossible to separate pregnancy and birth from religion. Physical human acts are necessary, but not sufficient to create a fetus; indeed it is God who decides when a woman gets pregnant. God is also seen as intimately tied to the outcome of one's pregnancy and birth. A conversation that I had with my neighbor in Santa Cruz is illustrative of this point. She had given birth during a year in which an unusual number of women had died during childbirth. "Were you ever scared?" I asked, "No," came the response. She told me that she felt completely at ease in her relationship with God. She had committed no sins. God would be there for her. Why would she be scared?

My neighbor's response illustrates how God's influence on birth is implicitly assumed to be a deciding factor of whether or not there is an obstetric complication. While the high numbers of maternal deaths made pregnancy-related mortality more real for me, my neighbor had no such reaction. Her response explained physiological problems as resulting from God's will. She felt confident in her relationship with God and, in turn, she felt confident that her birth would go well.

God's hand in determining the outcome of a birth is considered to be furthered by the *iyom*, or traditional midwife, who attends the birth. Unlike the way in which most biomedical providers choose their profession, a woman becomes a midwife in response to a divine calling. This view of midwifery as a "gift" has been well documented in Sololá and its environs (Paul 1975; Paul and Paul 1975). In this system, God sends a sign to a woman to let her know that she must start delivering babies. What this sign might be varies: many women fall ill and find no relief for their ailment until they begin attending births; others dream of delivering a baby and know that this is a sign; still others are born with the membranes around their heads still intact (this "cowl" indicating the baby's destiny as an *iyom*).

Indeed, it is these signs that are emphasized in relation to the vocation—not formal training.[8] My conversation with Cristina, an older midwife who had been practicing in a neighboring village for many years, illustrates how the connection between God and midwifery is typically underscored. When I asked her how she became a midwife, she told me that she dreamed of delivering a baby. When she woke up the next day, she told her neighbors. Soon thereafter, a woman went into labor and called for Cristina to come. I asked her if she had been nervous. She told me that she had not been nervous. Cristina said that she knew God had chosen her and that God would let her know what to do during the birth. And, as she anticipated, the birth went well.

The belief in a connection between God, pregnancy, and birth is fundamental to why the *iyom* is so trusted and sought out by her clients. God not only decides when a woman will get pregnant, but he chooses those whom he wants to deliver the babies he sends, and he guides each of these chosen individuals during the birth. In short then, having a home delivery with a midwife is, in some aspects, the culmination of God's will.

In Santa Cruz, religion and the institution of the church are pervasive in people's lives. Like most of Guatemala, in the past, the village was predominantly Catholic. Currently, however, there are more protestant evangelicals than Catholics. The population is small (~1,200) and families are large, so very few weeks pass when there is not a death, baptism, confirmation, marriage, or some other event physically observed in a church that one is invited to attend. Prayer is an important part of religious practice and every morning, one is woken to the sound of a congregation member greeting the new day over a portable loud speaker. Walking though the village, one frequently can hear the chanting of a group of women, either convening on their own or participating in a prayer intervention, pouring out from a house onto the street.

In this environment, one's spiritual connection to God is not esoteric or private and obeying God's will brings concrete benefits. One's status as sinner or saint is marked through everyday actions that simultaneously announce that status and remind the community of one's virtues or shortcomings. For example, some of the evangelical congregations divide their physical space of worship so that those who are doing penance are restricted to the back of the church, while those in God's good graces (or on a more skeptical note, in the pastor's good graces) have free reign of the church. These restrictions dictate that those who are doing penance are unfit to take on *"cargos,"* or voluntary service to the church, such as cleaning the church, or arranging the altar after hours. In everyday life, it is quite easy to distinguish who has free access to the sacred space of worship; they can be seen entering the church at any hour, or collecting flowers and plants to compose the altar. Their absence from other activities might also reference their presence in the church.

The pervasiveness of religion in everyday life heavily colors what sort of behaviors might make you be at odds with God. Fighting was a primary reason cited for complications in birth. One woman who I interviewed had labored for several days. Though the baby was fine, she told me that her troubles were the results of all of the fighting she had done with her sister-in-law while she was pregnant. Another woman told me that her own birthing complications were the result of her poor relationship with her mother-in-law, who was quite mean. She and her husband had tried to keep her mother-in-law from attending the birth. She told me that she had done much penance after the birth. A third woman, who had given birth to twins, expressed that her delivery problems were tied to her sinning husband, who had left her living with his parents for an affair with another woman. These types of explanations show how interviewees perceive that everyday social events are causally connected, though God's will, in determining birthing and pregnancy outcomes.

This intertwining of God with birth and the importance of religion and one's status with God in everyday life create concrete costs if a pregnancy or birth does not go smoothly. As my neighbor insinuated, a problem signals a poor relationship with God. This sign is available for all to interpret. In the realm of church, having problems in birth is just the sort of event that has the moral weight to change one's categorization from saint toward sinner, potentially changing a woman's and her family's social landscape. Such social pressures might keep a woman from running to the hospital at the first sign of an emergency.

The Safe Motherhood campaign assumes that pregnancy-related problems are, first and foremost, physical. The best way to resolve physical problems is to seek the care of a biomedical provider. In this context though, physical problems are not perceived by their bearers to be random or blameless occurrences. They are symptomatic of a deeper, spiritual problem. For many women, their families and midwives, the proper way to deal with a spiritual problem is to pray. Those who resort to the hospital may be able to alleviate their physical ailment, but in doing so may reveal their lack of willingness (or inability) to engage the more central issue: the sin or offense to God that resulted in a complicated birth.

The *Iyom* and the Problem of Referral

The reasons why women did not go to the hospital at first sign of an obstetric problem were further complicated by the dependence on the *iyom* as the trusted provider. As alluded to earlier, *iyoma* were preferred over biomedical personnel: quite simply *iyoma* could boast that they had God on their side, while biomedical providers could make no such claim. In Santa Cruz, where pregnancy and birth were perceived as dependent on God's will, the purported alliance between God and the *iyom* was paramount to her credentials. Since the *iyoma* attended almost all of the births in the district, getting a woman with problems to the hospital depended, to a large extent, on the *iyoma* making a referral (Berry 2006). Toward this end, health workers employed in the Safe Motherhood campaign were popularizing "danger signs" in pregnancy and birth by educating women during prenatal visits to government health posts and educating *iyoma* during monthly meetings. Most of the danger signs reviewed were physiological: bloating, leaking water, fever, and so on (MSPAS, Union Europea/Guatemala, MotherCare, and USAID 1996). They also included rules of thumb, such as anyone experiencing more than 20 minutes of postpartum bleeding or 24 hours of labor should be transported to the hospital. This aspect of the Safe Motherhood campaign revealed that the Ministry of Health and its partners imagined that birthing problems would be evaluated by their physical manifestations, and referrals made accordingly. I found, however, that *iyoma* were very unlikely to use the biomedical criteria they were being taught to decide when a woman needed to go to the hospital. I now turn to explain several reasons why it was unrealistic to expect *iyoma* to change their referral behaviors in response to the Safe Motherhood campaign.

Both the women and midwives whom I interviewed emphasized the variation in reproductive women's experiences. Some women find pregnancy draining while others feel energized. Some women have relatively easy births, while others must work harder. Physical "problems" were contextualized within this normal variation. Some women bleed for hours after a birth and were fine. Others bleed and were dead within 20 minutes. Likewise, some women labored for 2 days and eventually delivered healthy babies. Other labored for 2 days with no such luck. *Iyoma* specialized in providing individualized attention. The idea that one-size-fits-all guidelines should be used to decide when to refer a woman to the hospital challenged both the *iyom* and her client's understanding of reproductive experiences.

At least part of the differences in how difficulties in birth are understood and treated can be accounted for by different causal understandings of these difficulties. The Safe Motherhood campaign viewed problems as physiological malfunctions that a skilled biomedical provider could most likely remedy (if addressed in time). Birthing women, *iyoma*, and their families, however, tended to perceive physiological problems as symptomatic of underlying social and spiritual problems. Thus, while a problem might look bad, God could provide almost instantaneous relief. While collecting birthing histories, I heard countless stories of such miraculous recoveries—where women on the verge of death got down on their knees and prayed, and when finished, their problem had been alleviated, allowing them to give birth. It was, therefore, difficult for *iyoma* or their clients to blindly accept the "danger signs" as guidelines for action.

Another part of the differences alluded to earlier reflects a discrepancy in what counts as a source of knowledge. The biomedical guidelines that the Safe Motherhood campaign depended on were reflective of population-based, epidemiological studies. Midwives in this region, as Jordan (1978) pointed out, are empirical learners. This means that they glean their knowledge from lived experiences rather than abstractions (e.g., theory-based classroom learning). It is not at all surprising then that a midwife's lived experience might contradict, rather than reflect, the findings of population-based studies upon which the biomedical guidelines for referral are based. Indeed, some of these contradictions are the direct result of the "vertical" nature of the SMI. In the SMI, knowledge is produced far away from the places where women actually die, like Guatemala. This knowledge inspires SMI policies and interventions, which are subsequently implemented uniformly throughout the globe. The danger signs and guidelines that were promoted in Sololá reflected the most common sources of direct obstetric complications discussed in the safe motherhood literature.[9] Yet what constituted the top pregnancy-related complications internationally was not necessarily reflective of the most important pregnancy-related complications in Sololá. In Sololá, postpartum bleeding and retention of the placenta were top killers (MSPAS and JHPIEGO 1999, 2000, 2001, 2002, 2003). Uterine rupture, which may result when a scar from a C-section gives out during a subsequent pregnancy or delivery, was not an issue. As discussed, the number of women giving birth in facilities where they would have access to a C-section was minimal. Not all who went to the hospital received a C-section, so the number of women having post-cesarean deliveries was a small subset of those who went to the hospital. This risk of uterine rupture is likewise minimal.[10] Given the small populations of villages (in the district I worked in, all were fewer than 2,500 people), years would have to pass before a midwife would likely see a uterine rupture, and it would be highly improbable for her to see multiple uterine ruptures (the kind of empirical reinforcement needed to make a connection between the C-section scar and uterine rupture). Indeed, during the 6 years I had access to the causes of maternal mortality in the department, there was not 1 recorded uterine rupture. Despite its lack of importance in the local setting, the guidelines concerning referring every client with a C-section scar back to the hospital to prevent a potential uterine rupture were provided to midwives with the same emphasis as guidelines concerning referring a patient whose placenta was retained for more than 20 minutes. Yet in practice, midwives continually delivered the rare client with a C-section scar without problems. The contradiction between the recommendation of the guidelines and their own experience only served to cast doubt on the usefulness of all of the biomedical guidelines as a source of knowledge. Unfortunately, it made *iyoma* far less likely to pay attention to the specific guidelines that really could help save lives locally, such as making timely referrals of clients with retained placentas or hemorrhage.

The *iyoma* were at odds with the Safe Motherhood campaign's recommendations of who should be referred to the hospital for yet another reason. The guidelines were in place to try to prevent a maternal death by having *at-risk* cases referred. The populace in question, however, seemed to prefer sending only those who definitely needed treatment to a biomedical provider. A concrete example might make this point more clearly. After Olga had been evacuated to the hospital with a life-threatening postpartum infection, the nurse at the health post had a conversation with the *iyom* who attended her. The nurse challenged the *iyom*, asking her why she had not referred Olga earlier, when clearly fever was one of the danger signs that recommended referral. The *iyom* scoffed at the nurse's assertion. She saw fevers after birth routinely, and a fever definitely did not predict that a woman was going to have an infection. For the health workers, it made sense to use the symptom of fever to isolate a pool of parturients who were at risk for a postpartum infection. While some women who were in no danger would surely be referred, those who were in danger would get the help they needed. From the *iyom's* perspective, the guidelines could not be used to cast a small enough net to really predict exactly who would have big problems and who would not. The material in the previous section prepares us to understand some of the reasons why *iyoma*, their clients, and families would not be likely to preventively send women to the hospital when they might be able to get better at home.

Planning Safer Motherhood: Global Public Health versus Local Maternal Mortality

This case study concerning improving safe motherhood in Sololá demonstrates some of the planning challenges faced by global public health campaigns. As alluded to previously, the Ministry of Health had partnered with international and bilateral organizations for over a decade in their attempt to decrease maternal mortality. The policies and interventions that were promoted put Sololá on the cutting edge of global SMI policy.

The shifts that have occurred in how safe motherhood is approached in Sololá have been vertical in nature. None of the changes were in response to what those implementing safe motherhood policy in Sololá believe would be effective. Rather they reflected shifts in the global SMI policy. These global shifts determined what activities John Snow, Inc. was willing and enthusiastic to fund, and in doing so, determined the funding priorities for the Safe Motherhood campaign in Sololá. Cooperative agreements between the

Ministry of Health, MotherCare, and JHPIEGO meant that the Ministry's own Safe Motherhood budget was tied up in assisting the globally determined goals.

As I worked in Sololá, it was obvious to me that those in charge of carrying out the Safe Motherhood campaign, in both public and private sectors, were well aware of the pitfalls of globally dictated policy. I first visited Sololá only 6 months after funding priorities had shifted away from midwives and toward investing in biomedical care. Nevertheless, the director of the Sololá branch of the Ministry[11] already foresaw that women were not going to use the hospital.

The Sololá director of JHPIEGO[12] also struggled with the shift away from attention to the midwife. For the previous 10 years, the relationship between the campaign, the Ministry, and the local *iyoma* had been a major focus of activity. All of a sudden, there was no more money to work with midwives. Despite changes in global funding priorities, in Sololá, midwives were still important, trusted, and relied-upon providers for pregnancy care and childbirth. Biomedical providers still had little, if any, contact with potential obstetric patients. The health workers in the Safe Motherhood campaign had worked to collaborate with *iyoma*, but suddenly when funding priorities shifted, not only were they no longer encouraged to take this approach, but no money could also be dedicated to supporting it. This put health workers in an untenable position. They had spent years building trust with *iyoma*, and leaving those relationships and obligations would not only stop any progress, but could also create a setback.[13] In addition, health workers' own experiences in the department made many feel that maintaining their working relations with *iyoma* was fundamental to making progress on the issue of safe motherhood. Unfortunately, the only funding available for working with *iyoma* in the Safe Motherhood campaign involved continuing their biomedical education in the form of working with the "danger signs" guidelines.

The Safe Motherhood campaign in Sololá highlights the conflict that can exist between "testing" global policy and working to improve health outcomes. Structures of funding have restricted safe motherhood policy in Guatemala, dictating that internationally sanctioned approaches be the keystone of efforts to lower maternal mortality in Sololá. This vertical approach to policy making abandons the expertise of health professionals in charge of implementing a program, not to mention the communities at which interventions are aimed. In Sololá, health professionals were put into a difficult position, as they frequently perceived a divide between implementing the program they have been given on the one hand, and working toward decreasing maternal mortality on the other.

Attention to the quality of emergency obstetric care that a woman receives at a state hospital can undoubtedly play a part in making pregnancy and childbirth safer. However, channeling investment into the delivery of biomedical care when women prefer to give birth at home—and almost exclusively do so with non–biomedically trained attendants—is misguided. Empirical midwives, like those in Sololá, will never be the purveyors of such care, and have, therefore, been left to play a tangential and undefined role in the Safe Motherhood campaign. I now turn to look at some of the ways that local providers creatively addressed this lacuna in the Safe Motherhood campaign and to emphasize other areas of the campaign that could be strengthened.

Suggestions for Making Pregnancy Safe in Sololá

In Sololá, midwives are the primary birth attendants not because there is a lack of biomedical providers, but because women trust and esteem their spiritual credentials. Working with midwives, therefore, is a necessity for any Safe Motherhood campaign in the department. Despite the shift in funding priorities away from working with midwives, most factions discussing safe motherhood agree that midwives need to be included in the Initiative (de Bernis, Sherratt, AbouZahr, and Van Lerberghe 2003; Kruske and Barclay 2004; Sibley and Sipe 2004, 2006; van Roosmalen, Walraven, Stekelenburg, and Massawe 2005). Involving midwives in the Safe Motherhood effort in Sololá must entail more than just "educating" them.

During the years of this study, the local head of JHPIEGO informally spearheaded an initiative to integrate midwives into the State health system (Asowa-Omorodion 1997). The divide between "traditional" and "biomedical" providers runs deep, and building respect and tolerance among the different camps is a critical first step (Cosminsky 2001; Davis-Floyd and Sargent 1997; Jolly 2002). They began a pilot program that staffed the maternity ward with an *iyom* 24 hours a day, 7 days a week. This program was as important as it was innovative and necessary. Finding a place for midwives in the biomedical system is difficult, because they are being asked to participate in a place where their biomedical colleagues define them as "unskilled." Yet, in the end, the midwives were willing to staff the maternity ward and withstand even the initial disdain and rudeness of some of the hospital personnel, because they felt that their presence was important to the patients. Many of the women who came to the hospital seeking care were monolingual in indigenous languages and had no experience with biomedical obstetric care (Berry 2008). Hospital policy dictated that family members were not allowed to stay in the hospital with them. For these women, having an *iyom* present on the maternity ward was like having an ally there. Providing the *iyoma* with responsibilities in the hospital also served to increase their status with many of the biomedical staff, who were able to break through stereotypes about ignorant midwives.

Despite the importance of this program, the professionals working on safe motherhood found it difficult to fund. While they were able to pay for an evaluation of the program by slipping it into an exit interview concerning obstetric patients' hospital experiences, they were not able to use Safe Motherhood campaign funds to pay the honorarium that each *iyom* received for completing her shift. The Ministry of Health's budget was also tied up in the international agenda. Armed with the data showing the importance of the program to patients, they looked for funding from local mayors, who refused to participate. They used their own personal money to bridge the program until they could secure a constant source of funding.

The health workers who championed the midwives working on the maternity ward dreamed of having midwives throughout the hospital where pregnant women were attended, and I would concur that bringing *iyoma* into the ER is a critical next step. In addition to the comfort that seeing an *iyom* in the ER could bring to patients and their families, the ER is an excellent venue for empirical learners, since it is the easiest place to get lots of experience in obstetric complications. *Iyoma* who worked in the ER could witness the same complications over and over, shoring up an association between some symptoms and a referral—for example, fever and swelling postpartum means a bad infection. They would also get to see how easily and successfully some of the pregnancy-related complications can be resolved—for example, the manual extraction of a placenta. Knowing what would happen to a client in the hospital might make them more willing to refer. Building personal relationships between the *iyoma* and doctors would also be an essential ingredient in building trust between the hospital and the communities.

Though midwives are autonomous in how they chose to provide care, many midwives are eager to adopt new, useful practices. In my fieldwork, I found that local midwives built trusting relationships with private doctors and pharmacists, who would keep them abreast of the latest drug, or help them with a client who had a problem. Foster, and colleagues (2004) have likewise found that traditional, Guatemalan midwives are keen on sharpening their skills. Rather than abandoning midwife education, more attention needs to be focused on the types of pedagogy used. Jordan (1989) expertly details many of the pitfalls from which biomedical programs to teach Mayan midwives suffer. Theoretical classes need to be replaced with experience-based learning. For example, one of the more useful exercises that I participated in during the monthly midwife education classes that the Ministry held concerned postpartum bleeding. The objective of the exercise was to provide a guide as to what constituted excessive bleeding after birth. We started the class by mixing water with red dye and then pouring it onto a dry cloth. One of the cloths was saturated with an amount of water that represented excessive postpartum blood. We not only got to see what that cloth looked like immediately after it was doused, but we also returned to it throughout the class to notice how it looked. This is one area where the decades of experience of working with midwives around the world can help in Sololá. Health workers should teach such hands-on approaches, and steer away from trying to impart wisdom verbally or theoretically.

Another important reform for the Sololá campaign involves tailoring educational materials to make them more useful and more credible. Only the "danger signs" and guidelines that are important to tackling the most common pregnancy-related complications in Sololá should be included. Complications that are rare, such as uterine rupture, are essentially irrelevant to practice, and should be eliminated. Agreement between *iyoma* beliefs and "danger signs" and guidelines should be used to maximize *iyoma's* perceptions of the inclusion of their own knowledge in the "danger signs." For example, transverse lie—when a baby is in a horizontal position rather than engaged head first in the pelvis—is considered by midwives to signal a problematic or abnormal birth. This agreement in diagnosis between *iyoma* and biomedical providers could be taken advantage of by showcasing it both conceptually and visually in didactic materials.

The Safe Motherhood effort in Sololá has benefited from a skilled cadre of health professionals who are committed to lowering maternal mortality and has also enjoyed a comparatively ample budget. However, the Safe Motherhood campaign also demonstrates some of the pitfalls associated with relying on top-down intervention design. In short, better tailoring of the campaign to more closely reflect the realities of the local context might help the effort to reduce maternal mortality.

Conclusion: Using the Example of Sololá to Make Pregnancy and Birth Safer

The international health community is at a crossroads with regard to making pregnancy and birth safer for women in the Third World. The commemoration of the second decade of the SMI has provided another opportunity for the problem of maternal mortality to be in the spotlight and for resources to be garnered to reevaluate the problem. I would argue that anthropological work, such as the case study presented here, can be used to recommend important directions for future initiatives aimed at making pregnancy and birth safer.

This case study suggests that while adopting a specific focus for safe motherhood has helped garner resources for the effort, it has also backed us into a corner by excessively narrowing our understanding of maternal mortality. Maine and Rosenfield (1999) provided an important critique of the early SMI when they pointed out that it advocated such wide-ranging policies that safe motherhood programs were both everything and nothing. Most governments believed that they already had safe motherhood programs in place (e.g., family planning, women's education, etc.), so while they may have embraced the cause, they frequently took no additional measures to reduce maternal mortality. From this critique has sprung a more focused SMI that has suggested concrete safe motherhood programs to be carried out and evaluated, such as bolstering emergency obstetric care or, now, increasing skilled attendance at birth (de Bernis et al. 2000; Safe Motherhood Initiative Interagency Group 2000). One of the perhaps unintended consequences of this focus has been a narrowing of our understanding of maternal mortality that concentrates on its direct (physical) causes. Thus, the problem of maternal mortality itself is understood as a battle to address obstetric pathology. This perspective is illustrated by the fact that, in addition to monitoring maternal mortality ratios, the only other indicator of how close we are to achieving Millennium Development Goal Five is assessing the number of births attended by biomedically trained attendants.

Anthropological work, however, reinforces the idea that maternal deaths are frequently just as much the result of social and political processes as physiological pathologies. Both Davis-Floyd (2003) and Kaufert and O'Neil (1993) have helped demonstrate how the relative privileging of biomedical knowledge and concomitant denigrating of other knowledge and practices (e.g., women's own intuition about their bodies or midwifery, etc.) keeps women out of biomedical settings, away from care that they may need. Anthropologists have written extensively on how local understandings of risk can largely determine the care-seeking behavior of pregnant and birthing women (Allen 2002; Chapman 2003; Hay 1999; Obermeyer 2000) and how the meaning of risk assumed by the SMI can shape the care available. Janes and Chuluundorj (2004) show how political/economic trends and changes can affect family organization and cooperation, resulting in a change in rates of maternal deaths. The crux of the case study that I present here is that an understanding of maternal mortality that takes into account the perceived social reasons why women die is important to designing future interventions and deciding which policies to endorse.

A broad understanding of maternal mortality that encompasses both its direct physical and social causes should, however, not be confused with the lack of focus that characterized the beginning of the SMI. Advocating for a specific agenda to help make pregnancy safer will undoubtedly continue to be an important part of the solution (Anonymous 2006). Yet, focus in the SMI should not be restricted to narrowly endorsing and funding policies and interventions that necessarily privilege a biomedical solution to maternal mortality. In other words, we do not yet know what needs to be done (see Campbell and Graham 2006; Fauveau and de Bernis 2006; Maine and Rosenfield 1999).

While we have the biomedical knowledge necessary to prevent a vast majority of pregnancy-related deaths, we do not yet understand how to design and implement programs that work on a global scale (Costello, Azad, and Barnett 2006; Filippi et al. 2006). This ethnographic case study supports the conclusion that the contexts in which the issues surrounding maternal mortality play out are so variable (Hussein and Clapham 2005) that we will probably not find a one-size-fits-all solution to decrease global maternal mortality.

While the specificities concerning the relationship between religion and birth might be particular to Santa Cruz, the lesson that understandings of birthing complications often involve a deeper social understanding of maternal mortality than that offered by the medical model is quite generalizable. While changes in biomedical practice and biomedical infrastructure undoubtedly are important to lowering global ratios of maternal mortality, we cannot be complacent in thinking that advocating these changes alone constitutes sufficient policy. Globally, while the direct obstetric causes of maternal mortality may be uniform, the contexts in which these complications occur are not. Each obstetric problem or emergency manifests itself as but one aspect of a woman, who will be found in the midst of her own social, cultural, and political circumstances. We must, therefore, take into account these circumstances in order to meaningfully understand how women, families, and midwives respond to obstetric emergencies. Only through attention to the social and cultural details of women's lives will we be able to come up with policies that make sense.

Notes

1. The accepted convention is to measure the "maternal mortality ratio," which is expressed as the number of maternal deaths per 100,000 live births.

2. I use "safe motherhood" in this chapter in three distinct ways: (1) capitalized to refer to the Safe Motherhood Initiative (SMI), (2) not capitalized to refer to the concept of safe motherhood that was derived from the SMI, (3) capitalized to refer to the local Safe Motherhood campaign in Guatemala, which is modeled on the SMI's recommendations.

3. "Auxiliary" refers to the training that the nurse gets, which is less than that received by a "professional" nurse.

4. Both of these women were very old. In this area, the vast majority of the women who become midwives are older, often at the end of their reproductive lives.

5. I worked with 3 different women from 3 different villages. All were mothers who had finished high school, so their comparative educational level was high. We met several times before beginning our work to both talk about the project and rehearse.

6. We also tried to decrease the self-consciousness of the interview by not taperecording the interviews. We did record a subset of three different interviews ($n = 121$) with women who were well known to my assistant and who were trusting and comfortable with her. We did not solicit any others to be taperecorded.

7. We found that interviewees were far more comfortable talking to someone they knew than a stranger.

8. Nevertheless, as mentioned above, most midwives begin practicing when they have ended or are close to ending their own reproductive lives. By this time, they have probably given birth themselves a number of times and attended a number of other births of their sisters, sisters-in-law, daughters, and so on. There are, however, no formal apprenticeships.

9. Maine and Rosenfield's (1999) article is iconic in representing the shift toward improving obstetric care, and provides a good summary of the major direct causes of maternal mortality globally.

10. The Guatemalan Ministry of Health does not provide a statistical estimation of the likelihood of uterine rupture due to a previous C-section. However, the Ministry of Health (MSPAS 2002) does estimate that the risk of uterine rupture during pregnancy is about one in 1,500 to 2,000. This number is an estimate that includes all risks—car accidents or knife wounds, and so on—not just rupture of a C-section scar. The number for rupture of C-sections scars then is even smaller.

11. This individual began his career as a health post doctor in Sololá, traveling by foot from village to village. He spent his entire career in the department, eventually being promoted to the top job.

12. While the international organizations administrating the grant for Safe Motherhood in Sololá over the decades have changed, the funding organization insisted that the personnel implementing the policies remain the same. While I was working in Sololá, the director of the international organization was a doctor who had been working on Safe Motherhood for many years.

13. Sololá is littered with deteriorating buildings that tell the story of one or another development project that received a cycle of funding and then was abandoned. Indeed, as I heard over and over during my fieldwork, this sort of "flavor of the day" development approach has left bitterness in the mouths of many villagers. They expressed a lack of incentive to collaborate with any program, because history has shown them that the program will be abandoned and their effort will probably come to naught.

References

AbouZahr C (2003) Safe motherhood: A brief history of the global movement 1947–2002. *British Medical Bulletin* 67:13–25.

Allen DR (2002) *Managing Motherhood, Managing Risk: Fertility and Danger in West Central Tanzania.* Ann Arbor, MI: University of Michigan Press.

Anonymous (2006) Constantly shifting policy on safe motherhood an obstacle to progress. *Reproductive Health Matters* 14:195.

Asowa-Omorodion FI (1997) Women's perceptions of the complications of pregnancy and childbirth in two Esan communities, Edo State, Nigeria. *Social Science and Medicine* 44:1817–1824.

Bernard HR (1994) *Research Methods in Anthropology: Qualitative and Quantitative Approaches.* Thousand Oaks, CA: Sage Publications.

Berry NS (2005) Incorporating cultural diversity into health systems: An example of midwives teaching midwives. *Women in International Development Forum* XXVII:1–9.

Berry NS (2006) Kaqchikel midwives, home births, and emergency obstetric referrals in Guatemala: Contextualizing the choice to stay at home. *Social Science and Medicine* 62:1958–1969.

Berry NS (2008) Who's judging the quality of care? Indigenous Maya and the problem of "not being attended." *Medical Anthropology* 27:164–189.

Bullough C, Meda N, Makowiecka K, Ronsmans C, Achadi EL, Hussein J (2005) Current strategies for the reduction of maternal mortality. *BJOG: An International Journal of Obstetrics and Gynaecology* 112:1180–1188.

Campbell OM, Graham WJ (2006) Strategies for reducing maternal mortality: Getting on with what works. *Lancet* 368: 1284–1299.

Carlough M, McCall M (2005) Skilled birth attendance: What does it mean and how can it be measured? A clinical skills assessment of maternal and child health workers in Nepal. *International Journal of Gynecology and Obstetrics* 89:200–208.

Chapman RR (2003) Endangering safe motherhood in Mozambique: Prenatal care as pregnancy risk. *Social Science and Medicine* 57:355–374.

Cosminsky S (2001) Midwifery across the generations: A modernizing midwife in Guatemala. *Medical Anthropology* 20:345–378.

Costello A, Azad K, Barnett S (2006) An alternative strategy to reduce maternal mortality. *Lancet* 368:1477–1479.

Davis-Floyd R (2003) Home-birth emergencies in the US and Mexico: The trouble with transport. *Social Science and Medicine* 56:1911–1931.

Davis-Floyd R, Sargent CF (1997) *Childbirth and Authoritative Knowledge: Cross-Cultural Perspectives.* Berkeley, CA: University of California Press.

de Bernis L, Dumont A, Bouillin D, Gueye A, Dompnier JP, Bouvier-Colle MH (2000) Maternal morbidity and mortality in two different populations of Senegal: A prospective study (MOMA survey). *British Journal of Obstetrics and Gynaecology* 107:68–74.

de Bernis L, Sherratt DR, AbouZahr C, Van Lerberghe W (2003) Skilled attendants for pregnancy, childbirth and postnatal care. *British Medical Bulletin* 67:39–57.

Fauveau V, de Bernis L (2006) "Good obstetrics" revisited: Too many evidence-based practices and devices are not used. *International Journal of Gynecology and Obstetrics* 94:179–184.

Filippi V, Ronsmans C, Campbell OMR, Graham WJ, Mills A, Borghi J, et al. (2006) Maternal survival 5. Maternal health in poor countries: The broader context and a call for action. *Lancet* 368:1535–1541.

Foster J, Anderson A, Houston J, Doe-Simkins M (2004) A report of a midwifery model for training traditional midwives in Guatemala. *Midwifery* 20:217–225.

Hay MC (1999) Dying mothers: Maternal mortality in rural Indonesia. *Medical Anthropology* 18:243–279.

Hinojosa SZ (2002) "The hands know": Bodily engagement and medical impasse in highland Maya bonesetting. *Medical Anthropology Quarterly* 16:19.

Hinojosa SZ (2004a) Authorizing tradition: Vectors of contention in highland Maya midwifery. *Social Science and Medicine* 59:16.

Hinojosa SZ (2004b) Bonesetting and radiography in the southern Maya highlands. *Medical Anthropology* 23:263–293.

Hussein J, Clapham S (2005) Message in a bottle: Sinking in a sea of safe motherhood concepts. *Health Policy* 73:294–302.

Janes CR, Chuluundorj O (2004) Free markets and dead mothers: The social ecology of maternal mortality in post-socialist Mongolia. *Medical Anthropology Quarterly* 18:28.

Jolly M (2002) "Birthing Beyond the Confinements of Tradition and Modernity?" In: *Birthing in the Pacific: Beyond Tradition and Modernity.* V Lukere, M Jolly, eds. Honolulu, HI: University of Hawai'i Press, pp. 1–30.

Jordan B (1978) *Birth in Four Cultures: A Crosscultural Investigation of Childbirth in Yucatan, Holland, Sweden, and the United States.* St. Albans, VT: Eden Press Women's Publications.

Jordan B (1989) Cosmopolitan obstetrics: Some insights from the training of traditional midwives. *Social Science and Medicine* 28:925–944.

Kaufert PA, O'Neil J (1993) "Analysis of a Dialogue on Risks in Childbirth: Clinicians, Epidemiologists and Inuit Women." In: *Knowledge, Power, and Practice: The Anthropology of Medicine and Everyday Life.* S Lindenbaum, MM Lock, eds. Berkeley, CA: University of California Press, pp. 32–54.

Krause EL (2005) Encounters with the "peasant": Memory work, masculinity, and low fertility in Italy. *American Ethnologist* 32:593–617.

Kruske S, Barclay L (2004) Effect of shifting policies on traditional birth attendant training. *Journal of Midwifery and Women's Health* 49:306–311.

Mahler H (1987) The safe motherhood initiative: A call to action. *Lancet* 1:668–670.

Maine D (1999) "What's So Special about Maternal Mortality?" In: *Safe Motherhood Initiatives: Critical Issues.* M Berer, TS Ravindran, eds. London: Blackwell Science, pp. 175–182.

Maine D, Rosenfield A (1999) The Safe Motherhood Initiative: Why has it stalled? *American Journal of Public Health* 89:480–482.

Medina-Giron H (1989) *Estudio de Mortalidad Materna en Guatemala: Estimacion de Subregistro.* Guatemala, Guatemala: Ministerio de Salud Pública y Asistencia Social Departamento Materno-Infantil.

Miller S, Sloan NL, Winikoff B, Langer A, Fikree F (2003) Where is the "E" in MCH? The need for an evidence-based approach in Safe Motherhood. *Journal of Midwifery and Women's Health* 48:10–18.

MotherCare, MSPAS, USAID (1999) *Proyecto MotherCare II Guatemala: Informe de 5 años 1994–1999.* Guatemala: USAID.

MotherCare, USAID (1994) *Lograr La Maternidad Sin Riesgo.* Washington, DC: USAID.

MSPAS (2002) *Vigilancia y Control Epidemiologico Consolidado de Sololá: Memoria Anual de Vigilancia Epidemiológica.* Sololá, Guatemala: Ministerio de Salud Pública y Asistencia Social.

MSPAS (2003) *Línea Basal de Mortalidad Materna para el año 2000.* Guatemala, Guatemala: Ministerio de Salud Publica y Asistencia Social.

MSPAS and JHPIEGO (1999) *Registro de Muerta Materna Sololá.* Sololá: MSPAS.

MSPAS and JHPIEGO (2000) *Registro de Muerta Materna Sololá.* Sololá: MSPAS.

MSPAS and JHPIEGO (2001) *Registro de Muerta Materna Sololá.* Sololá: MSPAS.

MSPAS and JHPIEGO (2002) *Registro de Muerta Materna Sololá.* Sololá: MSPAS.

MSPAS and JHPIEGO (2003) *Registro de Muerta Materna Sololá.* Sololá: MSPAS.

MSPAS, Union Europea/Guatemala, MotherCare, USAID (1996) *Señales de peligro de embarazo, parto y recién nacido.* Guatemala: MSPAS.

Muhr T (2004) *User's Manual for ATLAS.ti 5.0.* Berlin: ATLAS.ti Scientific Software Development GmbH.

Obermeyer CM (2000) Risk, uncertainty, and agency: Culture and safe motherhood in Morocco. *Medical Anthropology* 19:173–201.

Partnership for Maternal NaCH (2007) *Ten-Year Strategy: The Partnership for Maternal, Newborn and Child Health.* Geneva: World Health Organization.

Paul L (1975) Recruitment to a ritual role: The midwife in a Mayan community. *Ethos* 3:449–467.

Paul L, Paul BD (1975) The Maya midwife as sacred specialist: A Guatemalan case. *American Ethnologist* 2:707–726.

Paxson H (2004) *Making Modern Mothers: Ethics and Family Planning in Urban Greece.* Berkeley, CA: University of California Press.

Ronsmans C, Graham WJ (2006) Maternal survival 1. Maternal mortality: Who, when, where, and why. *Lancet* 368:1189–1200.

Rosenfield A (1997) The history of the Safe Motherhood Initiative. *International Journal of Gynaecology and Obstetrics* 59:S7–S9.

Rosenfield A, Maine D, Freedman L (2006) Meeting MDG-5: An impossible dream. *Lancet* 368:1133–1135.

Rosenthal C (1987) Santa Maria De Jesus: Medical choice in a highland Guatemalan town. PhD dissertation, Department of Anthropology, Harvard University, Cambridge, MA.

Safe Motherhood Initiative Interagency Group (2000) *Skilled Attendance at Delivery: A Review of the Evidence.* New York: Family Care International.

Schieber B, Stanton C (2000) *Estimación de Mortalidad Materna en Guatemala Período 1996–1998.* Guatemala: GSD Consultores Asociados/Measure/Evaluation Macro International Inc.

Sibley L, Sipe TA (2004) What can a meta-analysis tell us about traditional birth attendant training and pregnancy outcomes? *Midwifery* 20:51–60.

Sibley L, Sipe TA (2006) Transition to skilled birth attendance: Is there a future role for trained traditional birth attendants? *Journal of Health Population and Nutrition* 24:472–478.

Starrs AM (2006) Safe Motherhood Initiative: 20 years and counting. *Lancet* 368:1130–1132.

United Nations Development Group (2003) *Indicators for Monitoring the Millennium Development Goals: Definitions, Rationale, Concepts and Sources.* New York: United Nations.

Uzendoski M (2005) *The Napo Runa of Amazonian Ecuador.* Urbana, IL: University of Illinois Press.

Van Roosmalen J, Walraven G, Stekelenburg J, Massawe S (2005) Integrating continuous support of the traditional birth attendant into obstetric care by skilled midwives and doctors: A cost-effective strategy to reduce perinatal mortality and unnecessary obstetric interventions. *Tropical Medicine and International Health* 10:393–394.

World Health Organization (2006) *The World Health Report 2005: Make Every Mother and Child Count.* Geneva: World Health Organization.

World Health Organization, United Nations Children's Fund, United Nations Population Fund (2004) *Maternal Mortality in 2000: Estimates Developed by WHO, UNICEF, UNFPA.* Geneva: World Health Organization.

16

Counting on Mother's Love: The Global Politics of Prevention of Mother-to-Child Transmission of HIV in Eastern Africa

KAREN MARIE MOLAND AND ASTRID BLYSTAD

Introduction

HIV transmission through pregnancy, birth, and breastfeeding presents the international community with one of the most pressing and ethically sensitive public health issues today. According to WHO updates, about 700,000 infants become infected with HIV every year, mainly because of mother-to-child transmission (MTCT). Of these, an estimated 300,000 children are infected through breast-feeding (UNAIDS 2005). Ninety percent of the MTCT of HIV worldwide occurs in sub-Saharan Africa where the AIDS epidemic in many areas has reversed the gains in life expectancy and child survival achieved during recent decades.

The child at risk of HIV infection, whether in the mother's womb or at her breast, has caused immense concern in the public at large, among health personnel, and policy makers. Throughout the region, programs for prevention of mother-to-child transmission (PMTCT) of HIV are presently being rolled out, but so far these programs only reach a very small minority of the target group. According to Joint United Nations Programme on HIV and AIDS (UNAIDS) estimates, less than 6% of the pregnant women in sub-Saharan Africa were offered services to prevent MTCT in 2005 (UNAIDS 2006:133).

The pregnant women who are reached through PMTCT programs and who test HIV-positive learn that they may transmit the virus to their infants during

447

pregnancy, birth, and breastfeeding. Through counseling they also learn that they may avoid infecting their infants if they take certain precautions and carefully observe instructions related to safe sex, birth care, and infant feeding. Even though the programs are welcomed by the mothers because they carry hope for an HIV-negative child, they have encountered enormous challenges of adherence.

A fundamental predicament of the standard PMTCT concept is that it does not offer treatment or follow-up of any kind for the HIV-positive mother, which implies that she will herself remain with an untreated HIV infection. The program, the aim of which is an HIV-negative child, is defined as one of prevention only. The health and survival of the mother is not an issue that the program addresses, even though the program's success is critically dependent on her efforts as a mother, carrying and nurturing her child.

International policy guidelines aimed at reducing the risk of transmission from mother to child specify methods of infant feeding that are safe (or safer) in terms of HIV transmission. The modifications required in infant feeding practices present particular challenges and concerns that have located infant feeding counseling at the very center of the PMTCT program. The purpose of infant feeding counseling is to prepare the mother to make an informed choice of a feeding method that is appropriate to her particular situation. In sub-Saharan Africa, where breastfeeding is normative and prolonged breast-feeding and early supplementation are customary, any alteration in infant feeding practice is, however, a complex issue that raises a number of collateral questions. Breastfeeding involves more than infant nutrition, and attempts to deviate from established infant feeding practices will engage power relations, social obligations and, we argue, fundamentally challenge customary ideas and values surrounding motherhood.

In this chapter, we seek to explore the experiences of HIV-positive mothers related to choice of infant feeding method, and problems of adherence to that choice in different PMTCT programs in Ethiopia and Tanzania. In an attempt to understand the challenges of the infant feeding component in PMTCT, we ask what is at stake for the individual mother, and why adherence to infant feeding prescriptions in PMTCT programs is so difficult to achieve. Furthermore we discuss how the talk about risk and informed choice define child survival as the responsibility of the HIV-positive mother. We set out not only to identify constraints to the local acceptability and feasibility of the PMTCT program in general and the infant feeding component in particular, but also to discuss the political and ethical conditions on which the PMTCT concept is based. We argue that PMTCT programs may, under particularly favorable circumstances, achieve the goal of an HIV-negative child, not the least because the program, with its emotional and moral appeals to "mother's love," articulates well with local values. But, as we will discuss below, counting on mothers' love without enhancing her survival chances is not an adequate public health response to the problem of MTCT. Neither is it an ethical response to one of the most disturbing public health problems of our time.

Background

Transmission of HIV through Pregnancy, Birth, and Breastfeeding

The problem of MTCT has stimulated considerable research aiming to reduce the HIV transmission risk to the baby in the womb, during delivery, and during breastfeeding. Clinical trials to test the effectiveness of antiretroviral (ARV) prophylaxis to mother and child at the time of birth have been promising in bringing down the transmission rate during labor and delivery. According to De Cock et al. (2000) ARV prophylaxis can reduce the perinatal transmission risk from 20% to 10%. A major problem, however, is that these simple medical regimes do not address the problem of HIV transmission through breastfeeding, which is responsible for as much as 5% to 20% of the pediatric HIV infections (De Cock et al. 2000). Hence, many infants who are HIV-negative at birth become infected during the period of breastfeeding.

The exact transmission risk during breastfeeding has been difficult to estimate because it is connected not only to the viral load in mother's milk but also to the duration of breastfeeding. Coutsoudis et al. (2001) found that the transmission risk is maintained throughout the period of breastfeeding, and estimated the postnatal transmission rate as 15% if women practice prolonged breastfeeding for about 2 years. Furthermore the risk of transmission has been found to be connected to the ways in which breastfeeding is practiced. An increasing number of studies document that exclusive breastfeeding, i.e., giving only breastmilk and no other liquids or solids, not even water, involves a lower risk of MTCT of HIV than mixed breastfeeding (feeding a combination of breastmilk and other foods or liquids) (Coutsoudis, Pillay, Spooner, Kuhn, and Coovadia 1999; Iliff et al. 2005).[1] A recent study by Coovadia et al. (2007) found that infants who received formula milk in addition to breastfeeding were almost twice as likely to be infected as infants who were exclusively breast-fed, and infants who received solid foods in addition to breastmilk were almost 11 times more likely to acquire HIV infection than infants who were exclusively breastfed.

The customary prolonged breastfeeding pattern in sub-Saharan Africa with early supplementation of fluids such as water and animal milk and solids of various kinds has thus been documented to strongly increase the HIV transmission risk to the baby. This adds to the concern about the HIV burden of the region. The knowledge of the risk of HIV transmission through breastfeeding has caused considerable uncertainty and confusion and may threaten the well-established culturally entrenched position of breastfeeding in sub-Saharan Africa. The international guidelines, which are meant to provide mothers and health workers with guidance on how to make infant feeding safer in terms of HIV transmission, have emerged as problematic and have probably added to, rather than reduced, this uncertainty (de Paoli, Manongi, Helsing, and Klepp 2001; Leshabari, Blystad, and Moland 2007).

Policy Guidelines

WHO's policy guidelines issued in 2000 have informed infant feeding counseling in PMTCT programs currently being set up in antenatal clinics in hospitals and health centers in sub-Saharan Africa. These guidelines on HIV and infant feeding have promoted replacement feeding as the first choice of infant feeding method for HIV-positive mothers. They state that "when replacement feeding is acceptable, feasible, affordable, sustainable, and safe, avoidance of all breastfeeding by HIV-infected mothers is recommended. Otherwise exclusive breastfeeding is recommended during the first months of life" (WHO 2000b:12). The guidelines also state that if these prerequisites are not met, exclusive breastfeeding should be practiced until 6 months, and at 6 months there should be rapid cessation of breastfeeding (WHO 2003a:12). Mixed breastfeeding, meaning mixing breastfeeding and any other nutrient, is strongly discouraged. The guidelines state further that the HIV-positive mother should be enabled to make an informed choice about the infant feeding method based on the information provided by the counselor and the so-called AFASS criteria that assess the acceptability, feasibility, affordability, sustainability, and safety of the various methods in the individual woman's situation.

The programs commonly offer a standard package of services consisting of voluntary counseling and testing services (VCT), ARV prophylaxis to the infected woman at the onset of labor[2] and to the infant within 72 hours after birth, and infant feeding counseling. The feeding options for HIV-positive mothers suggested in local PMTCT programs usually include exclusive replacement feeding or exclusive breastfeeding with early cessation (4–6 months). Exclusive replacement feeding is either commercial infant formula or home-modified animal milk. Although the options suggested by WHO include wet-nursing and expressed and heat-treated breastmilk also, these methods are generally not considered acceptable and feasible in the context of high HIV prevalence in sub-Saharan Africa, and are hence usually not adopted into local PMTCT programs.

Enhanced PMTCT Programs

In standard PMTCT programs, which do not address the survival chances of the mother, many of the children lose their mother to AIDS before they reach 1 year. Hence a highly ethically charged scenario characterized by an escalation of an already massive orphan challenge has been brought to the forefront through PMTCT programs. This sensitive problem has created an outcry calling for more comprehensive approaches. Initiatives that link prevention of infant HIV infection with care and treatment for the mothers are currently being tried out in a WHO coordinated multicenter clinical trial and in so-called MTCT+ projects. The aims of these initiatives are not only to increase prevention efficacy and improve the child's survival chances through exclusive breastfeeding, but also to improve the mother's health and her survival chances through HAART (highly active antiretroviral treatment) to her and her partner (WHO 2003b). Apart from a very limited number of ongoing clinical trials and interventions, PMTCT and HAART programs are, however, to date run separately, and are based in different departments (antenatal and medical departments), with limited client overlap.

The Infant Feeding Controversy

Promotion of exclusive feeding (either exclusive breastfeeding or exclusive replacement feeding) of infants born to HIV-positive mothers has proved to be a very controversial issue (Rollins 2007). The problem is connected to the fact that the global burden of HIV lies in sub-Saharan Africa where the major cause of infant death is malnutrition and infectious diseases (Coutsoudis, Goga, Rollins, and Coovadia 2002). At the same time as breastfeeding involves a considerable risk of HIV transmission, *not* breastfeeding is known to imply a considerable risk to infant survival in low-income countries (Black, Morris, and Bryce 2003). The promotion of breastfeeding has been ranked the most effective intervention for child survival internationally (Jones Steketee, Black, Bhutta, and Morris 2003). The physical benefits of breastfeeding are well documented (Coutsoudis et al. 2002), and breastfeeding, in particular during the first 6 months of life, reduces the risk of morbidity and mortality associated with infections diseases (WHO 2000a) and protects against deaths from diarrhea and pneumonia. The United Nations International Children's Emergency Fund (UNICEF) estimates that not breastfeeding is responsible for 1.5 million child deaths per year (UNAIDS 2000), and presents us with figures that by far outnumber the risks associated with HIV transmission through breastmilk.

How to weigh the benefits of breastfeeding against the risk of HIV infection is an issue that is presently vigorously debated. Some have maintained that considering the risk of infection through breastfeeding, replacement feeding should be the first choice as it is in high-income contexts, and could be made safer through a close follow-up during the infant feeding period (Brahmbhatt and Gray 2003). Others have maintained that even in the event of HIV transmission through breastmilk, breastfeeding is still the best option for HIV-infected women because of its immunological and nutritional advantages (see e.g., Coutsoudis et al. 2002; Piwoz and Ross 2005). In a study in South Africa, Thior, Lockman, and Smeaton (2005) found that even if breastfeeding with ARV prophylaxis (zidovudine) was not as effective as formula feeding in preventing postnatal HIV transmission, it was associated with a lower infant mortality rate at 7 months. The study brought renewed attention to the complexity of dangers related to formula feeding in low-income settings.

In view of the customary infant feeding pattern in sub-Saharan Africa and the dangers involved in not breastfeeding, a major challenge has become how to make breastfeeding safer (Rollins 2007). A significant step forward emerged through the intervention (cohort) study from South Africa by Coovadia et al. (2007) which aimed to assess the HIV transmission risks and survival associated with exclusive breastfeeding as compared with formula feeding and mixed feeding. In contrast to the study by Thior et al. referred to above, this study found that infants who were exclusively breast-fed did not run a greater postnatal risk of HIV transmission than infants who were formula fed. Mortality at 3 months was in fact almost double in the group that received formula feeding compared with the exclusively breast-fed infants. The reason for the diverging findings could be linked to the close follow-up offered in the latter study (Rollins 2007).

On the basis of recent findings, WHO concluded that exclusive breastfeeding involves a 2- to 4-fold lower risk of HIV transmission than mixed feeding, and updated the recommendation on HIV and infant feeding accordingly. It now reads, "Exclusive breastfeeding is recommended for HIV-infected women for the first 6 months of life unless replacement feeding is acceptable, feasible, affordable, sustainable and safe for them and their infants before that time" (WHO 2006:4).

The Problem of Choice and Adherence

However, the debate on infant feeding is not only on medical risk, safety, and feasibility but also on choice and women's rights to knowledge. The concern about the right to knowledge about risk and risk reduction and the right to choose among alternative infant feeding methods is reflected in the international guidelines that advocate informed choice of infant feeding method (WHO 2000b). The implementation of informed choice in concrete PMTCT settings is, however, very complicated in a situation where the actual risk of MTCT of HIV through breastfeeding is uncertain (Iliff et al. 2005). Furthermore, none of the infant feeding methods available (exclusive breastfeeding and exclusive replacement feeding) can guarantee the prevention of MTCT and at the same time ensure the good health of the child. Kuhn, Stein, and Susser (2004) hold that a fundamental recognition of these facts makes infant feeding counseling a very challenging task. Infant feeding is also an issue of decision-making power.

Not the least, a fear of disclosure of HIV-positive status works to undermine women's ability to resist the social pressure from kin and neighbors to feed the infant in the customary manner (Doherty, Chopra, Nkonki, Jackson, and Greiner 2006). Several studies that have investigated the relevance of the global guidelines in local contexts conclude that infant feeding choice and adherence to that choice cannot be understood in isolation from the social and cultural context in which the woman feeds her infant (see e.g., Moland 2004; Leshabari et al. 2007; Thairu, Pelto, Rollins, Bland, and Ntchangase 2005). Several studies furthermore fundamentally criticize the anticipated global validity of the international infant feeding guidelines and advocate approaches that are more locally informed (see e.g., Kuhn et al. 2004; Leshabari, Koniz-Booher, Åstrøm, de Paoli, and Moland 2006).

Through an exploration of what is at stake for the individual HIV-positive mother nurturing her infant we seek to examine the broader social and moral concerns that are raised through PMTCT. We explore not only conditions that work to hinder safer infant feeding practices among HIV-positive women, but also conditions that enhance the possibilities for women to adhere to safer infant feeding practices.

The Research Setting

The authors have carried out long-term community work and fieldwork in eastern Africa since the 1980s. The research, on which the present chapter is based, was carried out in Ethiopia and Tanzania. The choice of these 2 countries for the present study was linked to the authors' research experience and language competence and to their knowledge of the national and local contexts in which the PMTCT programs were implemented. Furthermore, for a study that investigates the impact of a global health policy measure in local contexts, the different sociopolitical and epidemiological history of the 2 countries appeared potentially interesting. In terms of health and development indicators both the countries are rated among the poorest in the world. Very high maternal mortality rates (reported as 870 per 100,000 live births in Ethiopia and 580 in Tanzania in 2005 [UNICEF 2005]) are commonly used as indicators for poor general health standards as well as for malfunctioning health systems. Tanzania provides an HIV scenario that is relatively "typical" in an East African context, with a prevalence of around 6.5% in the adult population (Kenya 6% and Uganda 6.7%) and a prevalence of 7% among women attending antenatal clinics. Ethiopia, by comparison, has a lower overall national prevalence estimated at 1.4% (UNAIDS/WHO 2006), but the urban prevalence is above 10% and the prevalence among women attending antenatal clinics between 2003 and 2004 was as high as 8.5% (UNAIDS 2006).[3]

With a population of more than 80 million, the total number of HIV-positive individuals is however similar to that of Tanzania—a frightening 1.5 million people (UNAIDS/WHO 2006; HAPCO 2004). The very high number of people living with HIV presents both countries with enormous challenges in terms of prevention, treatment, and care. PMTCT initiatives have a slightly longer history in Tanzania than in Ethiopia. Although the number of PMTCT sites is quickly expanding to both hospitals and health centers in both countries, the service coverage is still limited. The policies and programs on PMTCT are very similar across the two countries, not the least because of the fact that they are guided by the same international guidelines.

The studies were linked up with various health institutions in the 2 countries—namely, Haydom Lutheran Hospital and Kilimanjaro Christian Medical Centre in Tanzania; Arba Minch Hospital and Yirga Alem Hospital in Southern Ethiopia; and Zewditu Hospital and 3 urban-based health centers in Addis Ababa (Bale, Tekleheimanot and Addis Ketema). Our study informants represent diverse ethnic and religious affiliation. Moreover, they differ in terms of age, educational- and occupational background and rural/urban residence. In the present research, the geographical location did not seem to have substantial impact on the general level of confusion regarding the WHO recommendations among staff and patients. The differences that emerged were rather linked to the particularities of the PMTCT programs and to factors linked to the individual woman such as economy and social support. For these reasons and to ensure anonymity, we will, with a few exceptions, not explicitly mention the health institution to which the informants were linked. All names used in the presentations are pseudonyms to further ensure confidentiality.

The Fieldwork

The present chapter draws upon material collected on PMTCT programs during several study periods of fieldwork in Ethiopia and Tanzania from 2002 to 2007. Fieldwork took place for a period of 7 months in Addis Ababa in Ethiopia, and for shorter periods in Arba Minch and Yirga Alem in Ethiopia and Haydom/Mbulu and Moshi in Tanzania.[4] Case studies, in-depth interviews, focus group discussions, and observation were used as prime data collection methods. The main groups of informants were HIV-positive women—primarily pregnant women and women with infants—and nurse counselors who were recruited from standard PMTCT programs (in Addis Ababa, Arba Minch, Yirga Alem and Moshi) and from one enhanced PMTCT program (in Haydom/Mbulu).

Data collection in the Addis Ababa study (2005–2007) was linked up with Tesfago, a local People Living with HIV (PLHIV) organization, and 3 health centers and 1 hospital running PMTCT programs in the city. The 3 health centers were all part of a pilot PMTCT initiative run by Addis Ababa Health Bureau in collaboration with an international NGO (Intrahealth International) that was started in 2003. The 4 PMTCT sites offered a standard package of services (as described in the background). Infant feeding counseling presented the mothers with a choice of exclusive breastfeeding with early cessation or exclusive replacement feeding with either cow's milk or manufactured infant formula. None of the programs provided free infant formula or any kind of material support. The PMTCT programs were located in different subcities (*woreda*), and the women recruited to participate in the study were spread in many different urban communities (*kebelles*). This fact, combined with the very confidential nature of the study topic and the risk of disclosure of HIV status as a result of research attention, made it impossible to locate the study in one community and employ a traditional ethnographic approach.

Data collection in the Mbulu/Haydom study was carried out in the catchment area of Haydom Lutheran Hospital in September/October 2005 and October 2006. The extensive HIV-related activity based at Haydom Lutheran Hospital (HLH) was the vantage point for this part of the research. The PMTCT+ program was 1 of the 5 major pillars of the Haydom HIV program and was based on pre- and posttest counseling of the woman, disclosure of HIV status to a "guardian" (who accompanies the woman to the hospital), ARV treatment of the mother, and a single-dose Niverapine to mother and child at the time of birth. Exclusive breastfeeding with rapid cessation at 4 to 6 months was promoted, and material support in the form of a few free food items during the period of breastfeeding as well as free cow's milk after weaning was provided. The PMTCT+ package also included weekly support by community home-based care providers, occasional home visits by PMTCT counselors and monthly meetings for HIV-positive women.

To the extent possible, the research at the 2 main research sites, Haydom/Mbulu and Addis Ababa, used the same data collection methods. These consisted of in-depth interviews with HIV-positive women during pregnancy and/or during the infant feeding period, and with some of their partners. The interviews were carried out at the hospital and during home visits. At Haydom/Mbulu, the hospital-based interviews were tape-recorded and transcribed, but the interviews in Addis Ababa were translated by a research assistant and recorded in handwritten notes because informants were skeptical about having their voices and stories taped. Another issue that varied was follow-up. The home visits were characterized by more informal talk. In the Addis Ababa study, 21 informants were followed up at home or other convenient places during the critical phase of infant feeding—the first 6 months after birth. Furthermore, counselors, home-based care providers (HBCP) (Haydom only), members of HIV-positive organizations, as well as diverse groups of community members were interviewed.

The fieldwork was also drawing upon observation of various HIV-related settings including pre- and posttest VCT and PMTCT counseling, meetings for HIV-positive pregnant and breastfeeding women and village based outreach meetings. Focus group discussions were carried out with HIV-positive women, nurse counselors, traditional birth attendants, and home-based care providers.

The research in Arba Minch and Yirga Alem in southern Ethiopia was carried out jointly during 2 shorter fieldwork periods between 2005 and 2006. The data collection primarily consisted of individual interviews with HIV-positive hospital staff and patients as well as with counselors and physicians linked to the HIV programs at the major hospitals in the 2 areas. Brief periods of fieldwork were also carried out in Moshi, northern Tanzania, where HIV-positive mothers enrolled in PMTCT programs and traditional birth attendants as well as regular community members were interviewed informally.

Research Ethics

Research with a highly sensitive thematic focus requires particular caution regarding disclosure of information, in this case the threat of disclosing the HIV-positive status of women in a highly vulnerable situation, which had to be taken very seriously. Substantial effort was placed on ensuring the research participants' confidentiality. Recruitment of the HIV-positive women was done by PMTCT counselors, extension workers, and hospital staff living with HIV. The principle of informed consent was strongly emphasized. Quite a few women did not agree to participate in the study because of fear of disclosure. In some cases women agreed to participate on the condition that we did not visit them at home. An alternative location was chosen by the mother in such cases.

Concerns with Infant Feeding in a Time of AIDS

We will, in the following section, present study findings through glimpses of the multi-faceted, contradictory, and troubling scenarios that emerged surrounding HIV and infant feeding in the 5 study areas. All the narratives and quotes in the following cases are derived from interviews with HIV-positive women aged between 18 and 35 years and with nurse counselors in PMTCT programs. Where nothing else is mentioned, the material presented is from one of the standard PMTCT programs mentioned earlier.

Confusion over Choice of Infant Feeding Method

Making a choice about infant feeding method emerged as an issue of great concern to the HIV-positive mothers in the study. As individual counselors and HIV-positive women sought to make sense of and relate to the PMTCT prescriptions, a variety of complex responses emerged. A finding across the material, however, was a bewilderment regarding the information the nurse counselors presented about infant feeding options as the following 2 cases indicate.

"There Is Virus in the Milk." Mariam is 25 years old and is married. Her husband is also HIV-positive. When they learned about the PMTCT program, they decided to try to have a child together. Mariam was highly motivated to follow the PMTCT program, the take the medication, give birth in the hospital, and practice safe sex and safe infant feeding. She enrolled in the PMTCT program nearby and was counseled on infant feeding during pregnancy. Having considered the different options together with her husband, she ended up planning to exclusively breastfeed. It was only after delivery that she got confused. When the nurse gave Mariam her child after delivery, she warned her that "there is virus in the milk," and asked her if she knew that the virus can be transmitted through breastfeeding. She asked if Mariam was willing to feed her baby by the breast. The nurse also told her that if she could manage she should not breastfeed. Mariam was exhausted after the delivery and did not know what to do. Her major concern was to not transmit the virus to the child. She had set her mind on solely breastfeeding, but now became very uncertain, and told the nurse: "I cannot decide, ask my husband." The husband responded that if HIV is transmitted through breastmilk, the child should not be breastfed. He should get cow's milk. When we visited the following morning we found Mariam in tears. She was feeding her child with a bottle, but told us that the child had vomited several times and was unsettled. Her breasts were tense and uncomfortable, yet she was not supposed to breastfeed. A friend who was there cooking complained about Mariam's decision to give cow's milk since she and her husband did not have a regular income and did not even have enough food for Mariam to eat during her confinement period. She thought it would be better for Mariam to breastfeed. Mariam said she wished to breastfeed her child, but since the nurse and the husband were against it she became confused. Her friend resolutely took the bottle and threw it in the bin. Then she gave the baby to Mariam to breastfeed. In view of the warning that "there is virus in the milk," the father later said that he felt that it had been difficult to insist on breastfeeding. But when Mariam changed to breastfeeding the day after, he accepted it because he knew that providing cow's milk for 6 months was going to be very difficult. To Mariam the issue was a very emotional one. As her breasts filled with milk, she experienced a bodily urge to breastfeed and she felt strongly that she was doing the right thing when she started to breastfeed her baby.

This case shows a confused decision-making process where the nurse–midwife in the delivery room adds doubt and uncertainty about the safety of breastfeeding. Related to her fear of the virus in the milk, she promotes formula feeding without discussing the mother's wishes and possibilities. With the aim of bringing down the HIV transmission rate, a majority of the counselors in the studies kept a substantial focus on the risk of HIV transmission through breastmilk, and left out information about the nutritional and immunological benefits of mother's milk. Similarly, when they counseled women on replacement feeding, many nurses tended to focus on risk reduction in terms of HIV transmission, leaving out the risks of childhood infections and malnutrition. Hence, breastfeeding was commonly promoted as an alternative for the unfortunate mother who cannot afford the best and safest infant feeding option, as the subsequent case indicates.

"You Are Poor—You Should BreastFeed." In contrast to Mariam, Worknesh, a 24-year-old single mother, had not voluntarily disclosed her HIV status to anybody in her family or in the compound where she rented a room. When she was told about her HIV status, Worknesh offered to take part in a PMTCT research program where she would get close follow-up of her child if she was willing to breastfeed. She told us: "They informed me about exclusive breastfeeding and told me I should breastfeed because I am poor, but I nonetheless decided to feed the child NAN [infant formula]. It was my choice because it is safer." But despite her decision to replacement feed, Worknesh ended up breastfeeding, as she did not manage to secure enough formula. She experienced feeding her baby as a big burden because of the constant fear of HIV transmission. She explained: "I did not have a choice, so I breastfed the child for 2 months. I was very nervous when I breastfed and I was crying a lot. I worried about my child."

The 2 conflicting counseling messages that the women in the examples above refer to, namely "there is virus in the milk" and "you are poor–you should breastfeed," spring out of the infant feeding guidelines highlighted by the so-called AFASS criteria and powerfully reveal the ambiguity and uncertainty pervading infant feeding counseling. Whereas the first message implies that breastfeeding is risky and should be avoided, the second message implies that, "in your situation" you have no choice but to take the risk. This experience is powerfully summed up in several similar statements from a focus group discussion with traditional birth attendants in Addis Ababa who stated that: "If the mother is poor she has to breastfeed and let the child die."

The 2 examples also demonstrate how the awareness of risk takes on different bodily expressions in the experiences of the 2 women trying to secure the health and survival of their babies. Whereas Mariam expressed a bodily urge to breastfeed, Worknesh expressed a deep bodily discomfort in having to breastfeed. How the knowledge of MTCT is embodied in the desire or repugnance to breastfeed varies with the individual woman, and is not the least related to her experiences with infant feeding counseling and the knowledge and information exchanged with the counselor and with individuals in her immediate social surroundings.

Women's initial intention to choose one or the other infant feeding method was found to be considerably influenced by the particular message presented during individual counseling sessions. Being exposed to different sources of knowledge and having different experiences with infant feeding, counselors would gain their own thoughts and preferences related to the issue. Some counselors would strongly promote exclusive breastfeeding because they believed it was the only feasible and acceptable option for poor HIV-positive mothers. Others would primarily promote replacement feeding because they felt it was ethically wrong or difficult to advise women to expose their infants to HIV transmission through breastmilk. The preferences tended to follow institutional lines, but would sometimes also vary between individuals within the same institution.

The substantial differences in terms of actual infant feeding messages presented during counseling sessions became quite noticeable when we moved among the different research locations. Indeed, at 3 of the 5 major study sites, different PMTCT programs located in close geographical proximity to each other would promote divergent infant feeding methods as first choice. Whereas one health facility in a location would promote exclusive breastfeeding on a routine basis, another health facility in the vicinity would promote replacement feeding to the same population.

Family Pressure

Our study demonstrates that the actual choice of infant feeding method a woman makes is strongly influenced by the limitations as well as opportunities that prevail in her wider social environment. Indeed, her choice will be strongly influenced by actual or sensed inputs or pressures from significant others, such as partners, parents, mothers-in-law or neighbors as the next examples indicate.

While she was pregnant Nigist, told us, "After being counseled I decided to feed my baby breastmilk for four months. I cannot afford to buy milk anyhow and I like to feed him by the breast."

After delivery she had changed her mind however:

> I considered breastfeeding, but people told me that since the virus is in the milk I should not. I bought NAN and gave that the first months before I continued with cow's milk. But it was difficult; the baby vomited a lot as I did not know how to dilute. He did not put on weight and got very sick. We were admitted in hospital only 6 days after delivery and the nurse taught me how to dilute the powder. Then I understood ... When my mother came from the countryside to see me and the baby after birth she was shocked to see that I did not breastfeed. She asked me how I expected this child to grow and told me that I harm my

baby. She told me that I should breastfeed. So I gave in and started breastfeeding. But it did not last for long. When she left I went back to NAN and kept him on that for 4 months.

Nigist explained that her mother had come a long way to visit her. She had to pay her respect and felt obliged to yield to her wishes, but it was a great relief when she left and Nigist was able to reassume sole responsibility for feeding her baby.

In the case of Absera, the husband became deeply involved in the infant feeding issue. Both learned about their HIV-positive status during the pregnancy, and the husband was very concerned about the risk of disclosure to his family who lived nearby. Absera told us:

> I was counselled to give powder milk if we could afford it, but when I told my husband he said that if I would do that the family would become suspicious. He said that I'd better give both, breast and powder, as they would then not suspect anything ... Finally I have decided that I will breastfeed. After delivery I will be in the house of my mother in law. I think she will accept that I do not want to give the child any water.

When a couple has discordant HIV status and the HIV status is disclosed between the partners, the husband's voice on infant feeding emerges as crucial. If he can afford to buy infant formula he may insist that his infant should not be breastfed as the following example illustrates.

> Lakech did not feel that she had a choice regarding infant feeding. She is married to an HIV negative man. She told us, "My husband does not want to hear the word breastfeeding. He wants me to feed the baby NAN. He has a salary and we can afford it. Our first-born died. I would like to be able to breastfeed, but I do fear the virus."

In an HIV context where customary feeding is increasingly interpreted as a threat to child survival, the social nature of infant feeding decisions is clearly demonstrated. All the examples above show that choice of infant feeding method is not an issue that is left to the mother alone. On the contrary, it raises considerable concern among close kin in general and among husbands in particular. Furthermore, the examples demonstrate the difference between intention and actual choice. They show how the mother's intention to choose one or the other method of feeding is often compromised by a variety of contingencies related to counseling services and to the social environment in which the mother feeds her infant.

The impact of a constraining or conducive social environment surrounding HIV-positive women will further emerge in the next section where we shift our focus from the situation of choice of infant feeding method to the experiences presented by the women as they move through the phase of trying to comply with the chosen method.

The Struggle to Observe Infant Feeding Prescriptions

Even though the PMTCT programs are guided by the principles of informed choice of infant feeding method, not all counselors openly present the various options for the women to consider, as was seen in examples mentioned earlier. Irrespective of whatever is presented and recommended, the challenges related to following the infant feeding instructions proved to be numerous. Eliwayda's story introduces us to some of the challenges related to the exclusive breast-feeding regime. She is linked to a so-called PMTCT+ site where only exclusive breastfeeding with rapid cessation at 3 to 6 months is promoted. The program offers HAART for treatment of the mothers and extended support from nurse counselors and home-based care providers. A major concern common to most women enrolled in this program as well as in standard PMTCT programs is that they fear social stigma and exclusion and, hence, choose not to disclose their HIV status to other family members and/or in the communities where they live.

The Instruction to Infant Feed "Exclusively." Eliwayda is 32 years old, is married, and has 5 live children, the youngest being 4 months old. One child died at birth 9 years ago, whereas another died during the first year some 3 years back. Eliwayda learned about her HIV infection during an antenatal checkup in her last pregnancy, and was at that point introduced to the dangers of transmission of HIV to her infant. Four months after delivery she told us the following story:

> I struggle with the feeding of the baby. I make an effort to follow the instructions given to me by the counselors. They tell me to breastfeed without giving the baby anything else for 6 months and then to stop abruptly and start with other foods. But I worry. Will I really have milk enough to solely breastfeed the child for 2 more months? I breastfed my other children for almost 2 years, but I gave them water and soup from when they were 3 months old. The sister of my mother-in-law tells me to give the baby at least some drops of cow's milk and water. But I don't give him any. Since I have this problem I have been told I am not allowed to give even a drop of water. My other children are often tempted to give the baby some liquids, but I tell them that he can die if he gets water, and it is not a lie. Even though he is getting heavy I bring him to the fields now, and never leave him with others. I am so afraid that he will be infected by this vicious virus. People ask me: "Eliwayda do you really manage to cultivate when you bring your child along? I answer that his siblings cannot yet take properly care of him."

The nurses continue to encourage me and tell me that I will manage. They explain how I shall cope with the situation, they laugh together with me, and tell me that I can depend upon their support. They even like us I think. Sometimes I become confused. Really, there are times when I want to run away and leave the child with mama Neema (counselor at the hospital).

A home-based care provider comes to our home by bike twice a week, and brings vegetables, a little flower, a couple of eggs or some fruits to help me increase the milk production. She comes home to me, and I continue to live. She tells me: "What are you thinking about Eliwayda? Don't think, live with hope, this is now a common illness." Several months back we decided to tell people that this baby has a stomach problem that makes it dangerous for him to get anything but my milk. But after 6 months we must plan the whole thing carefully again, because at that point the baby can suddenly have no more milk from me, and then I need to say the opposite … I need to find a reason I can tell people for feeding my child in such a strange way. I thank God that until now I have not fed the baby anything but my own milk.

Eliwayda managed to follow the recommendations, as did apparently many other women at this particular PMTCT site. This was found to be closely related to a number of particular features of the PMTCT+ program: Only exclusive breastfeeding was promoted, that is, the women were not presented with infant feeding choices; treatment to ensure the mother's survival was provided (HAART); there was close follow-up by health care providers; and some limited material support was provided during the infant feeding period. This particular package of services offered seemed to greatly influence a mother's possibilities of adhering to the recommended feeding methods. This is however far from the standard PMTCT package offered at most sites in sub-Saharan Africa. Our findings indicate that without comprehensive inputs including continuity of care and close follow-up, major problems of adherence will occur, producing mixed feeding patterns, the least favorable option in terms of risk of HIV transmission, as expressed in the following cases:

Elisabeth, who knew about her HIV-positive status before she got pregnant with her first-born child, told us:

I chose exclusive breastfeeding because I had nothing else to give, so for the first 2 weeks after birth I only gave breastmilk. When I went for follow up in the clinic after birth I met a nurse who reminded me that there is virus in the milk and said that it was better to stop breastfeeding. I was also worried about feeding my child bad milk, so I decided to stop. I started feeding the baby with the bottle, but soon did not have enough money to buy the powder, so I gave a little bit of each. When I went back to the clinic for the third visit I met a different nurse who said: "Are you bottle feeding? You should breastfeed!" So I went home and tried to breastfeed only, but I was so tired. I was exhausted. I was very skinny and could not eat. I could not feed my child. I hated myself, and fed him whatever milk I had.

Sara, who is in her mid 20s and was recently left by her HIV-positive husband, recalls:

> The first day after birth I had no milk so the hospital staff gave me powder to give the baby. I was very sick and I could not take care of my child. I suspected that the child was positive already at birth. I started breastfeeding, but I got very stressed. He was so small. He could not suck. I did not have enough milk. He was starving. His stool was very dry, so I gave him water. I also gave him "camomilla" to relieve abdominal cramps. After 40 days I gave up and started giving powdered milk again. I was informed not to mix; but when I did not have enough powder, what could I do? After 1 year and 6 months, the child was tested. He was like me, HIV positive.

Both Elisabeth and Sara were informed by their counselors that they should not mix breastfeeding with other milk or food, but circumstances worked otherwise. Their major and immediate concern was to relieve the pain of a hungry child. The risk of HIV infection, though a major worry, was not the number one concern.

The Instruction to Stop Breastfeeding Early and Rapidly. A further major obstacle was experienced in relation to the requirement of rapid discontinuation of breastfeeding at the age of 6 months, or earlier if necessary, to reduce the likelihood of mixed feeding. For some women the early weaning in fact turned out to be the most hazardous requirement of all, as for Aster:

> I breastfed my child for 55 days without giving her anything else but some water. At that point I had to go back to my work. I left the house in the morning and came back late, and therefore had to introduce cow's milk. I gave her breastmilk at night only the first days because breastfeeding is good for the child, but after 60 days I stopped completely. The baby wanted the breast. I used to cry with the child at night. I was alone. This was the most difficult part for me. I was away all day working and could not make my child grow. I had to give up my job.

Although rapid cessation is a major challenge both because it is emotionally and practically difficult and because it commonly raises a lot of questions and suspicion, some do succeed as the following example illustrates.

After delivery, Agnes moved into the house of her mother-in-law as is customary in the area where she lives. She did not disclose her HIV-positive status to anybody, and was very nervous that the mother-in-law would give the baby other foods and fluids. She therefore kept a constant eye on her and the baby. Apart from a few incidents where her mother-in-law had given the baby water, Agnes told us that she managed to stick to exclusive breastfeeding. At 4 months, her husband, her mother-in-law, and her neighbors complained that the child was crying during the night and that it was not putting on weight. They advised her to start giving other foods. When she did not do as she was advised, her husband threatened that he would start giving the child porridge. The pressure was so great that Agnes decided to stop breastfeeding so that she could start giving other foods. However, she would not do it while at home, as she feared people's questions. She rather went to stay with her mother for 2 months and with her support managed to stop breastfeeding rapidly. When she came back the child was 6 months and was doing well on other foods. At that point nobody bothered to ask her any more about it.

The very real doubt about actual observance of the exclusive feeding regimes emerged strongly in relation to both exclusive replacement feeding and exclusive breastfeeding, and was related, as we have seen, to a complex scenario of everyday obstacles. The counselors themselves would indeed, at times, voice frustration over the challenging new infant feeding prescriptions. As one counselor who had earlier worked with the promotion of exclusive breastfeeding put it:

> In this part of the world it has been the breast since time immemorial. Now, people ask what kind of a sickness this is that can prevent women from breastfeeding? ... In our community campaigns we have told women to breastfeed their children properly, and now suddenly comes news about the dangers of breastmilk and warnings against breastfeeding. She herself feels healthy, the baby is healthy, but she should not breastfeed her child!?

Striving to be a Good Mother

A common concept in all four project areas is that "a real mother is a mother who breastfeeds her child." As one woman told us: "I like to breastfeed because of love itself—as a mother." Having good and enough milk was located at the heart of women's nurturing concerns. Many mothers worried that the milk they produced would not be enough for the child to thrive. A counselor was concerned that the customary mixed feeding pattern that was practiced was linked to the idea of mother's milk not being enough for an infant to grow:

> It is not necessarily right that their [women's] milk production is insufficient. You will find that many actually have enough milk. It is the thought that their milk will not satisfy the child, that there will be too little milk that frightens them. This is a fear among all women, whether HIV positive or not, because then they won't fulfill the expectations of mothers as the ones who secure the healthy growth of their child.

But mother's milk is more than food. The HIV epidemic and the problem of HIV transmission through mother's milk has made this very clear. Abebesh was constantly worrying about what she transfers to her newborn infant through breastfeeding. She told us:

> The child gets everything from his mother's milk. If the mother is a patient, the child will get the disease, if she is healthy and clean, the child gets cleanliness, if she is

well fed, the child will be well fed. If she is healthy or sick the child will be the same. Breast milk is made from blood—it is the same, it is produced by the same body.

The child mirrors the state of the mother and the responsibility for the health of the child unquestionably rests with the mother. Hence, HIV-positive mothers are often overwhelmed by a feeling of guilt for posing such an overt bodily risk to the child's health. Abebesh, who struggles hard to exclusively breastfeed, sees adherence to the exclusive breastfeeding regime as a penitence for her mistake of becoming pregnant while being HIV-positive. She feels that she has to make this sacrifice for her "unlucky child" whom she has unwillingly exposed to risk: "I do not want to harm my child so I have to breast-feed him up to 6 months. I tell myself that instead of him having a problem, I better have the problem. I was the one who brought the problem."

The experience of guilt pervades both the period of pregnancy and breast-feeding as expressed by Mulu in the following quote.

> During the time of pregnancy I was thinking a lot about the bad things that could happen to the baby inside my womb. It was hard to carry the child because I did not know. When I was counselled on infant feeding, the nurse told me to breastfeed because I am poor. But I do not want to breastfeed. I will never give him my breast. I know the milk is coming from my body. I do not want him to grow by my body.

When Mulu had practiced replacement feeding for a few months she was still convinced that she did the right thing not to breastfeed her baby, but she was uncertain about the bonds created between herself and the baby. She said "I wish I had been able to breastfeed. I wonder when my son grows up, whether he will see me as his real mother." Mulu expressed not only lack of confidence that her body could produce good milk but also experienced her body as a threat to the survival of her child. At the same time, however, she questioned if close motherly bonds would develop in the absence of breastfeeding.

The location of breastfeeding in the center of the mothering experience and the sense of loss if not breastfeeding are clearly expressed also by Tarikwa who is married to an HIV-negative man and who ended up formula feeding her baby: "My only thought is not to infect my baby so I give powder milk, but my own interest is to feed him by my breast. I am a mother, so I want to breastfeed. I'd like to love him more."

Testing the Child: The Great Ordeal

The significance placed on the HIV test of the child at 18 months is immense and is experienced as a fatal moment that decides the future of the child. It also decides how a woman will be judged by herself and others as a mother. Counselor informants pointed to the responsibility placed on a woman for her child's survival. It is not the child alone that is tested, they noted. The mother Grace, in the example below, interpreted the event also as a test of herself as a committed mother observing the instructions of the nurse to feed her child breastmilk only. When she came to the hospital for the test she had told the counselor, "Today I have come. Today I have come for the big exam, I don't know if I have failed or if I have passed." The counselor recalled, "We tested the child and her fear was so huge that she could not stand up nor talk. When she got the result that her baby was HIV-negative she cried out: 'Is it true or do you fool me?'"

The concept of "failing or passing the exam" as a mother clearly describes the emotional stress and the sole responsibility felt by women struggling to get an HIV-negative child. The close connection between carefully observing the instructions of the counselor to exclusively breastfeed and getting an HIV-negative test is also pointed to by the counselor honoring Grace for her success. The counselor recalls the conversation: "Well didn't you do as I told you?" She answered "Yes! If I went to my neighbors I said, 'Don't feed my child. You may even be witches, don't give him even a drop of water, do you hear?'"

To others who may not have been able to adhere so strictly to the infant feeding instructions, the test carries no less importance. Elisabeth knew that she had exposed her child to additional risk through mixed feeding giving "whatever milk she had" and she had a friend whose child tested positive. Recognizing the importance of the test, and at the same time the haphazard nature of the test result, she said, "Getting a child and then getting an HIV-negative child was a lottery, a *tombola*. It was God's *tombola* and I won."

Regaining Control

The possibility of actively pursuing exclusive feeding methods as a way of getting an HIV-negative child appears for some to be experienced as an opportunity to regain some control and take charge of the situation. Women who are suspected to be HIV-positive or women who are declared as HIV positive are carefully monitored throughout pregnancy and after childbirth. Getting an HIV-negative child is in these cases is understood as an achievement on the part of the mother and enhances her social standing. As expressed by a traditional birth attendant in a focus group discussion: "People show respect to a mother who grows her child well."

The fundamental respect met by women who successfully manage to bring up children gains an additional dimension in an HIV context. Elisabeth has disclosed her HIV status on TV, and has had to tolerate a lot of scorn from family and neighbors, but as they have observed her child grow up healthy, their attitude toward her is changing, "When people got to know that I have an HIV-negative child they started showing me respect. Nobody insults me now. I have become useful—I am the mother of a healthy child. I have someone to replace me. People see me as an example."

This was also strongly emphasized by Mariam (in the first case presented) who named her baby "Yedenkachew," meaning "let them be surprised." She explained that although her HIV status has been known in the neighborhood, people have started to doubt that she is HIV-positive since her child is healthy and grows well. They have started to approach her with respect.

Failing and Blaming

Although women with HIV-negative children regain respect, it is common to blame the mother if the child turns out to be HIV-positive. They blame her for becoming pregnant and for exposing her child to the virus in her body. Eliwayda told us:

> Some really don't manage to exclusively breastfeed. I told one among us at Haydom: "If you are told by Mama Upendo to continue to breastfeed for 6 months, and the child is now 3 months and you feed him soup here and breastfeed him there, you surely give him a problem. I can't feel sorry for her even in front of God. Who is she to blame but herself?"

The baby focus in PMTCT programs reinforces the idea that it is the mother who carries the responsibility for the health of the child. The way to save your child from infection is presented as dependent upon a mother's proper follow-up of counselors' instructions. This was demonstrated by the following statements by women enrolled in the PMTCT+ program:

> The counsellor asked me, "Would you like your child to become like yourself?" I answered no. She then replied, "Well if you don't want the child to get the virus, make great effort to swallow the pills properly." I pray intensely that the child does not get this problem.
>
> I will follow this program because they [the nurses] have promised that if I follow the instructions my child will not be infected. The mother who truly loves her child and wants him to have good health must adhere to these rules given to us. Since I have got this problem I just have to follow the instructions in the way I have been given them.

A counselor commented upon the child focus in PMTCT programs saying, "These women make up an entirely different category of sick people, because they first and foremost fear for the health of their child. It becomes very different from people with other diagnoses."

The idea of a mother's individual responsibility for the health of the baby is a very explicit strategy in promoting commitment to exclusive feeding regimes and, when successful, may give vulnerable women a sense of control. This demanding concept places a huge additional burden on exposed and vulnerable women as revealed in many of the examples above.

Concerned about the undue pressures placed upon the HIV-positive mothers in PMTCT programs, a nurse counselor reflected:

> This is so difficult for a new mother to carry through. Some don't manage because of all the pressures. Why can't they just get HAART to reduce the viral load, and continue to breastfeed as usual while they take the medicine—if it is possible. It is too taxing on them as mothers to struggle with these demanding infant feeding regimes.

Global Politics and Local Lives

PMTCT is a global program promoted internationally by the WHO in an effort to actively address the huge problem of MTCT of HIV in a sustainable and cost-effective manner in health systems characterized by severe shortages of human and material resources. At a time when thousands of babies were born HIV-positive with the sole prospect of sickness and early death, the PMTCT initiative represented a timely response to the international claim that the child should be protected from MTCT. Not only that but the PMTCT programs also responded to HIV-positive women's yearning for an HIV-negative child.

However, on the basis of our empirical evidence from different PMTCT programs in eastern Africa, we argue that the standard PMTCT approach is charged with 2 fundamental problems. One of them is that the concept of PMTCT focuses only on the child and neglects the health and life of the mother. The second problem is that the "one size fits all" design of the standard PMTCT package does not necessarily mesh well with local realities. As in many other public health programs the top-down approach of the PMTCT program meets a number of challenges when confronted with people as they live in particular social and cultural circumstances. The tension between the global PMTCT program and local realities is brought to the surface through the promotion of informed choice of infant feeding method, which is basic to the international guidelines of HIV and infant feeding and hence, to infant feeding counseling.

In the following sections, we will discuss the concept of informed choice of infant feeding method and the cultural conditions on which it is based against the possibilities for women to make an informed choice, in the context of the PMTCT programs in eastern Africa. We argue that a fundamental problem is that the medical knowledge on which PMTCT is based addresses infant feeding in a discourse of risk and responsibility without due consideration to the close coupling between breastfeeding and motherhood that prevails in large parts of the world where postnatal MTCT is a major public health problem.

The Discourse of Choice

The international guidelines on HIV and infant feeding introduce a new discourse of "choice" to an area in sub-Saharan Africa where infant feeding has not been a subject of choice (Seidel 2000). Breastfeeding has by and large been taken as "the (only) way to feed an infant" (see e.g., Leshabari et al. 2007). Alternative methods have been used only in the case of a crisis, such as maternal death. However, the PMTCT program promotes alternative infant feeding methods as safe or safer in an HIV context and presents HIV-positive women with a choice. The problem of choice pervades the literature on infant feeding in PMTCT programs, but very few studies discuss the particular conditions for and implications of the central location of informed choice in PMTCT.

A fundamental problem in the implementation of PMTCT, we argue, is that the program is grounded in an individual-oriented approach to disease prevention. It is based on the assumption that choice is a cognitive process and that the mother is capable of making an autonomous decision about how to feed her infant if she is provided with sufficient information. However, this assumption ignores the social environment of the individual. It fails to take into account the fact that a pregnant woman lives her life in the midst of many social relationships that influence her sense of self, her experiences as an expectant mother, and the decisions that she makes (see also Thachuk 2007). As our examples illustrate, infant feeding is an issue that is culturally entrenched and subject to considerable social pressure and control. What runs through many of the cases described in this chapter is the conflict between the intention of choice of infant feeding method in pregnancy and actual feeding practices. The various contingencies (such as values, social pressure, and emotions) that intervene in the decision-making process tend to make the choice of infant feeding method to be based in social processes rather than in an autonomous informed choice.

In their study of informed choice, Young, and colleagues (2006) point out that the framing of an issue as one of informed choice places the choosers in empowered positions. But, as they argue, this is a highly problematic assumption for several reasons. Patients may lack the appropriate knowledge to make an informed choice; not all choices are available to everybody; and the professional–patient relationship may not be empowering (Young et al. 2006). As we have seen above, HIV-positive mothers' knowledge about HIV and infant feeding is often rather confused. This obviously reflects confusing counseling messages and probably also the general uncertainty of the biomedical knowledge on the risk of HIV transmission through breastfeeding (Coutsoudis et al. 2001).

Furthermore, the complicated mechanisms behind the increased risk of HIV transmission through mixed feeding may be rather difficult to understand and, not the least, to convey in a simple manner to the uninformed mother. Besides, the competing risks associated with replacement feeding are substantial (see e.g., Kuhn et al. 2004). On the basis of this uncertainty, which is reflected in the ambiguity of the infant feeding guidelines, the information given to HIV-positive mothers is often biased toward the particular knowledge, preferences, and beliefs of the individual counselor. A proper AFASS assessment to identify the feeding method that is most appropriate, and hence most likely to be adhered to, in each case is commonly not done.

PMTCT counseling involves the exchange of information between the HIV-positive mother and her counselor. The mothers are presented with expert-defined truths where risk calculations have been translated into expert advice on behavior. This raises the question of the link between expertise and power (Murphy 2000:318). Considering the substantial social and cultural inequalities between the trained nurse–counselor and the HIV-positive, often poor and uneducated mother, the counselor may be expected to exert considerable power over infant feeding decisions. Their infant feeding messages are no doubt important in shaping women's knowledge about and attitudes to HIV and infant feeding, but to what extent their impact is heavy enough to overrule other competing concerns varies.

The power of expertise, then, may not primarily be linked to direct control over infant feeding decisions forcing women to feed their infants in particular ways, but in shaping the moral context in which women make their choice (Murphy 2000). The PMTCT program is based in a risk rationality that links health behavior to concrete manifestations of good or ill health. It follows that the discourse of risk and risk taking is, as Lupton (1993) has pointed out, a very moral one that raises the issue of responsibility. In her article on infant feeding Elisabeth Murphy (2000) argues that the moral judgment arising from the discourse on risk and responsibility "acquires a particular force when the consequences of risky behavior are borne not by self, but by others" (Murphy 2000). In PMTCT programs, the potential victim of risky behavior on the part of the mother is the child. Whereas the child is constructed as innocent and vulnerable, the mother is constructed as responsible for the outcome. As asserted by Murphy (2000:320), "[the] discourse on risk and responsibility [in infan t feeding] is particularly heightened where it intersects with the ideology of motherhood."

Motherhood at Stake

To understand choice of infant feeding method and adherence to that method among women in PMTCT programs we need to understand what is at stake. Throughout this chapter we have demonstrated that in addition to the concern linked to infant survival and freedom from HIV infection, motherhood concerns emerge as prominent in the decision-making process and not the least in adhering to the particular infant feeding method chosen. Infant feeding choice, we argue, is closely connected to what is considered acceptable and unacceptable mothering behavior in particular contexts.

In eastern Africa, where infant mortality is high and the infection pressure great, breastfeeding has commonly been considered vital to child survival. In this context it is the mother who is held responsible for child growth and development, and motherhood is basically constituted as carrying and nurturing the child (Figure 16.1). Failure to thrive on the part of the child raises questions about how the infant is being fed and about the mother's ability to care for the child. Breastfeeding is located at the very centre of the motherhood ideology and, as we have shown, is often perceived as inseparable from the mothering experience. A very telling quote in this context is "A real mother is a mother who breastfeeds her child." The experience of not breastfeeding is commonly perceived as a threat to the development of the close bodily and emotional bonds between mother and child—sometimes to the extent that the status as mother could be questioned if breastfeeding is not practiced.

Since breastfeeding is so closely associated with maternal love and commitment, not breastfeeding is experienced as failing to be a good mother. As such, not breastfeeding may be seen as a "significant failure of motherhood" (Howard and Millard 1997; Moland 2004) pointing to the substantial failure to live up to practices deeply embedded in a culturally constituted moral universe. A mother who replacement-feeds her baby may accordingly find herself in "moral danger" (Lupton 1993; Murphy 2000), and is left potentially vulnerable to criticism and blame for not maximizing the health outcomes of her child (see Murphy 2000).

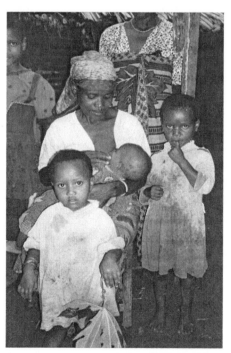

Figure 16.1. A rural Tanzanian woman breastfeeding, while her other children pose for the photographer (Photo by Karen Marie Moland).

In her article on breastfeeding and HIV in South Africa, Seidel (2000) asks whether the social construction of motherhood is changing in the wake of the HIV epidemic. The discourse on risk and responsibility in PMTCT reproduces an ideology of motherhood where women are held responsible for the health outcomes of their babies. At the same time, as the examples given in this chapter indicate, the interpretation of risk of MTCT may transform the experience of childbearing and in particular infant feeding and the perception of self as a mother. Our findings suggest that with its focus on the maternal body as a threat to infant survival, the PMTCT program may work to change ideas about the nurturing maternal body and, in particular, of breastfeeding as the socially sanctioned way to feed an infant.

The Issue of Rights

Global programs in general and PMTCT in particular raise a discussion about the relationship between universal validity and cultural appropriateness. In some contexts informed choice of infant feeding method is not offered because it has been seen as culturally inappropriate. In the PMTCT program at Haydom Lutheran Hospital, one of the sites of the present study, women have not been exposed to a choice of infant feeding method. On the contrary, only exclusive breastfeeding is promoted. With good follow-up this one-method strategy seems to have been rather successful in terms of adherence. Our results from the other study sites aiming to implement informed choice were far less convincing. In fact, infant feeding choice and adherence are experienced as extremely confused. The problems and doubts created by the emphasis on exclusive replacement feeding as the first option indicate that women living in poverty situations may manage better if they are not presented with alternative infant feeding methods and hence with a difficult choice.

On the basis of these observations, combined with the recent results on the safety of exclusive breastfeeding in sub-Saharan Africa by Coovadia et al. (2007), it would be tempting to suggest that the promotion of informed choice to women in resource-poor settings is not appropriate, and that in these areas, exclusive breastfeeding should be promoted. However, restricting the opportunity to choose also means restricting information. In terms of universal health care ethics, restricting information and thus restricting choice is extremely problematic. How ethical is it not to inform HIV-positive women about the risk of HIV transmission through breastfeeding? (Seidel 2000:25). The issue has raised the voices of human rights advocates, African feminists, and PLHIV, who have stressed the right of the woman herself to be informed about the benefits and the risks of both replacement feeding and breastfeeding and to make her choice on that basis (see e.g., Kaijage 1995).

But, as Seidel (2000) argues, in the PMTCT context, the assumption of relative patient autonomy inherent in the concept of informed choice is linked to the assumption of a culture of women's rights and access to resources. To what extent these assumptions reflect social reality varies with culture and with the social and economic status of the individual. However, in poverty-ridden areas in sub-Saharan Africa where the bulk of MTCT is found, a mother's autonomy is often restricted not only by economic factors, but as we have demonstrated, also by social hierarchy.

Counting on Mother's Love

Mother's love is presumably a universal phenomenon and is an implicit condition in numerous health promotion and disease prevention programs targeting children. The PMTCT strategy, we argue, also counts on mothers' love. Without a mother's commitment to prevent MTCT, the PMTCT strategy will fail. In this chapter we have demonstrated that counting on mother's love is a promising strategy also in PMTCT. HIV-positive mothers across the 5 study sites suffer and make sacrifices both in terms of their own health and social life and in terms of the family economy to secure an HIV-negative child. Through a number of cases and narratives we have also demonstrated that many women, despite their dedication to the course and despite their maternal love, do not manage to adhere to the demanding infant feeding prescriptions. The question then is not whether "counting on mother's love" is an effective and acceptable strategy in PMTCT, but whether it is effective and acceptable in the absence of treatment and support to secure the health and the survival of the mother.

The weak position of the mother in mother-and-child health programs is not a phenomenon characterizing PMTCT programs only. In an article in the Lancet in 1985 Rosenfield and Maine (1985) criticized the neglect of maternal mortality in mother and child health care services (MCH) and asked "Where is the M in MCH?" Following the Nairobi conference on safe motherhood in 1987, the Safe Motherhood Initiative was launched, putting maternal mortality on the international agenda. It was argued that maternal mortality and morbidity was a neglected problem because its victims were poor—rural peasants and women— the least powerful and influential in society (Mahler 1987). Twenty years later, maternal morbidity and mortality remains a big problem, and the M in PMTCT is defined mainly as a threat to infant survival (see also Inhorn 2006).

Conclusion

This study of PMTCT initiatives in Tanzania and Ethiopia has demonstrated that the challenges related to the infant feeding prescriptions are enormous, and there is nothing that indicates that the programs we have studied are unique cases in this regard. On the contrary, we believe that the knowledge presented in this chapter related to obstacles to the WHO infant feeding prescriptions is valid to quite some extent in other settings also where breastfeeding is normative and where low income hinders exclusive use of replacement feeding products. The results from 1 of our study sites, a PMTCT+ project in Tanzania, however, indicate fairly good adherence to an exclusive breastfeeding regime. This positive finding supports other studies documenting that it is possible to enhance PMTCT adherence within particularly favorable frames, not the least within research settings. Even the culturally contested concept of expressed "heat-treated breast milk" has been favorably evaluated in a clinical trial (e.g., Israel-Ballard et al. 2006). But a clinical trial is not "real life," and it is very far from well-functioning, high-input initiatives to viable public policy. The vast majority of HIV-positive mothers do not live in the vicinity of high-input PMTCT trials, nor will they do so in the foreseeable future.

What is then the way forward? As pointed out by Fowler and colleagues (2007), the optimal strategy for infant feeding among HIV-positive mothers has yet to be outlined, and we can merely present a few reflections here, based on our research experience.

A first premise is to secure follow-up and, if necessary,[5] treatment of the HIV-infected mother, that is, maternal HAART. One can neither medically nor morally handle the issue of MTCT of HIV and the related orphan challenge without taking the mother's health fundamentally into account. A second premise in a PMTCT context must be to direct the prescriptions away from illusionary choices of infant feeding method and to reintroduce breastfeeding as the obvious and natural source of infant feeding and as the first choice for everyone. As Fowler et al. (2007:8) put it, "This strategy has the benefit of reducing the risk of HIV acquisition while maintaining breast milk as a source of life-saving nutrition." These concerns are also reflected in the updated guidelines on PMTCT issued in 2006 (WHO 2006).

A third premise lies in moving the attention away from the HIV-positive woman, which causes little but suffering among a group of highly vulnerable women. We hence believe that the work ahead lies in making mothers' milk safer for every child, where an exclusive breastfeeding regime (documented to be the best infant feeding method) is promoted among all women. Our material has demonstrated that culturally exclusive breastfeeding regimes are highly uncommon, and that outside of high support programs the adherence is very low. It is, however, difficult to envisage that support programs (in terms of material and human resources) are a feasible and realistic measure for the vast majority of HIV-positive mothers. This makes us and many others anxiously await improved medical regimes in the form of infant prophylaxis or HIV vaccines.

We close with a few reflections on what anthropological approaches can add to public health in relation to the PMTCT challenge. A large number of writings on the global MTCT problem recognize and point out financial and sociocultural challenges implied in preventive initiatives. Fowler et al. (2007:3), for example, write that PMTCT programs are hampered by "a variety of factors such as inadequate funding and cultural, social, and institutional barriers." The vast majority of the writings on the topic, however, do not move beyond such broad statements. This is rather problematic as the so-called AFASS criteria—the evaluation of whether nutritional substitutes to breastmilk are "culturally acceptable, feasible, affordable, sustainable, and safe"—are located at the core of the PMTCT challenge. Indeed, adherence to one of the exclusive feeding regimes is critical to "treatment success," which in PMTCT is an HIV-negative child. But as we have seen in this chapter adherence is no simple matter. Since infant feeding is an activity that is practiced at home and out of reach of continuous health care surveillance, getting reliable adherence data is very tricky even in clinical trials with regular follow-up of the study participants. Assessment of sensitive issues is always charged with potential bias, but in this case researchers are confronted with challenges of new proportions. A mother who admits that she has failed to adhere to the infant feeding instructions given by the counselor indirectly admits putting her infant at severe risk of a life-threatening and stigmatized infection through her breastmilk. The potential of anthropological methods to generate knowledge that is socioculturally, politically, and experientially sensitive therefore seems to be of particular value in a PMTCT context.

As we have seen in this chapter, the PMTCT concept is founded on the premise that individual women can make infant feeding choices that enhance their infants' survival chances. However, what has become overwhelmingly clear in our work is the limited degree to which the individual mother can modify deeply meaningful nurturing practices without being the victim of particularly close unwanted scrutiny. The cultural significance attached to breastmilk and breastfeeding is in most communities extensively elaborated upon in ways that will impact an individual's potential for modification and maneuver. This social and cultural habituation of human thought and practice is brought to the forefront in the account discussed.

The close attention anthropology can give to people's practical lives and their experiences generate substantial knowledge of the political–economic, and by extension, the moral–ethical dimensions of the topic at hand. The morally challenging scenario produced by the WHO guidelines is brought to our awareness through the incomprehensible burden of responsibility for infant survival that is placed on the poor, usually untreated, HIV-positive mothers.

Acknowledgments

We would like to sincerely thank all informants, both patients and staff, who took part in the present study. The following health institutions welcomed us to carry out research: Haydom Lutheran Hospital and Kilimanjaro Christian Medical Centre, Tanzania; Arba Minch Hospital and Yirga Alem Hospital, Southern Ethiopia; Zewditu Hospital, Bale; and Tekleheimanot and Addis Ketema Health Centers in Addis Ababa. The Centre for International Health, University of Bergen, Norway; Commission for Science and Technology (COSTECH); and National Institute of Medical Research (NIMR) in Tanzania, as well as the Addis Ababa Health Bureau and the medical faculty at Addis Ababa University and Debub University in Ethiopia facilitated the studies administratively and secured research permits and ethical clearances. The study was financed by the Research Council of Norway and the faculty of medicine at the University of Bergen, Norway. Sincere thanks go to all the aforementioned institutions. Finally, we would like to thank Marcia Inhorn and Robert Hahn for very valuable comments on chapter drafts.

Notes

1. Although the exact mechanism behind the increased risk associated with mixed feeding is not known, it is anticipated that additional liquids and fluids may compromise intestinal integrity, resulting in small lesions in the immature gut where the virus can pass to infect the infant (Coutsoudis et al. 1999).

2. An increasing number of programs now also offer prophylaxis for the mother during the last trimester of pregnancy.

3. The prevalence among antenatal attendees may be considerably overestimated. Antenatal clinic attendance in Ethiopia is well below 50%. Attendance is particularly low in rural areas where the HIV prevalence is low.

4. The authors received grants for the present research from the Research Council of Norway in collaboration with the Medical Faculty at the University of Bergen (Moland 2005–2007, Blystad 2005–2006). The projects were granted research/ethical clearance by The Tanzania Commission for Science and Technology (COSTECH) and the National Institute for Medical Research (NIMRI) in Tanzania, and by Addis Ababa University and the Regional Health Bureau in Addis Ababa and Awasa, Ethiopia.

5. This depends on the CD4 count of the mother. The cut-off point varies, but most commonly HAART is not considered feasible in sub-Saharan Africa if the mother's CD4 count is above 200.

References

Black RE, Morris SS, Bryce J (2003) Where and why are 10 million children dying every year? *Lancet* 361:2226–2234.

Brahmbhatt H, Gray RH (2003) Child mortality associated with reasons for non-initiation. *American Journal of Obstetrics and Gynecology* 189:1398–1400.

Coovadia HM, Rollins NC, Bland RM, Little K, Coutsoudis A, Bennish ML et al. (2007) Mother-to-child transmission of HIV-1 infection during exclusive breastfeeding in the first 6 months of life: An intervention cohort study. *Lancet* 369:1107–1116.

Coutsoudis A, Pillay K, Spooner E, Kuhn L, Coovadia HM (1999) Influence of infant-feeding patterns on early mother-to-child transmission of HIV-1 in Durban, South Africa: A prospective cohort study. South African Vitamin A Study Group. *Lancet* 354(9177):471–476.

Coutsoudis A, Pillay K, Kuhn L, Spooner E, Tsai WY, Coovadia HM (2001) Method of feeding and transmission of HIV-1 from mothers to children by 15 months of age: Prospective cohort study from Durban, South Africa. *AIDS* 15(3):379–387.

Coutsoudis A, Goga AE, Rollins N, Coovadia HM (2002) Free formula milk for infants of HIV-infected women: Blessing or curse? *Health Policy and Planning* 17(2):154–160.

De Paoli MM, Manongi R, Helsing E, Klepp KI (2001) Exclusive breastfeeding in the era of AIDS. *Journal of Human Lactation* 17(4):313–320.

De Cock KM, Fowler MG, Mercier E, de Vincenzi I, Saba J, Hoff E (2000) Prevention of mother-to-child HIV transmission in resource poor countries. *Journal of the American Medical Association* 283:1175–1185.

Douglas M (1966) *Purity and Danger: An Analysis of Concepts of Pollution and Tabu.* London: Routledge and Keagen Paul.

Douglas M (1970) *Natural Symbols.* New York: Pantheon Books.

Doherty T, Chopra M, Nkonki L, Jackson D, Greiner T (2006) Effect of the HIV epidemic on infant feeding in South Africa: "When they see me coming with the tins they laugh at me." *Bulletin of the World Health Organization* 84(2):90–96.

Fowler MG, Lamp MA, Jamieson DJ, Kourtis AP, Rogers MF (2007) Reducing the risk of mother-to-child immunodeficiency virus transmission: Past successes, current progress and challenges, and future directions. *American Journal of Obstetrics and Gynecology.* Supplement to September 2007.

HAPCO (National HIV/AIDS Prevention and Control Office) (2004) *Ethiopian Strategic Plan for Intensifying Multi-Sectoral HIV/AIDS Response.* Addis Ababa: Federal Ministry of Health.

Howard M, Millard AV (1997) *Hunger and Shame: Poverty and Child Malnutrition on Mount Kilimanjaro.* New York: Routledge.

Iliff PJ, Piwoz EG, Tavengwa NV, Zunguza CD, Marinda ET, Nathoo KJ (2005) Early exclusive breast-feeding reduces the risk of postnatal HIV-1 transmission and increases HIV-free survival. *AIDS* 19:699–708.

Inhorn MC (2006) Defining women's health: A dozen messages from more than 150 ethnographies. *Medical Anthropology Quarterly* 20(3):345–378.

Israel-Ballard KA, Maternowska MC, Abrams BF, Morrison P, Chitibura L, Chipato T, et al. (2006) Acceptability of heat treating breast milk to prevent mother-to-child transmission of human immunodeficiency virus in Zimbabwe: A qualitative study. *Journal of Human Lactation* 22(1):48–60.

Jones G, Steketee RW, Black RE, Bhutta ZA, Morris SS, for the Bellagio Child Survival Study Group (2003) How many child deaths can we prevent this year? *Lancet* 362:65–71.

Kaijage TJ (1995) HIV and breastfeeding: The health of mother and infant. *Reproductive Health Matters* 3(5):124–126.

Kuhn L, Stein Z, Susser M (2004) Preventing mother-to-child transmission in the new millennium: The challenge of breast feeding. *Paediatric and Perinatal Epidemiology* 18:10–16.

Leshabari SC, Koniz-Booher P, Åstrøm AN, de Paoli MM, Moland KM (2006) Translating global recommendations on HIV and infant feeding to the local context: The development of culturally sensitive counselling tools in the Kilimanjaro Region, Tanzania. *Implementation Science* 1:22.

Leshabari S, Blystad A, Moland KM (2007) Difficult choices: Infant feeding experiences of HIV positive mothers in Northern Tanzania. *Journal of Social Aspects of HIV/AIDS* 4(1):544–555.

Lupton D (1993) Risk as moral danger: The social and political functions of risk discourse in public health. *International Journal of Health Services* 23:425–435.

Moland KM (2004) Mother's milk: An ambiguous blessing in the era of AIDS: The case of the Chagga in Kilimanjaro. *African Sociological Review* 8(1):83–99.

Murphy E (2000) Risk, responsibility and rhetoric in infant feeding. *Journal of Contemporary Ethnography* 2000:291–325.

Mahler H (1987) The Safe Motherhood Initiative: A call to action. *Lancet* 1(8534):668–670.

Piwoz EG, Ross JS (2005) Use of population-specific infant mortality rates to inform policy decisions regarding HIV and infant feeding. *Journal of Nutrition* 135:1113–1119.

Rollins NC (2007) Infant feeding and HIV: Avoiding transmission is not enough. *British Medical Journal* 334:487–488.

Rosenfield A, Maine D (1985) Maternal mortality: A neglected tragedy. Where is the M in MCH? *Lancet* 13:83–85.

Seidel G (2000) Experiences of breastfeeding and vulnerability among a group of HIV-positive women in Durban, South Africa. *Health Policy and Planning* 15(1):24–33.

Thachuk A (2007) *Midwifery, Informed Choice, and Reproductive Autonomy: A Relational Approach*. Thousand Oaks, CA: Sage Publications.

Thairu LN, Pelto GH, Rollins, NC, Bland RM, Ntchangase N (2005) Sociocultural influences on infant feeding decisions among HIV-infected women in rural Kwa-Zulu Natal, South Africa. *Maternal and Child Nutrition* 1:2–10.

Thior I, Lockman S, Smeaton LM (2005) Breastfeeding with 6 months of infant zidovudine prophylaxis vs formula-feeding for reducing postnatal HIV transmission and infant mortality: A randomised trial in Southern Africa. Paper presented at the Retroviruses and Opportunistic Infections. 22–25 February, Boston.

UNAIDS (2000) Report of the Global HIV/AIDS epidemic. Geneva: UNAIDS. UNAIDS/00.13E.2000

UNAIDS (2005) Global Summary of the AIDS epidemic. AIDS epidemic update, December 2005.

UNAIDS (2006) Report on the Global AIDS epidemic 2006:133. health/New_Publications/NUTRITION/consensus_statement.pdf

UNAIDS/WHO (2006) AIDS Epidemic Update December 2006 Sub-Saharan Africa http://www.unaids.org/en/KnowledgeCentre/HIVData/EpiUpdate/EpiUpdArchive/2006/Default.asp

UNICEF (2005) www.unicef.org/index.php

WHO (2000a) Collaborative study team on the role of breastfeeding on the prevention of infant mortality. Effect of breastfeeding on infant and child mortality due to infectious diseases in less developed countries: A pooled analysis. *Lancet* 355:451–455.

WHO (2000b) New data on the prevention of mother-to-child transmission of HIV and their policy implications. Conclusions and recommendations. WHO technical consultation on behalf of the UNFPA/UNICEF/WHO/UNAIDS Inter-Agency Task Team on Mother-to-Child Transmission of HIV. Geneva, October 2000.

WHO (2003a) WHO/UNICEF/UNFPA/UNAIDS. HIV and Infant Feeding: Guidelines for Decision-makers. Geneva: World Health Organization 2003.

WHO (2003b) Impact of HAART during pregnancy and breastfeeding on MTCT and mother's health: The Kesho Bora study. Project summary 2003.

WHO (2006) HIV and Infant Feeding Technical Consultation held on behalf of the Inter-agency Task Team (IATT) on Prevention of HIV Infections in Pregnant Women, Mothers and their Infants. Geneva, October 25–27, 2006. www.who.int/child-adolescent-health/New_Publications/NUTRITION/consensus_statement.pdf

Young A, Carr G, Hunt R, Skipp A, Tattersall H (2006) Informed choice and deaf children: Underpinning concepts and enduring challenges. *Journal of Deaf Studies and Deaf Education* 11:3.

17

The Brazilian Response to AIDS and the Pharmaceuticalization of Global Health

JOÃO BIEHL

Introduction

Brazil is known for its stark socioeconomic inequalities and for its persistent challenges in development. Yet, against all odds, Brazil has invented a public way of treating AIDS. In 1996, it became the first developing country to adopt an official policy that provided universal access to antiretroviral drugs (ARVs), about 5 years before global policy discussions moved from a framework that focused solely on prevention to one that incorporated universal treatment (Biehl 2004; Galvão 2000; Levi and Vitória 2002). The AIDS treatment policy was made possible by an unexpected alliance of activists, government reformers, development agencies, and the pharmaceutical industry. About 200,000 Brazilians are currently taking ARVs that are paid for by the government, and this policy is widely touted as a model for stemming the AIDS crisis worldwide (Berkman, Garcia, Muñoz-Laboy, Paiva, and Parker 2005; Okie 2006).

This chapter examines the Brazilian response to AIDS, revealing the possibilities as well as the inequalities that accompany a magic-bullet approach to health care. It moves between a social analysis of the institutional practices shaping this therapeutic policy and an account of the experiences of people affected by it, particularly in impoverished urban settings where the epidemic is spreading most rapidly. I draw from open-ended interviews I carried out with activists, policymakers, health professionals, and corporate actors in both Brazil and the United States between 2000 and 2005. I also draw from my longitudinal study of the lives of marginalized AIDS patients and of the work of grassroots care services in the northeastern city of Salvador. I chronicled the activities of Dona Conceição, a philanthropist helping homeless AIDS patients, and I carried out participant observation at a "house of support" called Caasah. I undertook this study between 1995 and 2005 for a total of 20 months. In 1997, I collected the life stories of 22 AIDS patients who lived at Caasah and I have charted their life trajectories before and after access to antiretroviral therapies (Biehl 2006). All these materials are part of my ethnography *Will to Live: AIDS Therapies and the Politics of Survival* (2007).

Some of the questions that guided my investigation include which public health values and political and technological practices make this therapeutic policy possible, and what guarantees its sustainability? How has the AIDS policy become a kind of public good, emblematic of the state's universal reach, even though it is not enjoyed by all citizens? What networks of care emerge around the distribution of lifesaving drugs? How do the poorest understand and negotiate medical services? How do their lifestyles and social support systems influence treatment adherence? What happens to poverty as these individual sufferers engage the pharmaceutical control of AIDS? What do these struggles over drug access and survival say about politics, citizenship, and equity on the ground and globally?

Universal Access to Lifesaving Therapies

Amidst denial, stigma, and inaction, AIDS became the first major epidemic of present-day globalization. Of more than 33 million people estimated to be HIV-infected worldwide, 95% live in middle- or low-income countries, causing life expectancy to drop dramatically in those countries worst hit. In late 2003, with only about 400,000 people receiving treatment, the World Health Organization (WHO) and the Joint United Nations Programme on HIV/AIDS (UNAIDS) announced their goal of having 3 million HIV-positive people on antiretroviral therapy by 2005 (known as the "3 by 5" campaign). The results have been mixed, but by any account Brazil has been a leader in the effort to universalize access to treatment. By the end of 2004, the number of people on ARVs had increased to 700,000 globally—in the developing world, this figure stood at 300,000, of which half the people lived in Brazil. And when the deadline arrived at the end of 2005, with an estimated 6.5 million people requiring treatment, 1.2 million were on ARVs—encouraging, but still short of the target. Brazil, with less than 3% of the world's HIV/AIDS cases, still accounted for nearly 15% of people on ARVs.[1]

Brazil is the epicenter of the HIV/AIDS epidemic in South America and accounts for 57% of all AIDS cases in Latin America and the Caribbean.

The country's first AIDS case was diagnosed (retrospectively) in 1980 and through mid-2002 the Ministry of Health had reported nearly 240,000 cumulative cases. HIV prevalence in Brazil is higher than in most of its neighbors, although this is in part due to more accurate reporting (Berkman et al. 2005; Castilho and Cherquer 1997). At the end of 2001, an estimated 610,000 individuals were living with HIV/AIDS (an adult prevalence of 0.7%, about half of what had been projected). Social epidemiological studies show considerable heterogeneity in HIV infection rates, with large numbers infected among vulnerable populations and a fast-growing number of heterosexual transmissions (Bastos and Barcellos 1995). In 1998, 18% of sex workers tested in São Paulo were HIV-positive, and in certain areas of the country, intravenous drug users contributed almost 50% of all AIDS cases. Since 1998, the death rate from AIDS has steadily declined, an achievement attributed to the country's treatment policy (Dourado, Veras, Barreira, and de Brito 2006).

Throughout the 1990s, a range of different groups and institutions—activists and local nongovernmental organizations (NGOs), central and regional governments, and grassroots organizations, along with development agencies such as the World Bank—came together, helping to address what was earlier perceived to be a hopeless situation (Bastos 1999; Parker 1994; Parker, Galvão, and Bessa 1999). This combination of social organization and education, political will (at various levels of government), and international cooperation made it possible for Brazil to overcome AIDS denial and to respond to an imminent crisis in a timely and efficient way. AIDS activists and progressive health professionals migrated into state institutions and actively participated in policy making (Parker 1997). They showed creativity in the design of prevention work and audacity in solving the problem of access to AIDS treatment. In their view, the prices pharmaceutical companies had set for ARVs and the protection they received from intellectual property rights laws and the World Trade Organization (WTO) had artificially put these drugs out of reach of the global poor. After framing the demand for access to ARVs as a human right, in accordance with the country's constitutional right to health, activists lobbied for specific legislation to make the drugs universally available.

The Brazilian government was able to reduce treatment costs by reverse engineering ARVs and promoting the production of generics in both public- and private-sector laboratories (Cassier and Correa 2003). Had an infrastructure for the production of generics not been in place, the story being told today would probably be different. For its part, the Health Ministry also negotiated substantial drug price reductions from pharmaceutical companies by threatening to issue compulsory licenses for patented drugs. Media campaigns publicized these actions, generating strong national and international support (Galvão 2002; Serra 2004). The result—a policy of drugs for all—has dramatically improved the quality of life of the patients covered. AIDS treatment has been incorporated into the country's ailing unified health-care system (Sistema Único de Saúde, SUS) and, according to the Health Ministry, both AIDS mortality and the use of AIDS-related hospital services have subsequently fallen by 70% (Ministério da Saúde 2002). Brazil's treatment rollout has become an inspiration for international activism and a challenge for the governments of other poor countries devastated by the AIDS pandemic. This policy challenges the perception that treating AIDS in resource-poor settings is economically unfeasible, and it calls our attention to the possible ways in which lifesaving drugs can be integrated into public policy even in the absence of an optimal health infrastructure.

By 2000, the Brazilian AIDS Program had been named by UNAIDS as the best in the developing world, and in 2003 it received the Gates Award for Global Health. Brazil is now sharing its know-how in a range of ways. It has taken on a leadership role in the WHO's AIDS program and it is supporting international networks aimed at facilitating treatment access and technological cooperation on HIV/AIDS. In the past years, the Brazilian government has also been leading developing nations in WTO deliberations over a flexible balance between patent rights and public health needs. Practically speaking, Brazil opened channels for horizontal collaborations among developing nations, and devised political mechanisms (as fleeting and fragile as they may be) for poor countries to level out some of the pervasive structural inequalities that place their populations at increased risk and continued ill health.

Persistent Inequalities and Grassroots Health Services

The medical accountability at stake in this innovative policy has drastic implications for Brazil's 50 million urban poor, either indigent or making their living through informal and marginal economies. By and large, they gain some public attention during political elections—even then only in the most general terms—and through the limited aid of international agencies. Through AIDS, however, new fields of exchange and possibility have emerged.

I was in the coastal city of Salvador (the capital of the northeastern state of Bahia) conducting fieldwork when AIDS therapies began to be widely available in early 1997. Considered by many as "the African heart of Brazil," Salvador was the country's capital until 1763. A center of international tourism, today Salvador has an estimated population of 2.5 million, with more than 40% of families living below the country's poverty line. At the time of my fieldwork, local health officials claimed that AIDS incidence was on the decline in both the city and the region, ostensibly in line with the country's successful control policy. But the AIDS reality one could readily see in the streets of Salvador contradicted this profile. A large number of AIDS sufferers remained epidemiologically and medically unaccounted for, thereafter dying in abandonment (Biehl 2005). Meanwhile, community-run initiatives provided limited care for some of the poorest and the sickest.

Every Wednesday at noon, Dona Conceição, a 50-year-old nurse, cooked large pans of food and, with the help of her religious friends, handed it out to dozens of poor people and families who lived with AIDS and very little else in the abandoned corners of the city's historical compound known as the Pelourinho (*Pillory*)—once a place where African captives were auctioned and rebellious slaves punished. Today it is a lively cultural heritage center. She provided free meals and some care (medication, clothing, and rent aid) to a total of 110 adults, most of them involved in prostitution and drug dealing, and to their children. As Dona Conceição put it, "Medical services never meet the demands and civil society has abandoned them. They are at the margins of law and life. I give them a little comfort and help alleviate things a bit. I am tied to them in spirit." Even though she had some support from her extended family and friends, Dona Conceição had to generate money for her AIDS work on her own (mostly through handicrafts sales and donation campaigns).

I talked to Dona Conceição's "street patients" on several occasions. Soft-spoken Jorge Araújo said that he was born on January 1, 1963. "I will not lie to you, I injected drugs, and I have AIDS," he told me without hesitation. "I abused drugs and myself. I had to amputate my left leg. When I got to the hospital it was too late. And on top of losing the leg they told me I had AIDS." Jorge had lived by himself and on the streets since the age of 14: "I left home because of my stepfather; we didn't get along. I did little jobs, here and there, sold drugs. I think it is a thing of destiny, right?" At some point, he lived with an older woman and had a child, but he eventually left them. "If I kept thinking about AIDS, I would already be dead. I carry out my life as God wants it. One must forget. One cannot put in one's mind that one is the disease. If we dwell on the disease, then one starts to say 'Maybe I should not do this or eat that for it will harm me' and then one is left with even less. To be a patient one needs things. What is there here to have?"

One should not expect these patients to adhere to medical treatments, says Dona Conceição, because "they just use medication until they recover." And she did not blame them: "How can they comply if they live on the streets? Until they have a home, no treatment will work." Dona Conceição did not judge her street patients and their actions in terms of right or wrong, in terms of normality or pathology; she understood that structural violence[2] compounded substance- and self-abuse. In doing so, she implicitly made their condition a public affair, a Brazilian social symptom, I thought. But to complicate things further, she refused to treat them as a collective, and that's what drew them to her. She helped them individualize, and she literally struggled in their place: "Each one has a history, a life left behind. Jorge suffers emotionally—all the discrimination he goes through, and he is unable to overcome his personal failures. He does not struggle for health; I struggle for him." How, I wondered, would the antiretroviral rollout fare in this context of multiple scarcities and spurious regional politics? How would the most vulnerable transform a death sentence into a chronic disease? What social experimentation could make such medical transformation possible?

Caasah, a focal point of my research, was founded in 1992, when a group of homeless AIDS patients, former prostitutes, transvestites, and drug users (Jorge was among them) squatted in an abandoned hospital formerly run by the Red Cross. "Caasah had no government," recalled Celeste Gomes, Caasah's president.[3] "They did whatever they wanted in here. Everybody had sex with everybody, they were using drugs. There were fights with knives and broken bottles, and police officials were threatening to kick us out." Soon, Caasah became a nongovernmental organization (NGO) and began to receive funding from a World Bank loan disbursed through the Brazilian government. By 1994, eviction threats had ceased, and the service had gathered community support for basic maintenance. Caasah had also formalized partnerships with municipal and provincial Health Secretariats, buttressed by strategic exchanges with hospitals and AIDS NGOs. Throughout the country, other "houses of support" (casas de apoio) like Caasah negotiate the relationship between AIDS patients and the haphazard, limited public health-care infrastructure. By 2000, at least 100 of the country's 500 registered AIDS NGOs were houses of support. To belong to these grassroots services, people must break with their old habits, communities, and routines as they forge new lives.

By the mid-1990s, the unruly patients in Caasah had been ejected. "I couldn't stand being locked in. I like to play around," Jorge told me. A smaller version of the group began to undergo an intense process of resocialization mediated by psychologists and nurses. Jorge and about 80 other outpatients remained eligible for monthly food aid. Patients who wanted to stay in the institution had to change their antisocial behaviors and adhere to medical treatments. Caasah now had a reasonably well-equipped infirmary, with a triage room and a pharmacy. Religious groups visited the place on a regular basis and many residents adopted religion as an alternative value system. As Edimilson, a former intravenous drug user and petty thief, put it, "In Caasah we don't just have AIDS—we have God." According to Celeste, "With time, we domesticated them. They had no knowledge whatsoever, and we changed this doomed sense of 'I will die.' Today they feel normal, like us, they can do any activity, they just have to care not to develop the disease. We showed them the importance of using medication. Now they have this conscience, and they fight for their lives."

Rose's left hand was atrophied, and she limped. "It is all from drug use. I was crazy. I went to the street, to a bar, left with a client, did his game, and drugged myself with the money". Rose and other healthy patients in Caasah repeatedly pointed to the marks on their bodies as images of past misdeeds, as if they were now in another place, seeing and judging their past selves from a photographic distance. "Ah, now I see. If I only had thought then the way I think now."

Rose grew up in the interior and was expelled from home at the age of 13, after she became pregnant. She moved into a red light district at the Pelourinho. By the end of 1993, Rose learned that she was both pregnant and HIV-positive. A physician who did volunteer work among prostitutes arranged Rose's move to Caasah. One by one, Rose gave up her children for adoption. The newborn girl was adopted by Naiara, Caasah's vice president, and her little boy was adopted by Professor Carlos, the chief nurse. "What else could I have done? I couldn't give them a house. I also thought that I would not live much longer." But Rose has lived longer than she expected. For 4 years, she had been off illegal substances. She had remained asymptomatic, had become literate, and had learned to make handicrafts. At that time, she was involved with Jorge Ramos, another resident, and was beginning to take ARVs. "I take life in here as if it were a family, the family I did not have," she stated.

Caasah's residents and administrators constituted a viable public that effectively sustained itself in novel interactions with governmental institutions and local AIDS services. Instead of succumbing to the factors that predisposed them to nonadherence to treatment (such as poverty and drug addiction), residents used their "disadvantages" to create the AIDS-friendly environment that is necessary to accumulate health.[4] In this "proxy family" people did not have to worry about the stigma that came with having AIDS "on the outside," and there was a scheduled routine and an infrastructure that made it easier to integrate drug regimens into the everyday life (Abadia-Barrero and Castro 2006). The right to health was group-privatized, and an intense process of individuation—"salvation from my previous life," as some put it—and a spirit of competition with fellow residents motivated treatment adherence as well.

"Did you ever see an AIDS patient in here hoping for the other's good?" Evangivaldo asked me as he was being quarantined because of his scabies. Residents constantly denounced each other's faults and demanded the rigorous application of the law: "Is there a law? Where is it? Why is it not being applied?" The others' misbehavior was also a measure of their own progress, a measure of their own change and self-control. "I am not like him." "He did it to himself, and now wants another chance." Money was also at stake. The administration was mediating the extremely bureaucratized application for AIDS disability pensions, and priority was given to those residents who showed change. Well-behaved and compliant patients were also allowed to help in the storage room, where they then had priority in choosing clothing for themselves and for family members living outside.

I have chronicled life in and out of Caasah for more than 10 years, and at the end of the chapter I will take the reader back there to see what has happened to this "house" and its residents over time. AIDS therapies are now embedded in local worlds, and hundreds of medico-pastoral institutions of care similar to Caasah help to make AIDS a chronic disease also among the poor. Medicines have indeed become key elements in state–civil society relations. But this is not a top-down biopolitical form of control. The government is not using AIDS therapies and houses of support as "techniques ... to govern populations and manage individual bodies" (Nguyen 2005:126). Poor AIDS populations are rather temporarily organized through particular and highly contested engagements with what the state has made pharmaceutically available. And as I will show at the end of the chapter, the political game here is one of self-identification, and it involves a new economics of survival.

A Political Economy of Pharmaceuticals

Brazil's response to AIDS "is a microcosm of a new state-society partnership," Fernando Henrique Cardoso, Brazil's former president (1995–2002) and the country's most prominent sociologist, stated in an interview with me in May 2003: "I always said that we needed to have a porous state so that society could have room for action in it, and that's what happened with AIDS."[5] I met with Cardoso in Princeton, at the Institute for Advanced Study, where he was participating in a meeting of the board of trustees. After leaving the presidency, Cardoso had been traveling the international lecture circuit and had taken a professorship at Brown University. He had no qualms about extrapolating, using the AIDS treatment policy as evidence of the "success" of his state reform agenda—a state open to civil society, decentralized, fostering partnerships for the delivery of services, efficient, ethical, and, if activated, having a universal reach. "Government and social movement practically fused. Brazilian society now organizes itself and acts on its own behalf."

This new state–society synergy reflected in the country's AIDS Program has developed in the wake of Brazil's democratization and the state's attempt to position itself strategically in the context of globalization. Cardoso argued, "We cannot do politics as if globalization did not exist. One must see and decide in practice what is good and what is bad about it. This new phase of capitalism limits all states, of course, including the United States, but it also opens up new perspectives for states." Cardoso said that both he and the new president Luis Inácio Lula da Silva from the Workers' Party (Partido dos Trabalhadores) "in the end say the same thing." That is, "that globalization is asymmetric and that it does not eliminate the differences imposed on nations. So we have to take concrete steps toward decreasing this asymmetry, mainly at the trade level so that we can have access to markets, and also to the control financing mechanisms." He made the case that Lula's government was basically following the same "ultra-orthodox" economic line of his administration—but that, "surprisingly," the new government lagged in social program innovation: "The proposals they have are centralized, very vague, mismanaged, and don't match with what Brazil already is." Cardoso was proud of the ways the AIDS Program—with its multisectoral partnerships and high-tech delivery capacity—had pushed the envelope of what was governmentally possible.

"The idea that nothing can be done because rich countries are stronger is generally true, but not always," stated Cardoso. "You can fight and, in the process, gain some advantages. You must penetrate all international spheres, try to influence and branch out. The question of solidarity must be continuously addressed." Brazil's struggle for drug price reduction, he says, "shows that under certain conditions you can gain international support to change things. All the nongovernmental work, global public opinion, change in legislation, and struggle over patents are evidence of new forms of governmentality in action … thereby engineering something else, producing a new world." The rhetoric of state agency and the abstractions that Cardoso articulated—mobilized civil society and activism within the state—are part of a new political discourse. This language belongs to a public sphere strongly influenced by social scientists, as well as by politicians who do not want to take responsibility for their decisions to conform to the norms of globalization. For example, Cardoso makes no specific reference to the measures his administration took to open the economy such as changes in intellectual property legislation and the privatization of state industries. This political discourse does not acknowledge the economic factors and value systems that are built into policy making today.

As with all things political and economic, the reality underlying the AIDS policy is convoluted, dynamic, and filled with gaps. The politicians involved in the making of the AIDS policy were consciously engaged in projects to reform the relationship between the state and society, as well as the scope of governance, as Brazil molded itself to a global market economy. And one of my central arguments is that behind the concept *model policy* stands a new political economy of pharmaceuticals. Just a few months before approving the AIDS treatment law in November 1996, the Brazilian government had given in to industry pressures to enshrine strong patent protections in law. Brazil was at the forefront of developing countries that supported the creation of the WTO, and it had signed the Trade-Related Aspects of Intellectual Property Rights treaty (TRIPS) in December 1994. Parallel to the new patent legislation, pharmaceutical imports to Brazil had increased substantially. Between 1995 and 1997, the trade deficit in pharmaceutical products jumped from $410 million to approximately $1.3 billion (Bermudez, Epsztein, Oliveira, and Hasenclever 2000).

Moreover, in his pragmatic approach to globalization, Cardoso articulates a market concept of society. For him, citizens are consumers who have "interests" rather than "needs." The government does not actively search out particular problems or areas of need to attend to—that is the work of mobilized interest groups. "There has never before been so much NGO action within the government as has occurred in the past ten years. In all our social programs there was some kind of social movement involved." According to Cardoso, these elements of cooperation and nongovernmental involvement are key for maximizing the state's regulatory power and equity in the face of the market's agency in resource allocation and benefits. The work of NGOs and their international counterparts gives voice to specific mobilized communities and helps to consolidate public actions that are "wider and more efficacious than state action."

In these conditions, lawmaking is the main arena of state action—and putting new laws into practice is an activist matter. Cardoso lauds the signing of the AIDS treatment law, given that "They said nothing would pass." In mobilizing for a law and approving it, the state realizes its social contract. In Cardoso's vision, specific policies and legislation replace a wider social contract. In practice, people have to engage with lawmaking and jurisprudence to be seen by the state and the implementation of the law remains subject to a whole range of exclusionary dynamics related to economic considerations and specific social pressure. The AIDS treatment policy, one can argue, illuminates what was at stake in past political decisions and economic maneuvers and how they are being remediated by novel state–medical–market initiatives.

The Pharmaceuticalization of Public Health

Global pharmaceutical sales reached $602 billion in 2005—a growth of 7% from the previous year. According to IMS Health, the world's leading market intelligence firm: "As growth in mature markets moderates, industry attention is shifting to smaller, developing markets that are performing exceptionally well."[6] This is the case of Brazil, now the 11th largest pharmaceutical market in the world (see Bermudez 1995). Currently, some 550 pharmaceutical firms (including laboratories, importers, and distributors) operate in Brazil and compete for a slice of its lucrative pharmaceutical market, which in 2005 reached $10 billion. By 2010, the developing world is expected to account for approximately 26% of the world pharmaceutical market in value, compared with 14.5% in 1999.

Dr. Radames, a Brazilian infectious disease specialist and adviser to the WHO explained to me: "Pharmaceutical companies had already recouped their research investment with the sell-off of AIDS drugs in the United States and Europe and now with Brazil, they had a new fixed market and, even if they had to lower prices, they had some unforeseen return. If things worked out in Brazil, new AIDS markets could be opened in Asia and perhaps in Africa" (personal communication, August 2000).

Dr. Jones, an executive of a pharmaceutical multinational that sells ARVs to the Brazilian government, does not put things so explicitly, but he asserts that "patents are not the problem. The problem is that there are no markets for these medications in most poor countries. Things worked out in Brazil because of political will" (personal communication, June 2003). For him, "no markets" in Africa, for example, dovetails with poverty *and* with local governments' lack of a holistic vision of public health in which the public and private sectors work in tandem: "AIDS lays bare all the inadequacies of a country's approach to public health. We see an evolution in countries that have coordinated efforts, a strong national AIDS program, partnership with private sectors, and the country's leader supporting intervention."

Dr. Jones continued: "Health is not an area that the Brazilian government allowed to deteriorate anywhere near the degree of what we see in other developing countries. You had an existing structure of STD clinics and World Bank funding helped to strengthen the infrastructure." In this rendering, Brazil's "massive political will" to treat AIDS coincides with the country's partnership with both international agencies and the pharmaceutical industry:

> Different than in Africa, in Brazil we had a successful business with our first antiretroviral products. And we will continue to have tremendously successful businesses based on our partnership approach with the government. Brazil continues to be an example of how you can do the right thing in terms of public health, understanding the needs of both the private sector and the government and its population. The government was able to take advantage of existing realities. There was no intellectual property protection for our early products, and given Brazil's industrial capacity, they were able to produce the drugs.

I asked Dr. Jones how the pharmaceutical industry reacted to this strategy. "We were angry," he said. But rather than withdraw from Brazil, the company used the incident over pricing and generics to negotiate broader market access in Brazil.

> The downside could have been "why bother and continue to invest in Brazil?" But anti-HIV products are not the sole bread and butter of most companies. So from a portfolio perspective, any private company balances its specific activities vis-à-vis the entirety of what it is doing. This one sector was being affected but our company had been in Brazil for a long time and we continued to be ranked as a top company there. So we had to look at it in a much broader perspective than an action taken in one product category.

By juxtaposing the arguments of both corporate actors and policymakers one can identify the logic of such a pharmaceutical form of governance. Here, political will means novel public–private cooperation over medical technologies. Once a government designates a disease like AIDS "the country's disease," a therapeutic market takes shape—the state acting as both the drug purchaser and distributor. As this government addresses the needs of its population (now supposedly contained in the "country's disease"), the financial operations of pharmaceutical companies are taken in new directions and enlarged, particularly as older lines of treatment (generic ARVs) lose their efficacy, necessitating the introduction of newer and more expensive treatments (still under patent protection) that are demanded by mobilized patients. Patienthood and civic participation thus conflate in an emerging market. Development agencies (such as the WHO, UNAIDS, and the World Bank) assist this process, which has crucial ramifications for the nature and scope of national and local public health interventions.

Magic-bullet approaches (i.e., delivery of technology regardless of healthcare infrastructure) are increasingly the norm, and companies are themselves using the activist discourse that access to medicines is a matter of human rights. This pharmaceuticalization of public health has short- and long-term goals, as Dr. Jones puts it:

> At what point does it get to the government that today citizens put a huge premium on access to health? And it is not just a matter of guaranteeing access to the available medications but to the new ones being developed. If you don't have the capacity to produce this new medication, then you have to find a way to align yourself and trade with those who are doing it. With a global disease like AIDS, you must play together and not on your own.

I asked former Health Minister José Serra (an economist and now governor of the state of São Paulo) whether the state had the capacity to address other large-scale diseases pharmaceutically. "Without a doubt," the economist said.

> But the problem does not lie in government. The government ends up responding to society's pressure, and with AIDS, the pressure was very well organized. See the case of tuberculosis. It is easier to treat than AIDS, and much cheaper. The major difficulty lies in treatment adherence. But you are unable to mobilize NGOs and society for this cause. If TB had a fifth of the kind of social mobilization AIDS has, the problem would be solved. *So it is a problem of society itself* (personal communication, June 2003).

For Cardoso, too, the management of AIDS is clear evidence that politics have moved beyond the control of parties and ideologies. "There is no superior intelligence imposing anything ... a party, a president, an ideology. Rather there are assemblages, alliances, strategies," he stated in the interview in 2003.

> Today Brazilian society is much more open than people imagine and very mobilized. In reality, people do not live in a state of illusion as intellectuals and journalists generally think of them; they have learned to mobilize and know how to make pressure and activate those in congress with whom they have affinities.

This is also true for the pharmaceutical industry and its powerful lobby, I added. Cardoso replied,

> Indeed, they also mobilize because there is a struggle going on. A bet on democracy leads to this kind of diversity. The government has to navigate amid all these pressures. It must set some specific objectives and develop directives that end amid this confusion. It cannot just be on this or that side, it must more or less pilot.

The ARV rollout was implemented across the country through an ailing universal health-care system. This specific policy was aligned with a pharmaceutically focused form of health delivery that was being articulated by the Cardoso administration. Indeed, Brazil has seen an incremental change in the concept of public health, from prevention and clinical care to community-based care and medicating—that is, *public health is increasingly decentralized and pharmaceuticalized.* As part of a policy of rationalization and decentralization of assistance, in the mid-1990s the government began to recast the costly and inefficient basic pharmacy program whereby municipalities distributed state-funded medicines to the general population (this program preexisted the ARV rollout). Provinces and municipalities were urged to develop their own epidemiologically specific treatment strategies and to administer federal and regional funds in the acquisition and dispensation of medicines. According to government officials, the policy would contribute to reducing hospitalizations (which tended to dominate state funding) and to making families and communities stronger participants in therapeutic processes (Cosendey, Bermudez, Reis, Silva, Oliveira, et al. 2000).

Overall, as I discovered in my fieldwork in the southern and northeastern regions, the availability of essential medicines has been subject to changing political winds; treatments are easily discontinued, and people have to seek more specialized services in the private health sector or, as many put it, "die waiting" in overcrowded public clinics. Even though the responsibility for distributing medicines has become increasingly decentralized, the lobbies of patient groups (modeled after AIDS treatment activism) and of the pharmaceutical industry have kept the federal government responsible for the purchase of medication classified as "exceptional," as well as medication for disease populations that are part of "special national programs" such as the AIDS program. An increasing number of patients are filing legal suits, forcing regional governments to maintain the inflow of high-cost medicines that are entering the market. According to public health expert Jorge Bermudez "an individualized rather than collective pharmaceutical care" is being consolidated in the country (Bermudez et al. 2000). A critical understanding of the AIDS policy's success must keep in sight this mobilization over inclusion and exclusion as global drug markets and certain forms of "good government" are being realized.

Global Health Politics

The AIDS crisis in the developing world is finally on the radar of transnational organizations, governments, and citizens alike. Many public- and private-sector treatment initiatives are being launched, and the international debate has now shifted to how this can be most effectively done in contexts of limited resources. According to activist groups, the Global Fund to Fight AIDS, TB, and Malaria "represents the globalization of Brazil's model of harnessing the forces of government and civil society to confront the AIDS challenge."[7] More than 100 countries have together committed a total of $3 billion to the Global Fund—an international health financing institution—with the United States pledging to donate the most, $2 billion. Here, governments and civic organizations focus on funding rather than implementation. The development of aid projects (mostly aimed at helping women and vulnerable children) is left to local groups. When the United Nations' AIDS Program was founded in 1996 it had $300 million available for loans to middle- and low-income countries. This budget increased to $4.7 billion by 2003. The World Bank, which has supported the development of the Brazilian AIDS program, has played the largest role in financing UNAIDS.

This increase in AIDS funding in recent years "is largely a fruit of the well-coordinated activism of the international community," stated Dr. Paulo Teixeira, Brazil's former AIDS coordinator, in a Global Health Governance Workshop in São Paulo in June 2005 (see Wogart and Calcagnotto 2006). "We have changed the discourse and paradigm of intervention," he told me. "It has become politically costly for development agencies and governments not to engage AIDS." Yet, the operations of global AIDS programs and their interface with governments and civic organizations "reflect and extend existing power relations, and this synergy can be quite negative," Dr. Teixeira added. "The negotiating power of developing countries is simply too low, be it at the United Nations or at the WTO. AIDS gave poorer countries a small window of opportunity to intervene in global governance and to try to recast the uneven correlation of forces."

Dr. Paulo Teixeira is an insider to these emergent forms of transnational (pharmaceutical) governance. Alongside Dr. Jim Yong Kim, he helped coordinate the joint WHO and UNAIDS "3 by 5" campaign, aimed at providing ARVs to 3 million people by 2005. In June 2005, the WHO reported that approximately 1 million people were on ARVs in low- and middle-income countries, in contrast to 400,000 in December 2003. Dr. Kim reflected on falling short of the desired target: "We didn't do enough, and we began to deal with the problem too late." Yet, "before '3 by 5' there was no emphasis in saving lives," he said. "Many world leaders thought that we had to forget this generation of HIV-infected people and to think only of the next generation. We did something to change this."[8] Indeed, increased availability of ARVs averted an estimated 250,000–350,000 premature deaths in the developing world in 2005 alone (WHO 2006). Yet, funding bottlenecks, personnel shortages, and continuing debates on drug pricing and patents have limited this and many other AIDS initiatives. As Dr. Teixeira put it, "In the name of their own interests, private foundations, rich governments, and pharmaceutical companies keep putting all kinds of obstacles to a more rapid scale-up of AIDS treatments. Interventions of the pharmaceutical companies are paralyzing the WHO."

In October 2005, I talked to Dr. Jane Walker, the executive vice president of a U.S.-based pharmaceutical company. For her, the Brazilian AIDS treatment program worked "not so much because of politics, but because of a good allocation of resources." As for treating AIDS in poorer regions, Dr. Walker insisted that "drug price is not the problem; the problem is infrastructure." Dr. Walker was now leading her company's efforts to "not just" bring ARVs to women and children in hard-hit places in sub-Saharan Africa, "but to build up local treatment capacity." This medical care and research endeavor was carried out in partnership with global AIDS initiatives, local health-care groups, and NGOs. For this executive, it seemed matter-of-fact that public–private partnerships did better infrastructural work than state institutions alone. This discourse of state replacement, I thought, added an activist and morally urgent spin to a central tenet of neoclassical economics: the idea of a self-regulating market. The challenge, Dr. Walker told me, "is to find treatment models that can be inexpensively scaled up. Every one of the estimated 40 million people living with HIV is a person. We must do something as a world. We must save every one of these lives. The solution is not medicine as we practice and as we know it. We must save every one of these lives."

In this philanthropic discourse, one saves lives by finding new technical tools and cost-effective means to deliver care: that is, medicines and testing kits. The civil and political violations that precede disease are apparently out of sight in this pharmaceutical humanitarianism, and the economic injustices reflected in barely functioning health-care systems are depoliticized (Farmer 2003). In the end, governments function on the business side, merely purchasing and distributing medicines, while nurture—now a technological endeavor—is left to communities and patients.

The U.S. president's $15 billion Emergency Plan for AIDS Relief (PEPFAR) reflects this global pharmaceutical frame of assistance. Announced in early 2003, PEPFAR aims to bring therapy to 2 million people and to prevent 7 million new infections by 2008 in 15 of the neediest countries in Africa and the Caribbean. However, there is a catch: rather than subscribing to the WHO's drug-approval process, PEPFAR requires separate approval from the U.S. Food and Drug Administration (FDA). Officials claim that this is to protect the safety and quality of drugs. But critics have accused the Bush administration of delays and of actually reserving money for expensive brand-name drugs, thus reducing the number of potential recipients.[9] Defying these and other criticisms, in May 2004 PEPFAR began buying generics, and in July 2006 the FDA approved a generic 3-in-1 combination ARV made by the Indian manufacturer Aurobindo Pharma. According to Dr. Mark R. Dybul, acting U.S. global AIDS coordinator, it is unclear if the generic drug will significantly cut costs, but by requiring patients to only take 1 pill 2 times a day the combination drug "should facilitate better therapies and better adherence."[10] Global ARV rollouts rightly open the door to drug access, but they also exemplify the inadequacies of a magic-bullet approach to health care. The methodological designs of AIDS treatment programs (pilot and otherwise), as well as the models they employ need to be carefully scrutinized by policymakers and politicized by activists. PEPFAR, for example, has an expeditionary quality, implemented from without, and is designed to save lives. It favors large-scale drug distribution but does not adequately address the issue of public health-care infrastructure improvements, or, for that matter, prophylaxis and treatment of opportunistic diseases. This focus on drug delivery and supply chain management stretches far beyond ARV rollout and has recently contributed to popularizing blanket treatment approaches for many tropical diseases, including preventive medications for conditions such as childhood malaria and river blindness, as well as antibiotic treatments that have no preventive function in national deworming campaigns for schoolchildren. Critics have rightly pointed out that, generally speaking, the strategies underlying new global health interventions are not comprehensive and are ultimately of poor quality (Epstein 2007; Ramiah and Reich 2006). Many question their sustainability in the absence of more serious involvement of national governments and greater authority for international institutions to hold donors and partners accountable. With health policy's success largely re-framed in terms of providing and counting the best medicines and newest technology delivered, what space remains for the development of low-tech solutions (such as community development or the provision of clean water) that could prove more sustainable and ultimately more humanistic?

Drugs are ancillary to the full treatment of the disease. Alone, neither money nor drugs, or even a sophisticated pilot model guarantee success. Healing, after all, is a multifaceted concept, and healing is no more synonymous with treatment than treatment is with drugs. Large-scale treatment programs tend to miss cultural systems and the interpersonal networks that link patients, doctors, and governments, which are especially important in resource-poor settings, where clinical infrastructures are not improving (Whyte, Whyte, Meinert, and Kyaddondo 2006). This elision of the local from the planning framework leaves unaddressed the clinical continuity necessary for successful AIDS treatment. As a result, extremely well-endowed efforts—facing the humanitarian paradox of lifesaving drugs versus caregiving infrastructure—are by and large falling short of the mark, without effecting the changes hoped for.

The work of anthropologist-physician Paul Farmer and Partners in Health provides a contrasting community-based model for AIDS treatment. The HIV Equity Initiative in Haiti does not operate like a traditional NGO, that is, removed from people. A pragmatic solidarity with the ill and destitute is its starting point. It uses the local clinic as the nexus of care within integrated prevention activities and ARV administration. "Improving clinical services can improve the quality of prevention efforts, boost staff morale, and reduce AIDS-related stigma," states Farmer (n/d; see also Walton, Farmer, Lambert, Léandre, Koenig, et al. 2004). In this holistic approach, accounting for individual trajectories and staying with patients through the progression of the disease (the work of *accompagneteurs*) is considered as important as tackling the social factors that affect patients' families and mitigating the decays of clinical infrastructures.

While Partners in Health's treatment initiative is by no means accepted as a gold standard, its presence has created dents in the prevailing rationalities that guide the treatment of AIDS in resource-poor settings. In challenging the view that comprehensive care of this sort is unsustainable, the project has gained a kind of iconic role/value, expressing unforeseen possibilities and articulating a new human rights imperative. However, its expansion also begets an array of questions concerning the ethical grounds for prioritizing AIDS over other diseases of poverty (malaria and diarrhea, for example), as well as political questions regarding its operationalization and sustainability over time (Das 2006). The WHO's difficulties in pushing forward with the "3 by 5" campaign leave no doubt that even the noblest of efforts are inherently political and must be understood in relation to the strategies of both national governments and global initiatives. Nonetheless, Partners in Health has opened up new spaces and redefined the perceived boundaries of feasibility.

Drug Resistance and the Sustainability of ARV Rollouts

In our conversation in June 2005, Dr. Teixeira expressed concern about the sustainability of Brazil's AIDS treatment policy. "I had high hopes in this government. But for reasons that have not been made public, the government has been reluctant to make bold moves as far as generics, patents, and international relations are concerned." By early 2004, for example, the national AIDS program had taken the technical and legal measures that were needed for the government to issue compulsory licenses for the production of 2 patented drugs that took up almost 60% of the country's AIDS treatment budget. "We had preliminary agreements with Indian companies to provide us the necessary chemical materials, and I was at the WHO to provide international support," Dr. Teixeira stated. "It was just a matter of the health minister appearing on national television and announcing it, but he did not." Other public health scholars at the Global Health Governance Workshop told me that the AIDS policy had actually lost some of its political currency, as it was taken as a "success story of the previous administration." The current administration wants to construct "its own success stories." As is always the case in Brazil's political culture, electoral motives take priority over policy continuity. Besides political factors, "there is also confusion and administrative incompetence," pointed out Michel Lotrowska, an economist working for Doctors Without Borders' research program on neglected diseases in Rio de Janeiro. Given new budgets and bureaucracies, for the first time in 2005 there were shortages of ARVs in the health-care system, Lotrowska stated.[11]

"The vigilance that was in place is being compromised," Dr. Teixeira added. "We are lagging in technology."[12] The ARV reverse engineering program at Farmanguinhos (the state's main laboratory) has been partially dismantled and generic drug development is not keeping pace with the market. Lotrowska gave the example of Tenefovir, an important rescue drug (used in case of treatment resistance):

> Brazil is one of the few emerging markets in which companies make money with ARVs. So they isolated Brazil in terms of pricing. It is a very expensive drug, it takes a lot of the AIDS budget, and there is nothing to replace it. India never got interested in producing it, and Brazil did not think prospectively. The government cannot issue a compulsory license for it. Things are disorganized, and people at various levels of government are fighting each other. The country's machinery of AIDS drug development is stalled. Of course, all this is good for big pharma.

Brazil is now experiencing what other countries treating AIDS will soon face. It has very inexpensive first-line ARVs, but a growing number of people are going into new drug regimens (either because earlier combinations did not work or because patients and doctors are demanding access to more sophisticated drugs, with fewer side effects) that are entering the market. With patients taking advantage of new treatments, Brazil's ARV budget has increased to nearly $500 million in 2005. In spite of the country's generic production, about 80% of the medication in the budget is patented. Lotrowska concluded:

> We are moving toward absolute drug monopoly. In a few years, the price of AIDS treatment will increase significantly. Given patent restrictions and all the bilateral agreements that are in place, we have less and less competition regarding generics. We have to find a mechanism that can lead to price reduction without this competition. Without such a mechanism, medics will soon have to tell patients "I can only give you first-line treatment, and if you become drug resistant then you will die."

In the meantime, as I have been arguing throughout this chapter, a pharmaceutically centered model of public health is being consolidated worldwide, and medicines have become increasingly equated with health care for afflicted populations. As with other disease entities, pharmaceutical companies have operated astutely within legal and regulatory windows of opportunity in the case of AIDS, redirecting activist and political gains to their own advantage—be it as public relations gains through corporate philanthropy, as financial profits from global treatment projects, or as market expansion via developing states that have made AIDS "the country's disease" (as it is with Brazil, now a captive purchaser of ARVs).

Consider Roche's recently introduced drug, T-20 (Fuzeon, enfurvirtide). This drug is the first of a new class of drugs—called fusion inhibitors, which keep HIV particles from fusing with lymphocytes—that will undoubtedly have great impact in preventing or coping with drug resistance. In Brazil, some 1,200 patients were prescribed T-20 immediately after the drug's debut, with a yearly cost of $20,000 per patient. "When the starting price of a drug is as T-20's, it is evident that after some time you will get a 30 to 50 percent price reduction," Lotrowska told me. "But even with this reduction, what will happen to the country's AIDS budget when thousands more will need it or want it?" While back in Salvador in June 2005, I learned that pharmaceutical representatives were training local infectious disease experts to make T-20 a first-line treatment rather than simply a rescue drug. This is a common practice, according to Bart Kroger, a Dutch medical researcher now living and working in Salvador. "These opinion-makers are extremely well paid, and they present the drug and treatment options in local congresses," he said, astounded by the global reach of medical science and ethics.

> The specialists take on a 'neutral' position, generally presenting positive aspects of the drug in question but also criticizing less important aspects of the drug. They don't want to sound as if they had been bought by the company. This is important for them not to lose credibility among peers and also to keep open the possibility of working for other companies in the future.

I also heard of cases where doctors began prescribing the rescue drug Kaletra (lopinavir/ritonavir) at the time of its 2002 launch in the United States, before its registration in Brazil. These doctors referred patients to a local AIDS NGO and to public-interest lawyers, forcing the government to provide medication not yet approved by the country's National Health Surveillance Agency. For better or worse, such developments compromise the sovereignty of the state in the fields of biological and pharmaceutical governance. In the face of pervasive pharmaceutical marketing, enmeshed with patient mobilization, regulatory incoherence thrives. And these local "medical sovereigns" are now also market operators. They mediate the introduction of new drugs in the public health-care system and, as we will in the next section, in the name of adherence and concern over drug resistance, they triage away patients who could benefit from the system's caregiving capacity, dismal as it is. Meanwhile, policymakers have to ceaselessly invent new political strategies to keep the country's pharmaceutical policy in place. In May 2007, Brazil crossed a new threshold when for the first time it broke the patent of an AIDS drug. The government stopped price negotiations with Merck over Efavirenz, which is used by 75,000 Brazilians, and decided to import a generic version from India. Officials claim that this will save the country some $236.8 million by 2012. Activists praise this move as an important advance in the widening of access to the newest and most expensive therapies.

Local Economies of Salvation

Just as the complex Brazilian response to AIDS must be understood within the wider context of the country's democratization and the restructuring of both state and market, so too it must be seen in light of its interaction with local worlds and the subsequent refiguring of lives and values. On the ground, health programs do not work in tandem and administrative discontinuities abound. Different provinces allocate public health resources differently according to the pressure of interest groups. And the AIDS NGOs that were supposed to have taken over assistance "have long lost idealism and passion," as activist Gerson Winkler bitterly told me in September 2005 in his hometown of Porto Alegre. "They keep selecting their clientele and find all kind of ways to pretend that they are fulfilling their projects' goals." Thus, against the background of budgetary constraints, regional politics, and the "professionalization and industrialization of the nongovernmental sector" (in Winkler's words), a multitude of interpersonal networks and variations in AIDS care have emerged, creating uneven levels of quality of life for patients—the underside of the pharmaceuticalization of public health. Only a few manage to constitute themselves as patient citizens, and this brings me back to Caasah.

When I returned to Caasah in December 2001, things had changed dramatically. Caasah had been relocated to a new, state-funded building. Located in a residential area near the famous *Igreja do Bonfim* (the church of the good end), the new facility was gated all around. With treatment regimens available, long-term residents had been asked to move out, and Caasah had been redesigned as a short-term care facility (a "house of passage," *casa de passagem*) for ill patients and a shelter for HIV-positive orphans. The triage room had been closed, and a team of social workers and nurses now worked directly with local hospitals and admitted to Caasah the patients who "fit into the institution and its norms," in the words of Celeste Gomes, still presiding over Caasah. Disturbingly, there was no systematic effort to actively track these patients and their treatment once they left.

"This is a beautiful building, but that's all the state gave us," stated Celeste. Institutional maintenance was a daily struggle. "We owe more than $1,000 to local pharmacies. Our patients come from the hospital with their ARVs but nothing else. No vitamins, no pain-killers, no bactrim to treat opportunistic diseases." As AIDS became more chronic than fatal, local programs were not necessarily readjusting themselves to meet the new needs of patients. The national ARV rollout was supposed to be matched by regional government's provision of treatments for opportunistic infections. But it was clearly up to proxy health services such as Caasah or to the patients themselves to arrange treatment beyond ARVs.

At the state hospital I learned of the existence of a triage system that Caasah is part of. "Homeless AIDS patients remain outside the system," one of the hospital's social worker told me. "Doctors say that they do not put these patients on ARVs for there is no guarantee that they will continue the treatment. They are concerned about the creation of viral resistance to medication." The hospital's leading infectious disease specialist confirmed that "if a patient is a drug user we tell him that he has to come back. If he demonstrates a strong will then we put him on treatment. But they never, or rarely, come back." Against an expanding discourse of human rights and pharmaceutical possibilities, we are here confronted with the limits of the on-the-ground infrastructures whereby accountability and the right to envision a new life with AIDS are realized, but only on a partial basis.

I looked for my former collaborators and tracked down those who had left Caasah. Of the 22 residents I had gotten to know in-depth in 1997, 10 were alive. Only Tiquinho, the hemophiliac child who had been raised there, was allowed to stay. All of the adult survivors created new family units. They lived with other AIDS patients, reunited with estranged relatives, married, and some even had children. All of them had disability pensions and were entitled to a monthly food basket at Caasah. By charting the trajectories of these AIDS survivors—those who lived pre- and post-ARV rollout—we can identify some of the everyday mechanisms that, despite the existence of medical technology, make AIDS a chronic disease.

"Today is another world," Luis Cardoso told me. "One Luis has died and another has emerged. A person has to think differently, forget the past." First diagnosed with AIDS in 1993, Luis lived in Caasah from 1995 to 1999. "One Luis has died and another has emerged. I have nothing to say against the antiretrovirals. Celeste and the psychologists motivated me a lot. But I don't live here anymore, and I must take care of myself. I got used to the medication. Medication is me now."

For Celeste, "Luis is like a son." He represents Caasah and the state of Bahia in national meetings of people living with AIDS, and he runs HIV/AIDS prevention workshops in the interior. Even Dr. Nanci, Luis' doctor, calls him "my teacher." As she told me: "I find this fantastic. The patient had a history of self-abuse, remains poor, but rescues himself and teaches others to do the same." Besides his AIDS disability pension, Luis also earned a salary as Caasah's office assistant. This allowed him to rent a shack with a friend, to eat well, and to save a little, because, as he put it, "I want to have my own corner." Open about his homosexuality, Luis insinuated he was dating. He also proudly told us that he had adopted an AIDS orphan in Caasah and was paying for the boy's grandmother to take care of him. "The world is a school in getting lost. But it is up to me to take life forward. I always believed in God, but religious talk does not help if you don't have the will to live inside you."

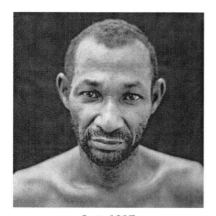 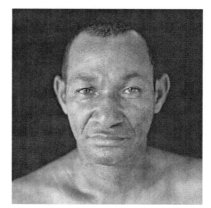

Luis 1997   Luis 2001
(Photo by Torben Eskerod)

Luis is an amazing person, hard-working, witty, *and* a master of a moral discourse. He speaks of a new economy of life instincts organized around AIDS therapies. "I face my problem. I take advantage of the help I get. I struggle to live." He is indeed the representative of a new medical collective, and his discourse conveys present-day forms and limits of society and state: "I have nothing to do with society," he says. "From my perspective, society is a set of masters deciding what risk is, and what is bad for them. I have never participated in that. As for the government, I must say that I am thankful for the medication. This is the good aspect of the state. The rest is for me to do."

Luis made treatment adherence seem too easy. As much as I admired his resilience, I also found his righteousness disturbing. For him, individual conscience was the apriority of a healthy existence, and mourning a loss, any kind of loss, was a defect to be overcome. Moreover, the overemphasis on individual responsibility was self-serving. It clearly reflected Caasah's house of passage modus operandi and, more broadly, the predominant discourse that one has to ever more be lord of oneself, upbeat, and upward. The institutional and interpersonal forces that have thrown Luis into action in the first place were absent from his life-extending account, particularly as he spoke of noncompliant *marginais*. It was evident from his recollection that without belonging to Caasah, ARVs wouldn't have had the same kind of efficacy they had for him, and that he kept harnessing strength from being the object of regular public attention. His narrative of regeneration remains built on the exclusion of those who cannot conform:

> It is not a matter of getting them [homeless AIDS patients] help. For they already have it [in the form of medication]. They use their social condition as an excuse to keep their habits. It is a question of self-destruction. As I see it, these people are more for death than for life. But I also know many people who struggle to live and to earn their money honestly and don't surrender. See Rose and Evangivaldo ... It is your mind that makes the difference.

"Welcome to the end of the world," Rose said jokingly as I entered her brick shack, located at the lower end of a muddy hill in the outskirts of Salvador. "I am sold on the antiretrovirals," she told me. "I am part of this multitude that will do whatever is necessary to guarantee our right to these drugs. I am proud of Brazil." Caasah helped Rose to get the shack from the government, and she was living there with her 1-year-old daughter. She had also taken in her now teenage son who had been under the custody of Professor Carlos, Caasah's chief nurse. "I am always struggling to pay the bills and raise my children, for I am mother and father."

Tearful, she recollected the death of her partner Jorge from AIDS-related diseases, a few months before the girl was born. She had done all that was medically possible. "Jessica got AZT, but the last exam showed that she is still seropositive." Rose knew that the child's HIV status could change until she reached the age of 2: "She has never been ill and we hope for the best." Rose was proud to be "a good patient, but not a fanatic one," she added.

> I drink a beer and have some fun on the weekends, but I know my limits, what my body can take. I don't live better for I lack material conditions. I tell you, I want to be alive to see a cure. In the name of Jesus, I want to be a guinea pig

when they test the vaccine. Yes, people are still dying with AIDS in the streets, but I am no longer there.

The political economy of AIDS, spanning both national and international institutions, engenders local therapeutic environments within which individuals and AIDS organizations are codependent and must recraft positions in every exchange. Their transactions are legitimated by a humanitarian and pharmaceutical discourse of lifesaving and civic empowerment. In adhering to drug regimens and making new and productive lives for themselves, patients are—in this discourse—saved. However, merely guaranteeing existence in such dire contexts, amid the dismantling of institutions of care, involves a calculus that goes well beyond numbers of pills and the timing of their intake. The political grounds of existence have been increasingly individualized and atomized, and poor AIDS patients rarely become activists. Even as they search for employment, AIDS survivors work hard to remain eligible for whatever the state's paternalistic politics and remedial programs have made available—renewal of disability benefits, free bus vouchers, and additional medication at local health posts, to name a few. Being adopted by a doctor and becoming a model patient greatly facilitates this. And this material calculus becomes all the more important as patients form new families and resume a life considered normal, which was previously impossible to them.

"What a joy you give me by coming back," beamed 38-year-old Evangivaldo. His face was barely recognizable, but the aesthetic side effects of antiretrovirals were the least of his concerns. I met him by chance, as he came by Caasah, looking for help: "Today I woke up anguished. We had no gas to cook. I hope you can help me." Evangivaldo and his partner Fatima left Caasah in 1999 and they had a 2-year-old daughter Juliana. "A child is what I wanted most in life. Juliana fulfilled my desire, a dream I had. I thought I would die without being a father." He said he was on antipsychotic medication and then added: "It is the financial part of life that tortures me." Evangivaldo showed me a piece of paper in which he had listed how his income was allocated and the debts he had to pay.

> When Fatima cannot do the work, I am the man and woman of the house. Sometimes I wake up at 4 A.M., leave everything ready, and ride my bike for 2 hours, to get downtown. I go door to door, asking for a job. There are days when I cannot get the money we need and I panic. My head spins, and I fall down. I hide in a corner and cry. Then I don't know where I am. But I tell myself, 'Focus Evangivaldo, you will find your bike and your way home.'

"And do you know why I manage to do this?" Evangivaldo asked me. "It is because my daughter is waiting for me." Indeed, to have someone to live for and to be desired by seemed to be a core element in the account of the AIDS survivors with whom I worked.

Understanding the Nexus of AIDS, Poverty, and Politics

"If you look carefully, nothing has changed. Things are the same as you saw last time," a tired Celeste told me in June 2005 during my last trip to Salvador. Caasah was still the only place in Salvador that provided systematic care to poor AIDS patients who have been discharged from public hospitals.

> They recover here, but medication for opportunistic diseases is difficult for us to get. Some patients return to their families. Others go back to the streets. I would say that half of people living in the streets are HIV infected. The situation remains the same: disease keeps spreading, and the government pretends not to know of it, so that it does not have to intervene.

At the state's main AIDS Unit, Dr. Nanci also told me that "things here have not changed." As she put it: "The reality of our Unit is the same as it was in the beginning of the epidemic: full of miserable and wasted patients. The difference is that they now come from the interior, where no new services have been created. Access to therapies has been democratized, but health has not."

I asked Celeste for news about the patients I had followed over the years. Out of the initial group of 22 patients with whom I had worked in 1997, 7 were still alive in 2005—among them, Luis, Rose, and Evangivaldo. This life extension is obviously a result of technological advancements, argued Celeste, "but it would not have happened if they had not learned to care for themselves." In the end, treatment adherence "is relative to each person. It requires a lot of will." Subjectivity—a person's manufactured will to live—had become a fundamental cog in the ARV adherence machine. Yet, as I would soon learn, all of the former residents who were still alive also possessed a place they called home, a steady if meager income, and a social network. And, in case of an emergency, they could still resort to Caasah. This tie to Caasah, as momentary and uncertain as it now was, remained vital to them.

Luis was still working at Caasah. He was in charge of the institution's fundraising activities. "I am not concerned with HIV. What I want is to live. If there is medication, let's take life forward. Life is to fight for." In the previous year, Luis had experienced kidney failure and had been hospitalized for 2 weeks. "Work keeps my mind occupied and one needs to have projects and objectives to meet—if not life has no meaning." Becoming a father, he said, "is the best thing that ever happened to me." Davi, his adopted son, was now a healthy 7-year-old—"He is a prankster. He is my passion. He makes it all worthwhile."

"I don't have the aid of a father and a mother, and I can only count on the tenderness of Fatima and Juliana," Evangivaldo told me as we met again. "When I see them with no food, it makes me ill. But when I find a job or get a donation, and there is nothing lacking at home, and all is normal, then for me it is another life, and it is all good." I asked Evangivaldo whether he had told his doctor all he has to go through in life. "Yes," he had once mentioned to his doctor that he routinely rode his bike for 2 hours "with only coffee and medication in the body" to get to downtown Salvador in search of a job. "Dr. Jackson said that he did not believe it, that my HIV was almost undetectable and that I acted as if I did not have AIDS. I told him that my bike was parked outside the hospital, that I would show it to him. He was amazed. He then called his superior and some residents and asked me to tell them my story."

After the spectacle Evangivaldo had become, "The doctors said that they were proud of me, and that if all HIV-positive people had the same will to live that I have then no one would have to be hospitalized. They said that I was an example for other patients." Evangivaldo took the opportunity to ask the doctors for advice on where to go to actually find a job, to which Dr. Jackson replied: "I feel bad for not being able to help, but I am sure that God will show a path for you to get where you want to." Meanwhile, Evangivaldo had to take 12 pills a day, and his doctor never considered putting him on a newer medication already made available by the government (fewer pills and fewer side effects).

Poor AIDS patients such as Evangivaldo continuously interact and trade with AIDS NGOs and civic groups that channel assistance, albeit minimal, from regional and national programs. The NGOs, which depend on their clientele to back up reports and authorize new projects (now mostly related to treatment adherence and income generation), become venues for some patients to access food, rent aid, and specialized medical consultations, among other things. Overwhelmed with assistance demands and concern for their own institutional survival, NGOs rarely succeed in placing the person in the market, but they do successfully differentiate politicized patients who defend their rights from those who passively circulate in the medical service system. Only a few, such as 30-year-old Sonara, manage to become "AIDS workers." She was Caasah's new poster person. A nurse introduced me to Sonara—"She was a drug user, but she now takes the medication, eats well, and takes care of her daughter, who is also HIV positive"—as she was running a candle-making workshop for a group of 12 patients. Sonara was the only white person there. Her style of dress, manners, and speech were characteristic of the Brazilian middle-class. As much as I admired Sonara's transformation, I could not have been more disturbed by her moral reasoning: "Today, people only die of AIDS if they want to."

A recent survey on mortality in the state of São Paulo revealed that AIDS is 2 times more fatal among black patients than it is among white patients. According to researcher Luís Eduardo Batista, "The majority of blacks have less formal education, lower income and live in the peripheries."[13] On average, a white person in São Paulo earns almost double of what a black person earns.

From Batista's perspective, "racism impacts health" because blacks receive substandard care and go unaddressed in prevention campaigns. The violence of daily life is reinforced in this case by interlocking and discriminatory organizational contexts, which overdetermine AIDS as a medical failure. The AIDS survivors I interviewed acted coldly toward fellow patients. For many, I thought, health corresponded to a measure of moral uprightness. Mutual empathy was rare. I will never understand why, for example, Luis did not let us take Rose's food basket to her as we were heading back to her shack in the Cajazeiras district in early June 2005. The previous day, over the phone, Rose had asked me to do just that. She would save a long trip and transportation expenses, I told Luis. But my request met a series of obstacles, both external and internal: "The baskets are not ready. Professor Carlos is not here to release them. I don't have much time. I must be back no later than 11 A.M. We have to go."

Rose was euphoric to see us. She was doing great. I was particularly happy to learn that her daughter had turned HIV-negative. Ricardo, her 15-year-old son, was helping 2 workers to finish the house's second floor: "It is my skyscraper. Water was infiltrating, and in the long run I plan to rent it out." She was disappointed that we had not brought her basket. I offered Rose a ride back to Caasah, but she said that she couldn't leave the construction unattended: "That's life. Each one is on her own." Rose intelligently navigated the local circuits of AIDS care. She had garnered the support of other NGOs and opened up a little business she called "*Rose tem de tudo*" (Rose has it all), and had also devised a construction fundraising campaign among religious philanthropists. She was proud of having been able to enroll her son in project Teenage Citizen (*Adolescente Cidadão*), which Dona Conceição was running with World Bank funds.

Later that week, I met with Dona Conceição. She had accomplished much and now headed IBCM (the Conceição Macedo Assistential Institute). With the help of a local sociologist, she had designed a project to employ 120 children of AIDS patients in local industries. She kept working with homeless and poor AIDS patients. "In the morning I am at IBCM, and in the afternoon I am in the streets." Dona Conceição aided a total of 200 families, she said: "Once a month, I also hold a general meeting for these AIDS patients to share experiences. I offer breakfast and they get their food baskets." Dona Conceição regretted that she remained the only institution to address AIDS in the streets; her funds from the World Bank would only last a year: "We cannot meet all the demand for help. It's a disgrace."

Pauper patients are not the problem in themselves. With no political voice, they have been both disregarded and made invisible. This is not due to governmental inability or ignorance. Where there has been active HIV research, testing, and care—in maternity wards, for example—infection has been curtailed.

If this is ethically acceptable and technologically possible, why not tinker with the HIV testing apparatus and organize alternative forms of on-site testing, side-by-side with medical care? To ensure quality care, policymakers would need to discuss interventions with particular vulnerable groups and make adequate medical information and technology available to them, along with sustained assistance. A deliberate engagement by AIDS NGOs in local politics might break open some new ground on this front.

Conclusion

Brazil's bold, multiactor, and large-scale therapeutic response to AIDS has made history. In this chapter, I have explored the broad economic and political effects that treating AIDS had on health services, both national and local, and how this lifesaving policy influenced international efforts to reverse the pandemic's course. I have also illuminated communal and individual modes of life that have emerged around ARVs among the country's most vulnerable urban populations. In highlighting the successes, failures, and complexities of the Brazilian response to AIDS, I have revealed significant structural, logistical, and conceptual changes in governance and citizenship—groundbreaking in their own right.

The Brazilian AIDS policy is emblematic of novel forms of state action on and toward public health. Pressured by activists, the democratic government was able to negotiate with the global pharmaceutical industry, making ARVs universally available to its citizens and also opening up new market possibilities for that industry. The sustainability of the policy has to be constantly negotiated in the marketplace, and one of the unintended consequences of AIDS treatment scale-up has been the consolidation of a model of public health centered on pharmaceutical distribution. This intervention gains social and medical significance by being incorporated into infrastructures of care that are themselves being reshaped by state and market restructuring.

There has been a striking decrease in AIDS mortality in Brazil, but seen from the perspective of the urban poor, the AIDS treatment policy is not an inclusive form of care or citizenship. Many are left out, saddled with categorizations such as drug addict, prostitute, beggar, and thief. Burdened by these labels, it is difficult for individuals to self-identify or to be identified as AIDS victims deserving of treatment and capable of adherence—they largely remain part of the underground economy and a hidden AIDS epidemic. As my ethnography shows, local AIDS services triage quality treatment, and wider rights for the poor and sick to housing, employment, and security remain largely unavailable. Therapy access reveals the urgency of improving people's basic living conditions. Moreover, damaging side effects should not be diverted to the afflicted themselves but should be guarded against by more and not less prevention-oriented policy making. Local politics matter and public institutions are indeed co-functions of successful AIDS treatment. This calls for ongoing self-examination by those who implement policies of their own effects on events and a search for ways to break open the widespread societal deafness to those most vulnerable, people who remain unheard despite all they have to say. It also involves a rethinking of how to reach the afflicted in their own terms, acknowledging self-destructiveness and human struggles for recognition in a largely hostile world. Likewise, at issue is a reconsideration of the systemic relation of pharmaceutical research, commerce, and public health care. We should think about a more sustainable solution to the obstacles posed by patentability and the pharmaceutical industry. The solution may indeed lie in comprehensive knowledge and technology sharing among southern countries already under way, a paradigm that would allow poorer countries to pool their manufacturing know-how and unite in the fight for fair prices, among other things. As Dr. Paulo Picon, a Brazilian academic scientist, told me: "If we don't find intelligent ways to counter this profit extraction from public health we will be left with insurmountable indebtedness, a wound that will not heal."

Caasah's former residents are the new people of AIDS. After experiencing social abandonment, they have come into contact with the foundational experiences of care and biotechnology. Refusing to be overpowered, they plunged into new environments. They have by all standards exceeded their destinies. Now receiving treatment, Rose, Luis, Evangivaldo, and many others refuse the condition of leftovers; they humanize technology, and redo themselves in familiar terms. And they face the daily challenge of translating medical investments into social capital and wage-earning power. They live between moments, between spaces, scavenging for resources. At every turn, they must consider the next step to be taken to guarantee survival.

Acknowledgments

In doing the research from which this chapter draws, I had generous support from the John D. and Catherine T. MacArthur Foundation, the Wenner-Gren Foundation, and the Committee on Research in the Humanities and the Social Sciences of Princeton University. I also acknowledge the support of Princeton's Grand Challenges research cooperative on Global Health and Infectious Disease. I am deeply grateful to Adriana Petryna, Tom Vogl, Amy Moran-Thomas, Alex Gertner, Marcia Inhorn, and Robert Hahn for their insightful comments and editorial help.

Notes

1. According to the World Health Organization, by early 2007 some 2 million patients in low- and middle-income countries were receiving AIDS therapies.

2. By "*structural* violence" I mean the way in which society's organization and institutions systematically deprive some of its citizens of basic resources and rights (Farmer 2003).

3. Caasah means Casa de Apoio e Assistência aos Portadores do Vírus HIV (House of Support and Assistance for Carriers of the HIV Virus). Caasah is pronounced like "*casa*," which means house in Portuguese.

4. Several studies in Brazil have uncovered a variety of factors associated with poor adherence to ARVs, and these findings have bearing on how we understand particular hardships and the possibilities for positive treatment outcomes in a place such as Caasah. See Abadia-Barrero and Castro 2006; Brigido, Rodrigues, Casseb, Oliveira, Rossetti, Menezes, et al. 2001; Nemes, Carvalho, and Souza 2004.

5. States do not necessarily weaken amid economic globalization. As states reform, they develop new strengths and novel articulations with populations (Hansen and Stepputat 2006; Ong 2006).

6. http://www.imshealth.com/ims/portal/front/articleC/0,2777,6599_3665_77491316,00.html

7. http://www.sarid.net/health/healthdocs/050701-hiv.htm

8. M. Morris, "OMS admite fracasso em meta de combate ao HIV," Folha Online 11/28/2005.

9. http://www.avert.org/pepfar.htm

10. The New York Times July 6, 2006. See also http://www.un.org/ecosocdev/geninfo/afrec/vol19no1/191aids.htm

11. See the report "Laboratórios apontam atraso de repasses," *Folha Online*, February 24, 2005 http://www1.folha.uol.com.br/folha/cotidiano/ult95u106036.shtml

12. See the report "Brazil Again Seeks to Cut Cost of AIDS Drug," *The New York Times*, August 19, 2005, http://www.nytimes.com/2005/08/19/business/19abbott.html See the report "Programa do Brasil para Aids 'é insustentável'," *Folha Online*, May 31, 2006, http://www1.folha.uol.com.br/folha/bbc/ult272u53675.shtml

13. Mortalidade de negros é maior do que a de brancos Folha Online August 3, 2005 (9:44 am). See http://www1.folha.uol.com.br/folha/cotidiano/ult95u111617.shtml (downloaded on March 12, 2008).

References

Abadia-Barrero CE, Castro A (2006) Experiences of stigma and access to HAART in children and adolescents living with HIV/AIDS in Brazil. *Social Science and Medicine* 62(5):1219–1228.

Bastos C (1999) *Global Responses to AIDS: Science in Emergency.* Bloomington, IN: Indiana University Press.

Bastos FI, Barcellos C (1995) Geografia Social da AIDS no Brazil. *Revista de Saúde Pública* 29(1):52–62.

Berkman A, Garcia J, Muñoz-Laboy M, Paiva V, Parker R (2005) A critical analysis of the Brazilian response to HIV/AIDS: Lessons learned for controlling and

mitigating the epidemic in developing countries. *American Journal of Public Health* 95(7):1162–1172.

Bermudez J (1995) *Indústria Farmacêutica, Estado e Sociedade: Crítica da Política de Medicamentos no Brasil.* São Paulo: Editora Hucitec e Sociedade Brasileira de Vigilância de Medicamentos.

Bermudez JAZ, Epsztein R, Oliveira MA, Hasenclever L (2000) O *Acordo Trips da Omc e a Proteção Patentária no Brasil: Mudanças Recentes e Implicações para a Produção Local e o Acesso da População Aaos Medicamentos.* Rio de Janeiro: Escola Nacional de Saúde Pública, Fundação Oswaldo Cruz/Organização Mundial da Saúde.

Biehl J (2004) The activist state: Global pharmaceuticals, AIDS, and citizenship in Brazil. *Social Text* 80:105–132.

Biehl J (2005) "Technologies of Invisibility: The Politics of Life and Social Inequality." In: *Anthropologies of Modernity: Foucault, Governmentality, and Life Politics.* JX Inda, ed. London: Blackwell, pp. 248–271.

Biehl J (2006) Will to live: AIDS drugs and local economies of salvation. *Public Culture* 18(3):457–472.

Biehl J (2007) *Will to Live: AIDS Therapies and the Politics of Survival.* Princeton, NJ: Princeton University Press.

Brigido LFM, Rodrigues R, Casseb J, Oliveira D, Rossetti M, Menezes P, et al. (2001) Impact of adherence to antiretroviral therapy in HIV-1 infected patients at a university public service in Brazil. *AIDS Patient Care and STDs* 15(11):587–593.

Cassier M, Correa M (2003) "Patents, Innovation and Public Health: Brazilian Public-sector Laboratories' Experience in Copying AIDS Drugs." In *Economics of AIDS and Access to HIV/AIDS Care in Developing Countries: Issues and Challenges.* Paris: ANRS, pp. 89–107.

Castilho E, Cherquer P (1997) A epidemia da AIDS no Brasil. *Epidemia da AIDS no Brasil: Situação e Tendências.* Brasília: Ministério da Saúde, pp. 9–12.

Cosendey MA, Bermudez JAZ, Reis ALA, Silva HF, Oliveira MA, Luiza VL (2000) Assistência farmacêutica na atenção básica de saúde: A experiência de três estados Brasileiros. *Cadernos de Saúde Pública* 16(1):171–182.

Das V (2006) Power, marginality, and illness. *American Ethnologist* 33(1):27–32.

Dourado I, Veras MA, Barreira D, de Brito AM (2006) AIDS epidemic trends after the introduction of antiretroviral therapy in Brazil. *Revista de Saúde Pública* 40(Suppl.):1–8.

Epstein H (2007) *The Invisible Cure: Africa, the West, and the Fight against AIDS.* New York: Farrar, Strauss, and Giroux.

Farmer P (2003) *Pathologies of Power: Health, Human Rights, and the New War on the Poor.* Berkeley, CA: University of California Press

Farmer P (n/d) Introducing ARVs in resource-poor settings: Expected and unexpected challenges and consequences. www.pih.org/inforesources/Articles/intro-ARV-plenarytalk.pdf

Galvão J (2000) *A AIDS no Brasil: A Agenda de Construção de uma Epidemia.* São Paulo: Editora 34.

Galvão J (2002) A política Brasileira de distribuição e produção de medicamentos anti-retrovirais: Privilégio ou um direito? *Cadernos de Saúde Pública* 18(1):213–219.

Hansen TB, Stepputat F (2006) Sovereignty revisited. *Annual Review of Anthropology* 35:295–315.

Levi GC, Vitória MCA (2002) Fighting against AIDS: The Brazilian experience. *AIDS* 16:2373–2383.

Ministério da Saúde (2002) *A Experiência do Programa Brasileiro de Aids*. Brasília: Ministério da Saúde.

Nemes M, Carvalho H, Souza M (2004) Antiretroviral therapy adherence rates in Brazil. *AIDS* 18(Suppl 3):S15–S20.

Nguyen V (2005) "Antiretroviral Globalism, Biopolitics, and Therapeutic Citizenship." In: *Global Assemblages: Technology, Politics, and Ethics as Anthropological Problems*. A Ong, SJ Collier, eds. Malden, MA: Blackwell Publishing, pp.124–44.

Okie S (2006) Fighting HIV—lessons from Brazil. *New England Journal of Medicine* 354(19):1977–1981.

Ong A (2006) *Neoliberalism as Exception: Mutations in Citizenship and Sovereignty*. Durham, NC: Duke University Press.

Parker R (1994) *A Construção da Solidariedade: AIDS, Sexualidade e Política no Brasil*. Rio de Janeiro: Relume-Dumará.

Parker R, ed. (1997) *Políticas, Instituições e AIDS: Enfrentando a Epidemia no Brasil*. Rio de Janeiro: Jorge Zahar/ABIA.

Parker R, Galvão J, Bessa MS (1999) *Saúde, Desenvolvimento e Política: Respostas frente a AIDS no Brasil*. São Paulo: Editora 34 and ABIA.

Ramiah I, Reich M (2006) Building effective public-private partnerships: Experiences and lessons from the African comprehensive HIV/AIDS partnerships. *Social Science and Medicine* 63(2):397–408.

Serra J (2004) The Political Economy of the Struggle Against AIDS in Brazil. School of Social Science of the Institute for Advanced Studies, Occasional Papers.

Walton DA, Farmer PE, Lambert W, Léandre F, Koenig SP, et al. JS (2004) Integrated HIV prevention and care strengthens primary health care: Lessons from rural Haiti. *Journal of Public Health Policy* 25(2):137–158.

Whyte SR, Whyte MA, Meinert L, Kyaddondo B (2006) "Treating AIDS: Dilemmas of Unequal Access in Uganda." In: *Global Pharmaceuticals: Markets, Practices, Ethics*. A Petryna, A Lakoff, A Kleinman, eds. Durham, NC: Duke University Press, pp. 240–262.

World Health Organization (2006) Progress towards Universal Access: 3 by 5 and Beyond (Report). Geneva: World Health Organization.

Wogart JP, Calcagnotto G (2006) Brazil's fight against AIDS and its implications for global health governance. *World Health and Population* 8(1):1–16.

18

Anthropological and Public Health Perspectives on the Global Polio Eradication Initiative in Northern Nigeria

ELISHA P. RENNE

Such interventions, based upon the assumption that science is universal, o'er-leap the barriers of national borders and cultural boundaries. Indeed what is so powerfully attractive about this vision of scientific knowledge is precisely its universality: its accessibility to all and its applicability to all …. It is the culture of the infecting organism, not the patient, that is relevant.

S Kunitz (1990)

Introduction

In 1988, the World Health Assembly voted to implement a campaign to eradicate poliomyelitis by the end of the year 2000, following the successful eradication of smallpox in 1980 (Henderson 1999). Nineteen years later, the number of polio cases worldwide have declined considerably, from 35,251 cases in 1988 to 1,310 cases by the end of 2007 (WHO 2008). However, cases of polio caused by wild poliovirus (WPV) continue to be reported, mainly in India, Nigeria, Pakistan, and Afghanistan, although cases have also been reported in the Democratic Republic of Congo, Myanmar, Niger, and Somalia in 2007 (GPEI 2007; see also WHA 2007). While Nigeria reported the largest number of new confirmed cases caused by the wild poliovirus in 2006 worldwide, this number has declined considerably in 2007, from 1122 WPV cases in 2006 to 285 WPV cases in 2007 (WHO 2008; Table 18.1) Nigerian health officials predicted that the transmission of WPV would be broken by the end of 2007 (Idris 2006), although this was not possible. Nonetheless, the decline in the number of confirmed WPV cases has been accompanied by a significant increase in overall levels of immunization of early childhood diseases in Nigeria, which the interim coordinator of the National Programme on Immunization (NPI), Dr. Edugie Abebe, reported had risen from 35% to 75% coverage in 2006 (Olayinka 2007b). However, WHO/UNICEF reports an estimated overall national coverage of 54% for the same year (WHO/UNICEF 2007).

512

Table 18.1. Acute Flaccid Paralysis (AFP) and Confirmed Cases of WPV in Nigeria, 1999–2007

YEAR	AFP CASES REPORTED	NONPOLIO AFP RATE	AFP CASES WITH/ ADEQUATE SPECIMENS (%)	TOTAL CONFIRMED POLIO CASES	WILD-VIRUS CONFIRMED POLIO CASES
1999	1,242	0.5	26	981	98
2000	979	0.7	36	638	28
2001	1,937	3.8	67	56	56
2002	3,010	5.7	84	202	202
2003	3,318	6.0	91	355	355
2004	4,814	8.0	91	782	782
2005	4,836	6.3	85	831	830[1]
2006	5,175	6.5	88	1143	1122
2007	4,277	5.9	94	353	285

Source: WHO 2008 http://www.who.int/immunization_monitoring/en/diseases/poliomyelitis/case_count.cfm, accessed May 14, 2008.
[1]The difference between total confirmed polio cases and WPV cases reflects the number of cVDPV cases identified that year.

This chapter uses anthropological research methods to examine changes in the reception and implementation of the polio eradication initiative in Zaria City, one section of the larger town of Zaria, in Kaduna State, in Northern Nigeria (Renne 2006). Zaria City is a useful place to consider changes in the local reception of the polio eradication campaign and its implementation, since health personnel have apparently been successful in immunizing sufficient numbers of children with sufficient doses of oral polio vaccine (OPV) to achieve herd immunity, when disease transmission is slowed or stopped because of the large number of children immunized (Miller, Barrett, and Henderson 2006:1167). As of July 2007, there have been no confirmed cases caused by WPV (Anonymous 2007; WHO-Kaduna 2007), down from 2 confirmed cases in the City for the comparable periods from January to July 2006 and 4 confirmed cases from January to July 2005 (Table 18.2). This decline represents a noteworthy achievement, as there has been considerable resistance to the Global Polio Eradication Initiative (GPEI) by residents and to the house-to-house visits of polio immunization teams.

The chapter begins with a description of the historical and political context of immunization in Nigeria, the study setting, and research methods. The following 3 questions frame this study of the polio eradication campaign in Northern Nigeria:

1. What were local perceptions of polio and of polio vaccination efforts, and how did these views affect the implementation of the GPEI?

Table 18.2. Confirmed Cases of Wild Poliovirus, Zaria LGA, Kaduna State, January–July, 2005 and 2006

CASE ID[1]	AGE (MO)	SEX	NO OF DOSES[2]	ONSET PARALYSIS	VIRUS TYPE	ID RESULTS
2005 (n = 8)						
A	22	M	2	14/07/05	P1	W1
B	10	F	3	10/03/05	P1	W1
C	18	F	3	07/07/05	P1	W1
D	10	F	4	15/07/05	P1	W1
E	23	F	0	06/04/05	P1	W1
F	20	F	0	11/05/05	P3	W1
G	51	M	0	21/05/05	P1	W1
H	24	M	0	13/06/05	P1	W1
2006 (n = 4)						
A	16	M	0	26/02/06	P3	W3
B	35	M	1	5/03/06	P1	W1
C	41	M	0	24/04/06	P1	W1
D	42	F	0	12/05/06	P3	W3

Source: Kaduna State Wild Polio Virus Linelist (WHO, Kaduna State 2005, 2006).
[1] Cases A,B,D,G (2005) and cases A,B (2006) occurred in Zaria City.
[2] There are several possible explanations for the three children who had received 3–4 OPV doses including that (1) antibodies ingested through their mothers' milk inactivated the vaccine in breastfed infants under 6 months, (2) children were suffering from other enteroviral infections, (3) vaccine had become ineffective due to heat or mishandling, or (4) mothers misrepresented, in the absence of card records, the number of doses of vaccine received.

2. How did public health officials reassess and revise their implementation of the GPEI in 2006 and how were these changes received by parents?
3. How might the application of combined public health and anthropological perspectives have facilitated community participation and the implementation of the GPEI campaign, and what lessons may be learned from this campaign?

This examination of the particular trajectory polio eradication has taken in one area of Northern Nigeria also provides the basis for a discussion of the larger question of how such global public health initiatives might be appropriately framed in the future. Whether one favors eradication or control as the most appropriate means of addressing a particular infectious disease or parasite, in areas of the world where resistance to such initiatives is likely to occur or has occurred, both public health and anthropological perspectives and methods are needed to plan, implement, and assess these programs if they are to be effectively realized (Miller, Barrett, and Henderson 2006; Nichter 1995; Streefland, Chowdhury, and Ramos-Jimenez 1999).

Polio Immunization in Nigeria

Among the diseases considered as candidates for eradication, poliomyelitis was chosen because of the successful progress in the interruption of WPV transmission in the Americas (Miller et al. 2006) and because of the ease of administration of OPV.[1] Poliomyelitis has a particular history in the West, which also lent special credence to efforts for its eradication. Several large polio epidemics were recorded during the first half of the twentieth century, including an epidemic in the summer of 1916, when 27,000 cases occurred in New York City and in several adjoining states (Oshinsky 2005). The anxiety associated with polio led parents to keep their children from going to public gathering places—swimming pools, cinemas, and even churches—for fear of their contracting the disease. Despite these measures, during the 1940s and early 1950s, the incidence of polio increased in the United States, with rates of 16 cases per 100,000 in the period from 1945 to 1949 rising to 37 cases per 100,000 in 1952, when over 52,000 cases of polio were reported (Oshinsky 2005). Nonetheless, in most cases, polio is asymptomatic or is associated with a slight fever. In 1 out of 200 cases of polio, however, the poliovirus spreads from the intestine to the nervous system, leading to the paralysis of one or more limbs, which is irreversible (Parry et al. 2004). In extreme cases, this paralysis affects muscles involved in breathing so that children were placed in iron lung machines (Oshinsky 2005); some children died, although this represented a very small percentage of cases (Oshinsky 2005). There was also considerable publicity surrounding this disease in part because President Franklin Delano Roosevelt had contracted the disease (as an adult) and had become paralyzed. These factors contributed to the drive to develop a polio vaccine, and in 1954, a national drug trial was conducted with elementary school children, using the killed polio vaccine developed by Dr. Jonas Salk. With the successful conclusion of this trial, the injectable Salk vaccine was manufactured for widespread distribution. Six years later, a clinical trial of the OPV developed by Dr. Albert Sabin was carried out and by August 1960, trial manufacture began (Oshinsky 2005). These two vaccines continue to be used in polio immunization, with the Salk inactivated polio vaccine (IPV) being used in the United States, where new cases of polio are rarely seen and with the Sabin attenuated OPV being used in developing countries.

When the 1988 World Health Assembly resolution (WHA 1988a) to eradicate poliomyelitis was unanimously approved, it was with the understanding that this initiative would also contribute to the strengthening of sustainable health care in the developing world (WHA 1988b)—through training of immunization teams, establishment of laboratories for clinical testing, and improvement of routine immunization and disease surveillance methods. The fact that some of these goals were superseded by time constraints and economic pressures to focus on the eradication of polio shaped the subsequent conduct of the campaign in Nigeria, even though routine immunization was extremely low.

Indeed, the implementation of the GPEI in Nigeria cannot be understood outside of the context of childhood immunization programs, such as the Expanded Programme on Immunization (EPI), which began in Nigeria in 1979, shortly after the eradication of smallpox was certified. Earlier in 1974, the World Health Organization had begun the EPI, which had the goal of providing vaccines for diphtheria, tetanus, whooping cough, measles, polio, and tuberculosis to more than 80% of children worldwide (Ekanem 1988). By reaching these levels of coverage, health officials sought to provide herd immunity (Henderson 1999:S55). The goal of this ambitious program was attained in some countries, particularly those with well-developed health infrastructures and trained personnel. However, in Africa, where infrastructural as well as political and economic problems hampered routine EPI immunization, it was only in 1990, when UNICEF and WHO pushed to achieve high EPI coverage rates, that widespread immunization of African children was achieved. In many African countries, these high levels have not been sustained (Taylor, Cutts, and Taylor 1997:924; WHO 2000).[2]

In Nigeria, political instability and a weak economy hampered national immunization efforts until 1986, when General Ibrahim Babangida appointed Professor Olikoye Ransome-Kuti as Minister of Health. Ransome-Kuti, who supported the EPI program, established a system of Primary Health Care (PHC) centers throughout the country through which vaccines were made widely available (Olatimehin 1988). In March 1988, the first phase of a National Immunization exercise was held at PHC centers. By 1990, 95% coverage was achieved for antituberculosis BCG (Bacille-Calmette-Guerin) vaccinations of children aged between 0 and 11 months, while DTP3 immunization levels peaked at 65% coverage (National Planning Commission [NPC-Nigeria] & UNICEF 2001). The year 1990 is considered to be the high point in national immunization coverage in Nigeria. The vaccines used in an effort to achieve 80% coverage during the EPI drive in 1990 were provided by UNICEF and other NGOs via the federal government without charge to local governments. However, when federal responsibility for PHC services was transferred to local governments in 1991 (Umar 1989), the availability of vaccines drastically declined.[3]

By 1993, immunization rates were reported to be around 30% on the basis of government data (FBA 2005). This was also a year of considerable political turmoil, with General Sani Abacha coming to power in a bloodless coup in November 1993. It was not until the NPI (formerly known as the EPI program) was formally launched in 1996 as part of the Family Support Programme, a project run by the First Lady Miriam Abacha, that immunization efforts resumed. The NPI, which operated under the direction of Dr. Dere Awosika,

was responsible for the importation and distribution of vaccines to cold-store centers throughout the country as well as for promoting immunization in Nigeria, including the polio immunization campaign that began in earnest in 1998.

In Nigeria, the decline in immunization during the 1990s meant that the NPI needed to begin a program of mass immunization through National Immunization Days (NIDs). It also established a system for monitoring WPV through identification of children with acute flaccid paralysis (AFP)—and through the collection and transport of stool specimens (CDC 2005). During the 2001 and 2002 NIDs, health workers went from house to house to increase coverage. All children under the age of 5 were given OPV, regardless of whether they had received earlier doses to ensure universal coverage. However, not all parents allowed health workers to immunize their children, and resistance to the polio eradication campaign in Kano—based on fears that OPV was contaminated with antifertility substances or the HIV virus—led to the cancellation of NIDs in 2003 in several Northern Nigerian states (Anonymous 2007; Smallman-Raynor, Cliff, Trevelyan, Nettleton, and Sneddon 2006).

After new polio vaccines were imported from Indonesia in May 2004, the Governor of Kano State agreed to the resumption of NIDs there in July 2004 (Musa 2004), although not all parents agreed with the focus on polio immunization and some still refused to participate. While this resistance has largely been attributed to Islamic religious leaders (Altman 2004), recent social analyses of the polio campaign in Northern Nigeria have discussed this resistance in a broader sociocultural and political context. Obadare (2005) examined the historical and political situation in Northern Nigeria where many people were genuinely afraid to risk having their children vaccinated, in part because of distrust of the federal government. Olusanya (2004) noted that Northern Nigerians still remembered the drug trial of the antibiotic, Trovan® (trovafloxacin), which—like polio vaccine—had been given free of charge during the 1996 cerebrospinal meningitis (CSM) epidemic. Five out of nearly 100 infants and children who were given Trovan® died (Stephens 2006).

Furthermore, with measles outbreaks in several Northern Nigerian communities in 2005 (Schimmer and Ihekweazu 2006) and measles immunization coverage in the Northwest Region (of which Kaduna State is part) reported to be 15.6% in 2003 (National Population Commission [Nigeria] and ORC/Macro 2004),[4] some parents who were asked to allow their children to be immunized in repeated NID rounds questioned the focus on polio immunization. According to the 2005 Feilden Battersby Analysts (FBA) report:

> Polio "fatigue" has set in across much of the country, with widespread resentment at the quantity of human and financial resources being thrown at a single disease that, both in public health terms and in popular perception, is relatively unimportant in Nigeria. National Immunization Days (NIDs) take health staff away from

their regular work. Some key staff spend up to 35 days on each NID, and there are five NIDs plus one sub-NID planned for 2005. Thus NIDs contribute to the continuing dysfunction of the primary health care system (FBA 2005).

Thus, even with the resumption of polio immunization in July 2004, there were increases in confirmed cases of polio reported in 2005 ($n = 830$) and in 2006 ($n = 1124$) (Table 18.1). At the March 2006 meeting of the Expert Review Committee (ERC) on Polio Eradication (National Programme on Immunization, Nigeria 2006a), government and NGO health officials decided on a new strategy, which included "health incentives" distributed during Immunization Plus Days (IPDs) and additional programs including the provision of measles vaccinations at fixed sites, to bolster routine immunization (Anonymous 2007:106). It is believed that these efforts, which were introduced during the May 2006 NIDs, have led to increased participation and levels of polio immunization, as evidenced in the reduction of confirmed cases of polio from WPV in 2007 (Table 18.1). Before examining these changes in implementation and Zaria City residents' responses to them and to the GPEI more generally, the study setting and research methods used in this study are described.

Research Setting and Methods

It is against the backdrop of declining PHC and immunization levels during the period from 1990 to 1999 as well as of political instability (which included 5 different national political leaders during this period) that polio eradication efforts took place in the town of Zaria. Zaria is famous for its educational institutions, including many Islamic schools, a large polytechnic college, and one of the oldest tertiary educational institutions in Northern Nigeria, Ahmadu Bello University, which has a well-established teaching hospital. This study focuses on Zaria City, the old walled section of the larger town of Zaria, and the former capital of the old Hausa Emirate of Zazzau. It consists of approximately 40 neighborhoods dispersed over 10 square miles—with open stretches of land devoted to farming on the edges of the more congested city center (Urquhart 1970). The population of Zaria Local Government Area (LGA) was provisionally estimated from the 1991 census to be 277,187 although the population of Zaria City itself may only include up to one-third of this figure.

Zaria City is presently the headquarters of Zaria LGA and local government offices, and the main local government clinic, along with the Emir's palace and the adjacent Friday mosque, dominate the central area of the city. This central section has paved roads, a relatively regular supply of electricity, and until recently, pipe-borne water, while the outlying, more rural neighborhoods are served by winding dirt roads, household wells, and kerosene lanterns. The City

has several Islamic schools, a number of private clinics, a local government clinic, and a large public hospital, along with traditional healers and several markets where traditional medicines are sold.

While the presence of 2 large institutions of higher education has given Zaria a certain cosmopolitanism, in other ways Zaria is similar to other Northern Nigerian towns and cities in which the majority of the population is of Hausa-Fulani ethnicity, among whom live many "strangers," including people whose origins are in Southwestern Nigeria, who are of Yoruba ethnicity and in Southeastern Nigeria, who are of Igbo ethnicity. The ethnic composition in Zaria is made even more complex by the presence of people from the southern part of Kaduna State itself, where there are many small ethnic groups—for example, the Kagoro, Kaje, and Kataf—who have also moved to Kaduna, the state capital, and to Zaria. These different ethnic identities are further complicated by religion, which is sometimes represented in Nigeria as a simple Muslim North–Christian South divide. However, while most Northern Nigerians are Muslims and most Southeastern Nigerians are Christians, there are approximately equal numbers of Christian and Muslim Yoruba in Southwestern Nigeria (Eades 1980). Indeed, there are many Muslim Yoruba fluent in Yoruba, Hausa, and sometimes, English, living in Hausa communities (Olaniyi 2006), including within Zaria City itself. This ethnic and religious complexity and the mobility of the population are compounded by size. Nigeria is the most populous country in sub-Saharan Africa, with a provisional population of 140,003,542, based on the 2006 census figures (Yishau 2007:18), dispersed over a land mass of 356,669 square miles (923,768 sq km), connected by a system of roads in varying states of repair on which people are constantly traveling—to trade, to visit relatives, to attend schools and conferences, and at times, to seek cure.

The size of the country—both in terms of people and space—and the complexity of people's social connections and identities are reflected in the range of choices available to people seeking medical treatment. For example, in Zaria, "modern" Western, Islamic, and "traditional" Hausa medicines may be used in child health care. In cases of high fever (*zazzabi*)—often associated with malaria—children may be taken to one of the local clinics or to Kofar Gayan Hospital, where they are given injections and Western pharmaceuticals for treatment. Alternately, sick children with high fevers may be given *rubutu*, verses from the Qur'an which are written in ink that are then washed off with water which is drunk, or traditional herbal medicines, such as an infusion of mahogany bark, *madaci* (*Khaya sengalensis*; Wall 1988), as treatment. They may also be taken to Islamic scholars (*mallamai*) or traditional healers (*boka*) for consultations. Indeed, the Hausa term for polio, *Shan Inna*, reflects traditional ideas about health, in which the spirit, Inna, of the spirit possession healing cult known as *bori*, was believed to cause paralysis

(Besmer 1983) by drinking (*shan*) the blood of the victim's limbs, causing withering, paralysis, and sometimes, death. However, *bori* is now practiced primarily in rural areas in Northern Nigeria. In towns such as Zaria known for Islamic education and where the majority are Muslims, *bori* spirit possession is dismissed as traditional religious belief and hence as an un-Islamic practice (Last 2005).[5] Consequently, other medical treatments for paralysis, Western, as well as Islamic, have come to be seen as more appropriate (Etkin, Ross, and Muazzamu 1990).

This study utilized 3 research methodologies including (1) participant observation; (2) qualitative open-ended interviews with individuals selected by a snow-ball sample based on type of participation in the immunization campaign; and (3) the review of polio-related documents, including newspaper articles about polio immunization, WHO and UNICEF materials in Nigeria (including NID information and promotional materials), mass media materials, relevant academic journals, archival materials in Nigeria, and WHO and CDC online polio data.

My residence in a family house in Zaria City for at least 2 weeks a year over the past 12 years has facilitated the observation of neighborhood house markings indicating NID visits and inquiries about whether polio immunizations had actually been administered. This long-term community residence made possible the initial snow-ball sampling conducted in summer 2005 of individuals associated with polio, which included parents who did or did not have their children vaccinated for polio ($n = 17$, including 10 parents who had polio themselves), students (without children) who had polio ($n = 2$), immunization workers ($n = 2$), and local government health officials ($n = 2$), as well as with Ahmadu Bello University Teaching Hospital (ABUTH) public health professors ($n = 2$), pediatricians ($n = 2$), 1 ABU pharmacologist, and 1 professor emeritus who specialized in polio research at the University of Ibadan. Two members of the WHO GPEI team, and the head of the Kaduna State NPI, both headquartered in Kaduna, were also interviewed.

In summer 2006, follow-up interviews with 18 individuals identified in the 2005 interviews were conducted, including interviews with traditional healers ($n = 3$), health workers, including USAID and WHO personnel in Kaduna ($n = 4$), religious scholars ($n = 3$), people who had polio ($n = 2$), parents of children with AFP ($n = 2$), and community leaders ($n = 2$). In addition, 2 mothers of children under 5 years of age who had not previously had their children immunized for polio were interviewed in summer 2007 about their assessment of the revised 2006 immunization plus campaign and other initiatives. A total of 52 open-ended interviews were conducted in Hausa or in English, 32 from July to September 2005, 18 from July to August 2006, and 2 in June 2007. Hausa interviews were conducted with the assistance of Hassana Tanimu and when possible, were recorded, transcribed, and translated, if in Hausa.

In addition, residing in a family house in the area where I was conducting fieldwork allowed me to discuss health concerns with women and men informally, to participate in activities of importance to them such as naming ceremonies, and to observe their responses to illness first hand.

Finally, during August 2004, articles on the polio campaign boycott published in 2 Northern Nigerian newspapers, *The Weekly Trust* and *The Daily Trust*, for the period from May 2003 to July 2004, were collected. These articles, along with archival newspaper clippings and unpublished materials held in the ABU Department of Community Medicine library, Arewa House, Kaduna (a Northern Nigerian research center), and the Nigerian National Archives, Kaduna, amassed during the summers of 2005 and 2006, provided background information on earlier immunization efforts in Nigeria.

Dynamics of Acceptance and Rejection of Polio Immunization in Zaria City

In 2003 and 2004, health workers associated with the NPI, WHO, and UNICEF attempted to meet the newly assigned global December 2004 deadline through additional house-to-house sub-NID exercises in Zaria. During house-to-house visits, immunization teams worked in groups of 6 (and sometimes 8) people— 2 recorders, 2 vaccinators, a crowd controller, and a ward head—along with a supervisor. One woman who worked on a team described the etiquette of entering a house and seeking permission to vaccinate:

> If I enter a house, I will do *salama alaikum* to them as Hausa people are doing. I will tell them we came to do polio vaccine to immunize their children. [I will tell them that] there is a need to eradicate this disease in Nigeria—just like smallpox was eradicated.
>
> I will ask them if any of their children have *sanyi kafa*, cold, a pain in their legs or if they have high fever. We will tell them the symptoms, and if they don't have the symptoms, then I will ask them to bring the children so we can look and see. Some brought their children and some did not.

For those parents who agreed to have their children vaccinated, the children's thumbs were stained with gentian violet. On leaving the house, a team member would make marks above the doorway—whether vaccine was administered or not—to indicate that the house was visited.

For some parents, the appearance of immunizing teams at their homes was seen as an intrusive imposition that they refused to accept:

> There was a time I nearly slapped one of those polio workers who came to the house. She [told] me to bring the children, but I said I didn't like the polio vaccine

and refused. She began talking and tried to convince me. But I nearly slapped her and asked her to go.

However, by 2006, immunization workers in Zaria City saw less resistance to polio vaccination and were optimistic that they might be able to complete their work:

> I have experienced a lot, because there are a lot of problems. Because [before] most of the people rejected it, but now some are receptive ... now most of the people are accepting, they have been enlightened ... Maybe this year we will finish it because some of the people who resisted before are accepting it now.

Yet for those who resisted in the past and for those who continue to resist immunization, there was a genuine fear that the polio vaccine is possibly harmful, which they had heard from various sources including Islamic schoolteachers, university professors, traditional healers, friends, and family members. One woman described how women attending Islamiyya schools in her neighborhood were discouraged to allow their children to be immunized:

> ... In Islamiyya school, they would tell people not to give their children the vaccine because there is something bad in it. It is because of this, that here in Locus [her neighborhood], in 1 in every 5 houses, you will find people who refuse to immunize their children.

Another woman, who had refused to have her children immunized, learned about polio vaccine informally:

> ... I heard the rumor that there was something bad in it. It is said that there is family planning in it. And I heard it when there were weddings, I heard people talking, and also at the mosque. They said we should not accept it .... Nothing can change my thinking about this polio vaccine. I don't like it at all. I heard a drama on polio on the radio and also on television. They didn't change my mind.

At the same time, there were others for whom the numerous radio and television spots emphasizing the importance of polio vaccination were convincing:

> The reason why I accepted the polio vaccine—it is said that prevention is better than cure. You say you would like to have it because you are afraid the disease will catch you. To avoid that you will take the vaccine. When you immunize [a child], even if the disease catches the child, it will not catch them very well. And another reason, I have seen parents taking their children for vaccination so it makes me accept it .... I used to encourage my relatives about the vaccine ... When you have seen it on TV and heard it on the radio all the time, even those who do not agree with it, later they will agree. Because they will see children given the vaccine, nothing happened to them.

Among those who feared that polio vaccine was unsafe, some believed that the vaccine contained substances that would make their daughters infertile, saying that it "killed the eggs of the woman" or that it contained the HIV virus. Others questioned the singling out of polio and the repeated doses of polio vaccine to the exclusion of other forms of PHC. The suspicion of the free and exclusive provision of polio vaccine was further explained by one man:

> No, I don't allow my children to have the vaccine because I don't trust the vaccine. Because they said they are going to do it free of charge. And if we go to the hospital, we have to buy medicine and it is costly there. But this one is free of charge—in the hospital, your child can die or your brother can die if you don't have money.
> My children have had measles vaccine, but this polio vaccine, I won't allow it. I took them to the hospital to do the measles vaccine, they didn't come to my house. And I never took my children for any immunization except this measles vaccine …. If I believe in polio or go to the hospital and have medicine free of charge, like this polio, I can accept the polio vaccine. But if I have to pay for medicine in the hospital, I will not accept this one.

This man's point differs from that of those who believed that the OPV was contaminated with substances that will cause infertility. Rather, he is opposed to the single focus of an eradication campaign that excludes the provision of affordable PHC for children. In other words, he does not approve of nor will he participate in a top-down approach to the health care of his children in which he has no say.

In another example, one Zaria City woman explained that she refused the polio vaccination because she had stopped immunizing her children after one daughter contracted measles after being vaccinated:

> Yes, I did take my children for immunization—I even took one of my daughters until she was 5 years old. But at last I stopped taking them. For example, the measles immunization, I took my children but they had measles and it was very dangerous, more than those who hadn't gotten immunized. Really, it changed [affected] my thinking. That was why I stopped taking the other children, the immunization had no use.

Indeed, the idea that immunization is the cause of illness was expressed by several people, although they gave different reasons for this belief. One physician noted that on receiving multiple doses of polio vaccine, for some " … the belief is … that they contract polio from the vaccine." For example, in 2007, a story was published in a local newspaper about the outbreak of 69 cases of paralysis caused by vaccine-derived poliovirus (Rabiu 2007). One woman whose daughter became paralyzed by polio attributed her condition to having received up to 10 doses of polio vaccine. Furthermore, 1 university professor, who cited cases of vaccine-derived poliovirus among children with immunodeficiency syndrome in the United States, questioned the safety of the OPV. As he put it, "In trying to intervene and prevent a disease, you should not introduce a more dangerous disease."

While this professor was concerned with the safety of the vaccine, 1 popular traditional healer (*boka*) in the area argued that "the 'spirit' that causes polio now—unlike the spirit Shan Inna in the past—is an *allura*—injection ... Children get polio through the injection, they are getting paralyzed from injection ... . Only doctors can give it." This man may have been referring to the way that injections may occasionally damage nerves, causing temporary paralysis, or to an association between the appearance of boils (abscesses that may develop at the injection site) and paralysis.

However, this man's hostility toward Western medical professionals and Western pharmaceuticals is not shared by all. Taking Western medicines such as chloroquine tablets to treat malaria fevers may be acceptable and indeed, chloroquine injections are a preferred method of treatment (Wall 1988). Yet immunization—taking something to prevent disease—has had a mixed reception. Etkin et al. (1990) observed that medicine is thought to work when disease is brought out from, not into, the body. When there is an imminent danger, such as a CSM epidemic, immunization is viewed as beneficial (Streefland et al. 1999) and in 1996, there was a high demand for CSM injectable vaccines (Ejembi, Renne, and Adamu 1998). However, routine immunization has been seen by some, but not all Zaria residents, as unnecessary or even possibly dangerous for infants and children who are not experiencing health problems.

A House in Zaria City

While uncertainty about the safety of immunization is not uncommon in Zaria, a more in-depth sense of how some parents weighed the benefits and risks of polio immunization may be seen in the actions of 2 mothers and their 2 small sons living in 1 house in Zaria City. From the markings over the door leading to the family compound, one might be led to believe that all children under 5 years living in the house, including these 2 boys, had been vaccinated for polio. However, until recently, this was not the case. My fieldnotes, from September 14, 2005, illustrate the process by which I came to understand how house markings that were meant to document vaccination visits could merely mean that a house had been visited. This information came from the house where I lived in Zaria City:

> There is a marking for the National Population Commission (NPC) census survey chalked on the wall near Alhaji's front door which I finally noticed. It made me revise my assumption that they hadn't taken polio vaccine in the house here.

There was even a faint SNID [sub National Immunization Day] written near the NPC mark and also a check mark that [I was told] meant that they'd visited the house. So I was thinking that Hassana Asibiti [a family in-law who is a nurse] had talked to Mallam and he'd agreed to let them come [in the house to vaccinate the children there]. However, when Mallam's wives were asked, they said, 'No, we didn't allow them in the house, they only put the marks there when they came.' This was last year [2004].

In the beginning of 2006, the young boys' mothers' resistance to house-to-house immunization was countered in 2 ways. First, polio vaccines were administered in nursery and primary schools providing Western education (boko) and second, through a mass immunization program that occurred in front of the Emir of Zaria's palace in early 2006. The 2 young mothers heard of the mass immunization from radio announcements and the house head (mai gida) told them to attend. One mother, dressed in hijab and wrapper skirt, took her 4-year-old son to the palace, but did not stay because there were so many women already there and she did not have time. Furthermore, her son had been immunized in nursery school (although this was done without her permission). The other young mother took her 4-year-old son for immunization at the palace, where he received 1 of the 4 necessary doses of OPV. However, she subsequently refused to allow health workers to vaccinate him when they came to the house. In both cases, their children were given OPV drops outside of their house. Indeed, according to one mother, the vaccine given in the house was contaminated with medicine (magani) that destroys their children's fertility (yana kashe kwayoyi haihuwa, literally, it kills the eggs of childbearing), while vaccine given in public—at school or at mass immunization programs authorized by the Emir of Zaria—did not. This explanation also suggests that when given in public, in venues which women trusted, these public programs imparted confidence in the vaccine, whereas private immunization by strangers in their homes did not.

Why Some Parents Resisted the House-to-House Campaign

Thus, there were several reasons why some parents did not allow health workers to administer the OPV in their houses. For some, it was distrust of the motivations of those promoting a Western health intervention or product, which has frequently been expressed in terms of fears of infertility. In Northern Nigeria, for example, "a Rotary Club immunization project in Zaria City in March 1995 was abandoned after the second visit because parents refused to bring their children out. They complained of boils around the site of immunization and of a loss of hearing" (Renne 1996). Rumors of infertility induced by vaccines have also occurred in other parts of Africa, for example, in a 1990 anti-tetanus vaccination campaign in Cameroon (Feldman-Savelsberg, Ndonko, and Schmidt-Ehry 2000). This fear has also been associated with Western products including Panadol® and Maggi® bouillon cubes (Renne 1996). There is a belief that "... Christian countries' concern to export bio-medicine to all parts of Africa is ... not as a charitable gesture but as self-interested and dangerous" (Last 2005). For others, it was distrust of the Federal Government, under the former President Olusegun Obasanjo, and the heads of both the Ministry of Health and the NPI, all of whom were southern Nigerians, who were held responsible for the deteriorating health conditions in Northern Nigeria (Obadare 2005). For some, it was distrust of immunization team members who sometimes behaved inappropriately, some refusing to follow local practices, such as veiling, which would have increased their local acceptability, and some who were so poorly trained that they could not answer parents' questions (see also Yahya 2007).

By focusing on polio, which many people did not see as a primary health problem for their children and by not improving PHC—including the provision of EPI vaccines[6] or free treatment for malaria, health officials and their international partners were seen by some as indirectly contributing to the deaths of their children. Yet for others, it was a genuine fear of the health consequences of the OPV on their children. Some had heard that the attenuated live vaccine used in the OPV could actually cause polio and some knew that IPV was being used in the West. The fact that IPV is used in the West, while the less costly and more easily administered OPV is used in Africa, has been discussed in the Nigerian press (Kazaure 2003). As with some parents in the United States, some Northern Nigerian parents "may prefer to make errors of omission ... rather than errors of commission" (Fredrickson et al. 2004; Nichter 1995; see also Blume 2006), and on hearing about the possibility of contracting vaccine-derived polio viruses, may have decided not to have their children immunized. Indeed, the news released by the CDC in late September 2007 that 69 children in Nigeria contracted paralytic polio from a type 2 circulating vaccine-derived poliovirus from July 2, 2005 through August 17, 2007 (CDC 2007a,b; Roberts 2007; WHO 2007b) may reinforce these parents' decision.

Public Health Perspectives

Public health officials in Nigeria noted several problems with the GPEI, which contributed to the resistance to polio immunization in Zaria City. According to 1 public health professor, there were 3 fundamental problems that affected the campaign: (1) the collapse of the PHC system, (2) low levels of immunization, and (3) mismanagement by the NPI. For example, only a portion of the monies allocated to local governments for NIDs were reaching health departments, with money "being siphoned off, all along the way." Funds were also spent for foreign WHO consultants who had little knowledge of the Nigerian situation. Another problem was the recruitment of inappropriate local health workers who went house-to-house—some of whom had little education and some of whom had no commitment to the eradication effort. Some workers were cited as being particularly irresponsible and the dumping of unused vaccine was reported by 2 individuals working closely with immunization teams, although it is difficult to know precisely how often this practice occurred.

One public health professor mentioned the difficulties of managing the cold chain in remote areas of the country, inadequate record keeping at some local government clinics, and the lack of health cards that were a part of the initiative. Consequently, with each NID and sub-National Immunization Day (sNID) round, children would be given repeated doses of vaccine, wasting both vaccine and effort, as well as raising alarm among parents who worried about the consequences of doses beyond the required four. One WHO official also noted the problem of using OPV, which contains an attenuated live virus, as some people requested the IPV. Other NGO health workers mentioned the lack of government commitment at the state and local levels: "It will go a long way in solving the problem if the Federal, State, and Local Government would get involved." In March 2006, with the decision at the federal level to implement several new programs including IPDs (WHA 2007), overall immunization coverage and the acceptance of polio vaccination began to improve, as will be discussed in the following section.

Public Health Initiatives and Local Concerns

After the ERC meeting in March 2006, the NPI and the Ministry of Health, along with WHO/CDC and USAID health officials, sought to overcome resistance to polio immunization in Northern Nigeria through revised services made available during NIDs and sNIDs, beginning in May 2006 (Anonymous 2007). Three different programs were implemented, including the IPDs, Community Participation for Action in the Social Sector (COMPASS), and the Revive Routine Immunization (Table 18.3). The IPDs program provided parents with access to routine immunization at health posts and clinics as well as "add-ons" such as soap, anthelminthics, oral rehydration therapy packets, insecticide-treated bednets (ITNs), and Vitamin A supplement, which were distributed house-to-house (Anonymous 2007; National Programme on Immunization, Nigeria nd).

Table 18.3. Immunization Programs in Nigeria

PROGRAM NAME	SPONSOR(s)	DATE BEGUN	PROGRAM OBJECTIVES	SOURCE
Polio Plus Program	Rotary International	1985	Provide financial contributions, volunteer time, and networking expertise to eradicate polio globally	http://www.rotary.org, accessed October 25, 2007
Global Polio Eradication Initiative (GPEI)	World Health Organization	1988	Eradicate polio globally, support routine immunization and primary health care	http://www.wemos.nl/ documents/WHA41.pdf, accessed May 22, 2007
National Programme on Immunization (NPI)-Nigeria	Federal Government-Nigeria; MOH-Nigeria	1996	Provide immunization for early childhood diseases nationally, procure vaccines, organize polio eradication efforts	http://www.technet21.org/ backgrounddocs.html, accessed on September 2005
National Immunization Days (NIDs)	WHO, Ministry of Health-Nigeria, UNICEF, USAID	1998	House-to-house and fixed site provision of polio vaccines by immunization teams, according to annual schedules	http://www.technet21.org/ backgrounddocs.html, accessed on September 2005
Global Alliance for Vaccines and Immunization (GAVI)	Gates Foundation	2000	Provide support for vaccine provision and immunization delivery systems, with accountability requirements	http://www.vaccinealliance.org/, accessed September 30, 2007

Program	Organizations	Year	Description	Source
Immunization basics	USAID Global Bureau, Division of Health, Infectious Disease & Nutrition	2004	Collaborate with organizations engaged in routine immunization at the national and state levels—in Sokoto and Bauchi States, Northern Nigeria	http://www.immunizationbasics.jsi.com/Index.html, accessed November 10, 2007
Immunization Plus Days (IPDs)	WHO, Ministry of Health-Nigeria, UNICEF, Rotary, USAID/CDC, EU, COMPASS	2006	Provide routine immunization and "add-ons"—soap, anthelminthics, oral rehydration therapy packets, insecticide-treated bednets, and Vitamin A supplement, along with oral polio vaccine	http://www.polioeradication.org/content/meetings/10thERCMetingFinalReportJul2006.pdf, accessed May 15, 2007
Revive Routine Immunization (RRI)	Department for Intl Development (UK)	2006	Revitalize routine immunization for children and women of reproductive age in low coverage states in Northern Nigeria	http://www.dfid.gov.uk/countries/africa/nigeria_programme.asp, accessed November 10, 2007

IPDs were devised by public health officials to address some of the concerns of parents about the GPEI, including the single vaccination focus of earlier NIDs. For parents concerned about measles, measles vaccine—along with other vaccines (DPT3, BCG, yellow fever, and hepatitis B)—was made available at fixed sites free of charge. For parents concerned about malaria, ITNs were given to those whose children had completed the 4-dose polio sequence. The implementation of this program (of which Revive Routine Immunization was also part) was also meant to allay international concerns about low levels of immunization in Nigeria.

The COMPASS program has been developed to actively involve community members in health initiatives. While originally instituted in 5 states, the Federal Government and COMPASS/USAID health officials decided to introduce a COMPASS Polio program that focused on polio immunization in the 8 states in Northern Nigeria—Kaduna, Kano, Jigawa, Bauchi, Kebbi, Sokoto, Zamfara, and Yobe—where polio was endemic. One of the first steps taken by COMPASS Polio program in Kaduna State was to establish partnerships with local community groups, including the members of the Polio Victims Association (Figure 18.1), FOMWAM (a Muslim women's organization) and Sakefa (a youth organization), who were incorporated in various ways in IPDs.

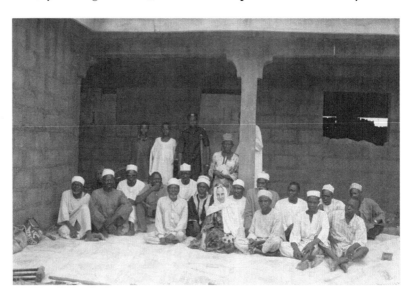

Figure 18.1. Members of the Kungiyar Guragu-Zazzau (Association for the Lame-Zaria), some of whom are also members of the Polio Victims Association (PVA), with Elisha Renne in front of the association's new workshop, which they worked together to roof. PVA members also worked with COMPASS personnel in the implementation of Immunization Plus Days in 2006 (Photograph by Hassana Tanimu, Zaria).

For example, members of the Polio Victims Association sometimes accompanied immunization teams:

> Their own responsibility is to jump-start the parents to ... bring their children if they want them to be well, but if they don't want and they want their children to be like us ... So then everyone will relax and feel the sympathy for the position they have and they will rush to bring their children ....

COMPASS personnel also met with political and religious leaders in communities where resistance to the GPEI was high in order to identify people who had influence with local people:

> We will invite them for a meeting, after we will briefly inform about the program, then we will ask them their own views, their perspectives on what they think polio immunization is all about. They will tell us ... their own perception of it and then we tell them that everybody has an equal right to say his own word and that he is not speaking for anyone but his own heart, that is the law and the rule. So after we go around about 7 or 10 of them, then we come into agreement and we will tell the situation of their own area, particularly on polio program, then they may decide on what to do. So that is the beginning of ownership.

These community leaders would then work together to talk with recalcitrant parents in their villages and some also went to other communities as part of a health education campaign. This community dialogue as well as the inclusion of extra IPDs (in which COMPASS was also involved) meant that in 2006, there were 3 rounds of NIDs and 6 rounds of IPDs, which continued into 2007 (WHO 2007a). These efforts, along with the mass polio immunization programs sponsored by traditional political leaders such as the Emir of Zaria, appear to have had a significant impact on the number of confirmed cases of WPV reported in Kaduna State in 2006 and 2007. As of July 1, 2007, only 4 confirmed WPV cases had been documented in Kaduna State, compared with 40 WPV cases at the end of June 2006 (WHO-Kaduna 2006, 2007). Furthermore, "an increase in population immunity against poliovirus infection is indicated by the substantial decrease in the proportion of non-polio AFP cases with zero doses of OPV," according to the Weekly Epidemiological Record (Anonymous 2007). While it is not altogether clear, from Zaria City parents' perspectives, how these changes influenced their decisions to allow their children to be immunized, they were strongly supported by one Zaria City woman interviewed in 2006 about ITN ownership: "Really, it is a good thing they are doing. If they are taking bednets house to house, it will be good because some they don't know they are distributing the bednet in the hospital. I will agree for the polio people to do polio for my child because I need the bed net."

While limited funds and a universal protocol may militate against tailoring global eradication efforts for local considerations, the apparent success of these

revised immunization programs, along with the advocacy of trusted community leaders in Zaria suggest the importance of taking community concerns
into account before such initiatives begin and during their implementation
(Taylor, Cutts, and Taylor 1997).

Protesting the Polio Eradication Initiative and Program Implications

Although some people refused to allow their children to be vaccinated because
they believed that the polio vaccine was contaminated with the HIV virus or
with antifertility substances as a plot to reduce Muslim populations, disputes
over the safety of the polio vaccine and the appropriateness of the polio eradication campaign were more complex than this single explanation for people's
refusal to participate suggests. These debates also raised the question of what
sorts of public health programs should be implemented and about the underlying ideologies associated with appropriate community health care. While the
belief that OPV was a form of anti-Islamic population control *was* a significant
reason for some, the decision to focus on polio alone through house-to-house
campaigns disturbed others, suggesting that these people questioned a top-
down government decision to promote a public health initiative for what was
perceived as a minor health problem, an initiative that came from outside
in which they had no input. Some also wondered about the wisdom of an
eradication program that appeared to them to reduce the resources and personnel available for PHC. While polio vaccines were given freely, medicines
for malaria had to be paid for, and other vaccines, when available, sometimes
incurred "incidental" expenses.

Having discussed these objections to the GPEI campaign in Northern Nigeria
and its subsequent revision using community dialogue and health incentives,
how might the application of combined public health and anthropologists' perspectives have facilitated community understanding and the implementation of
the GPEI campaign from the beginning?

First, one might look at the earlier smallpox eradication campaign and subsequent EPI initiative to identify areas where potential problems might arise.
During the 1967–1970 smallpox campaign in Nigeria (which coincided with
the beginning of the Nigerian Civil War), Northern Nigeria had the largest
number of smallpox cases in the country. Immunization efforts in Northern
Nigeria faced immense challenges—poor roads, lack of trained staff, limited
health centers, and an ineffective monitoring and reporting system. Despite
these challenges, traditional rulers were able to organize effective mass immunization efforts in Northern towns, cities, and villages; later outbreaks were
contained using mobile vaccination teams (Fenner, Henderson, Arita, Jezek,
and Ladnyi 1988). More recently, the successful mass immunization program

sponsored by the Emir of Zaria in 2007 suggests the wisdom of this strategy. Yet with increasing disparities in wealth following the 1970s oil boom years and disillusionment with successive military and civilian governments during the 1980s and 1990s, the EPI met with resistance, including rumors in Northern Nigeria that the vaccines included "family planning" (Renne 1996). While recurrent rumors about Western medicines and commodities laced with infertility drugs or the HIV virus were not the only reason for relatively low immunization coverage in Northern Nigeria, these rumors have been widely reported, even in the Western press, and suggest the possible resistance to the GPEI there.

Second, along with noting this earlier resistance to EPI efforts and taking it more seriously as a form of distrust of foreign intentions or of government programs, researchers might meet with parents to ascertain their perceptions of their children's main health problems and their assessment of the relative risks of illness and immunization. For example, measles was considered a life-threatening illness in Northern Nigeria, while polio was considered a minor problem. Yet before December 2005, only polio vaccine and Vitamin A supplement were available during NIDs and sNIDs, unlike the earlier smallpox eradication campaign when measles vaccine (for control) was also administered. Consequently, public health specialists working in Northeastern Nigeria noted that

> While three confirmed cases of poliomyelitis registered in Adamawa State in 2005 triggered massive resource mobilisation and action, hundreds of children dying due to measles during the same time frame did not elicit anything close to an appropriate outbreak response .... Sustained vaccine coverage for measles of below 40%, as in Nigeria, in an era of regular immunisation days for polio is highly disconcerting (Schimmer and Ihekweazu 2006).

By assessing and responding to local health concerns, the initial implementation of the GPEI might have been more effective.

Third, there was also need for culturally appropriate advocacy for the campaign and for meetings with a range of community leaders, from the beginning of the GPEI and continuing during its implementation. As 1 public health professor explained:

> The targets of this advocacy might not be traditional rulers alone [but] even religious leaders, so we need to make more comprehensive advocacy with plans to get to almost everybody who is important. We need to repeat and repeat the message and if the program could find a way of finding the ones who are [not accepting] ....

However, there was also a need for collaborative dialogue throughout the polio eradication effort, as ultimately introduced through the COMPASS program.

Conclusion

The Nigerian economic and political situation as well as the management of the NPI were obstacles which preemptive public health strategies and anthropological research might not have been able to overcome in any event. Yet, collaboration between public health specialists with detailed knowledge about the logistics of health campaigns and medical anthropologists with long experience in communities where resistance might possibly occur could provide important synergistic insights during the preparatory, implementation, and maintenance phases of health campaigns such as the GPEI (Heggenhougen and Clements 1990). Indeed, during the proposed maintenance phase of the GPEI in which the provision of IPV injections is being considered (Anonymous 2003), in order to limit further vaccine-derived poliovirus transmission, public health specialists and anthropologists might fruitfully work together to dispel beliefs about injections causing paralysis. Indeed, such beliefs surfaced recently at an January 2007 NID in Zamfara State where parents accepted OPV, saying "they could see no harm in dropping the liquid into children's mouths," while refusing the Hepatitis B injections on the grounds that "they could lead to paralysis" (Olayinka 2007a). It is important that anthropologists examine the logic underlying these associations, which could then be used in community discussions of immunization injections in relation to local concepts of disease, while public health specialists devise better vaccination techniques to reduce immunization site infections.

Kunitz (1990) has noted that disciplinary boundaries may impede the successful merging of public health and anthropological perspectives on global health initiatives. Yet thinking through the possibilities of resistance and how these potentialities might be addressed needs both the particularistic knowledge of anthropologists and the broadly based epidemiological knowledge of public health specialists to better implement public health campaigns.

Acknowledgments

This study was conducted, in part, with funding from the Advanced Studies Center, the International Institute, and from the Institute for Research on Women and Gender, University of Michigan, Ann Arbor. I would like to thank Hassana Tanimu, Mohammed Musa, Dakyes Usman, Rabiu Muhammad, Yau Tanimu, Charity Warigon, E.O. Musa, Hassan Yakubu, Mairo Bugaje, and Josiah Olubowale for their kind cooperation. I am also grateful to Alhaji (Dr.) Shehu Idris CFR, Emir of Zazzau, for permission to conduct research in Zaria City; and to the staffs of the Nigerian National Archives, Kaduna, and Arewa House, Kaduna, for their helpful assistance. Additional thanks go to Clara

Ejembi, Robert Hahn, and Marcia Inhorn for comments and corrections. Opinions expressed in this chapter are solely my own.

Notes

1. Other aspects of this vaccine, such as the need for multiple doses of heat-susceptible vaccine and the possibility that attenuated OPV could devolve into circulating vaccine-derived poliovirus, as happened in Nigeria in 2005–2007 (CDC 2007a,b; Rabiu 2007), have impeded eradication efforts.

2. One of the difficulties of maintaining broadly based programs is long-term financial sustainability. One recent approach to vaccine provision sponsored by the Gates Foundation is the Global Alliance for Vaccines and Immunization (GAVI) program (GAVI 2007; Table 18.3).

3. For a more detailed discussion of the politics involved in these immunization efforts, see Renne (2006).

4. There was considerable regional variation in measles immunization in Nigeria, with the Northwestern Region having the lowest coverage and the Southwestern Region, the highest (National Population Commission [Nigeria] and ORC/Macro 2004).

5. Belief in the spiritual source of polio is common in rural Hausa communities (Yahya 2007:196). The association of *bori* spirits with rural life was evident at a drama performance in Zaria in 2005, in which one actor referred to a small boy who had wandered on stage as a spirit, exclaiming, "I didn't realize they had spirits in town too!"

6. These vaccines were not always available. The 10th ERC report noted that for the period from January to May 2006, "95% of the LGAs reported BCG vaccine stock-out; 84% of LGAs reported OPV vaccine stock-out; 76% of LGAs reported Hepatitis B vaccine stock-out and 68% of LGAs reported DPT vaccine stock-out" (National Programme on Immunization, Nigeria 2006b).

References

Altman L (2004) Polio cases in West Africa may thwart W.H.O. plan. New York Times (January 11).

Anonymous (2003) Introduction of inactivated poliovirus vaccine into polio-virus vaccine-using countries. *Weekly Epidemiological Record* 78:241–252.

Anonymous (2007) Progress towards poliomyelitis eradication in Nigeria, January 2005 to December 2006. *Weekly Epidemiological Record* 82(13):105–111.

Besmer F (1983) *Horses, Musicians, and Gods: The Hausa Cult of Possession-Trance.* South Hadley, MA: Bergin & Garvey.

Blume S (2006) Anti-vaccination movements and their interpretations. *Social Science and Medicine* 62:628–642.

Centers for Disease Control (CDC) (2005) Progress toward poliomyelitis eradication—Nigeria, January 2004–July 2005. *Morbidity and Mortality Weekly Report* 54(35):873–877.

Centers for Disease Control (CDC) (2007a) Laboratory surveillance for wild and vaccine-derived polioviruses—Worldwide, January 2006–June 2007. *Morbidity and Mortality Weekly Report* 56(37):965–969.

Centers for Disease Control (CDC) (2007b) Update on vaccine-derived polioviruses—Worldwide, January 2006–August 2007. *Morbidity and Mortality Weekly Report* 56(38):996–1001.

Eades J (1980) *The Yoruba Today*. Cambridge, UK: Cambridge University Press.

Ejembi C, Renne E, Adamu HA (1998) The politics of the 1996 cerebrospinal meningitis epidemic in Nigeria. *Africa* 68(1):118–134.

Ekanem E (1988) A 10-year review of morbidity from childhood preventable diseases in Nigeria: How successful is the expanded programme of immunization (EPI)? *Journal of Tropical Pediatrics* 34:323–328.

Etkin N, Ross P, Muazzamu I (1990) The indigenization of pharmaceuticals: Therapeutic transition in rural Hausa Land. *Social Science and Medicine* 30:919–928.

Feilden Battersby Analysts (FBA) (2005) *The State of Routine Immunization Services in Nigeria and Reasons for Current Problems*. Bath: FBA Health Systems Analysts. www.technet21.org/backgrounddocs.html. Accessed September 2005.

Feldman-Savelsberg P, Ndonko F, Schmidt-Ehry B (2000) Sterilizing vaccines or the politics of the womb: Retrospective study of a rumor in Cameroon. *Medical Anthropology Quarterly* 14(2):159–179.

Fenner F, Henderson DA, Arita I, Jezek Z, Ladnyi ID (1988) *Smallpox and Its Eradication*. Geneva: World Health Organization.

Fredrickson D, Davis T, Arnold C, Kennen E, Humiston S, Cross J, et al. (2004) Childhood immunization refusal: Provider and parent perceptions. *Family Medicine* 36:431–439.

Global Alliance for Vaccines and Immunisation (GAVI) (2007) GAVI Alliance Strategy (2007–2010). http://www.gavialliance.org/resources/GAVI_Alliance_Strategy__2007_2010_.pdf. Accessed September 30, 2007

Global Polio Eradication Initiative (GPEI) (2007) Wild Poliovirus Weekly Update. www.polioeradication.org/casecount.asp. Accessed October 1, 2007.

Heggenhougen HJ, Clements CJ (1990) An anthropological perspective on the acceptability of immunization services. *Scandinavian Journal of Infectious Diseases* 76(Suppl):20–31.

Henderson DA (1999) Lessons from the eradication campaigns. *Vaccine* 17(Suppl 3):S53–S55.

Idris H (2006) NPI predicts eradication of polio by 2007. *Daily Trust* (July 20).

Kazaure M (2003) "We will not submit our children for vaccination." Emir of Kazaure. *Weekly Trust* (November 8–14).

Kunitz S (1990) "The Value of Particularism in the Study of the Cultural, Social and Behavioural Determinants of Mortality." In: *What We Know About Health Transition*, Vol I. J Caldwell, S Findley, P Caldwell, G Santow, W Cosford, J Braid et al., eds. Canberra: Health Transition Centre and ANU, pp. 92–109.

Last M (2005) "Religion and Healing in Hausaland." In: *African Religion and Social Change: Essays in Honor of John Peel*. T Falola, ed. Durham, NC: Carolina Academic Press, pp. 549–562.

Miller M, Barrett S, Henderson DA (2006) "Control and Eradication." In: *Disease Control Priorities in Developing Countries*, 2nd ed. DT Jamison, JG Breman, AR Measham, G Alleyne, M Claeson, D Evans, P Jha et al., eds. New York: Oxford University Press, pp. 1163–1176.

Musa, JN (2004) Polio: 60,000 kick-off immunisation in Kano. *Daily Trust* (July 29).

National Planning Commission (NPC-Nigeria) & UNICEF (2001) *Children's and Women's Rights in Nigeria: A Wake-Up Call: Situation Assessment and Analysis 2001*. Abuja: National Planning Commission and UNICEF-Nigeria.

National Population Commission (Nigeria) and ORC/Macro (2004) *Nigeria Demographic and Health Survey 2003*. Calverton, MD: National Population Commission and ORC/Macro.

National Programme on Immunization, Nigeria (2006a) 9th Meeting of the Expert Review Committee (ERC) on Polio Eradication in Nigeria. Kano, March 14–15. http://www.polioeradication.org/meetings.asp. Accessed May 15, 2007.

National Programme on Immunization, Nigeria (2006b) 10th Meeting of the Expert Review Committee (ERC) on Polio Eradication in Nigeria. Kano, July 12–13. http://www.polioeradication.org/meetings.asp. Accessed May 15, 2007.

National Programme on Immunization, Nigeria (nd) Basic Messages & Frequently Asked Questions on Immunization Plus (Muhimman Sakwanni Tare da Tamboyoyin da a kan yi Game da Sabon Tsarin Alluran Riga-kafin Cututtukan Yara) (obtained in Kaduna, July 2006).

Nichter M (1995) Vaccinations in the Third World: A consideration of community demand. *Social Science and Medicine* 41(5):617–632.

Obadare E (2005) A crisis of trust: History, politics, religion and the polio controversy in northern Nigeria. *Patterns of Prejudice* 39(3):265–284.

Olaniyi R (2006) "Approaching the Study of the Yoruba Diaspora in Northern Nigeria." In: *Yoruba Identity and Power Politics*. T Falola, A Genova, eds. Rochester, NY: University of Rochester Press, pp. 231–250.

Olatimehin O (1988) Accomplishing the goal of EPI. *National Concord* (April 27).

Olayinka C (2007a) Zamfara residents reject polio vaccines. *The Guardian* (January 29).

Olayinka C (2007b) Immunisation body, primary healthcare agency for merger. *The Guardian* (May 8).

Olusanya B (2004) Polio-vaccination boycott in Nigeria. *Lancet* 363:1912.

Oshinsky D (2005) *Polio: An American Story*. Oxford, UK: Oxford University Press.

Parry E, Godfrey R, Mabey D, Gill G, eds. (2004) "Poliomyelitis." In: *Principles of Medicine in Africa*. Cambridge, UK: Cambridge University Press, pp. 696–701.

Rabiu R (2007) Under-vaccination triggers another polio epidemic. *Sunday Trust* (October 7), www.dailytrust.com. Accessed October 9, 2007.

Renne E (1996) Perceptions of population policy, development, and family planning in Northern Nigeria. *Studies in Family Planning* 27(3):127–136.

Renne E (2006) Perspectives on polio and immunization in Northern Nigeria. *Social Science and Medicine* 63(7):1857–1869.

Roberts L (2007) Vaccine-related polio outbreak in Nigeria raises concerns. Science 317(5846):1842. www.sciencemag.org/cgi/content/full/317/5846/1842. Accessed September 30, 2007.

Schimmer B, Ihekweazu C (2006) Polio eradication and measles immunisation in Nigeria. *Lancet* 6:63–65.

Smallman-Raynor MR, Cliff DA, Trevelyan B, Nettleton C, Sneddon S (2006) *Poliomyelitis: Emergence to Eradication*. Oxford, UK: Oxford University Press.

Stephens J (2006) Panel faults Pfizer in '96 clinical trial in Nigeria. *Washington Post* (May 7).

Streefland P, Chowdhury AMR, Ramos-Jimenez P (1999) Patterns of vaccination acceptance. *Social Science and Medicine* 49:1705–1716.

Taylor CE, Cutts F, Taylor ME (1997) Ethical dilemmas in current planning for polio eradication. *American Journal of Public Health* 87(6):922–925.

Umar A (1989) No free EPI vaccines to states from '90. *New Nigerian* (October 27).

Urquhart A (1970) "Morphology of Zaria." In: *Zaria and Its Region*, Occasional Paper No. 4, Department of Geography. MJ Mortimore, ed. Zaria: Ahmadu Bello University, pp. 123–128.

Wall L (1988) *Hausa Medicine*. Durham, NC: Duke University Press.

World Health Assembly (1988a) Global Eradication of Poliomyelitis by the Year 2000, Resolution WHA 41.28. Geneva: WHO. www.wemos.nl/documents/WHA41.pdf. Accessed May 22, 2007.

World Health Assembly (WHA) (1988b) *Global Eradication of Poliomyelitis by the Year 2000: Plan of Action*. Geneva: WHO. http://whqlibdoc.who.int/hq/1996/WHO_EPI_GEN_96.03.pdf. Accessed May 21, 2007.

WHA (2007) Poliomyelitis: Mechanism for management of potential risks to eradication. Report to the Secretariat, April 12, 2007, WHA A60/11. www.who.int/gb/ebwha/pdf_files/WHA60/A60_11-en.pdf. Accessed May 22, 2007.

WHO (2000) EPI in the African Region 2001–2005: Situation Analysis and Action Plan. www.afro.who.int/ddc/jpd/epi_mang_course/pdfs/english/red.pdf. Accessed September 28, 2007.

WHO 2007a National Immunization Days Calendar. www.polioeradication.org/nid.asp. Accessed May 21, 2007.

WHO (2007b) Circulating Vaccine-Derived Poliovirus Count, 2000–2007. http://www.polioeradication.org/content/fixed/opvcessation/opvc_vdpv.asp.

WHO (2008) Polio Case Count, 2008. www.who.int/immunization_monitoring/en/diseases/poliomyelitis/case_count.cfm. Accessed May 14, 2008.

WHO-Kaduna (2006) Kaduna State Wild Polio Virus Linelist, 2006. Unpublished.

WHO-Kaduna (2007) Kaduna State Wild Polio Virus Linelist, 2007. Unpublished.

WHO/UNICEF (2007) Review of National Immunization Coverage, 1980–2006: Nigeria. www.who.int/vaccines/globalsummary/immunization/countryprofileresult.cfm

Yahya M (2007) Polio vaccines—"no thank you!" Barriers to polio eradication in northern Nigeria. *African Affairs* 106:185–204.

Yishau O (2007) Figures of controversy. *Tell* 5(January 27):16–19.

Part IV

ANTHROPOLOGICAL CRITIQUES OF PUBLIC HEALTH POLICY

19

"Sanitary Makeshifts" and the Perpetuation of Health Stratification in Indonesia

ERIC A. STEIN

Introduction

The 2006 UNDP Human Development report, noting that 2.6 billion people worldwide lack basic access to toilets, has called for the renewed prioritization of sanitation within global health and development agendas. Inadequate sanitation, combined with the lack of access to clean water, has contributed to the persistence of diarrheal diseases, dysentery, cholera, hepatitis, typhoid, parasitic infections, and skin rashes—diseases that have largely disappeared from the US and Europe since the early twentieth century but continue to define global disparities in health conditions. Access to sanitation, and to toilets in particular, can have a considerable impact on health outcomes. While access to basic pit latrines results in a 30% reduction in child mortality on average, the provision of flush toilets can have much greater benefits; for example, in Egypt and Peru families with access to flush toilets experienced a nearly 60% decrease in mortality for children in their first year (United Nations Development Program [UNDP] 2006). Despite the advantages of flush toilets, the UNDP report reigns in ambitions for providing such technologies globally, stating that "inadequate financial resources and technical capacity, allied in some cases with water shortages, make it unrealistic to assume that a developed country model could be extended rapidly across the developing world"

(UNDP 2006:112). Rather than insisting on developed country standards anytime in the near future, the UNDP—committed to reaching Millennium Development Goal sanitation targets by 2015—emphasizes steady increments on a ladder of improved sanitation, beginning with the construction of simple pit latrines for the majority of those without current access.

In *War against Tropical Disease* (1920), Andrew Balfour, one of the early twentieth century figureheads in the field of tropical medicine, described the "sanitary makeshifts" constructed in East Africa by British army hygienists during World War I. Balfour praised improvised technologies such as sliding drawer latrine buckets, petrol can manure incinerators, and urinals carved into ant hills, but also implied that such solutions were suitable only under the "exceptional circumstances" posed by the war (1920:99–142). Yet, the standards created under exceptional circumstances have often become the norm in developing contexts. Because of the reluctance of donor foundations, health organizations, and national governments to invest in sanitary infrastructure, "cost-effective" sanitary makeshifts have in many cases become permanent "appropriate technologies." Although such makeshifts often satisfy the "basic needs" requirements of development targets by reaching large numbers of people relatively cheaply, they often constitute unreliable, labor-intensive solutions that become social markers of poverty. What are the local, long-term consequences of "cost-effective" sanitary solutions? How might inadequate sanitary facilities further promote social inequalities? Given the critical importance of sanitation for improving morbidity and mortality as well as for fostering social status and practical convenience, what are the barriers that prevent the widespread distribution and use of more adequate technologies, such as flush toilets?

This chapter addresses these questions through an historical and ethnographic consideration of sanitation in rural Banyumas, Central Java, Indonesia. The first part examines sanitary makeshifts created in conjunction with Rockefeller Foundation hookworm prevention campaigns in the 1930s, during the time of the Netherlands East Indies colony. Rockefeller Foundation campaigns, responding to economic depression and funding constraints within the Dutch colonial state, emphasized a system of "costless" hygiene in which even the poorest villagers were expected to build latrines, water pipes, and toothbrushes from the palm leaves, bamboo, stones, and coconut husks that could be gathered from wooded commons. Village elites trained as hygiene technicians orchestrated sanitary work, showed public hygiene films, and made rounds of village houses giving educational speeches on disease transmission and latrine construction. After decolonization in the 1950s, certain characteristics of the Rockefeller Foundation approach remained salient in the work of the Indonesian national health services and continue to parallel general patterns within global health policy. Exploring these historical transitions and their implications for understanding social class in contemporary Java, the chapter considers how both technologies and health personnel constitute makeshifts within economically deficient sanitary programs.

Methodology

This study draws from the approach of historical anthropology, combining archival research, oral history, and ethnography to understand the long-term shifts in local Javanese experiences related to sanitary campaigns in the Banyumas region. Field reports, journals, correspondence, and other records at the Rockefeller Archive Center provided an overview of policy decisions, theories behind sanitary work, and activities in Java from the perspective of Dr. John Hydrick, the Rockefeller Foundation field officer in Java. While such sources show what health institutions and their agents intended to achieve, they rarely give a clear picture of what actually happened on the ground in public health work. Moreover, official documents are often sculpted for the benefit of aid organizations, which reward optimistic reports of development activities with continued funding. However, no written archive that records the perspective of Javanese villagers during the 1930s campaigns exists. What I know about rural Javanese experiences with Rockefeller Foundation hookworm projects is taken from the recollections of octogenarian Javanese villagers, whose memory fragments have enabled a piecing together of certain aspects of the past. From documents in the Rockefeller Archive Center, I identified a rural sub-district in Banyumas that was heavily invested in during the hookworm prevention campaigns in the 1930s. From 2002 to 2003, I lived in the sub-district and held extensive conversations with older villagers, numbering 15 in total, who could still recall the work of the hygiene technicians. Although such memories have been shaped by collective storytelling and resonate with the politics of present understandings of the past (Halbwachs 1992; Portelli 1991; Stoler and Strassler 2000), these narrative accounts provide an important contrast with official archives, revealing details that suggest the limits of sanitary policy. Certain data that would be particularly important from a public health standpoint are irretrievably lost: rates of hookworm and other diseases linked to poor sanitation, number of villagers with access to latrines, and the availability of clean water.[1] Yet, other details emerged regarding patterns of social deference to hygiene technicians and conditions of extreme poverty that provide an ethnographic understanding of life in late colonial rural Java.

During the period of fieldwork in Java, I also carried out 120 extensive, unstructured interviews with current health officials, sanitary workers, midwives, doctors, village volunteers, farmers, students, and others regarding their understandings of and experiences with public health. These interview conversations, carried out in a mixture of Indonesian and Javanese, centered on perceptions of existing health and development services, personal illness accounts, ideas about the body and pollution, and various forms of village gossip. The many conflicting narratives about health often indicated the socioeconomic fissures within the village, as wealthier, better educated villagers often held more biomedically oriented etiological models of disease and were more likely to seek hospital care than social subordinates.[2]

While much of my time was spent inside villagers' homes in rural Banyumas, I also participated in village development sessions, followed sanitary workers on village visits, attended meetings of the village women's Family Welfare Organization (PKK), attended village maternal and child health clinics, hung out on street corners with unemployed youth, and attended afternoon ping-pong matches in my neighborhood. As much as my fieldwork was ethnographic, I also strove to frame what was happening in rural Banyumas within the larger politics and history of the Banyumas region and in the sphere of the nation. Thus, when I was not in Karang Wetan I stayed in the city of Purwokerto, the Banyumas regional center, and met with health administrators at hospitals, the department of public health, the Environmental Health Academy (AKL) and General Sudirman University, also utilizing available library and historical materials from each location. I made several visits to Yogyakarta for similar meetings, traveled to the former School for Hygiene Educators in Magelang, and took a 2-week archival visit to Jakarta that included meetings with administrators in the Indonesian Department of Health. A portion of this chapter draws from materials I gathered at these locations as well as from the Royal Tropical Institute (KIT) in Amsterdam, the Royal Institute for Linguistics and Anthropology (KITLV) in Leiden, and the National Archives in the Hague in the Netherlands.

Colonial Era Rural Public Health

Throughout the nineteenth and early twentieth century the primary objective of colonial public health services had been to protect the lives and economic interests of European colonists through sanitation and quarantine in cities, ports, barracks, and plantation estates.[3] The rural expanse in Asia, Africa, and Latin America, where the vast majority of the world's population resided, was largely untouched by public health until the years after World War I, and even then only in patches.[4] In the Netherlands East Indies, rural public health was mainly limited to smallpox and other vaccination campaigns until the 1920s (Boomgaard 1986; Schoute 1937). Clinically focused, hospital- or laboratory-based Dutch physicians in the Public Health Service were largely unsupportive of sanitation and hygiene education for indigenous populations.[5] Such activities were deprioritized and underfunded within official policy, despite the general recognition among liberal politicians of the importance of such activities for "civilizing" colonial subjects (Benda 1958; Gouda 1995; Groeneboer 1998). By the late 1930s, however, the Netherlands Indies Public Health Services had warmed to such work, in part through the influence of the Rockefeller Foundation, which began hookworm prevention sanitary campaigns in the colony in 1924. In 1937, the Netherlands Indies hosted the League of Nations Intergovernmental Conference of Far-Eastern Countries on Rural Hygiene, which proposed "enrolling the local people themselves to cooperate in the task of their own improvement" (League of Nations 1937:42). This participatory approach foreshadowed the principles of Primary Health Care introduced at Alma Ata nearly 40 years later (WHO 1988).

The Rockefeller Foundation, a transnational philanthropic institution funded by the Standard Oil wealth of John D. Rockefeller, played a major role in the expansion of medical services and public health in 62 countries and territories, across Europe, Australia, Asia, Africa, Latin America, and the Caribbean since 1913. The initial work of the Rockefeller Foundation focused on hookworm eradication campaigns in the rural U.S. South, but expanded through the International Health Division to work on hookworm, malaria, and yellow fever, as well as on other forms of technical and educational assistance (Ettling 1981; Farley 2004). A primary supporter of the League of Nations Health Organization, one of the objectives of the Rockefeller Foundation was to multiply institutions of public health education and maintain global networks of disease surveillance (Manderson 1995; Weindling 1995). The Rockefeller Foundation used colonial networks to create vast laboratories, secure test subjects, disseminate biomedical principles, publicize its medical philanthropy, and also develop certain ideas of humanitarianism and rights that predicated the demise of colonialism and outlived the time of explicit colonization. As an external agency, the Rockefeller Foundation used the infrastructure and security of colonial states to sponsor a vision of public health based heavily on prevention, without taking the same risks as European governments that invested in the overall economy, security, and infrastructure of the colonies.

Hookworm was often the explicit rationale used by the Rockefeller Foundation to gain entry into the institutional space of foreign public health administrations (Lowy and Zylberman 2000). The Rockefeller Foundation selected hookworm as a model disease because of its chronic presence throughout much of the tropics, its ability to be easily purged from the body with vermifuge treatments, and its potential to be eliminated from the environment through the construction and use of latrines. Although the Rockefeller Foundation exhibited an interest in improving health conditions on a global level, the main purpose of the work by the International Health Board was primarily demonstrative. As John Farley (2004:5) states in his history of the Rockefeller

Foundation International Health Division, "The eradication of hookworm was a means to an end, not an end in itself." Hookworm prevention work provided initial inroads into various foreign health services, serving to demonstrate the effectiveness of Rockefeller Foundation public health methods for physicians abroad.

According to biomedical models, hookworm, a parasitic soil helminth, persists in warm environments through cycles of chronic infection linked to practices of outdoor defecation. Typically entering the body through pores or wounds in the feet when one steps on contaminated soil, hookworm larvae mature in the bloodstream, then travel from the alveolar capillaries into the lungs, where they are expectorated into the mouth and ingested, finally settling in the small intestines. There, the mature worms feed on blood from the walls of the small intestines and lay millions of eggs, which are expelled from the body through defecation, potentially repolluting the soil with future larvae, completing the cycle of infection. Severe and prolonged hookworm infection creates a distinctive body type, characterized by an emaciated, skin-and-bones frame with a protruding, swollen stomach. Hookworm disease, the outcome of protracted hookworm infection, produces anemia, contributes to growth stunting and mental retardation in children, and weakens the immune system, making the body more susceptible to infectious diseases. The debilitating effects of hookworm disease, though rarely fatal, are marked by a persistent lethargy, earning its designation by journalists in the early twentieth century U.S. South as the "germ of laziness" (Ettling 1981:36–38). Reforming hygiene practices through the construction of latrines and education campaigns held the potential for breaking cycles of reinfection. From the perspective of colonial governments and plantation owners reliant on indigenous labor, hookworm prevention was particularly attractive in areas with high rates of infection, as the disease caused a persistent and debilitating lethargy that hindered worker productivity (Hewa 1995). Such colonial concerns, although often secondary to Rockefeller Foundation objectives, provided an economic incentive for colonial governments to accept offers of Rockefeller Foundation aid.

Despite the potential benefits of hookworm eradication, the arrival of the Rockefeller Foundation in Java in 1924 was fraught with persistent tensions with physicians in the Netherlands Indies Public Health Service, who perceived the intervention as an encroachment on their own medical sovereignty. For the first few years, the Dutch assigned Dr. John Hydrick, the Rockefeller Foundation field officer, to Serang, an insurrectionary district in West Java. In Serang, rumors abounded among colonized populations over the nature of his activities, with some claiming that Hydrick and his staff intended to steal the souls of Muslims and convert them to Christianity.[6] Deaths from overdoses of Oil of Chenopodium, the vermifuge used in the curative treatment of hookworm disease, further escalated distrust.[7] Such tensions, coupled with the strict financial limitations on Hydrick's activities during the 1930s depression, led to his adoption of a particularly frugal model of health prevention that sought to ease tensions with rural populations and achieve compliance with Western standards of hygiene through the cheapest possible means. By 1933, Hydrick had chosen the area surrounding Poerwokerto in the Banyumas region of Central Java as the demonstration area for his Intensive Rural Hygiene projects, turning over 60 villages into health models for inspection by Dutch bureaucrats, Rockefeller field officers, foreign health administrators, indigenous medical students, Asian royalty, and other curious travelers. By the end of the 1930s, the head of the Dutch Public Health Service called Hydrick's Demonstration Unit in Poerwokerto the "center of rural hygiene" for all of the colony.[8]

The centerpiece of the Rockefeller Foundation Intensive Rural Hygiene projects was the hygiene *mantri*, or hygiene "technician," a low-level administrative figure trained to provide rudimentary health education and sanitary inspections within the village of his own origin. The Dutch had used other kinds of *mantri*—smallpox vaccinators, tax collectors, labor contractors, and farm administrators—as an extension of indirect rule, drawing on local elites to maintain order beyond the reaches of colonial governance. For Hydrick, the hygiene *mantri* constituted a critical means for reaching local populations not only in their own vernaculars but also through the social networks that made the hygiene *mantri* familiar, and status-superior, to those he visited on his rounds of the villages. In Karang Wetan, the Banyumas village in which I carried out much of my research, the hygiene *mantri* in the 1930s was the son-in-law of the village head and the son of the *Kayim* (chief Islamic leader) of a neighboring village. Although he died of malaria in 1942, he is well remembered in Karang Wetan because his daughter married his nephew, who became village head in the 1970s, and later remarried the son of the village secretary, who went on to become village head from 1996 until 2003. In rural Java, such dense concentration of authority around several interwoven village bloodlines is not uncommon. Hydrick, continuing the tradition of colonial indirect rule, tapped into such networks of authority though his policy of local assignments for the hygiene technicians with the aim of legitimating his projects among village populations.

In 1936 Hydrick established a Hygiene *Mantri* School in urban Banyumas, which produced several hundred graduates stationed across various parts of Java. The school expanded the previous hygiene *mantri* training program from 6 to 18 months, adding in laboratory technique and extensive field practice components. Yet, graduates of the Hygiene Mantri School were not comprehensive health professionals, but were, rather, highly specialized hygiene propagandists trained largely in persuasive methods and in techniques of basic sanitation. As George Strode, the associate director of the Rockefeller

Foundation International Health Division, observed during a 1938 visit to the Poerwokerto Demonstration Unit, the hygiene *mantri* was an inferior version of sanitary officers trained in the West:

> What is Poerwokerto? It is an attempt to develop constructively permanent health work among the teeming millions of illiterate and poverty-stricken natives at a cost within the capacity of local governments to pay ... the interesting thing is the instrument though which the objectives are reached and the care used in applying that instrument. The hygiene-mantri is the instrument. She, or he, is simply a health visitor but one who could not measure up to the standards considered necessary in the Occident ... nor would a hygiene-mantri be of great use if transplanted to a highly civilized community, as would a competent P.H. nurse from the West were she employed in the East. The Hygiene-mantri is a makeshift ...[9]

For Strode, a double standard was necessary to meet the health needs of the "teeming millions" within the financial limits set by penurious colonial welfare policy. Yet, the hygiene *mantri* was for Strode not a temporary "makeshift," but part of a permanent solution that supplanted colonial commitments for the provision of clinical care in rural areas.

In theory, the hygiene mantri's propaganda films, health speeches, and home visits were expected to cultivate desires among villagers to participate in and pay for the construction of their own sanitary infrastructure. Hydrick disputed the limits that poverty placed on the ability of village populations to fund sanitary works:

> The idea is everywhere prevalent that village populations never have any money and that it will be difficult to pay three or four guilden at once, but if the matter concerns an article that the native villager likes to have he can always find the money for it. Propaganda must create the desire ... .[10]

For those villagers who could not find the money to afford manufactured cement latrine pit linings and covers, Hydrick devised a system of "costless" sanitation and hygiene that could be constructed out of the plentiful natural resources within village yards and commons. The hygiene *mantri* taught school children how to make toothbrushes and fingernail brushes from the fibers of coconut husks, to drink from individual homemade bamboo cups, and to build bamboo piping to funnel water for hand washing and bathing. Diagrams on hygiene propaganda posters showed village women how to weave together food covers from bamboo fibers in order to prevent contamination from flies. Hygiene films demonstrated how the latrine, the most important element within the Rockefeller Foundation projects, could be made by digging a simple pit topped with a bamboo platform secured by stones and covered with thatch (Figure 19.1) (Hydrick 1937). At face, Hydrick's model seems

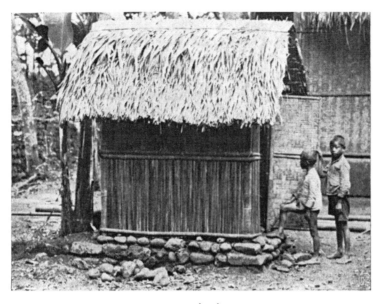

A sanitary costless latrine

Figure 19.1. 1930s hygiene propaganda image, with original caption (Hydrick 1937).

particularly empowering and utopian. It relied on communal participation to construct the essential sanitary implements necessary to prevent parasitic infections and other prevalent forms of disease in the rural tropics, drawing only from the free, available resources in the local environment. In that respect, the Intensive Rural Hygiene Projects might be seen as a prescient parallel of contemporary participatory development schemes.

Yet, the sanitary infrastructure produced out of such initiatives suffered from several critical problems. Although few archival data exist to document latrine coverage and use for the 1930s, several small landholders in rural Banyumas recalled that it was only "*wong sugih-sugih*," the wealthy, who could afford to construct the latrines. They also explained that some wealthy villagers owned latrines even before the time of the hygiene *mantri*, as status symbols that connected them to the modernity and convenience of the late colonial world. Many rural Banyumas families reported first having access to latrines or toilets only after the 1970s, if at all. Bu Lilis, a former female hygiene *mantri* active in the late 1930s, suggested that many people in Banyumas wanted to build latrines, but were forced (*terpaksa*) "*not* to make them" because of conditions of poverty. Those who did build latrines could rarely afford to finish the construction process. While some construction materials might have been freely obtained, the extensive labor for producing such works was never factored into Hydrick's economic equation. Banyumas villagers explained that it might take over a full week to dig the 3 meter deep latrine pit and complete the latrine cover.[11] The value of such intensive labor investments—which might have been used instead to secure family income through other productive activities—was offset by the ephemerality of the makeshift latrines, which, if they survived heavy monsoon rains, filled to capacity every several years and had to be replaced. In the absence of trained sanitary engineers planning their construction, makeshift latrines also had the potential to contaminate ground water and overflow into rivers. While sturdier concrete lined pit latrines might have proved more durable, no service existed in the 1930s to pump and discard the latrine contents.

In addition to these infrastructural problems, the particular social dynamics that governed interactions between elite hygiene *mantris* and subordinate villagers also shaped the possibilities for effective sanitary campaigns. Village elites in Java occupy a role as patrons who provide work and other benefits to subordinate clients, but they are also generally feared for the power they wield over the social order. A former hygiene *mantri* recalled that people would sometimes flee their homes or refuse to answer the door when they arrived for educational home visits. Part of this fear might have been linked to the hygiene *mantri's* association with other colonial authority figures, such as smallpox vaccinators (*mantri cacar*), who exercised some degree of coercive power over village life. The time of the 1930s in Banyumas was also particularly tense, as government transmigration programs led to rumors about "kidnapping *mantri*" (*mantri culik*), who abducted people from the villages and sent them off to Sumatra as forced plantation laborers.[12] In their social position as superior elites and within the climate of late colonial violence, hygiene *mantris*, though known in their own villages, were perceived with some distrust despite their commitment to persuasive methods of health education. Because of their association with latrines and polluting aspects of the body, the hygiene *mantris* were also the subjects of village mockery. In the present, Banyumas villagers refer to the hygiene *mantris* not by their Dutch title (*mantri higiene*), but by the humorous and derogatory term "*mantri kakus*," meaning "outhouse technician." One woman referred to the hygiene mantris as "technicians of messing up other folks' business" (*mantri orak arik*), suggesting that some villagers perceived their home inspections, intimate questionings, and probing into backyards as unwanted violations of privacy. The practice of using local elites mobilized the most educated and influential villagers into the field of public health, but also infused health work with the malevolent power dynamics of indirect rule within highly stratified village societies.

In the 1930s, Rockefeller Foundation rural hygiene projects worked within the extreme financial limits posed by depression economics and adjusted to the deprioritization of rural sanitation within national health agendas. The Intensive Rural Hygiene Projects in Java reflect the consequences of operating under such conditions. Partially trained, exclusively preventive health propagandists were paid a fraction of the wages of Dutch health professionals and expected to provide coverage to thousands of households each. On the basis of such fleeting visits, rural Javanese villagers, many uneducated and living at the threshold of subsistence, were expected to embrace biomedical etiologies and commit money and labor toward the construction of temporary sanitary facilities. Memories of older Javanese villagers suggest that the project of sanitary reform in rural Banyumas was largely unrealized except among wealthier, educated families who could better comprehend the hygiene messages and afford to invest in latrines, wells, and other implements of hygiene. Others relied on *"garam inggris,"* English salts, as a purgative to cure them of worms as they endured cycles of reinfection. As will be discussed subsequently, certain elements of the Rockefeller Foundation projects remained intact following decolonization in the 1950s and came to reflect general strategies within global health policy, reproducing the same kinds of village health stratification as those that occurred in the 1930s.

Postcolonial Transitions

The 1937 League of Nations Intergovernmental Conference of Far-Eastern Countries on Rural Hygiene in Bandung, influenced by the Rockefeller Foundation perspective, represented a global shift toward the increasing prioritization of sanitation and hygiene for rural populations across Asia. The conference expressed optimism for the possibility of indigenous cooperation and active participation in the project of "rural reconstruction," which was conceived as a holistic, integrated approach including health, economy, agriculture, and education (Litsios 1997:261). The World Health Organization, reflecting on the history of public health, noted the similarities between the objectives of the 1937 League of Nations conference and the goals of the 1978 Alma Ata Primary Health Care Declaration (WHO 1992:201). In the interim between the 1930s and 1970s, however, emphasis on the total welfare of rural populations, including sanitary reform, was largely displaced by other health and development objectives. The violence and dislocations of World War II and the wave of decolonizations that followed across Asia disrupted the growing trends of the 1930s. The World Health Organization, replacing the League of Nations as the key international health policy agency in the postwar period, invested heavily in malaria control strategies in the 1950s that largely proved to be unsuccessful (Packard 1997). Rather than emphasize drainage and sanitation as a way to eliminate the breeding grounds of anopheles mosquitoes, the malarial control programs relied on aggressive spraying with DDT and other insecticides, reflecting the technologically centered trends of other postwar development approaches (Litsios 1997).

In Indonesia, doctors trained under the Rockefeller Foundation continued to pursue the Intensive Rural Hygiene approach following the departure of Dr. Hydrick in 1939. Although activities of the projects were attenuated during the period of the Japanese occupation of the Netherlands East Indies colony in World War II, Indonesian doctors revived the Hygiene *Mantri* School after 1945. In 1947, when Dutch return to rule over the former colony instigated a revolutionary war, Indonesian doctors fled the Banyumas region and reestablished the Hygiene *Mantri* School to the East in Magelang, claiming rural hygiene for the emerging Indonesian nation. Dr. R. Mochtar, who had been Director of Health Propaganda under the Dutch at the end of the 1930s, was integral to these efforts linking rural hygiene with the project of nationalism. Following Indonesian independence, Dr. Mochtar served as Head of the Division of General Hygiene through much of the 1950s and attempted to expand the rural hygiene approach. Beginning during the revolutionary war in the late 1940s, hygiene *mantris* were renamed "hygiene educators" (*pendidik hygiene*) and presided over a system of village level "hygiene workers" (*djuru hygiene*) intended to carry out house visits, oversee latrine construction, and inspect sanitary conditions of village neighborhoods. Although the projects expanded the number and kinds of personnel involved with hygiene work, the postwar approach retained the economizing features of the earlier hygiene work, as rural health and sanitation remained deprioritized within national and international policy agendas. By the mid-1950s, fewer than 700 *pendidik hygiene* and *djuru hygiene* combined operated throughout the entire Indonesian archipelago out of a total population of over 100 million (Mochtar 1957:315). In 1961, an American NGO commissioned a survey of the Banyumas hygiene projects and found that they had only a minimal impact even in areas of long-term activity (Calhoun 1961). Pak Arif, a former *pendidik hygiene*, recalled that around 1960, "health centers were lacking" and that rather than concentrate his efforts on sanitation, he was "still caught up helping to look for areas with malaria and smallpox." The perpetual deferral of attention to conditions of poverty and the emphasis on "emergency" disease conditions thus complicated long-term efforts to transform sanitation in rural areas.

While the project of rural hygiene barely left an imprint upon the Indonesian archipelago across a 30-year period from the 1930s to the 1960s, the global shift to prioritization of family planning in the late 1960s led to the rapid mass mobilization of resources to limit population growth. Shortly after General Suharto displaced President Sukarno from power in 1966 following the mass killings of over 500,000 suspected "communists," Suharto redirected military, police, and other institutional resources toward intensive national birth control campaigns. At the village level, the majority of family planning work was carried out by female village volunteers called *kader*. Continuing the precedent of indirect rule set by the earlier hygiene projects, *kader* were drawn from the ranks of rural elites—typically they were obligated to carry out their duties as the wives of minor officials—enabling them to best influence reproductive decisions within the village. By the 1970s, the *djuru hygiene* position was dissolved and home visits regarding sanitation were replaced with home visits to enlist new IUD acceptors. *Kader* activities in the related Family Welfare Program (PKK) required female village elites to teach classes on cooking and nutrition, give demonstrations on child rearing, and to encourage women to sweep their yards and maintain clean homes. By the 1980s, the *kader* role expanded to include maternal and child welfare activities, which continue today in the form of monthly village clinics limited to the principles of Selective Primary Health Care. In the 1990s, there were approximately 1.5 million active *kader* in Indonesia (Ministry of Health 1994), up to 25 to 50 for each village, particularly in densely populated Java where family planning work has been most active. Aside from sub-district sanitation officials who each preside over 10 to 15 villages, the *kader*, who receive very little training and no pay, are most directly responsible for teaching principles of hygiene and sanitation as part of their village welfare work. In the following section I discuss contemporary sanitary conditions in rural Banyumas, Central Java, concentrating on the forms of stratification that characterize village access.

Stratified Hygiene

Banyumas villagers like to joke that the major irrigation canal through the region, part of which was built by the Dutch, is now the "longest toilet in Java." In the early mornings, people can be found wading in the canal to do the wash, bathe, and relieve themselves. In areas without regular access to running water, open yards are also used out of necessity. After over 70 years of sanitation and hygiene efforts, only about 50% of families in the Banyumas region have access to basic private toilet facilities in their homes as of 2002.[13] Karang Wetan, which has served as a model development village since the 1930s, has attained the highest level national village development ranking—*swasembada*, meaning "self-sufficient." The village has electricity, paved streets, and other official indicators of modernity. Yet, of the 536 households in Karang Wetan, over 100 have neither a latrine nor an indoor toilet, less than one-third of homes have piping for the disposal of waste water, and over 200 homes are without wells or other on-site sources of clean water.[14] Banyumas villagers without sanitary facilities are primarily landless sharecroppers, pedicab drivers and other day laborers, or small landowners farming remote hillside plots (*lading*) for cassava, potatoes, corn, and other low-value staples. The cost of installing a toilet and septic tank inside the home is approximately US$60 dollars—nearly double the local monthly wages—and the cost of wells runs many times higher. Government programs since the 1980s like the "Family Toilet" (*Jamban Keluarga*) campaigns and various rotating credit schemes (*arisan*) have provided some financial assistance, but fall far short of meeting the extensive needs of the rural populace. Even within model villages like Karang Wetan, considerable disparities persist, with possible ramifications for morbidity and mortality.

The reasons for such sanitary deficiencies are complex. Ways of accounting for these deficiencies, however, often shift blame for poor sanitation or mask the problem completely, which may further entrench existing patterns of exclusion. When I first arrived in Karang Wetan in 2002, village officials responded to my inquiries about sanitation by assuring me that *all* villagers owned and used toilets, which I soon learned to be untrue. Because of issues of village pride, shame over existing poverty, and desires to maintain high development rankings, usually well-intentioned officials were prone to lead me astray. I looked beyond such forms of sanitary subterfuge to the everyday practices that served as alternates to the use of indoor toilets in Karang Wetan and in the wider Banyumas region.

A common and widespread location for outdoor defecation in the Banyumas region is the many fishponds (*blumbang*) used to raise catfish, gurami, and carp for market sale and local consumption (Figure 19.2). This pattern also exists more widely across Indonesia (Mukherjee 2000). Bu Haryati, a house servant from Karang Wetan born in the mid-1930s, recalled that when she was a child a large fishpond behind the home of the village head was used as the latrine for most people in her neighborhood up until the mid 1940s, when the Japanese appropriated all of the fish and the pond was drained. Some Javanese consider defecating in fishponds to be essential for the economy, as carp, catfish, and gurami all feed on human feces. Thus, using the ponds is encouraged by local fish farmers, who build semi-private latrine platforms (*plangkrangan*) above them for squatting. From a public health perspective, such practices have the potential to spread parasitic infections to consumers of contaminated fish. Several villagers, appearing to recognize the potential dangers of oral–fecal transmission, claimed to never eat the fish from their own ponds, but sell it instead in public markets. The presence of convenient and semi-private fish pond latrines served as a deterrent for some villagers for investing in indoor toilet facilities, which failed to recycle potentially useful human wastes.

Ecological factors also foster the use of public waterways as locations for defecation outside the home. In Karang Wetan, the dry season between May and November can exhaust available sources of water that might be used for

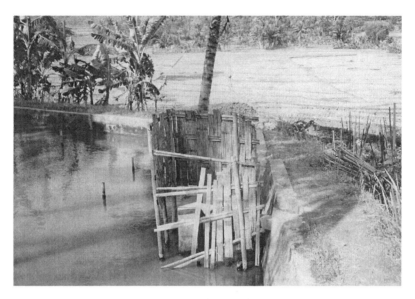

Figure 19.2. Latrine over a Banyumas fishpond, 2002. (Photo by Eric A. Stein)

hygienic purposes. By September, rice fields that flowed with water several months earlier are reduced to barren patches of cracked earth. Because of the uneven water table in Karang Wetan, many wells on the East side of the village dry up around that time, making washing, bathing, or using toilets inside the home very difficult. The severe drought creates a situation in which using the nearby river that borders the village becomes a necessity, even for those villagers who own toilets but lack sufficiently deep wells or servants to transport water into the home. Such limits on access to water are not absolute. Wealthier villagers who can afford to build deeper, better maintained wells with electric pumps continue to have access to clean water inside the home year round.

Yet, the use of the river cannot be reduced to a problem of drought. The river also serves as a space of public sociability where women converse as they bathe and wash clothing, children swim, and men fish or gather sand for use in construction work. When the water level was still low 10 years ago before the construction of a major dam downstream from Karang Wetan, young women washing in the morning would cross the river to meet up with the young men who lived in the village on the other side, taking some of them as husbands. Now, because the water level is high and the current much faster, the river is considered too dangerous for crossing, but people still do their washing and bathing at the edge, sometimes defecating into the water. There is also a particular aesthetic of purity that guides use of the river. For some, defecating in the river is considered refreshing (*sejuk*) and more comfortable than using a toilet in the home. Those who use the bamboo stands constructed over the river's edge report enjoying the satisfying *"Plung Lap!"* sound of the feces entering the water and disappearing, without any smell. The aesthetics of the river—coupled with the comforts of defecating in a familiar place—compels a few people to visit the water's edge even when the wells are full and the indoor toilets are flowing.

For wealthier, better educated villagers as well as sanitary officials, social subordinates' apparent pleasure in using the river is taken as evidence that unsanitary practices are the result of cultural backwardness rather than poverty. Such practices are perceived to be tied to the persistence of "primitive" behavior. Pak Satiman, a former hygiene educator who had recently retired from sanitary work, expressed "cultural backwardness" in terms of a generational gap:

> There are people from villages who when they defecate they must submerge their buttocks entirely underwater. Then at some point they go to visit their children in Jakarta. The bathroom has a sit-down toilet. For a full week they can't defecate, the river is too far. In the end by the time they get back to Purwokerto their feces is already hard and they need medicine for constipation. This is a true story, not a fable.

Pak Satiman attributed such behavior as well as fears over the home visits of sanitary personnel to the "stupidity" of rural villagers, who stubbornly resisted modernity and its associated hygienic practices. Pak Guru, a retired school teacher, explained that "hygiene has progressed" since the time of the *mantri*, "but there are still those who need to be straightened out [*benahi*]." This rhetoric of development, in which "backward" villagers need "straightening out," replicates an earlier colonial discourse on hygiene, in which Europeans defined "native" bodies as inherently dirty, open, and polluting (Anderson 1995, 2006; Burke 1996; Comaroff and Comaroff 1992; McClintock 1995; Stoler 1995). In postcolonial Indonesia, such perceptions of hygiene have shifted to the determination of class difference, where a similar discourse on hygiene casts the poor as predisposed to unclean lifestyles. This perspective blames sanitary deficiencies on individual ignorance and stubborn adherence to traditional ways, downplaying the economic and environmental factors that prevent access to toilets and other facilities.

Rural elites have a twofold stake in monitoring the sanitary conditions of subordinate villagers. Within dense village settlements, cement walled houses with wells and running water stand adjacent to dirt floored bamboo houses without toilet access. Aside from aesthetic concerns, wealthier villagers who tend to embrace biomedical conceptions of disease etiology fear that unsanitary practices will spread infection into their own homes. Pak Guru, the man who wanted unhygienic villagers "straightened out," complained that in his neighborhood there were 5 or 6 houses without toilets. During the rainy season people developed scabies and houses were infested with biting ants "because all of the yards were soiled with human feces." Pak Guru and other villagers who recognize uncontained waste as an epidemiological danger identify subordinate villagers who lack sanitary facilities as the primary cause of outbreaks of infectious disease.

Beyond the potential risks for his own family, Pak Guru was also a practicing Muslim and an elite landholder with ties of patronage to subordinate clients, who worked as sharecroppers in his rice fields and provided other forms of labor during the off-season. As such, he held a stake in the moral economy of village society, in which he was obligated to attend to the welfare of dependents (Scott 1976). For many village elites, volunteering in village governance activities or serving as Family Welfare *kader*, is treated as a way to discharge such obligations to the village poor. Through the Family Welfare Program (PKK), elite female *kader* run the maternal and child health clinic and hold monthly meetings open to the public to discuss matters of health, hygiene, sanitation, nutrition, development, home economy, and other areas of practical knowledge that might "empower" villagers in attendance. To some extent, these services displace more traditional expectations of patronage tied to moneylending, labor, and food redistribution. In effect, the makeshift approach to hygiene and sanitation has placed village elites in the role of "biological patrons" who are invested more in monitoring and cultivating the healthy bodies of subordinates than in seeing to their material well-being.

While the system of biological patronage mobilizes educated elites through unpaid volunteer work using existing systems of moral order, it also represents and reproduces problems inherent to the social stratification upon which it depends. Many village poor actively avoid public figures (*tokoh masyarakat*) like teachers, officials, *kader*, and wealthy landowners out of fear and deference to authority. This avoidance is compounded by elites' attitude that economically disadvantaged villagers adhere stubbornly to the past, living in unsanitary or "primitive" home conditions by choice. Consequently, Family Welfare meetings are largely comprised of *kader* themselves, so that sanitation and hygiene messages they might disseminate rarely reach the lower economic strata of village society directly. Certain exceptions exist. One woman in Karang Wetan who regularly attended the Family Welfare meetings lived in a dirt floor home without a toilet and relied on the income of her husband, a poor pedicab driver. I later discovered that she attended the meetings out of obligation to the neighborhood *kader*, who allowed the woman to watch television in her home.

Kader express frustrations that they are unable to do more through their work to benefit the poor. Some *kader* manipulate the data on Family Welfare surveys so that poorer villagers will gain added rice supplements or health insurance. Other *kader*, unsatisfied or bored with their obligations, fail to attend meetings or completely drop out. Recognizing that work as village volunteers almost never leads to government employment possibilities, many women leave their posts as soon as their husbands leave office. Finally, family welfare work is targeted exclusively toward women, who may heed sanitary messages, but have insufficient power within the household to demand that economic resources be dedicated to the construction of toilets and wells.

The gendered nature and exclusionary aspects of the Family Welfare system, which primarily benefits female *kader* and their peers, poses limits to the effectiveness of health education messages that have particular consequences for the transmission of infectious disease. During the dry season of 2003 I encountered numerous people who claimed to be suffering from typhoid fever. From a biomedical perspective, typhoid fever is caused by *Salmonella typhi* bacteria, which is transmitted primarily through a fecal–oral route by contaminated food or water. Untreated typhoid fever is associated with a case fatality rate as high as 10%, primarily caused by intestinal hemorrhaging and fatal peritonitis. Typhoid can be treated effectively with antibiotics; however, an incomplete course of antibiotics can increase the chance that an individual will become an asymptomatic carrier of *S. typhi* bacteria. Understanding both the etiology of typhoid and the effective cure is therefore critical for ending cycles of reinfection.

When I solicited villagers' explanatory models (Kleinman 1980) on typhoid—how they named the disease, accounted for its origins, described its symptoms, and proposed a cure—the majority explained that typhoid was caused by eating food that was too spicy. Other explanations of etiology included cigarette consumption, coffee, or bodily imbalances. Few Banyumas villagers identified typhoid as an infectious disease, fewer knew that it was spread by fecal contaminated water and food, and no one, not even health professionals, knew that one could become an asymptomatic disease carrier. When I asked a nurse who lived in Karang Wetan and worked as a *kader* in the Family Welfare Program about typhoid education campaigns, she complained that she had publicly explained the cause of typhoid numerous times and that she could not imagine that anyone in the village did not understand how it was spread. The misperception of some *kader* that they are reaching entire village publics with their speeches furthers the blaming of poor, excluded villagers for failing to heed warnings about washing hands and boiling water and causing their own infectious diseases.

The problem of typhoid fever goes beyond the level of village health education, to policy making on a global scale. Typhoid falls within the category of "neglected infectious diseases," yet remains largely under-represented even within this emerging field of epidemiological interest.[15] Although typhoid fever ranked fourth among 10 common diseases in Central Java hospitals during the 1980s, with a case fatality rate between 3.1% and 10.4% (Gasem, Dolmans, Keuter, and Djokomoeljanto 2001), it remains a low priority at multiple tiers of the health system. These seemingly high rates of sickness prompted me to inquire about local typhoid fever prevalence rates at the sub-district clinic (*Puskesmas*). The *mantri* in charge of clinic records informed me that no such data existed. Because typhoid fever is not considered to be as life threatening as other major tropical infections, it does not warrant a separate category within the clinic's system of disease recording. Instead, when someone is diagnosed as potentially having typhoid fever, it gets recorded as a "gastrointestinal disturbance" along with various other forms of diarrhea and intestinal distress. In part, this generalized category was due to the lack of available testing equipment at the clinic and the generality of typhoid symptoms, which complicates definitive diagnoses. The result is that typhoid fever epidemics may go unreported, unless a significant number of cases require hospitalization. Since the antibiotic used to treat typhoid fever is the same as what is given to treat a variety of other gastrointestinal infections, making the distinction matters little from the perspective of the health clinic staff. Although a relatively cheap and effective, yet short term, vaccine exists for typhoid fever, it is not included among the many other immunizations received in childhood or thereafter in Indonesia. Because of the emergency paradigm that governs which diseases become vital on an international level, particularly in terms of funding aid, certain infections receive extensive attention to the exclusion of others. The absence of an "emergency" status for typhoid fever allows a variety of conflicting local etiologies to flourish, which, from an epidemiological standpoint, miss the critical importance of preventing contagion from recently infected disease carriers. The misapprehension of typhoid fever also masks its essential structural component: typhoid fever is typically caused by inadequate water and food sanitation in places with a weak infrastructure for human waste disposal and hand washing. But because it is more often attributed to spicy food, and, with no health workers arriving to correct this belief, most people lack the motivation to avoid potential exposure and cannot complain that their routine suffering is caused by a lack of sanitary facilities.

Conclusion

Although ecological factors shape sanitary access, such limits are rarely absolute. The vast desert settlements throughout the Southwestern United States, served with flush toilets in almost every house, are a testament to the capabilities of sanitary technologies to provide adequate coverage in even the most water-scarce environments. The problem of sanitation is ultimately one tied to a range of disparities, not only in the economic differences among household incomes, but also in the global and national prioritization of sanitary policy, the differential provision of sanitary technologies, and the level of inclusion of impoverished families within health education campaigns. While the vital importance of sanitation has long been recognized within the field of public health, there has rarely been a prolonged commitment in policy for addressing sanitary needs within underdeveloped countries or adequate funding for carrying out the task.[16] The largely vertical determination of health priorities by global health agencies since the end of World War II has favored attention to a small number of diseases with high mortality rates over nationally contained everyday infections that cause routine suffering, such as those tied to lack of sanitation (Birn 2005; Farmer 1999; Litsios 1997; Packard 1997; World Health Organization 1992). Rather than the creation of sustainable sanitary infrastructure, emphasis has been on low-cost, "sanitary makeshifts" to provide temporary solutions to widespread lack of access. These may take the form of improvised or inadequate facilities—bucket latrines, unlined latrine pits, bamboo pit covers, or even flush toilets without a stable water source—that are sometimes labeled as "appropriate technologies" within development discourse.

Deficient technologies, however, only partially account for the perpetuation of health stratification. Poorly trained, underpaid or volunteer health personnel also constitute "cost-effective" solutions that ultimately fail to accomplish their objectives.[17] Hierarchies are exacerbated by conscripting village elites as often reluctant unpaid local health educators to teach about hygiene and sanitation, creating their biological patronage over low-status clients. Village elites heed the messages of public health and benefit from improved sanitation, but rarely convey such messages and benefits effectively to rural poor. Furthermore, continued emphasis on personal responsibility for labor-intensive sanitary construction and maintenance is conducive to an economy of blame, in which subordinate villagers are shamed by village elites for failing to meet sanitary expectations and also treated as dangerous and polluting. This effectively replicates the language of an earlier colonial discourse on hygiene, but places it within a framework of social class, reinforcing existing social inequalities.

While people in the upper economic strata of any society enjoy sanitary facilities built into their homes, schools, and places of work without effort, impoverished people, especially in the global South, are expected to remain persistently vigilant in guarding their own health conditions by expending their own labor and funds. Although some villagers receive indoor toilets, they may not have the time or money to keep them maintained or have access to water to put them to use. These partial sanitary systems are often counted in village development reports even though they offer no health or other benefits for their owners. Moreover, sanitary makeshifts, though only partial and temporary, may lift the health conditions of villages, slums, or countries just above the threshold of emergency concern, making them ineligible for further aid.[18] The emphasis of the UNDP Human Development Report on meeting Millennium Goal Sanitation targets by providing millions of people with pit latrines may serve to ameliorate the most severe sanitary deficiencies, but it may also mean those pit latrine owners will be passed over on the next round of funding and not climb higher up on development rungs, maintaining them in conditions of poverty.

The breadth of the field of anthropology—which recognizes history, ecology, health, economy, politics, culture, and power as interdependently contributing to the formation of social conditions in any given location—offers a unique and complex perspective from which to view problems of sanitation. Anthropological work on symbolic pollution (Douglas 1966) has provided a rich starting point for understanding human "waste" not only as a vehicle for the transmission of infectious pathogens, but also as a conceptual category tied to moral sentiment, religious principles, and ethnic, class, and national identities. Yet, an "anthropology of sanitation" has yet to emerge as a distinctive area of interest, despite increasing anthropological attention to public health and development. For the same reason that Javanese hygiene *mantri* became the subjects of village mockery, anthropologists may be reluctant to engage in research that casts them into the marginal field of "toilet studies." Historical anthropologists exploring the lasting imprints of colonial orders, however, may discover that hygiene, the body, and waste serve as a key to understanding mechanisms of social subordination and difference (Anderson 2006; Burke 1996; Comaroff and Comaroff 1992). Applying such understandings to address the contemporary inequities of sanitary conditions might be seen as less a niche topic than part of a larger project to come to terms with unequal power relations on a broader scale.

Notes

1. While older villagers' narratives provide a general outline of health conditions in the 1930s, such narrative knowledge does not meet the statistical criteria of epidemiological precision. Moreover, responses sometimes diverged about basic sanitary resources, such as access to clean water, with some villagers recalling a common practice of boiling drinking water and others remembering that water was consumed directly from the river. Such differences, I suggest, most likely reflect stratified forms of knowledge and practice around health and the body.

2. By "subordinates" I refer both to clients in direct subordination to economic and social patrons as well as the general differentiation of class and status in Java that entails everyday deference to educated social figures, professionals, officials, and wealthy landowners.

3. John Farley (1991:4) suggests that the "basic goal of tropical medicine was to render the tropical world fit for white habitation and white investment." See also Arnold 1988; Bashford 2003; Curtin 1989, 1996, 1998; Macleod and Lewis 1988; and Manderson 1995, 1996 for discussion of various aspects of the political economy of medicine in European colonies.

4. Several historians (Arnold 1988; Manderson 1996; Gardiner and Oey 1987) have noted the limited reach and effectiveness of colonial medicine within indigenous populations into the twentieth century.

5. Letter from Hydrick to Sawyer, December 17, 1935 RF RG1.1 Series 655J Box 1 Folder 5, Rockefeller Foundation Archives, Rockefeller Archives Center (RAC), Sleepy Hollow, New York.

6. John L. Hydrick, "Third Quarter 1925 Report," p. 53, box 228, series 655, RG 5.3, Rockefeller Foundation Archives, RAC.

7. John L. Hydrick, "Third Quarter 1925 Report," box 228, series 655, RG 5.3, Rockefeller Foundation Archives, RAC.

8. Letter from Dr. Offringa to the Minister of Colonies, January 3, 1936, No. 25, Ministerie van Kolonien 1900–1963, Openbaar Verbal, Algemene Rijksarchief, The Hague.

9. George Strode officer's diary, July 30, 1938, p. 25, RG 12.1, Rockefeller Foundation Archives, RAC.

10. Hydrick to Van Lonkhuijzen, November 5, 1930, p. 2, folder 3753, Series 655, RG 2, Rockefeller Foundation Archives, RAC.

11. It is unclear whether this estimated construction period also included the lengthy process of making the latrine liner, a woven bamboo tube 3 meters long that was sealed with pitch. It is likely that many latrines went without liners and deteriorated more rapidly.

12. One man in Banyumas claiming to be in his 90s reported having been himself a victim of such kidnapping until he returned from Sumatra in the 1950s after decolonization.

13. This figure was reported to me by a sub-district sanitation official and might be regarded as a general average estimate, though numbers vary widely from village to village.

14. The accuracy of such data, which I compiled from the annual village development report, is difficult to confirm. The tendency is to inflate such figures to increase village development rankings.

15. Although the World Health Organization has directed attention toward the problem of typhoid fever, other organizations, such as the Global Health Council and the Global Network for Neglected Tropical Diseases, do not include typhoid among their lists of "neglected" infections.

16. Renewed commitments to addressing sanitary disparities have been relatively recent, such as the UNDP 2006 report, the UN General Assembly declaration of 2008 as the "International Year of Sanitation," and the formation of the World Toilet Organization in 2001 (www.worldtoilet.org). These calls largely repeat the declaration of the "International Drinking Water Supply and Sanitation Decade" of the 1980s.

17. The designation of volunteer health personnel as "cost-effective" may be misleading, as their lack of training and motivation results in relatively ineffective health education and sanitation work that may defer costs to hospitals, clinics, and other treatment centers.

18. See Murphy 2004 on the notion of "sustainable peripheries."

References

Anderson W (1995) Excremental colonialism: Public health and the poetics of pollution. *Critical Inquiry* 21:640–669.

Anderson W (2006) *Colonial Pathologies: American Tropical Medicine, Race, and Hygiene in the Philippines.* Durham, NC: Duke University Press.

Arnold D (1988) "Touching the Body: Perspectives on the Indian Plague." In: *Selected Subaltern Studies*. R Guha, G Spivak, eds. Oxford, UK: Oxford University Press. pp. 391–426.

Balfour A (1920) *War Against Tropical Disease, Being Seven Sanitary Sermons Addressed to All Interested in Tropical Hygiene and Administration*. London: Baillière, Tindall & Cox.

Bashford A (2003) *Imperial Hygiene: A Critical History of Colonialism, Nationalism and Public Health*. London: Palgrave.

Benda H (1958) *The Crescent and the Rising Sun*. The Hague: W. van Hoeve Ltd.

Birn A (2005) Gates's grandest challenge: Transcending technology as public health ideology. *The Lancet* 366:514–519.

Boomgaard P (1986) The Welfare Services in Indonesia, 1900–1942. *Itineraro* 10(1):57–81.

Burke T (1996) *Lifebuoy Men, Lux Women: Commodification, Consumption, and Cleanliness in Modern Zimbabwe*. Durham, NC: Duke University Press.

Calhoun J (1961) *A Look at the Initial Health Education Project in Indonesia*. Djakarta: Ministry of Health.

Comaroff J, Comaroff J (1992) *Ethnography and the Historical Imagination*. Boulder, CO: Westview Press.

Curtin PD (1989) *Death by Migration: Europe's Encounter with the Tropical World in the Nineteenth Century*. Cambridge, UK: Cambridge University Press.

Curtin PD (1996) "Disease and Imperialism." In: *Warm Climates and Western Medicine: The Emergence of Tropical Medicine, 1500–1900*. PD Curtin, ed. Atlanta, GA: Rodopi. pp. 99–107.

Curtin PD (1998) *Disease and Empire: The Health of European Troops in the Conquest of Africa*. Cambridge, UK: Cambridge University Press.

Douglas M (1966) *Purity and Danger: An Analysis of Concepts of Pollution and Taboo*. New York: Praeger.

Ettling J (1981) *The Germ of Laziness: Rockefeller Philanthropy and Public Health in the New South*. Cambridge, MA: Harvard University Press.

Farley J (1991) *Bilharzia: A History of Imperial Tropical Medicine*. Cambridge, UK: Cambridge University Press.

Farley J (2004) *To Cast Out Disease: A History of the International Health Division of Rockefeller Foundation (1913–1951)*. Oxford, UK: Oxford University Press.

Farmer P (1999) *Infections and Inequalities: The Modern Plagues*. Berkeley, CA: University of California Press.

Gardiner P, Oey M (1987) "Morbidity and Mortality in Java, 1880–1940." In: *Death and Disease in Southeast Asia: Explorations in Social, Medical, and Demographic History*. NG Owen, ed. Oxford, UK: Oxford University Press. pp. 48–69.

Gasem H, Dolmans W, Keuter M, Djokomoeljanto R (2001) Poor food hygiene and housing as risk factors for typhoid fever in Semarang, Indonesia. *Tropical Medicine and International Health* 6(6):484–490.

Gouda F (1995) *Dutch Culture Overseas: Colonial Practice in the Netherlands Indies, 1900–1942*. Amsterdam: Amsterdam University Press.

Groeneboer K (1998) *Gateway to the West: The Dutch Language in Colonial Indonesia 1600–1950*. Amsterdam: Amsterdam University Press.

Halbwachs M (1992) *On Collective Memory*. Chicago, IL: University of Chicago Press.

Hewa S (1995) *Colonialism, Tropical Disease and Imperial Medicine: Rockefeller Philanthropy in Sri Lanka*. Lanham, MD: University Press of America, Inc.

Hydrick J (1937) *Intensive Rural Hygiene Work and Public Health Education of the Public Health Service of Netherlands India.* New York: Netherlands Information Bureau.

Kleinman A (1980) *Patients and Healers in the Context of Culture: An Exploration of the Borderland between Anthropology, Medicine, and Psychiatry.* Berkeley, CA: University of California Press.

League of Nations (1937) *Intergovernmental Conference of Far-Eastern Countries on Rural Hygiene: Report of the Preparatory Committee.* Geneva: League of Nations Health Organization.

Litsios S (1997) Malaria control, the cold war, and the postwar reorganization of international assistance. *Medical Anthropology* 17:255–278.

Lowy I, Zylberman P (2000) Medicine as a social instrument: Rockefeller Foundation, 1913–45. *Studies in the History and Philosophy of the Biological and Biomedical Sciences* 31(3):365–379.

Macleod R, Lewis M (1988) *Disease, Medicine and Empire: Perspectives on Western Medicine and the Experience of European Expansion.* London: Routledge.

Manderson L (1995) "Wireless Wars in the Eastern Arena: Epidemiological Surveillance, Disease Prevention and the Work of the Eastern Bureau of the League of Nations Health Organization, 1925–1942." In: *International Health Organizations and Movements, 1918–1939.* P Weindling, ed. Cambridge, UK: Cambridge University Press. pp. 109–133.

Manderson L (1996) *Sickness and the State: Health and Illness in Colonial Malaya, 1870–1940.* Cambridge, UK: Cambridge University Press.

McClintock A (1995) *Imperial Leather: Race, Gender, and Sexuality in the Colonial Conquest.* New York: Routledge.

Ministry of Health (1994) *Primary Health Care in Indonesia.* Jakarta: Ministry of Health.

Mochtar R (1957) Health Education in Indonesia. *Madjalah Kedokteran Indonesia* 7(10):315.

Mukherjee N (2000) *Myth vs. Reality in Sanitation and Hygiene.* Jakarta: Water and Sanitation Program East Asia and the Pacific.

Murphy E (2004) Developing sustainable peripheries: The limits of citizenship in Guatemala City. *Latin American Perspectives* 31(6):48–68.

Packard R (1997) Malaria dreams: Postwar visions of health and development in the Third World. *Medical Anthropology* 17:279–296.

Portelli A (1991) *The Death of Luigi Trastilli and Other Stories: Form and Meaning in Oral History.* Albany, NY: SUNY Press.

Schoute D (1937) *Occidental Therapeutics in the Netherlands East Indies during Three Centuries of Netherlands Settlement (1690–1900).* Batavia: Netherlands Indies Public Health Service.

Scott J (1976) *The Moral Economy of the Peasant: Rebellion and Subsistence in Southeast Asia.* New Haven, CT: Yale University Press.

Stoler A (1995) *Race and the Education of Desire.* Durham, NC: Duke University Press.

Stoler A, Strassler K (2000) Castings for the colonial: On memory work in new order Java. *Comparative Studies in Society and History* 42(1):4–48.

United Nations Development Program (2006) *Beyond Scarcity: Power, Poverty, and the Global Water Crisis.* Human Development Report.

Weindling P (1995) "Social Medicine and the League of Nations Health Organization." In: *International Health Organizations and Movements*. P Weindling, ed. Cambridge, UK: Cambridge University Press, pp. 134–153.

World Health Organization (1988) *Four Decades of Achievement: Highlights of the Work of WHO*. Geneva: WHO.

World Health Organization (1992) *Collaboration in Health Development in South-East Asia, 1948–1988*. New Delhi: WHO Regional office for South-East Asia.

20

Global Panic, Local Repercussions: Economic and Nutritional Effects of Bird Flu in Vietnam

STACY LOCKERBIE AND D. ANN HERRING

Introduction

In the wake of the deaths of 6 people in Hong Kong in 1997, which resulted from infection with the H5N1 strain of avian influenza, Hong Kong's entire chicken population was destroyed. The aim of this initiative was to stop the epizootic infection and thereby prevent the worrying possibility of the development of human-to-human transmission. The year 1997 thus captures the moment at which avian influenza, now referred to as H5N1 HPAI (highly pathogenic avian influenza), can be said to have emerged as a human disease. Since then, H5N1 viruses have been monitored closely to identify genetic and ecological changes that could signify the beginnings of a human pandemic. An upsurge of scholarly, public health, and media interest in the subject has heightened fears about an impending bird flu pandemic, centered in Southeast Asia, which will spread rapidly around the world (Herring in press; Herring and Lockerbie in press). It is no longer a matter of if, but rather a matter of when a pandemic will erupt: "pandemic influenza is imminent and severe acute respiratory syndrome (SARS) may reappear" (Webster, Plotkin, and Dodet 2005).

Most of the literature on avian influenza focuses on epidemiological and public health questions, such as surveillance and detection, the emergence of new strains, animal epizootics, and containment strategies. This chapter takes up problematic understandings of "the coming plague" and results from a collaboration between two anthropologists, one whose research focuses on the 1918 influenza pandemic (Herring) and the other who conducted research on development initiatives in Vietnam during the 2005 avian influenza crisis (Lockerbie). We examine ways in which the discourse on avian influenza contributes to notions of "the primitive other" and offer examples of how international initiatives to eradicate avian influenza pandemic are transforming the lives of ordinary people living at one of the epicenters.

Avian influenza is not simply a health issue; rural farmers, for whom chicken is often the cheapest animal protein, bear the brunt of drastic measures implemented for the sake of humanity. Anthropologists studying development issues therefore have much to contribute to the discussion (see Appadurai 2002; Ferguson 1994; Li 1999; Mitchell 1995). The unintended consequences of many development initiatives are well documented, such as unsustainable use of land, the growing divisions between the social classes and within communities (Crush 1995; Escobar 1995a,b; Farmer 1992; Ferguson 1994), and now, the emergence of disease.

This chapter begins with a short history of avian influenza and describes the circumstances that are creating a climate of panic about the possibility of a global pandemic among humans. We discuss how attempts to eliminate avian influenza in Southeast Asia have come to be framed within a discourse that reinforces dichotomies between "North" and "South," "modern" and "primitive," "hygienic" and "unhygienic." We then turn to consider H5N1 in Vietnam, government programs to stamp it out, and some of the impacts of these initiatives on food security, nutrition, foodways, the creation of "clean" and "dirty spaces," and the emergence of chicken as an elite food.

Avian Influenza

> You can't eat seafood because of the mercury, you can't eat ground beef because of mad cow—and now you can't eat poultry because of the bird flu. What's next? (CBC News 2005)

Since the Hong Kong outbreak in 1997, several waves of avian influenza have emanated from Southeast Asia. The World Health Organization's (WHO's) chronology for the first and most devastating wave of H5N1 avian influenza (2003–March 2004) locates "undetected and unreported outbreaks" among poultry in Asia; the virus was subsequently detected in poultry and mammals in China, Korea, Vietnam, Japan, Thailand, Cambodia, Laos, Indonesia and, later still, in Malaysia. At that time, a total of 35 human cases and 24 deaths, along with possible human-to-human transmission, were identified in Vietnam and Thailand. This wave of epidemics was linked to various avian influenza H5N1 genotypes, traced to the 1997 precursor virus (Horimoto and Kawaoka 2005). The almost simultaneous recognition of the disease in neighboring countries, coupled with the grouping of reports about them, suggests that the disease was actually widespread well before the outbreak (Martin et al. 2006).

Although human avian influenza is framed as an emerging disease in the international discourse, bird flu has been understood to be a severe disease in poultry since 1878 (Martin et al. 2006). Influenza viruses with the H5 surface antigen have been detected in human populations since the late 1950s (Wade 2006). The WHO has coordinated an international surveillance program for influenza for more than 50 years (Layne et al. 2001; Webster, Plotkin, and Dodet 2005) and Hong Kong has been a center for research on influenza ecology since the 1970s. This contributed to the early recognition of the 1997 outbreak (Shortridge, Peiris, and Guan 2003).

Avian influenza, evidently, has been endemic to poultry in many parts of Asia for a long time and it continues to evolve and spread. In 2003, concerns about a global pandemic were fuelled by the emergence of the highly patho-genic Z strain of H5N1 avian influenza, a series of outbreaks in Southeast Asian countries (Republic of Korea, Vietnam, Japan, Thailand, Cambodia, Lao PDR, Indonesia, and China), and the evolution of another deadly strain (H7N7) that resulted in one human fatality in The Netherlands. Unlike other previously known strains, the Z strain is pathogenic to a wider range of species, including mammals, and it is resistant to first-line antiviral drugs (Monto 2005).

With the emergence of the Z strain, it became evident that the ecology of avian influenza had shifted. The new strain infected bird species that normally harbor less pathogenic strains (Weir 2005). Worries about this new virus from Asia—and its ability to elude surveillance, containment strategies, and anti-biotic treatment—dominated media and reports (Herring in press; Herring and Lockerbie in press). In the United States, for example, there were 165 U.S. newspaper and wire service articles in 1997 that covered the threat of pandemic influenza. The volume of coverage changed little until 2003 when it rose to 746 items in association with the SARS outbreak and identification of avian influenza H7N7 in The Netherlands. In 2004, coverage doubled to 1,669 articles and then skyrocketed to an astounding 8,998 in 2005 (Trust for Health 2006).

It is, however, critical to distinguish between *outbreaks of avian influenza* (among birds) and *human cases of avian influenza*, an important difference often omitted in media reports. The majority of avian influenza outbreaks have occurred among poultry and wild birds, not among humans. As of October 27, 2007, there were relatively few laboratory-confirmed instances of highly path-ogenic avian influenza H5N1 among humans: 332 infections and 204 deaths worldwide over a span of 5 years. Human cases have been reported in 12 countries,[1] 7 of which each accumulated fewer than 20 cases[2] over 5 years (WHO 2007b). Important measures of the potential for a pandemic remain unknown, notably the infection rate, morbidity rate, and the incidence of mild and asymptomatic cases. However, a study of 224 confirmed human cases reported to WHO and extracted from Chinese official reports from 2003 to 2006 showed a high fatality rate of 56.7% (Chen, Chen, Dai, and Sun 2007). Person-to-person spread is suspected among cases from Vietnam (4 cases) and Indonesia (7 cases), but the majority of human cases have resulted from direct infection from live or dead birds (Chen et al. 2007; Kandun et al. 2006; WHO 2007a).[3] The distribution of 172 cases reported to WHO for which age and gender were known suggests that older people (>37 years old) are more immune to infection while children and young adults (<27 years old) are more susceptible to the virus (Chen et al. 2007).

Despite the small number of confirmed human cases ($n = 332$), and even smaller number of human deaths ($n = 204$), the conflation of epizootics and human cases in media reports of avian flu serves to exaggerate the threat of an emerging pandemic. Even when reports are careful to indicate that an avian influenza strain is not lethal to humans, we are warned that "the virus remains deep-rooted and can kill at any time" (Associated Press 2007) and that it *"will eventually mutate* so that it can easily be passed from human to human and become a pandemic" (Strain 2007, emphasis added). News stories include warnings from credible sources such as the WHO that "a great influenza pandemic of type A H5N1 could kill from one to more than 40 million people worldwide" (VietNamNet 2007).

The possibility of an avian influenza pandemic, moreover, has been anchored to the devastation of the 1918 influenza pandemic (Herring in press; Herring and Lockerbie in press). *Anchoring* is a mechanism whereby the understanding of a new disease is linked and configured in terms of past epidemics (Joffe 1999). This process of representation normally makes a crisis understandable and therefore less threatening because it connects the crisis to familiar historical events, metaphors, or symbols. In the case of a potential avian influenza outbreak among humans, the opposite effect has occurred because H5N1 HPAI has been anchored to the 1918 influenza pandemic. The 1918 pandemic is "the catastrophe against which all modern pandemics are measured," in which anywhere from 50 to 100 million people may have perished worldwide (Pandemics and Pandemic Threats Since 1900: 1; Johnson and Mueller 2002); it is the "mother of all pandemics" (Taubenberger and Morens 2006). This is all the more noteworthy because other less sinister and more recent anchors for bird flu are available (Herring in press), notably 3 other influenza pandemics that occurred since 1918: 1957, "Asian influenza pandemic," H2N2; 1968, "Hong Kong pandemic," H2N2; and 1977, "Russian flu" or "Russian threat," H1N1.

Anchoring avian influenza to the 1918 pandemic *augments* the climate of viral panic in the same way media representations of SARS increased fear when it too was anchored to the 1918 influenza pandemic and the Black Death (Washer 2004).

Publication of the genome of the 1918 virus in October 2005 further escalated concerns when it was revealed that the 1918 strain appeared to be almost entirely avian (Taubenberger, Reid, Lourens, Wang, Jin, and Fanning 2005). Commentators noted, "they have constructed a virus that is perhaps the most effective bioweapon known" (Nature 2005:794). Set against the backdrop of the unpredicted emergence of SARS in China in 2002 (Webster, Plotkin, and Dodet 2005), the destructive potential of avian influenza was reported to be "short of a nuclear holocaust of unbelievable proportions" (Branswell 2004:1). A WHO flu spokesperson in 2005 estimated that it is realistic to expect 7.4 million deaths globally should pandemic avian influenza emerge, scaled down from the 5 to 150 million deaths mentioned only days earlier by a spokesperson for the United Nations (Trust for Health 2006).

In keeping with these concerns, the WHO has made the prevention and control of influenza a top priority, instituting a pandemic preparedness plan in 1999. In 2002, WHO further developed a global agenda on influenza to guide, support, and coordinate influenza research, control, and surveillance (Webster, Plotkin, and Dodet 2005). Many nations have invested heavily in pandemic planning and are developing protocols, should one occur (WHO 1999).

Apart from the real possibility of an influenza pandemic in the future, avian influenza has come to embody the fears of contemporary Western societies gripped with "germ panic," echoing a similar response to infectious disease in the early twentieth century (Tomes 2000) but now framed within a more generalized anxiety about potential dangers-at-a-distance, yet to be experienced, but threatening nonetheless (Joffe and Haarhoff 2002). The mutability of avian influenza strains, their zoonotic origins, shifting antigenic coats, ability to spread rapidly across boundaries, evade surveillance and antiviral technology, and connection to the 1918 pandemic, all serve to amplify worries that a global cataclysm lies just beyond the horizon, waiting to emerge (Herring in press; Herring and Lockerbie in press).

Situating Avian Influenza

A much less visited part of the story of avian influenza is the way in which Asia has been situated in the international media discourse. Bird flu has come to be represented as an "Asian problem" both in etiology and in fatality (GRAIN 2006), even though avian epizootics occur outside the region. Likewise, free-range and backyard farms in rural regions have become a target of international scrutiny. What is striking about the media discourse is the understanding of Asia as a homogenous place "over there," which contrasts with the substantial differences between, for example, Vietnam, Indonesia, Korea, and China. Headlines such as "Bird flu heats up Asia with five new cases" (Associated Press 2007) facilitate this misunderstanding; the article features news about recent avian flu activity in Vietnam and yet proceeds to address this as an "Asian" phenomenon. The media coverage fosters a divide between "us" and "them" and "here" and "there" in a way that shifts the blame for an emerging pandemic on this part of the world. It ignores the interplay of global processes and reverts to old modes of thinking about a linear progression from primitive to modern and from underdeveloped to developed. In many ways, portrayals of the threat of a human pandemic of avian influenza can be understood as an expression of anxieties about globalization (see Joffe and Haarhoff 2002).

Contrary to media images of avian flu sweeping across Asia, nations such as the Philippines, Singapore, and Brunei have been disease free since 2003. Accordingly, these nations have made very public attempts to protect this status and to challenge the notion that they are plagued by influenza. The Philippines, for example, banned imports of poultry or live birds from countries with known cases, such as Britain, Korea, and Canada. In the latter case, this trade prohibition stems from one bird found carrying the H7N3 strain on a farm in Saskatchewan in October 2007 (Reuters 2007a).

While the potential for a global pandemic is reported and debated, the cost to animals, the poultry industry, and Asian economies has been large. Market shock quickly ensued in the wake of the 2003 avian influenza outbreak; poultry prices rose and international demand dropped in the face of consumer fears and import bans on trading partners affected by HPAI in 2003 and 2004. Asian nations, especially Thailand and China, lost market share as purchasers shifted to South American sources and as worried consumers replaced chicken with other protein sources (FAO 2007). Investors were warned that avian influenza could precipitate a global financial crisis and advised, "to have a prudent degree of balance in portfolios to help you ride out the storms that can occur in investment markets" (Cooper and Coxe 2005:4). By 2006, avian influenza had cost Asian economies more than $15 billion (Anand 2005–2006). That same year it was estimated that perhaps 85% of known avian species had been affected by H5N1 bird flu (Waltz 2006). Over 250 million chickens have either died from avian influenza or been exterminated to stop the spread of infection (FAO 2007).

Little attention has been paid, however, to the effects of extermination programs on the livelihoods of rural farmers. The 250 million chickens that have been culled have come primarily from family farms in rural communities because chicken is often the cheapest animal protein in developing countries. Avian influenza eradication policies therefore place a large economic burden on rural farmers who are the most vulnerable to economic failures and to nutritional inadequacies (FAO 2007; Pfeiffer 2006; Waltz 2006).

At the Epicenter: Avian Influenza in Vietnam

Shortly after the onset of the avian influenza outbreak in Vietnam, one of us (SL) spent 4 months from September 2005 to January 2006 living in Hue city and traveling to rural fishing communities bordering the Tam Giang lagoon in Thua Thien Hue Province of Central Viet Nam (Figures 20.1 and 20.2). The research was part of a project funded by the Canadian International Development Agency (CIDA) and it benefited from the partnership between researchers at Dalhousie University, Hue University of Science (HUS), and the Center for Social Science and Humanities (CSSH) in Hue city, Vietnam. Placed against her earlier work in the region during the SARS scare in 2002, the climate of panic during the avian influenza outbreak came to frame SL's research focus on the recent transition to aquaculture and the creation of an export economy. The bulk of our observations about bird flu in Vietnam stems from candid conversations in these rural and urban settings.

Tam Giang Lagoon is a central feature of the province and the largest lagoon system in Southeast Asia. Thirty percent of the province's population lives in the lagoon regions. Most of the fieldwork was conducted in Vihn Ha commune, 1 of the province's 7 communes, and a region identified to be especially marginalized and poor. Vihn Ha commune consists of 2,010 households and is divided into villages made up of farmer and fisher families (Lam 2005). SL observed and

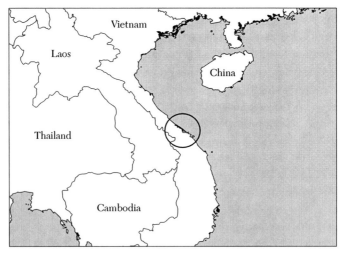

Figure 20.1. Map of Vietnam showing the location of SL's study area and Vihn Ha Commune.

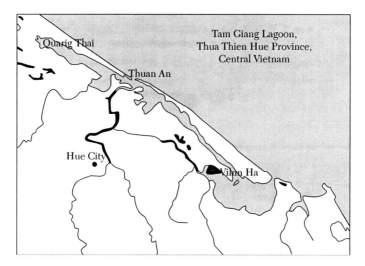

Figure 20.2. Location of Tam Giang Lagoon, the largest lagoon system in Southeast Asia.

interviewed fisher families in Vihn Ha Commune about their daily eating habits, preferences, and livelihood strategies. Aside from these primary research activities, she also taught English to students and faculty at HUS, and volunteered at the CSSH, editing various documents and proposals and presenting the findings of her research. Participating in a range of social activities and residing in a Vietnamese household created an ideal setting for contact with a wide variety of people and for learning about people's reactions to bird flu.

The alarm created by avian influenza in 2005 and the ensuing spectacle of mass chicken slaughtering merged into conversations about bird flu. Discussions of the pending pandemic naturally fit into research questions about a changing economy and the health and well-being of the population, and conversations on avian influenza emerged without prompting. People spoke openly about food and eating and their connections to bird flu because local understandings of the disease are deeply enmeshed in narratives of chicken—many people have lost their household flock or stopped buying chicken to feed their families. Our discussion of avian influenza, therefore, is community driven and guided by the fears and concerns of local people, rather than the product of a deliberately planned research agenda devised in Canada. Questions about avian influenza became part of the daily research agenda in the final phases of fieldwork, in the context of planning the next steps of the project. The support and enthusiasm for this research by Vietnamese people is also worth noting. In a conversation with the director of the CSSH about the possibility of studying bird flu, she responded excitedly, "I support you one hundred percent!"

The discussion presented in this chapter draws on this 4-month period of fieldwork, but is supported by ongoing correspondence with friends, former students, and colleagues in Vietnam through e-mail and Internet chat media. We draw from observations and informal "conversations with a purpose" (Burgess 1993) during trips to the field site or while going about a daily routine that involved buying food from street vendors, shopping in markets, or eating in restaurants. *Vietnam News* items (an English daily newspaper that amalgamates and translates headlines from other Vietnamese daily print), monitored from October 2005 until January 2006 for articles pertaining to avian influenza, also inform this chapter. To monitor the interplay between the global discourse and local reactions, we incorporate media and scientific research between the years 2003 and 2007.

Government Responses to Avian Influenza

Vietnam was among the first countries affected by avian influenza H5N1 when its first human infection was identified in December 2003. At the time of writing this chapter, 100 laboratory-confirmed human cases (30% of all cases) and 46 deaths (23% of all deaths) had been identified in Vietnam (Figure 20.3), placing it second only to Indonesia among countries most severely affected by HPAI (WHO 2007b). Since its first appearance on Vietnamese soil in 2003, Vietnam has been and continues to be in the spotlight of the discourse on avian influenza. Particular animal husbandry practices, especially free-range poultry (chicken and ducks) raising (Figure 20.4), coupled with local and national trade practices, have been identified as playing an important role in disseminating the infection beyond reservoir species (Martin et al. 2006).

The international strategy to address the threat of a human pandemic of avian influenza focuses on controlling HPAI in poultry (FAO 2007). In

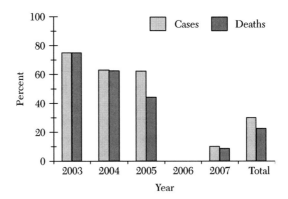

Figure 20.3. Proportion of worldwide laboratory-confirmed human cases and deaths from avian influenza, Vietnam 2003–2007. (Source: Cumulative Number of Laboratory-Confirmed Human Cases of Avian Influenza A/(H5N1) Reported to WHO, By Country 2007).

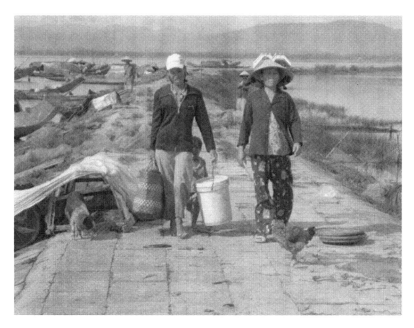

Figure 20.4. Free-range poultry are an important hedge against food insecurity. (Photo by Stacy Lockerbie).

response to the outbreaks of avian influenza, the Vietnamese government took far-reaching measures to protect its international image, to preserve trade and foreign investment, and to rid itself of the stigma of avian influenza. As the host country for the FAO/OIE Regional Meeting on Avian Influenza Control in Asia in Ho Chi Minh City in 2005 (FAO 2007:ix), government officials instituted a stringent policy of culling and vaccinating flocks, along with an intensive disease surveillance program that continually monitors and checks poultry at every stage: where it is raised, transported, and traded (People's Daily Online 2007). In 2004, approximately 66 million birds were culled— Vietnam's primary response to the avian influenza outbreak among poultry— and after 2005 Vietnam was the first nation to implement mandatory poultry vaccination (McKenna 2006a). The incidence of avian influenza was reduced significantly through a rigorous program of culling poultry, mass vaccination of its mostly small-holder poultry sector, closing live bird markets, banning duck breeding, public education programs, and a shift to centralized slaughtering (FAO 2007). Chicken rearing is banned in cities; country-raised chicken is inspected twice before it crosses into a city and, if necessary, killed, and incinerated. In 2005, a 2 shot vaccination program was mandated by the agriculture ministry, and was believed to have captured about 80% of all birds that year (McKenna 2006b).

These policies could not have succeeded without "the willingness of... thousands of small farmers... to follow the government's orders" (McKenna

2006b:1). Despite these efforts, some of which have profound costs for the daily lives, economic prosperity, and well-being of local Vietnamese (including those who cultivate and those who consume poultry), avian influenza continues to appear in new locations across the country. In September 2007, Vietnam was officially declared disease free after 2 months without any reported cases and more than a year without a human case. This respite was short-lived, however, because 1 month later the virus was discovered in the duck population in Vihn Tra province in Southern Vietnam and 5 people fell ill. The reappearance of the virus promptly undid the hard work and vigilance of Vietnamese people who were then chastised in the media for "show[ing] little fear of bird flu." Experts such as Peter Cordingley, the spokesperson for WHO's Western Pacific region, asks whether "the people [in Vietnam] have begun to drop their guard?" Hoang Van Nam, deputy director of the animal health department in Vietnam mirrored this sentiment when he said, "the last time we managed to control it, so people have become too confident" (Associated Press 2007; People's Daily Online 2007; Reuters 2007b).

The practice of keeping poultry is widespread in Vietnam, which enhances the challenge of controlling HPAI. The poultry sector is an important feature of its domestic economy, and small-scale poultry production is, moreover, a strategy for reducing poverty (Riviere-Cinnamond, Cuc, and Wollny 2005). Poultry keeping is found in about half of all rural and urban households in Vietnam; in the northern regions, 90% or more households keep poultry. Before the HPAI epidemic, flocks averaged about 16 birds. Most poultry keeping was, and still is, conducted in small backyard settings by low-income families that fall into the UN Food and Agriculture Organization's lowest category of 1 to 50 kg of poultry production per annum. Poultry density varies across the nation, but is closely linked to poverty; the highest densities of both, for example, occur in the Red River Delta area (Otte, Roland-Holst, and Pfeiffer 2006).

It comes as no surprise, therefore, that small-scale subsistence farming families have been the hardest hit by government policies aimed at preventing the spread of avian influenza because of the continued policy of culling infected chickens reared outside of government-sanctioned farms. The direct costs to farmers of culling and disinfecting birds in Vietnam from January 2004 to February 2005 were considerable: US$121.6 million, with farmers bearing 76% of the costs (Riviere-Cinnamond, Cuc, and Wollny 2005).

Slaughtering infected flocks avoids the considerable expense of vaccination programs and uses dramatic measures to display Vietnam's commitment to the control and eradication of avian flu to its populace and to the international community. The justification for culling stems in part from difficulty distinguishing infected birds from the vaccinated birds. Vaccinations, it is argued, do not secure immunity because the flocks "roam free" and therefore need to be immunized repeatedly (Bangkok Post 2007; Butler 2005a). Freely roaming poultry, also known in a Western context as "free range" and sold at a higher price, are the targets of viral spread, and are thus considered to be a major impediment to efforts to curb or eradicate the spread of avian influenza. In many rural villages, however, families rear a small number of birds and can easily monitor their vaccination record. One of SL's interviewees commented, "we know our birds are safe, we vaccinated them ourselves." This contrasts with the perception that backyard farms are by nature difficult to control because they are "small scale, free range, scattered and informal" (GRAIN 2006).

The culling of chickens, and spraying with disinfectant farms and humans in contact with infected chickens, reassures a panicked public and also serves to depict certain places and spaces as "clean" and "modern" and others as "unclean" or "polluted" (Anderson 1995; Chakrabarty 1991; Douglas 1992). Culling is only a temporary solution, however, and does not guarantee elimination of the virus (FAO 2007:xi), especially when "there are significant gaps in our understanding of the H5N1 HPAI virus and technologies and tools to control it" (FAO 2007:xiii). In many settings, moreover, there is insufficient knowledge or capacity to achieve "safe and humane culling and disposal of infected poultry" (FAO 2007:x). Medium- and long-term strategies beyond culling are needed to ensure that the burden of avian influenza (and the cost) does not fall solely on farmers (Riviere-Cinnamond, Cuc, and Wollny 2005).

Avian Influenza and Economic Development

In the midst of avian influenza and widespread poultry culling, food-rearing practices promoted for decades as the solution to economic development in Vietnam, including small-scale poultry holdings, are now in question. The Vietnamese government's drive for economic growth has been fuelled by an export-based economy introduced to reduce poverty and broaden the base of income-generating activities among the rural poor. As part of this national development program, individual regions have concentrated on farming a particular food item for export. Newspapers regularly feature articles about new development initiatives introduced to concentrate regional farming on a particular item for export, such as rice, dragon fruit, farmed shrimp, chicken, and fish sauce. These items, once grown and consumed within a regional or at least national radius, are all now grown intensively in their respective regions and are moving into the global market (*Vietnam News* 2005). As local farmers willingly accept and engage in these new subsistence activities, such as the fishers in Vihn Ha commune who converted to aquaculture, they simultaneously become good citizens of the country (in raising income-generating activities) and bad citizens of the world (in creating an environment characterized by many animals in small spaces that allows disease to flourish).

As part of the Vietnamese government's program to reduce avian influenza and sanitize the Vietnamese poultry industry, there is a proposal to get rid of backyard operations and reorganize production into large, biosecure farms (McKenna 2006b:2). This is in keeping with *The Global Strategy for Prevention and Control of H5N1 Highly Pathogenic Avian Influenza*, which identifies countries with high poultry population densities and large small-holding poultry sectors as one of the major risk factors for HPAI (FAO 2007).

In Vietnam and elsewhere, small-scale subsistence fishing and farming are regarded as inefficient, and the development discourse often includes recommendations that it be replaced by larger income-generating enterprises that incorporate the global market (Lockerbie 2006; Menzies 2002). Government-sanctioned and commercial farms are promoted as "safe" and "clean" spaces even though these are the very farms in developed countries where avian influenza erupts. Viruses spread slowly among small village chicken flocks and die out under low-density conditions; in contrast, they spread quickly in densely packed factory farms. Furthermore, even though migrating birds have transmitted avian influenza over long distances, less attention has been paid to the role of integrated trade networks in the transboundary spread of avian influenza. The trade in chicks, eggs, live birds, meat, and secondary products, such as manure, feathers, and animal feed, allows avian influenza to spread within regions and across international borders (Butler 2005b). The illegal bird trade has been implicated in human cases of avian influenza. "Safe trade" in birds and poultry products is part of the FAO strategy to reduce HPAI (FAO 2007), but modifying international trade regulations is a far more complicated and long-term process than the seemingly more expedient and immediate action of killing infected flocks.

In Vietnam, intensive fishing and farming practices are promoted by various development firms to take the pressure off intensively used resources and to add a new source of revenue to the community. Local fishers throughout the regions bordering Tam Giang lagoon were using environmentally damaging fishing techniques such as electric currents to catch more fish with fewer inputs. Aquaculture has been introduced to a variety of regions to actively discourage these practices. It seems, however, that one issue of sustainability simply replaces another. Fish farms have become the central economic activity of villages and regions, are used beyond sustainable levels, and become paired with the threat of disease. Similarly, economically focused proposals to prevent avian influenza in Vietnam by introducing large-scale "biosecure" poultry farms ignore the important function served by small-scale poultry operations as a hedge against food insecurity, and as a supplementary source of protein for poor families. They also fail to take into account gendered effects that will ensue from dismantling backyard operations; women directly control small-holder poultry production and income, income that is often used to feed and educate their children (FAO 2007).

Eating Chicken in Vietnam: Global Health Politics and Food Security

Fear of a global pandemic is having a significant impact on the landscape of food and eating in Vietnam. Food is both a popular topic of conversation and a window on life as it supports national, regional, and gendered identity, demarks social class, mediates social relationships, and is closely connected to feelings of health and well-being (Lockerbie 2006). There is a large body of literature about the ways in which food has significance well beyond its nutritional value (Caplan 1997; Lupton 1996; Mintz 1986, 1999; Watson 1997). This literature is especially salient in Vietnam where SL was told, "Vietnamese food is very simple and low in fat ... we do not like to eat anything else but Vietnamese food." Each region is carefully delimited by the taste of the broth or the size of the noodle, as SL learned by eating with others in restaurants, street stalls, or in private homes.

To elaborate on the first point, food is an important facet of Vietnamese identity. Vietnamese people living and traveling abroad take great pride in the quintessential Vietnamese dishes such as Hanoi's beef noodle soup, known locally as *Pho*, and eating this food is what "makes them Vietnamese" while living away from Vietnam (Thomas 2004). This sensation seems only to be heightened in a food's absence. In the context of avian flu, chicken becomes more deeply entrenched in ideas of national identity. Like the case of beef in Britain during the BSE scare (Washer 2006), chicken in Vietnam is described with special emphasis with comments such as "Vietnamese chicken is the best chicken in the world." Yet, SL's host family responded to her interest in bird flu with strong statements about the need to avoid all poultry products. The family also expressed regret in doing so, exemplified by the father's dismay, "it's too bad you cannot enjoy Vietnamese chicken, it is Quyen's [his son's] favorite." To those who no longer consume it, chicken affects notions of identity as people long for its return to their diet.

Beyond the loss of chicken in the diet, other initiatives aimed at "cleaning up" the poultry industry are interrupting local foodways. One proposal, in place in Ho Chi Minh City and in northern Vietnam, replaces live bird markets with Western-style supermarkets where dead birds, killed in centralized slaughterhouses, can be bought (McKenna 2006b). Supermarkets, however, are elite spaces where very few Vietnamese people shop. Food items are expensive and these Western-style markets are located in urban centers. They are inaccessible, by virtue of location and cost, for the large portion of the Vietnamese population that lives in rural communities—the people most directly affected by restrictions on poultry. Supermarket culture also cancels meaningful connections to food created by caring for and raising the very food one is eating. In the cities, it also eliminates the ability to forge symbolic and social connections to the food by establishing relationships with the vendors who raise it.

In Vietnam eating chicken has important ceremonial functions over and above its nutritional benefits. Birds are slaughtered to commemorate special occasions, such as weddings or festivities that honor deceased ancestors. The subtle effects of avian influenza on such practices are exemplified by a meal SL attended with her host family in honor of a deceased relative. A wide range of food was served while each family member said a silent prayer and lit incense in his honor. Chicken was not served on this occasion because of bird flu, although it was noted that it typically would have been an important part of the ceremony. The residents of Vihn Ha commune mourned the omission of poultry at such occasions, more so because their daily diet has little variety and rarely strays beyond rice and fish. There are few alternatives for celebratory food once villagers lose their poultry so it is difficult to sustain festive occasions like the one described here. Chicken is also an important element in observing *Tet*, the Lunar New Year. On successful days of fishing and selling to middlemen, the villagers of Vihn Ha Commune often buy chicken or beef with the extra money they earn. Even in fishing villages, where the ban on raising chickens has little impact on the daily diet, it is greatly missed as a ceremonial and supplementary food.

Worries about bird flu are also framed within ongoing concerns about food safety throughout Vietnam. Local residents often suffer from gastroenteritis because of contaminated food or water. Those who routinely visit the market establish trading relationships with particular vendors not only to ensure a fair price, but also for assurance that they are purchasing quality food, free from contamination. SL observed Mrs. Hanh, the mother of the household in which she was living, walk past dozens of vendors selling many of the things she was looking for only to buy them from the same women and the same stalls every day. The vendors worked hard to obtain Mrs. Hanh's unflagging business and to ensure that she always received quality goods. Live bird markets are centers for social life in rural communities; replacing them with Western-style supermarkets dismantles a long-standing system of trust and obligation among market sellers and market goers.

In response to the exigencies of a potential avian influenza pandemic, government-imposed restrictions on chicken in Vietnam have made it much more difficult to obtain for rural and city dwellers. The former are subject to the forcible culling of their family's poultry and have limited access to markets that lie far beyond the village confines. Many urban dwellers have become wary of buying chicken in the marketplace because it is impossible to ensure that it comes from a safe and reliable source. Government-sanctioned farms produce chicken officially identified as "safe and clean" but it passes through a long chain of hands by the time it reaches the market. In particular, urban markets are disconnected from the original source on chicken farms and it is well understood that vendors can claim that their birds come from a government farm. Indeed, it is in urban settings, where raising chickens has been banned and where the commodity chain separates consumers from producers, that people are afraid of eating chicken. In rural communities people can speak with confidence about the source of their meal. Ironically, it is the residents of rural communities who suffer the greatest threats to their livelihoods.

Akin to the striking historical shift in the use and meaning of sugar (Mintz 1986, 1999), in the shadow of avian influenza, chicken is emerging as a status food in Vietnam because it is difficult to obtain. It is not the food itself that is important, but the demonstration that one possesses the knowledge and personal connections necessary to obtain it. During a holiday celebration among the elite of Hue city, for example, it was evident that guests shared an assumption that the chicken they were served was safe to eat in this prestigious setting. The host who made the catering arrangements, it was understood, must have had the requisite connections to ensure its quality because most of Hue's local elite and foreign residents were in attendance. Similarly, weddings and other catered events are considered to be safe places to eat chicken. These are occasions when rice is not even served because it is considered to be ordinary food; instead, meats and vegetables and plenty of beer are served as much for display as for nourishment. Chicken seems to have taken on heightened importance in these settings. Special occasions therefore are spaces in which a host displays privileged access to quality chicken. Through webs of social connections these elite spaces decontaminate food, and accordingly, chicken emerges as status food.

Urbanites who are confident about eating chicken in their daily routine are those who can afford to eat in more expensive restaurants. Eating poultry becomes a symbol of education and demonstrates connections to knowledge and regular association with Westerners. One of SL's contacts, working for a local NGO, explained that she and her coworkers have been given bird flu insurance, where their medical bills will be covered in the case of contact or infection with bird flu; the work involved in traveling to rural villages is believed to put them at a higher risk of exposure to the disease.

Aside from the more abstract processes that serve to redesign the landscape of food and eating in Vietnam, bird flu has more concrete and more realized consequences as many people have lost access to poultry products, even in communities where chicken is not a primary or even secondary source of livelihood. Rural households, even those with only a handful of chicken and ducks raised for personal consumption, have lost their flocks in the wake of avian influenza. One fishing family of 12[4] in Vihn Ha commune, for example, kept 5 or 6 ducks for special occasions such as weddings and major holidays, and as a measure of food security. The household lacks a stable food base year round and is particularly vulnerable to shortages during the rainy season when fishing is less lucrative and more dangerous due to storms. Days and sometimes weeks passed without a successful day of fishing. Over the years, the family has carefully managed its resources and met its nutritional needs during hard times through the judicious consumption of its household ducks. When bird flu eradication programs target rural communities, they pose a great threat to households such as this, even when only a few birds are lost. For this family of 12, and others like it, the culling of backyard poultry flocks has the potential to upset the delicately balanced subsistence strategies that have sustained them over the years.

It is not only chicken but also other poultry products, such as ducks, quail, and eggs that have come to embody the set of fears linked to avian flu. Duck and quail farming also have been restricted. As was the case for the Vihn Ha family mentioned earlier, ducks are kept by some families to supplement their diet. Eggs are also a significant and potentially detrimental omission from the Vietnamese diet. They are inexpensive, high in protein, and a major component of street food. While wealthy and educated urban dwellers continue to have access to these foods, it is precisely those who need it the most who are kept from it; inequities in access to these types of food reinforce discrepancies between the social classes.

The nutritional qualities of food, however, are not separate from its symbolic meanings as both values are closely intertwined. Certain foods, for example, are eaten according to the lunar calendar. Twice each month, at the new moon and the full moon, people purchase food, especially fruit, to offer to their ancestors, and then can consume it themselves the next day. All Buddhists in Vietnam refrain from eating meat on such days. On other occasions like weddings or anniversaries, foods that poorer families rarely consume, such as beef or chicken, are served. Holidays therefore have distinctly functional qualities. They create occasional but regular opportunities for people, especially children, to make up for long-term nutritional deficiencies.

Conclusion

International attempts to eliminate avian influenza in Southeast Asia have come to be framed within a discourse characterized by viral panic, anchored to the imagery of the 1918 influenza pandemic, the experience of SARS, and worries about bioterrorism. In this climate, the relatively small number of human deaths from HPAI has gained enormous significance while less attention is being paid to its impact on food security, nutrition, and the health of people living in its epicenters. In Vietnam, and elsewhere, it is the rural poor, whose livelihoods are sustained or supplemented by small household flocks, who bear the brunt of policies aimed at improving global biosecurity. These consequences are contradictory to development goals to reduce poverty that have actively promoted the farming practices—including the keeping of small backyard poultry flocks—now blamed for fostering the ideal conditions for avian influenza to spread.

Avian influenza has been framed primarily as a health issue but it is clearly a much broader problem and speaks of the unintended consequences of development initiatives. Rural farmers now face the triple burden of the loss of their flocks, the stigma for creating the spaces within which H5N1 HPAI can flourish and spread, and the burden of risk associated with living at the epicenter of the disease itself.

Raising and eating chicken has become a dangerous undertaking in Vietnam. It widens a divide between rural and urban, elite and poor, primitive and modern, clean and unclean spaces. Efforts to sanitize and control poultry production by eliminating backyard operations and reorganizing the industry into government-sanctioned farms have a profound impact. They undermine the symbolic importance of poultry as celebratory food for auspicious events, take away an important hedge against income and food insecurity, and rupture intimate economic and social relationships nurtured over many years between poultry buyers and sellers. The campaign against highly pathogenic avian influenza, aimed at preventing a global pandemic on the horizon, is undermining the health and well-being of farmers in Vietnam and other parts of Asia. Rural farmers, for whom poultry is often the cheapest animal protein, have borne the brunt of drastic measures against avian influenza that are being implemented for the sake of humanity.

Notes

1. Azerbaijan, Cambodia, China, Djibouti, Egypt, Indonesia, Iraq, Lao People's Democratic Republic, Nigeria, Thailand, Turkey, Vietnam.

2. Azerbaijan, Cambodia, Djibouti, Iraq, Lao People's Democratic Republic, Nigeria, Turkey.

3. Human-to-human transmission is also suspected during the H7N7 outbreak in The Netherlands (van Boven et al. 2007).

4. The household consisted of a married couple, 8 young children, and 2 grandparents.

References

Anand NN (2005–2006) The economic impact of a flu pandemic. *Lab Business* Winter 2005–2006:18–21.

Anderson W (1995) Excremental colonialism: Public health and the poetics of pollution. *Critical Inquiry* 21(3):640–669.

Appadurai A (2002) "Disjuncture and Difference in the Global Cultural Economy." In: *The Anthropology of Globalization: A Reader.* JX Inda, R Rosaldo, eds. Oxford, UK: Blackwell Publishing, pp. 46–64.

Associated Press (2007) Bird Flu heats up in Asia with five new cases. MSNBC (22 June).

Bangkok Post (2007) Bird Flu cases in Vietnam, Indonesia. www.bangkokpost.net/ breaking_news/breakingnews.php?id=122552

Branswell H (2004) Flu pandemic would wreak social devastation. http://www. medbroadcast.com/channel_health_news_details.asp?news_id=3228&channel_ id=1006&relation_id=0&acomment=submit_article_comment

Burgess RG (1993) *Studies in Qualitative Methodology*, Volume 4. Greenwich, CT: Jai Press Inc.

Butler D (2005a) Vaccination will work better than culling say bird flu experts. *Nature* 434:810.

Butler D (2005b) Bird flu moves towards Europe. www.nature.com/news/2005/050801/ full/news050801-1.html

Caplan P (1997) *Food, Health and Identity.* New York: Routledge Press.

CBC News (2005) Billion bird flu? The hour with George Stroumboulopoulos. www.cbc.ca/thehour/video.php?id=739 (November 22).

Chakrabarty D (1991) Open space/public space: Garbage, modernity and India. *South Asia: Journal of South Asian Studies* 14:15–31.

Chen J-M, Chen J-W, Dai J-J, Sun Y-X (2007) A survey of human cases of H5N1 by the WHO before June 2006 for infection control. *American Journal of Infection Control* 35(7):467–469.

Cooper S, Coxe D (2005) *An Investor's Guide to Avian Flu.* Toronto: BMO Nesbitt Burns Research.

Crush J (1995) "Introduction: Imagining Development" In: *Power of Development.* J Crush, ed. London: Routledge pp. 1–26

Douglas M (1992) *Risk and Blame.* New York: Routledge.

Escobar A (1995a) *Encountering Development: The Making and the Unmaking of the Third World.* Princeton, NJ: Princeton University Press.

Escobar A (1995b) "Imagining a Post Development Era." In: *Power of Development.* J Crush, ed. London: Routledge pp. 211–227.

Farmer P (1992) *AIDS and Accusation: Haiti and the Geography of Blame.* Berkeley, CA: University of California Press.

Ferguson J (1994) *The Anti-Politics Machine.* Minneapolis, MN: University of Minnesota Press.

Food and Agriculture Organization of the United Nations (FAO) (2007) *The Global Strategy for Prevention and Control of H5N1 Highly Pathogenic Avian Influenza.* Rome: FAO.

GRAIN (2006) Fowl play: The poultry industry's central role in the Bird Flu crisis. GRAIN Briefing, February 2006. http://www.grain.org/briefings/?id=194 (March 15, 2006).

Herring DA (in press) "Viral P panic, Vulnerability and the Next Pandemic." In: *Health, Risk, and Adversity: A Contextual View from Anthropology.* C Panter-Brick, A Fuentes, eds. Oxford, UK: Berghahn Press.

Herring DA, Lockerbie S (in press) "The Coming Plague." In: *Plagues: Models and Metaphors in the Human "Struggle" with Disease.* DA Herring, A Swedlund, eds. Oxfordshire and Gordonsville, VA: Berg Publishers.

Horimoto T, Kawaoka Y (2005) Influenza: Lessons from past pandemics, warnings from current incidents. *Nature Reviews Microbiology* 3:591–600.

Joffe H (1999) *Risk and the Other.* Cambridge, UK: Cambridge University Press.

Joffe H, Haarhoff G (2002) Representations of far-flung illnesses: The case of Ebola in Britain. *Social Science and Medicine* 54:955–969.

Johnson NPAS, Mueller J (2002) Updating the accounts: Global mortality of the 1918–1920 "Spanish" influenza pandemic. *Bulletin of the History of Medicine* 76:105–115.

Kandun IN, Wibisono H, Sedyaningih ER, Yusharmen DPH, Santoso H, Septiawati C, et al. (2006) Three Indonesian clusters of H5N1 virus infection in 2005. *New England Journal of Medicine* 355:2186–2194.

Lam Thi Thu Suu (2005) Report on a Participatory Study of Livelihood at Vihn Ha Commune: Vietnam.

Layne SP, Beugelsdijk TJ, Kumar C, Patel N, Taubenberger JK, Cox NJ, et al. (2001) A global lab against influenza. *Science* 293(5536):1729.

Li T (1999) Compromising power: Development, culture, and rule in Indonesia. *Cultural Anthropology* 14(3):295–322.

Lockerbie S (2006) Diary of an ethnographer: Following fish from the local to the global. MA thesis. Dalhousie University.

Lupton D (1996) *Food, Body and the Self.* Thousand Oaks, CA: Sage Publications.

Martin V, Sims L, Lubroth J, Kahn S, Domenech J, Benino C (2006) History and evolution of HPAI viruses in southeast Asia. *Annals of the New York Academy of Science* 1081:153–162.

McKenna M (2006a) Vietnam's success against avian flu may offer blueprint for others. Special report. University of Minnesota: Center for Infectious Disease Research and Policy. www.cidrap.umn.edu/cidrap/content/influenza/avianflu/news/oct2506vietsuccess.html

McKenna M (2006b) When avian flu control meets cultural resistance. Special report. University of Minnesota: Center for Infectious Disease Research and Policy. www.cidrap.umn.edu/cidrap/content/influenza/avianflu/news/oct2606vietculture.html

Menzies C (2002) "Red Flags and Coiffes: Identity, Livelihood, and the Politics of Survival in the Bigoudennie, France." In: *Culture, Economy, Power: Anthropology as Critique, Anthropology as Praxis.* W Lem, B Leach, eds. Albany, NY: State University of New York Press, pp. 235–249.

Mintz SW (1986) *Sweetness and Power.* New York: Penguin Books.

Mintz SW (1999) *Tasting Food, Tasting Freedom—Excursions into Eating, Culture and the Past.* Boston: Beacon Press.

Mitchell T (1995) "The Object of Development." In: *Power of Development.* J Crush, ed. London: Routledge, pp. 129–157.

Monto AS (2005) The threat of an avian influenza pandemic. *New England Journal of Medicine* 352(4):323–325.

Nature (2005) The 1918 flu virus is resurrected. *Nature* 437:794–795.

Otte J, Roland-Holst D, Pfeiffer DU (2006) HPAI control measures and household incomes in Viet Nam. Food and Agriculture Organization of the United Nations. Pro-Poor Livestock Policy Initiative. http://www.fao.org/ag/AGAinfo/programmes/en/pplpi/docarc/feature02_hpaicontrol.pdf (July 7).

Pandemics and pandemic threats since 1900. U. S. Department of Health and Human Services. [Online]. Available: http://www.PandemicFlu.gov (May 23, 2006).

People's Daily Online (2007) Bird Flu returns in Vietnam. http://English.people.com. cn (October 11).

Pfeiffer DU (2006) "Avian Influenza in Viet Nam." In: Socio-economic Impact Assessment of Selected Control Strategies for Avian Influenza in Viet Nam and Thailand. Pro-Poor Livestock Policy Initiative, Bangkok, June 29, 2005. Rome: FAO, pp. 15–18.

Reuters (2007a) Philippines bans poultry, bird imports from Canada. http://ca.today.reuters.com/news/newsArticle.aspx?type=topNews&storyID=2007–10–10T114301Z_01_MAN206721_RTRIDST_0_NEWS-BIRDFLU-PHILIPPINES-COL.XML (October 20).

Reuters (2007b) Update 1-Bird Flu Returns to Ducks in Southern Vietnam. http://kr.itv.reuters.com/news/articlebusiness.aspx?type=health&storyID=nHAN201412&imageid=&cap= (October 11).

Riviere-Cinnamond A, Cuc NTK, Wollny C (2005) Support Policy Strategy for Avian Influenza Emergency Recover and Rehabilitation of the Poultry Sector in Vietnam. Conference on International Agricultural Research for Development, Stuttgart-Hohenheim, October 11–13.

Shortridge KF, Peiris JK, Guan Y (2003) The next influenza pandemic: Lessons from Hong Kong. *Journal of Applied Microbiology* 94(Suppl):70S–79S.

Strain J (2007) Banks preparing for bird flu, and so should you. thestreet.com (October 11).

Taubenberger JK, Morens DM (2006) 1918 influenza: The mother of all pandemics. *Emerging Infectious Diseases* 12(1):15–22.

Taubenberger JK, Reid AH, Lourens RM, Wang R, Jin G, Fanning TG (2005) Characterization of the 1918 influenza virus polymerase genes. *Nature* 437(7060):889–893.

Thomas M (2004) Transition in taste in Vietnam and the diaspora. *Australian Journal of Anthropology* 159(1):54–67.

Tomes N (2000) The making of a germ panic, then and now. *American Journal of Public Health* 90(2):191–198.

Trust for Health (2006) Covering the Pandemic Flu Threat. Tracking Articles and Some Key Events: 1997 to 2005. http://healthyamericans.org/reports/flumedia/CoveringReport.pdf

van Boven M, Koopmans M, Du Ry van Beest Holle M, Meijer A, Klinkenberg D, Donnelly CA, et al. (2007) Detecting emerging transmissibility of avian influenza virus in human households. *PloS Computational Biology* 3(7):e145.

VietNamNet (2007) Risk of bird flu outbreak remains on high alert. http://english.vietnamnet.vn (October 7).

VNS (2005) Seafood imports surge amid bird flu fears. *Vietnam News* (November 11).

VNS (2005) Food security fears trigger export ban. *Vietnam News* (October 14).

VNS (2005) Health Ministry identifies tasks for producing safe, hygienic food. *Vietnam News* (December 26).

VNS (2005) Agriculture exports to fetch $5b. *Vietnam News* (December 26).

VNS (2005) Minister rides to the rescue of chicken. *Vietnam News* (December 27).

VNS (2005) Quality, hygiene key to US market. *Vietnam News* (December 28).

VNS (2005) Agricultural sector overcomes difficult year. *Vietnam News* (December 30).

Wade N (2006) Studies suggest avian flu pandemic isn't imminent. *New York Times* (March 23).

Waltz E (2006) Pandemic prevention schemes threaten diversity, experts warn. *Nature Medicine* 12:598.

Washer P (2004) Representations of SARS in the British newspapers. *Social Science and Medicine* 59:2561–2571.

Washer P (2006) Representations of Mad Cow Disease. *Social Science and Medicine* 62:457–466.

Watson J (1997) "Introduction: Transnationalism, Localization and Fast Foods in East Asia." In: *Golden Arches East: McDonalds in Asia.* J Watson, ed. Stanford, CA: Stanford University Press, pp. 1–38.

Webster R, Plotkin S, Dodet B (2005) Emergence and control of viral respiratory diseases (conference summary). www.cdc.gov/ncidod/EID/vol11no04/05–0076.htm (April 22).

Weir E (2005) The ecology of avian influenza. *Canadian Medical Association Journal* 173(8):869–870.

World Health Organization (1999) Influenza Pandemic Plan. The Role of WHO and Guidelines for National and Regional Planning. Geneva, Switzerland.

World Health Organization (2007a) H5N1 avian influenza: Timeline. http://www.who.int/csr/disease/avian_influenza/timeline.pdf (July 8).

World Health Organization (2007b) Cumulative Number of Confirmed Human Cases of Avian Influenza A/(H5N1) Reported to WHO. www.who.int/csr/disease/avian_influenza/country/cases_table_2007_10_25/en/index.html (October 27).

21

Neoliberal Infections and the Politics of Health: Resurgent Tuberculosis Epidemics in New York City and Lima, Peru

SANDY SMITH-NONINI

Introduction

Few infectious diseases pose simultaneously such dangers to human beings and such a challenge to health-care systems worldwide as resurgent tuberculosis (TB), which kills 3 million people a year, and has been designated "a global health emergency" by the World Health Organization (WHO) (1997). As with Acquired Immune Deficiency Syndrome (AIDS) in the 1980s, the urgency of TB was brought into the public eye when it threatened U.S. citizens. In the 1990s, epidemics of TB dominated the news in New York City and several other U.S. inner cities, and the disease continues to crop up in settings of extreme poverty. The outbreaks in the 1990s were shocking to many who came of age in the 1960s and recalled the U.S. Surgeon General celebrating the medical conquest of infectious disease. But in reality the dreaded "white plague," which initially manifests as a persistent cough, night sweats, and weight loss, continues to be deadly if untreated.

TB has killed more people worldwide than any disease in history (Reichman 2002), and a third of humanity is estimated to have antibodies to the TB bacillus, indicating that the latent (inactive) form of TB remains prevalent. Among the poor, many stressors such as poor nutrition or an HIV infection may suppress the immune system and lead to active infection (Farmer 1999a; Ott 1996). Internationally—effective drugs notwithstanding—this neglected public health menace remains the largest preventable cause of adult disability and

death in the world, according to the WHO (1997). TB is also a major opportunistic infection affecting AIDS patients, and is the final cause of death for
many who succumb to the virus; so resolving the HIV epidemic also depends
on stemming the spread of TB.

Recent studies show that the multiple-drug resistant tuberculosis (MDRTB)
strains seen in recent epidemics have caused quiet epidemics in numerous
countries, particularly in settings where AIDS, warfare, or worsening poverty
have reduced immunity (Cohn, Bustreo, and Raviglione 1997; IAUTLD 1997;
Pablos-Mendez et al. 1998).[1] The resurgence of the disease has pointed up the
high cost of treating drug resistance and the potential for airborne spread of
MDRTB by patients who remain contagious for months or years.

With migration, global trade, and air travel linking nations ever more tightly
together, resurgent TB in poor countries rapidly becomes a First World health
problem—a third of the new United States TB cases were diagnosed in foreign-born patients (McKenna, McCray, and Onorato 1995). Also, MDRTB can
jump across socioeconomic divides. Although the TB epidemic in New York
remained "hidden" among the marginalized poor for nearly a decade, once
drug resistance became established, middle-class AIDS patients, nurses, and
prison guards were among those who became infected in institutional settings;
and MDRTB can kill a patient with active disease in a matter of weeks. So,
clearly, solutions to resurgent TB must cross over national borders and socioeconomic classes.

On the one hand, successful control of TB requires health workers to tran-
scend the dominant curative care paradigm of Western biomedicine—there
is no "magic bullet" for curing TB. Once patients are infected, drug therapy
must continue for 6 to 12 months, long after patients begin to feel better. Since
incomplete treatment leads to drug-resistant strains of the bacillus, patient
compliance remains one of the largest challenges. Public health authorities
consider the best model for TB control in epidemic situations to be supervised or directly observed therapy (DOT), where health aides actually observe
patients take their pills (WHO 1997)—an approach that calls for an unusually
high level of collaboration between physicians, patients, and health workers
(Fujiwara, Larkin, and Frieden 1997).

However, the spread of MDRTB has also demonstrated the shortcomings
of international public health models that are too rigid, or which over-rely on
standardized treatment protocols, and pay insufficient attention to cultural difference and diversity of needs at the community level. To work, DOT protocols
must be adapted to individual patients' needs and setting, and there must be
a comprehensive package of care, including food aid and support for transportation to clinics in the case of the poorest patients. These requirements pose
challenges to TB control programs in many poor countries that lack adequate
health funding for infrastructure or staffing (Farmer 1999b).

Methodology

In this chapter, I discuss findings from a qualitative comparative study of the role of health policy in 2 epidemics of resurgent TB—one in New York City, and the other in Lima, Peru, one of the "hot spots" of international MDRTB identified in the late 1990s. Unlike many medical anthropologists who focus on cultural models of disease and patient-centered analyses, my interests in this study were to explore the political and economic aspects of the makings of an epidemic. Many public health workers and medical historians refer to TB as a "social disease" because its outbreaks so often parallel shifts in economic and political policies that affect the poor. Yet, an interesting aspect of recent epidemics has been the ways they caught modern systems designed to track infectious outbreaks of TB by surprise. How, I wondered, is it possible that health divisions specifically tasked with tracking this disease failed to sound the alarm long after statistics indicating an outbreak were collected? My analytical gaze, therefore, needed to focus on those points where external forces, including levels of funding and political ideology, intersected with health policy.

This approach, which Laura Nader (1974) called "studying up," poses some classic problems, compared with the more common anthropological approach of training our gaze on "subaltern" (underprivileged or minority) populations. For example, highly educated professionals such as doctors are not accustomed to being asked to account for their actions, except to their peers and professional associations, and officials in government hierarchies likewise usually prefer to avoid public scrutiny over issues such as failures in public policy. Therefore, access for traditional ethnography in such settings is rare. Further, in this case, I needed to reconstruct events in the recent past, and some key informants no longer worked in the jobs they held during the period of the epidemics. For all these reasons, my methodology relied heavily on in-depth interviews with key individuals who were knowledgeable about these events.

In some ways, this methodology is similar to journalism, except that infectious disease policy is rarely covered in any detail in the media, and the historical perspective and cultural questions that drive an anthropological analysis are likewise usually outside the purview of newspaper or magazine accounts.

The study is based on 60 open-ended, in-depth interviews carried out between January and June 1999, with public health experts, current and former public health officials in TB control programs, health workers, and TB patients in both cities. Among those interviewed were TB specialists at the Centers for Disease Control and Prevention (CDC) in Atlanta and at the WHO in Geneva. Most interviews were done face-to-face, but some were conducted by telephone, with follow-up by e-mail. While in Lima, I visited and observed the TB programs at a government-run TB clinic and at a clinic run by a nongovernmental organization (NGO) that specialized in community-based TB care. Most informants spoke on the record, but I protected identities of individuals in a few instances, where their comments might prejudice relationships with supervisors, co-workers or colleagues.

Interview data were supplemented with a Lexus-Nexus search of media coverage of the New York epidemic, and a review of the TB literature in medical, social science, and health policy journals. I also attended a public health forum while in Peru, and read transcripts of several international conferences on MDRTB held in the late 1990s.

I will first discuss these 2 settings in light of the prevalent socioeconomic forces that, locally and internationally, hindered the capacities and political will of agencies to perceive and track the reemergence of TB. I argue that the reemergence of TB can be read in part as a biological marker for the human costs of the neoliberal movement, which began in the mid-1970s and became formalized with the backing of the World Bank and the International Monetary Fund (IMF) in 1980. The neoliberal ideology of shrinking government and deregulating capital flows shaped both national economies and international and development agendas for 3 decades, and has been heavily criticized for deepening economic inequality (Gandy and Zumla 2003; Kim, Shakow, Bayona, Rhatigan, and Rubin de Celis 2000). In the second half of the chapter I discuss how distinctive political traditions and cultures of biomedicine and international health development shaped responses to rising TB incidences, the adoption of the DOT strategy, and strategies for treating MDRTB in New York and Peru.

Economic and Political Origins of Resurgent Tuberculosis

The Dismantling of Tuberculosis Control in New York City (1965–1989)

Unlike outbreaks of "emerging" diseases like Ebola, Hanta Virus or AIDS, in the case of New York City's epidemic of resurgent TB, which emerged into the public eye between 1990 and 1991, the famous disease detectives of the CDC faced the challenge, not of identifying a new pathogen, but of developing policies to correct a breakdown in institutional disease control that had been more than a decade in the making. The few remaining TB specialists in the United States had warned for years that TB resurgence was likely due to the dismantling of the city's public health surveillance and treatment programs since the 1960s. One of those critics was Dr. Lee Reichman, Executive Director of the National Tuberculosis Center in Newark, NJ, who in 1992 described the upsurge in TB cases as "horrendous" to a *New York Times* reporter, remarking that, "This was a 100% preventable and curable disease." [2]

Many observers have noted that TB control was in some ways a victim of its own success. There was a general sense within the medical community that the advent of new drug therapies in the 1950s heralded the end of TB as a major public health problem, and physicians turned their attention to chronic problems such as cancer and heart disease, which had become more common causes of death among Americans (Garrett 1995; Lerner 1993). In 1972, categorical TB project grants were phased out and replaced by general federal grants that freed states and local governments to shift funds to other purposes.[3] Over the next few years, the breakdown in New York City's health infrastructure translated into the closing of 13 of the 21 TB clinics that had been operating citywide in 1970 (Brudney and Dobkin 1991). During the city's 1975 fiscal crisis, Health Department staffing was cut by a quarter and TB control was hit particularly hard—New York State, which had provided half of the TB budget, had terminated state support by 1979, and federal moneys for TB dropped by 80% (Lerner 1993). Dr. Reichman, who directed the city's TB Bureau in the early 1970s, Michael Iseman of Denver's National Jewish Medical and Research Center, and a handful of other TB experts, warned of future epidemics unless funds from the cuts in defunct TB inpatient programs were diverted to strengthening outpatient programs. A series of Congressional hearings was held in 1972 and periodically thereafter, but in general, the TB specialists' concerns went unheeded.[4]

An indirect cause of the hidden TB epidemic was an increase in poverty, linked to economic recession and to declines in social programs. From 1969 until 1982, the incidence of poverty rose by more than half (Lerner 1993). Wallace and Wallace (1998) documented that in the Bronx, where all but one TB clinic were closed, whole neighborhoods became devastated and abandoned, with arson and the expanding drug trade claiming entire blocks, while fire and police services were cut back. Homelessness was also on the rise; by the late 1980s the city's shelters resembled refugee camps in a war zone, with wall-to-wall cots filling armories and warehouses.[5]

These sites became focal points of TB transmission. Health Department surveys later showed that the city's TB patients were disproportionately male and non-White, and included high percentages of homeless persons, HIV-positive patients, recent immigrants, and IV drug users (Frieden, Fujiwara, Washko, and Hamburg 1995). The incidence of TB in the city began creeping upward again with small but steady increases each year after 1978, notably *before* the arrival of AIDS as a public health problem. Between 1979 and 1986, the incidence rose by 83% (Lerner 1993).

By the mid-1980s, health officials were preoccupied with the AIDS crisis and when new federal moneys became available, TB programs competed poorly for public health dollars. The marginalized populations affected with TB, many of whom were co-infected with HIV and needed drug rehabilitation, had few constituencies to advocate for new policies. As former New York City Health Commissioner Margaret Hamburg later put it, "until 1990, TB wasn't on the health department's radar screen."

The rightwing political climate had generated an atmosphere of retrenchment in the public health community. Every year from 1981 to 1987, the Reagan Administration called for repeal of the federal TB program (Ryan 1992). Ironically, in 1986, the year when New York City's TB case rates suddenly rose by 20% over the previous year, the federal-supported TB surveillance program for drug resistance was discontinued (Berkelman, Bryan, Osterholm, LeDuc, and Hughes 1994).

Dr. Dixie Snider, who headed the Division of Tuberculosis Control[6] of the CDC in 1986, became concerned about the rising TB case rates nationally, and led the development of a new plan for TB "elimination." Despite support from the American Thoracic Society and other TB researchers, requests for the necessary funds fell on deaf ears in Washington. Snider's eradication plan was not formalized by the CDC until 1989, after which it remained unfunded until 1992.[7]

Meanwhile the disease spread. In February 1990, after New York City health authorities had documented a dramatic rise in TB cases, budget officials at the Bush White House cut the CDC's TB control request from $36 million to $8 million.[8] In the first 6 months of that year the CDC received reports of 9 TB outbreaks nationwide, 5 of which involved MDRTB strains.[9] By June 1991, the City Hospital Center in Queens, NY, had treated 13 patients with MDRTB, and the CDC was called in to investigate. Eleven of those patients died; most had been co-infected with HIV.[10] Only after revelations of drug-resistant TB in New York and a flurry of publicity in local and national media did funding for TB control increase significantly.

Neoliberal Restructuring and the Collapse of Public Health in Peru (1975–1989)

The TB crisis that Peru faced in 1990 must be seen in relation to the prolonged economic crisis of the late 1970s and 1980s, which impoverished much of the population and decimated the public health system. In addition, the Shining Path rebellion and military repression from the government's counter-insurgency efforts resulted in massive refugee flows into urban areas and the loss of public services to large sections of the rural countryside.

At the heart of the prolonged crisis were neoliberal macroeconomic reforms that allowed the Peruvian government to restructure its external debt, conditional on currency devaluations and cutbacks in public services. Such reforms were initially put in place by a military regime, following a coup d'etat against a populist reform effort in 1975, but after 1978 the reforms became part of a package administered by the IMF. These policies, reinforced by the prevailing conservative bent in foreign policy of the Thatcher and Reagan administrations, unleashed high inflation, which led to a reduction in real wages by more than half between 1975 and 1985. The reforms eliminated trade barriers, leading to an influx of foreign consumer goods and the collapse of export revenues.

As the GDP declined and prices soared, levels of infant malnutrition increased dramatically. By 1985, food consumption had fallen by 25% as compared to 1975 levels (Chossudovsky 1997). Popular support for the Shining Path rebellion, which originated in one of the poorest areas of the Southern Highlands, was influenced strongly by the steep drop in income and subsistence levels experienced by rural peasants (McClintock 1989). From 1979 to 1983, the number of TB cases rose by 30%, making it the fifth most important cause of death in Peru (Ministry of Health 1983). In an evaluation of a 12-month TB therapy regimen used by the Peruvian Ministry of Health in 1981, Hopewell and colleagues (1984) reported that 41% of patients abandoned therapy before the tenth month. Only 47% were cured. Cure rates improved when the Ministry adopted a shorter 8-month regimen, according to a second survey (Hopewell, Ganter, Baron, and Sanchez-Hernandez 1985), but the economic situation made the gains difficult to sustain. The Ministry's underpaid and overworked staff were handicapped by shortages of TB drugs within the Health Ministry[11] and by the increasing rural violence due to the Shining Path war.

A short-lived respite came in 1985 with the election of President Alan Garcia of the reformist American Popular Revolutionary Alliance (APRA) party. Garcia promised to increase wages and control inflation by reducing the country's debt service. In retaliation, the IMF, the World Bank, and international commercial banks cut off financial support to Peru. Although real purchasing power did increase over the next year, by 1987, when local business elites also "declared war on the government," hyperinflation returned and earning power once again plummeted (Chossudovsky 1997).

In 1986, the World Bank suspended a $40 million loan for water and sewer improvements in Lima after the government had spent less than a third of the funds. After the cholera epidemic broke out in 1991 a U.S. Agency for International Development (USAID) mission cited the condition of the municipal water and sewer system, noting that the cholera outbreak was "a disaster waiting to happen" (Harantani and Hernandez 1991, cited in Cueto 1997:183).

Peru's health ministry was a highly politicized institution, with leadership appointed by the president and a well-established system of political patronage. Davíd Tejada de Rivero, a former subdirector of WHO, took over as

Minister of Health under García and became a strong promoter of primary health care for the poor in Peru. His campaign, however, met resistance from many doctors and hospital administrators. After Fujimori's election in 1990, the Ministry changed course and primary health care became "just another program" rather than a guiding philosophy.[12] But what health workers and officials interviewed about this period most remember is the steady decline in resources. By 1991, health worker salaries had declined to US$40 to US$75 per month and workers in both the education and health sectors were on strike. That year the country's health budget spending was less than a quarter of what it had been in 1980 (Cueto 1997).

Continued civil war eventually closed down scores of rural clinics, further damaging morale. After the collapse of the public health infrastructure in the *selva* (rainforest) region there was a resurgence of malaria, dengue, and leishmaniasis (Chossudovsky 1997). The only health program to continue functioning countrywide was vaccination against childhood diseases, thanks to intervention by UNICEF and the WHO and an accord with armed rebel groups permitting vaccination in regions they occupied.

Chronic undernutrition also contributed to the rise in TB during the 1980s. More than 83% of the population failed to meet minimum calorie and protein requirements by 1991, and the national rate of child malnutrition rose to the second highest in Latin America (Chossudovsky 1997). Only half of the TB patients received treatment in the late 1980s, and half of those eventually abandoned treatment and were lost to follow-up. Only a fifth of the country's clinics even offered TB treatment in 1989, and the country's information system for TB was in disarray.[13]

This was the situation when Peruvians elected Alberto Fujimori on a populist platform. Once elected, after consulting with IMF advisors, Fujimori reneged on his promises of improving quality of life for the majority and instituted his famous "Fujishock," further compressing wages and social expenditures, and laying off more public sector workers. Prices shot up overnight. Thousands of soup kitchens sprang up in *pueblos jovenes* (urban squatter communities) as families began pooling resources to make ends meet. To give just one example, the 30-fold increase in fuel costs in Lima made it difficult even for the middle class to boil water or cook, one of a combination of factors thought to have contributed to the 1991 cholera epidemic (Chossudovsky 1997). The epidemic drew international attention and overshadowed other health problems.

As cholera was being brought under control, a group of Peruvian physicians met with Fujimori about the country's TB problem and convinced him to make TB a national priority. Following the 1992 capture of Shining Path leader Abimael Guzman, effectively ending the civil war, the improvements in TB control from 1992 to 1996 paralleled restoration of resources to public health in general. Many health policy observers interviewed for this study believed this initiative, uncharacteristic for the neoliberal regime that had scoffed at most antipoverty programs, was influenced by the bad publicity the country received during the cholera epidemic.[14] The risk of contagion may have been seen as a further potential threat to tourism and foreign investment at this key moment when the government sought postwar funding for reconstruction. Another factor some observers cited was a series of demonstrations by TB patients and activists demanding access to lifesaving drugs.

Despite disparate epidemiological conditions and levels of development in New York City and Peru, an accounting of the socioeconomic causes of these 2 TB epidemics illustrates why, in the words of one Peruvian health expert, resurgent TB is a "social disease." In both settings, public health programs were dismantled along with other social services in the name of making the government more efficient and diverting capital to private sector concerns that stood to gain from investments in economic growth.

The role of poverty in the epidemiology of TB is an old story (Dubos and Dubos 1952). Also, the helplessness that many health professionals feel in the face of rising inequity has contributed to what some authors have called "public health nihilism"—or pessimism about the possibilities of controlling TB (Fairchild and Oppenheimer 1998). But as events in these 2 settings show, it is not only the incidence of the disease but also the incidence of public health funds that create epidemics. A more accurate account of the relations between poverty, public health programs, and TB should acknowledge that poverty is not just an unvarying fact of nature but is created by human beings in the form of economic policies (often backed by structural violence) that sacrifice the health of the most vulnerable to divert funds to profit more privileged classes, a process that is as transnational as the epidemiology of TB.

The Role of Medical and Public Health Cultures in Resurgent Tuberculosis

"Medicalization" of TB and the New York City Epidemic

Social studies of medicine have documented many historical cases of "medicalization" in which complex illnesses that had no easy cure suddenly became reframed from "social" pathologies to individualistic "medical" problems for which specialists sought one-shot solutions. In some cases, as with the rapid dominance that male obstetricians established over childbirth (to the detriment of midwifery) in the first 2 decades of the twentieth century, medicalization fit the needs of an expanding medical profession, as it sought to wrest the legal rights to practice medicine away from practitioners not trained in scientifically approved schools (Starr 1982). In the cases of mental health and

TB in the late 1950s, medicalization followed the development of new drug therapies that made older therapeutic regimens (such as institutionalization of schizophrenics or TB patients) obsolete. Unfortunately, the dominance of the medical model in the United States has often contributed to tossing the baby (of effective social interventions) out with the bath water (of ineffective therapies); such was the case with TB as effective programs of public education, outpatient care, and clinics for screening and surveillance were closed down in the same decade as funding was discontinued for obsolete sanitariums.

Although, as we have seen, political cutbacks in funding played an important role in creating the conditions for resurgent TB, the medical community was not without complicity in this process, and in many cases played a leading role in creating conditions for the return of the "white plague." Yet, other physicians, working within a different paradigm within the public health sector, played heroic roles in defending public health. The clashing health care paradigms at work in this story reveal much about the cultural fissures that must be overcome to build "integrated" approaches to health care.

No better moment epitomizes medical triumphalism than U.S. Surgeon General William Stewart's 1967 proclamation: "It's time that we close the book on infectious disease." In effect, Stewart was restating Louis Pasteur's 1870 prediction that someday disease-causing microbes would be eliminated across the globe (DeSalle 1999). The scores of outbreaks of emergent and resurgent infections worldwide since the 1960s point up the shortcomings of reliance on "magic-bullet" solutions that ignore the role of complex systems—including the biological, ecological, economic, technological, and cultural forces—that interact in the health of populations. But in the 1960s and 1970s, such triumphalism reigned, and in the case of TB there was relatively little opposition from the medical community to the dismantling of programs for a disease that was no longer a major cause of morbidity or mortality. In 1968, the National Tuberculosis Association changed its name to the National Tuberculosis and Respiratory Disease Association (Lerner 1993). During the 1970s, public health programs actually discouraged physicians from keeping newly diagnosed TB patients under their supervision (Nolan 1997).

TB had not gone away. The incidence in New York City began rising again gradually each year after 1978. But, physicians had an explanation. In 1979, an influential article identified "patient compliance" as the "most serious remaining problem of TB" (Addington 1979, cited in Bayer et al. 1998). The problem was a longstanding one: TB patients began to feel better after a few weeks of treatment and simply stopped taking their drugs long before the tuberculin bacteria were eradicated. This notion that the problem of TB centered on patients' failings (with no mention of poverty, access to health care, or the actual functioning of health services) held vogue throughout the 1980s in the mainstream medical literature.

And, the problem was ubiquitous. New York City Health Department statistics showed increasingly low rates of patient compliance in TB treatment programs beginning in the early 1980s. Published articles in the medical literature warned about the dangers of this. When such patients relapsed later and sought treatment again, the likelihood of a cure would be lower. The TB strains that had multiplied in their lungs since their initial bout of therapy would be more likely to be resistant to rifampicin and isoniazid, the most commonly used antibiotics. Further, when such patients got the active disease a second time they would be a source for spread of resistant strains.

Data existed from both international and US trials showing the effectiveness of supervised or directly-observed therapy (DOT) programs in such situations (Bayer and Wilkinson 1995). The CDC provided funds to New York City and two other cities for selective DOT as early as 1980—targeted at noncompliant patients. Although several hundred New York patients were identified as eligible for the program in the early 1980s, the number enrolled remained minuscule (Brudney and Dobkin 1991; Lerner 1993). The expense of DOT was one of the reasons officials did not seriously consider it, according to Dr. Jack Adler, a private respiratory medicine physician who in the mid-1980s directed the city's TB Bureau. Adler, who was a personal friend of the Health Commissioner, had no prior experience in public health, when he was appointed to the post, which, at the time, was only a halftime position. Like many physicians in the private sector, Adler had favored traditional approaches to TB treatment—which placed full responsibility for compliance with the patient, not health providers, and emphasized physician prerogatives in dealing with patients.[15] This stance reflected the predominant thinking about TB treatment by American physicians (Bayer and Wilkinson 1995).

The number of new research grants for TB had dropped significantly by 1979 (Ryan 1992). Compared to heart disease or cancer research, TB research lacked prestige in the medical world. Dr. Barron Lerner, who interned at Columbia Presbyterian Medical School in 1986, recalled that, "we started admitting a lot of TB patients, but when physicians saw a patient with the disease it was treated like a 'curio'. TB was thought of as an interesting disease that everyone thought had disappeared. It was a case of collective lack of memory." This inattention to TB in medical schools contributed to a decline in practitioners entering the field.[16]

Yet, signs of a problem were mounting. In 1985, Dr. Lloyd Friedman tested welfare applicants in New York City and found that one-third tested positive for TB and 1% had active disease.[17] In 1986, a large hike in the city's TB cases drew the attention of local health authorities and the CDC, but little was done, in part because health staffing levels had failed to keep up with the increase in cases (Fujiwara et al. 1997). Two years later, in 1988, only 93 patients were receiving supervised treatment (Bayer and Wilkinson 1995).

Karen Brudney, who directed TB clinics for the city's Bureau of Tuberculosis in Manhattan and the Bronx in those years, had noticed steady increases in patients with TB and became dismayed over how many fell through the cracks in the city's underfunded and overwhelmed public health facilities.[18] In 1989, she and coworkers at Harlem Hospital undertook a study of the hospital's TB program and found an alarming rate of noncompliance, with 89% of patients lost to follow-up (Brudney and Dobkin 1991). Since Brudney had directed the TB program in Managua, Nicaragua, from 1984 to 1986, she had a unique perspective on New York's program. She noted that while case finding was regarded as the main priority in TB programs in the developing world, in the United States health workers made the false assumption that all cases are reported. One problem she identified was the policy of relying on part-time physicians, who were responsible only to see patients who appeared during their shifts. At that time, the hospital had no organized review of lost or non-compliant patients.

In an article entitled "A Tale of Two Cities" that compared New York City's TB control (rather unfavorably) with Managua's innovative program in the mid-1980s, Brudney and Dobkin (1991) detailed the reasons why patients in New York had difficulty seeking care—not only socioeconomic issues such as homelessness and lack of transportation but also issues related to the health system such as long waits in clinic waiting rooms and hostile treatment of patients by overworked clinic staff. Despite ample staff and resources, New York's TB clinics' "organization and operation appear nearly calculated to alienate and frustrate patients .... The effect of New York's enormous staff and cascading statistics has obscured from the public as well as from the authorities the true nature and size of the problem," wrote Brudney and Dobkin (1991:269). Many of their observations were confirmed in a critical 1992 New York State Health Department review of the city hospitals' TB control.

Brudney and other health workers interviewed for this study in 1999 also pointed to a crisis of leadership within the health department during the late 1980s. In her article, Brudney wrote, "proven approaches" such as positive incentive programs to improve compliance "(have) been repeatedly suggested to the bureau's director and the health commissioner, but to date there is no such program." The TB Bureau's crisis of credibility began in 1987 when, following a 17% jump in the city's TB cases in 1 year, the CDC issued a highly critical review of the program, urging officials to reorganize the bureau, improve the computer system used for tracking patients, and hire additional outreach workers. It also recommended the establishment of a TB shelter for homeless patients, where infectious patients could be concentrated and their treatment supervised. This came as a slap in the face to Adler, the head of the TB bureau, who had made recent public statements claiming that TB was *not* a problem in the shelters.

Leadership was also lacking at higher levels. Mayor David Dinkins lacked the political backing he needed to reform the city's failing social and health services. And Dr. Woodrow Meyers, the Commissioner of Health for the city in 1990, resigned (after a short tenure) due to a controversy over public statements he had made about the possible quarantine of AIDS patients. In his efforts to leave on good terms, Meyers failed to defend programs such as immunization and correctional health and school health programs from municipal budget cutters.[19] During the late 1980s, in spite of the growing increases in TB incidence, the city's share of CDC funds for TB had actually declined slightly each year because the Health Department, caught in a citywide hiring freeze, was not spending all the funds it received, and unspent funds were carried over to the next year.[20]

Some observers blame the inattention to TB in New York in the mid-1980s to the distraction due to AIDS, which drew funds, researchers, and public attention away from older, more common threats like TB; however, this was mitigated to a degree when many AIDS researchers, aware of the risk TB posed to HIV-infected patients, began to advocate for TB control.[21] When federal funding failed to materialize for TB, the CDC obtained Congressional approval to transfer a portion of HIV funds to TB control to make up some of the shortfall.[22]

Throughout the 1980s, the medical leadership of New York's TB Bureau failed to respond to a significantly rising incidence in the disease the bureau was set up to control, and when confronted about the problems, found conservative "scientific" rationales to continue ignoring them. To be sure, Adler was able to find backing for a nonaggressive response to TB in the medical literature, where "noncompliance" was still cited as the major problem precluding a cure for TB. Yet, it is no coincidence that "medicalization" of TB took the route of least resistance, by requiring little in the way of new funding. Public health in the United States has long operated within the dominant medical paradigm, and when illness is explained as a problem of individuals, the solutions are far cheaper than solutions that involve public works or social reforms (Lerner 1993; Weiss 1997). Examples of this attitude prevailing in TB care date back to the early 1900s (Starr 1982).

New York City Turns to a "Third-World" Solution

At the end of 1990, when the extent of the city's TB problem was just beginning to gain public exposure, Meyers resigned and the mayor appointed Dr. Margaret Hamburg as acting Health Commissioner. Hamburg, who later became the permanent Commissioner, immediately lobbied (successfully) to get $20 million of cuts in basic health programs restored to the health department.

In 1991 Dr. Tom Frieden, a recently trained physician and Epidemic Intelligence Service officer on loan from the CDC, undertook a study of drug resistance in New York City. His research showed the presence of resistance to 1 or more TB drugs in 33% of patients diagnosed with positive cultures, and resistance to 2 or more TB antibiotics in 19% of the patients (Frieden et al. 1993). Later in 1991, news reports revealed that drug-resistant TB was associated with 13 deaths in the state prison system. A series of reports on infected hospital workers, prison guards, and HIV/AIDS patients over the next year sparked national media coverage, which drew widespread criticism of city authorities. New York City's TB funding rose sharply in the following 2 years. In 1992, Hamburg replaced Adler with Frieden as head of the TB Bureau, now a fulltime position.

With the backing of the CDC, Frieden undertook several reforms, including instituting mandatory surveillance for drug resistance, testing TB patients for drug susceptibility, a 4-drug regimen for all new patients, and a massive expansion of community-based DOT, with food supplements and incentives offered to low-income patients.[23] New York City's aggressive promotion of DOT, in particular, was widely credited for the rapid drop in TB cases that occurred between 1992 and 1995 (Frieden, Fujiwara, Washko, and Hamburg 1995; Fujiwara et al. 1997). However, it is important to keep in mind that New York City's practice of hospitalizing and curing patients with drug resistance also likely reduced spread of the disease (a strategy that cost millions of dollars and would be an unlikely option for a poor country).

Unlike the more mainstream physician leadership of the 1980s, those who were involved in reforming the city's TB program had a history as public health advocates who had gone against the grain of biomedicine's individualistic model. Brudney had previously run a TB program in Nicaragua; Frieden had been an advocate for health rights in Central America for a decade, and had edited *LINKS*, a small journal on community-based health care in the Third World. Hamburg recruited Dr. Paula Fujiwara (who later became Director of the city's TB Bureau) to New York from San Francisco to work with Frieden precisely because she had run a successful DOT program in that city.

Frieden and his staff had to take special initiative in overcoming bureaucratic and political constraints to put the new program in place rapidly—for example, special permission was sought to hire a large number of city workers in a short time. Hamburg and Frieden also worked out an arrangement with the city's Office of Management and Budget to coordinate TB-related operations across agency budgets. This ensured that health professionals, as well as administrators, were involved in prioritizing TB spending. In line with this goal, an effort was made to involve nontraditional actors in meetings on TB, including representatives from corrections, education, labor, and the quasi-public agency running the city's homeless shelters. Hamburg credits Frieden with much creative initiative in dealing with bureaucratic roadblocks. For example, in order to short-circuit routine bottlenecks—such as delays while all the prospective DOT outreach workers received physicals—Frieden and Fujiwara convened an "open clinic" for job applicants on a Saturday and did the physicals themselves.[24]

As New York City's reconstituted Bureau of Tuberculosis Control discovered, implementation of a labor-intensive program such as DOT in a developed country is very expensive.[25] In addition, frightened by publicity about drug-resistant strains of TB, community outreach workers, who delivered medicines to two-thirds of the city's TB patients after 1992, were initially fearful. Also, in New York City these workers were unionized. Fujiwara found herself meeting frequently, and not always congenially, with health worker union representatives who took an interest in every aspect of the new policies.

The rapid expansion of DOT in New York and new CDC guidelines recommending DOT in health jurisdictions where fewer than 90% of TB patients were completing therapy led to debates in the medical literature over the value of supervised treatment. A conference was held on the rights of TB patients in New York, led by physicians and social scientists whose views had been shaped by recent debates over the rights of HIV/AIDS patients. Many private physicians resented the intrusion of public health authorities into the physician–patient relationship through DOT programs which required their patients to come into clinics for their medicines (and in New York City private physicians treated a significant number of patients—especially those with Medicaid or Medicare coverage.) Advocates for DOT countered with data from the medical literature showing that physicians differ widely in diagnostic and prescribing practices regarding TB, contradicting the common belief among physicians that they can predict patient compliance (e.g., see Frieden et al. 1994; Kopanoff, Snider, and Johnson 1988; Liu, Shilkret, and Finelli 1998). Subsequent studies showed a high level of patient satisfaction among DOT patients in New York (Davidson, Smirnoff, Klein, and Burdick 1999).

Hamburg blames the inattention to TB in physician education, in part, for the differences that have emerged over this issue. She and Lerner both commented on the large amount of time Frieden devoted to responding to and educating physicians about the rationale behind the city's new policies. Frieden offered grand rounds on TB, developed diagnostic and treatment cards physicians could carry in their pockets, and distributed doctors' office charts with TB protocols.

In the aftermath of the crisis, New York City's DOT program has been emulated by many other cities. The TB Bureau's website is a model for public education on TB. Its leaders have emerged as public health heroes. Frieden went on to work with the WHO on TB in India, which has the second largest DOT program in the world, and returned to become Commissioner of Health in New York City. Hamburg later became assistant secretary for planning and evaluation at the U.S. Department of Health and Human Services, and has been called on often to give public talks on how her team saved New York from contagion.

We see several themes in New York City's response (and initial lack of response) to resurgent TB. The dominance of private practice and the individualized curative care medical model in the United States has balkanized health policy decision making. This shaped the cultural milieu in which the availability of new drug therapies for TB and the rise of neoliberal politics turned into a license to dismantle public health infrastructure. The lack of funds allocated to public health, further diminished the prestige of practicing or doing research in the field, a situation that makes for weak leadership, as the best and brightest seek more remunerative careers.

TB Control in Peru, 1992–1999: "The Program Is Good, but the Disease Is Better."

The availability of more effective drugs for TB in the developed world did not translate into better disease control in poor countries. Rather, efforts to fund adequate global distribution of TB drugs languished, and the apparent success in the fight against TB in the United States and Europe created complacency in the international health community about the disease in the 1970s and 1980s. The lack of access to quality medical care (and continuity of care) in the Third World contributed to 3 decades of a global TB epidemic that resulted in millions of preventable deaths and the outbreaks of drug resistance that plague us today. Only the decision of the World Bank to focus on diseases causing disability during adults' productive years (an offshoot of the Bank's 1993 introduction of economic criteria like productivity to health decision making) made TB programs, and particularly DOT, an international health priority.

Physicians who had a strong commitment to international public health played a leading role in designing the reform of Peru's TB program, and in promoting the program, which includes clinic-based DOT. However, classic problems of inadequate funding, professional dominance, bureaucratic intransigence, and government arrogance toward community-based approaches continued to plague Peru's TB program, and to interfere with a rapid response to the growing problem of drug resistance in urban areas. It is especially ironic, according to observers, that the relative success of the DOT program during the mid-1990s may have contributed to making physician leaders complacent and slow to acknowledge the problem with MDRTB strains discovered in Lima in 1996.

Before 1990, Peru's TB situation was in crisis, with 300,000 patients nationally who had active disease—half of them going untreated. There was no national system to track the many noncompliant patients. Dr. Cesar Bonilla, a pneumonologist at Daniel Carrion Hospital in Lima, recalled, "TB wasn't really seen as an emergency in the daily work of most health workers. Many had a fatalistic view—believing tuberculosis couldn't be cured as long as poverty persists—so what's the point of trying?"

Dr. Pedro Suarez, who directed Peru's National Tuberculosis Program for most of the 1990s, is widely credited for building a critical mass of supporters within the medical community and successfully lobbying the Fujimori administration to back the program. Bonilla recalled that beginning in 1990, Suarez invited scores of hospital physicians and university-based professors to meetings on TB, held all over country. The doctors were required to attend 3 to 4 meetings each year, dealing with both theory and clinical issues. At the end there were 200 to 300 health workers of all levels attending each meeting. Daniel Carrion Hospital became the center for training. "It was good that they started with physicians," Bonilla noted, "because the problem (with the TB program) had been the doctors, not the nurses. Many times doctors acted as obstacles to well-trained nurses. The specialists, particularly, had the attitude that nurses had to follow their orders, and even with a competent nurse, often the doctor wouldn't let her do her job."

Young MDs were especially important, according to Bonilla, because they criticized "false prophet" physicians who always talked "from my experience," relying on anecdotes. "We worked more from concrete investigations, and not only from studies done in the United States. We did studies of the situation in Peru. We adapted foreign models, but with a Peruvian slant. Our people became proud to work in such a program. Before this, to work in tuberculosis was to be marginalized. Today, other health programs are imitating the TB program."

Asked what he thought had convinced Fujimori to make TB a priority, Suarez responds diplomatically, calling the program "part of (the government's) struggle against poverty." He credited support and technical help from WHO, as well as fear of contagion in the aftermath of the cholera epidemic. One Ministry physician speculated that Fujimori's support of TB control was a response to protests about hunger and health conditions in Lima's *pueblos jovenes* since Fujimori needed "to give the impression internationally that he was very concerned about poverty."

After 1992, the state assumed almost all costs of TB medicines and other costs, and a nationwide clinic-based DOTS program was put in place (the "S" stands for short-course therapy). The national network of TB laboratories expanded from 2 in 1991 to over 45 sites. The number of cases dropped from 300,000 to around 46,000. In 1996 Peru's National Tuberculosis Program was honored by the WHO as a model DOTS program and it received high marks from many public health experts for bringing down the incidence of TB in only 4 years. It also stood out as one of the few programs in the Ministry with a reputation for efficiency.

However, despite the accolades and improvements, the TB picture was far from rosy in Peru. Even with the model DOTS program in place, the prevalence of TB remained among the highest in Latin America at 216 cases per 100,000 population (Farmer 1999b). Some critics of the Ministry complained that official methods of combining statistics from zones with disparate incidences of TB, tended to mask the concentration of TB in Lima's poor shanty-towns (Sanghavi et al. 1998). And, although the TB budget in Peru increased each year between 1992 and 1996, it stayed fixed after that, which meant a gradual decrease in real dollars allocated to the program.

Spiraling unemployment hamstrung the poor and middle class in Peru during the 1990s, and a further economic downturn in mid-1998 added insult to injury. Neoliberal proposals to reform public health while reducing government health spending generated widespread skepticism among public health experts. Even several years after restoration of health services funding, Peru's basic health indices remained among the lowest in Latin America (Cueto 1997).

Dr. Emma Rubin de Celis, a professor of health policy in Lima, said neoliberal reforms had pushed public health physicians to maximize numbers of consults, and process patients rapidly. Patients were urged to help finance care, "even to the extent of having family members of (poor) patients clean the hospital."[26] Meanwhile the value of physician and nurse salaries dropped, and the Ministry of Health began to contract with many physicians, instead of hiring them for permanent positions, a practice that caused high turnover and poor continuity of care, according to Dr. Rubin de Celis, who taught at the Cayetano Heredia University.

A major premise behind neoliberal health reform in Peru was to limit state responsibility in health to promotion and prevention, leaving most medical treatments in the private realm with costs falling on the individual patient (Kim et al. 2000). The state guaranteed direct health services only to the very poor, according to Dr. Julio Castro, a private physician and former legislator with the APRA party. But the problem, he noted, was that many studies showed that poor families made food and housing their top priorities, and tended to neglect health problems until they were serious.[27] The couching of public health problems in ways that blame the individual victims (e.g., for poor hygiene or poor compliance with treatment protocols) was prevalent within Fujimori's government even during the cholera epidemic, when public health messages emphasized hand-washing and ignored systemic causes of the outbreak (Cueto 1997).

Professors of public health at Cayetano Heredia University like to quote a phrase coined by Dr. Castro to describe Peru's TB program: "The program is good but the disease is better." Asked what he meant by this, Dr. Castro said, "The government is content in having a 'good program' for control of TB, but they are measuring the program, not the size of the TB problem. And the international agencies are content with this approach also." He blamed Fujimori's neoliberal policies for the continuing high rates of TB. "At the base of the problem is unemployment," said Castro, noting that since 1990, 1.5 million jobs had been lost in Peru.

Dr. Jose Santos, a 20-year veteran with the Ministry of Health, spent much of his time at ground-zero of Peru's TB epidemic—moonlighting in NGO-run health posts in northern Lima's shantytowns, where he was working during our interview. While talking about TB policy he examined a thin toddler with a runny nose, who had arrived at the clinic wrapped in a shawl slung over the shoulder of her mother, a small Indian woman who, like tens of thousands of Peruvians, recently immigrated to the outskirts of the capital fleeing rural poverty. Santos complained that for years he had watched patients' relapse after completing the Ministry's TB treatment program. With their energy sapped and their families' savings depleted, they went seeking in vain for expensive second-line antibiotics they could not afford. Santos claimed he had predicted that resistance to TB drugs was coming years ago. "The Ministry battles the bacillus, but it's the socioeconomic conditions of the people that cause TB," he said.

"The Ministry ought to ask: 'If we have such a good program, then why do we have so many patients?'" Santos argued that even patients who are cured of active TB would get sick again if they continued to be malnourished. He pointed to the growth charts for the toddler and her brother, who were once dangerously malnourished, but had steadily gained weight under the NGO's food supplement program. Santos had been a longtime advocate for better nutrition supplements for patients during the entire course of treatment. "You have children with TB and the Ministry has resources for pills, but not for food. What craziness is this!"

Similar recommendations came from a 1998 study of the National TB Program. The study, carried out by the *Proyecto Salud y Nutrición Básica*, (PSNB) found that patients in Lima, where the TB epidemic was most concentrated, had only received food supplements twice in the previous year, and a third of patients interviewed had never received food (PSNB 1998). Informants in the National TB Program confirmed that food supplements were no longer available for most patients, a problem that was blamed on cuts in foreign aid food programs. Such drops in funding, including cuts in the Title II food program of USAID, had forced many of Lima's "people's" kitchens to close. Whereas in 1993 about 7,000 such soup kitchens were in operation, by 1999 the number was closer to 500.[28] Malnutrition had improved since 1990, but a quarter of Peruvian children under the age of 5 remained chronically undernourished, with anemia affecting 60% of children under 2 years of age (Cortez and Calvo 1996–1997); so it was likely that inadequate nutrition continued to contribute to the incidence of TB.

The PSNB study found that, despite the Ministry's efforts, TB care was not integrated with other health services, and patients who came to a clinic with other health problems often did not get referred for TB symptoms. One of the study's strongest recommendations was to strengthen the clinic-based DOTS program with use of community-based promoters. To its credit, the Ministry did recruit lay health promoters from communities that its clinics served, but PSNB researchers found that their dedication to these unpaid positions varied greatly, and promoters played little role in TB care at most urban Ministry clinics. Partly as a result, home visits to follow-up on patient contacts who might be infectious tended to be perfunctory. A third of patients interviewed reported they had never been seen by a social worker. The study also found that the DOTS goal of supervised therapy was not met in many rural areas, where clinic staff gave patients a week's supply of pills at each visit.

An NGO-based community health worker I spoke with in a poor barrio of northern Lima agreed with the PSNB findings. She noted that one reason so many TB patients became noncompliant was because of the inconvenience and cost of taking public transport to a Ministry clinic to receive their pills. "Many enter treatment for 2 months and then disappear when they feel better because they have kids and have to work. If someone has to be at work by 7 AM, they can't just leave and go to the clinic when it opens at 8:30. Even if they did they'd find dozens of patients waiting to be seen and they'd have to wait," she said.

This theme came up later in a conversation I had with a Lima cab driver who revealed that he had an undernourished daughter in the hospital with TB-like symptoms. "Government clinics only offer bad service," he claimed. "They always tell you there are no more appointments, and that you have to come back another day." He complained bitterly about hospital costs, saying he had to go that very night to beg an administrator at the hospital to give him more time to pay a debt.

The lack of focus on community-based health work in Lima reflects, in part, the Health Ministry's reorganization after Fujimori's election. Dr. Cueto, a public health historian at Lima's Instituto de Estudios Peruanos, said that after 1990 "the community-based folks lost ground to vertical programs. You have to remember Fujimori was trained as an engineer. He favored single factor technical interventions and didn't tend to worry about those who get left out of the plan." Dr. Cueto noted that in recent years the Ministry of Health had tended to avoid encouraging public criticism and discussion of wider health problems (like those associated with causing the cholera or TB epidemics).

The tendency to avoid dealing with unpleasant realities that challenge the official description of a problem has peculiar consequences. A disturbing finding of the PSNB study was that some Ministry clinics kept a second set of records for patients who dropped out of TB treatment and then reentered the program later. Records for these "problem" patients were hidden and not reported to the central office, raising questions about the true failure rate of the National TB Program, which was officially reported at 15% (PSNB 1998). "These patients are a headache for the nurses. They don't like to deal with them. Many are addicts or drunks, so they try to turn them away. They mess up the statistics. Everyone thinks they will fail the program again," explained Beth Yeager, a researcher on the study. Two physicians with long-term experience with Peru's National TB Program also claimed in interviews that records for patients who abandoned treatment were not included with official government statistics.

Although Suarez attended planning meetings for the PSNB study, he showed no interest in the findings, according to a researcher who worked on the project. When asked about this in an interview, he dismissed the study as irrelevant. The PSNB recommendation to strengthen community-based health work, however, is in line with suggestions of many TB specialists who maintain that DOTS is only 1 element of a successful TB program (see, for example, Bayer 1998; Farmer 1999b; Farmer and Nardell 1998; Lerner 1993).

MDRTB and the Limits of International Public Health Models

Another Lima-based NGO played an important role in discovering and characterizing the city's TB drug resistance problem. Patients with MDRTB were first identified in early 1996 by Socios en Salud (SES), a health NGO based in Carabayllo, a poor barrio of northern Lima. An earlier survey of Latin American MDRTB clusters by Laszlo and Kantor (1994) had also identified a poor neighborhood on the outskirts of Lima as having the highest level of drug resistance in the survey at 54.5% of patient sample isolates evaluated.[29]

Drs. Paul Farmer and Jim Yong Kim, of SES's parent organization, Partners in Health (PIH), of Cambridge, MA, also held doctorates in medical anthropology, and had begun PIH with a commitment to a "social justice" approach to health work. Influenced by liberation theology in Latin America, both physicians had departed from traditional public health policy, which always involved a cost–benefit analysis in determining how to achieve the best results for a population with limited funds. The PIH philosophy was one of a "preferential option for the poor," and this meant that if they encountered sick patients, they made every effort to cure them, even if this involved high cost. Although curing patients no matter the cost is hardly a radical idea in the First World, it certainly was radical to apply this standard in health development work in poor countries.

Since the PIH doctors had gained experience with TB and drug-resistance in other settings, PIH/SES undertook drug susceptibility testing and began to treat the MDRTB patients they encountered in northern Lima (Farmer 1999a, 1999b; Farmer and Kim 1998). Dr. Jaime Bayona, Medical Director of SES, first approached Peru's Ministry of Health in May 1996 for help to obtain expensive second-line drugs for treatment of 10 MDRTB patients. The Ministry declined to participate. In an interview, Bonilla, speaking for the Ministry, explained that in 1996 government health authorities elected to concentrate their limited funds on drug-susceptible TB. "The way to stop MDRTB is to prevent it. This is a poor country, and there are low success rates for treating MDRTB everywhere."

The potential costs for treating MDRTB were indeed formidable. In the program that PIH/SES developed to treat MDRTB patients, the estimated costs to cure a patient with resistance to 2 drugs ran around $1,000, but treatment of patients resistant to 4 to 6 drugs might cost between $5,000 and $8,000 each to cure. In contrast, the cost of curing drug-susceptible TB in Peru was only about $50 per patient.[30]

The SES/PIH physicians continued to meet with Suarez, and share their data with the Ministry on the rates of drug resistance they were encountering in northern Lima. Of 160 TB patients tested who had failed to be cured in the National TB Program, 93.8% had active MDRTB (Becerra, Bayona, Freeman, Farmer, and Kim 2000). More than two-thirds of the drug-resistant patients SES identified were resistant to all 4 of the drugs used in Peru's National TB Program (Becerra et al. 2000). Many had been treated with an incomplete regimen of the drugs used in the country's "standard" treatment protocol before 1992, and that is how Farmer (1999b) believed most acquired their initial drug resistance. Later patients who relapsed were reenrolled in the Ministry program after the reforms and retreated with the same drugs and others. The PIH/SES researchers became convinced that WHO-approved DOTS strategies of reenrolling patients who formerly dropped out of therapy and treating them with the same drugs a second time was actually amplifying drug resistance (Becerra et al. 2000; Farmer and Kim 1998). Although Ministry officials continued to maintain that the MDRTB threat was minimal, they agreed to refer patients from northern Lima who abandoned TB treatment in Ministry clinics to the PIH/SES program.

Significantly, it was only in 1997 that the Ministry in Peru began using a 4-drug retreatment program for patients who had failed the initial regimen. Before that, all patients who had failed or abandoned treatment and reentered the program were retreated by the same drugs they had initially received—a practice well known for generating drug resistance.

Marcos Espinal, head of Communicable Diseases at the WHO, said the Peruvian Ministry had done the right thing from a public health standpoint in declining to treat MDRTB patients. In a May 1999 telephone interview Espinal said, "Most cases of TB in the world are drug-susceptible; it would be a major mistake to give the message to developing countries that MDRTB is a higher priority." He maintained that the SES model of community-based treatment was too expensive and too dependent on close physician oversight to be replicable on a larger scale.

Health policy analysts in Lima, however, noted that issues of prestige may have also been a factor in the Ministry decision. When confronted by the PIH/SES evidence of drug resistance, officials in the National TB Program were basking in the approval generated by WHO's 1996 designation of Peru's TB program as a model for the Third World and tended to dismiss criticisms of the program.

Realizing that the cost of second-line drugs would rapidly become prohibitive for their NGO undertaking, Farmer and Kim began lobbying WHO, USAID, and other international health institutions to draw attention to the need for affordable second-line drugs and international funding for MDRTB. PIH hosted several small conferences on drug resistance and pulled together a multi-institutional working group on MDRTB to advise international agencies.[31]

Their efforts were boosted when a new survey of drug resistance in the world commissioned by WHO and the International Union against Tuberculosis and Lung Disease was published in 1998. The survey, conducted from 1994 to 1997 in 35 settings, found drug resistance in every country and region surveyed, and identified MDRTB "hot zones" in Russia, Estonia, Latvia, the Dominican Republic, and Argentina (Pablos-Mendez et al. 1998). Peru also ranked high on the list. The WHO estimated that 50 million people were infected with drug-resistant TB strains by the late 1990s, with drug resistance developing in 10% of the 8 million new TB infections occurring each year.

In fall 1998, the Peruvian government, with WHO approval, began its own pilot program, using a standardized drug regimen to cure drug resistance, which was designed to cost no more than $1,500 per patient. "We became convinced we had to do something because each of these patients was a focus for transmission," recalled Bonilla. There were big differences between the Ministry's model and the PIH/SES model for treating MDRTB. The medical team from the 2 NGOs found they had to tailor regimens for no less than 34 drug-resistance profiles in the cohort of patients (Becerra et al. 2000). To manage this, SES health workers met daily, with follow-up communication by e-mail with Boston-based PIH to monitor each patient's progress, and adjust dosages and drugs as indicated.[32]

Although potential patients for the Ministry trial were given drug susceptibility tests to determine if they had MDRTB,[33] in initial trials the Ministry did not use the test results to tailor treatments to individual resistance patterns, as did PIH/SES. Instead, the Ministry sought to test a more affordable, and replicable "one-size-fits-all" drug regimen. A health worker in the Ministry's TB division attributed the decision not to individualize treatment in part to the difficulties of training doctors and nurses in a system in which so many now work on contract and often move from one post to another. In interviews, several TB experts with experience dealing with drug resistance expressed concern that, given the variety of MDRTB drug susceptibility profiles (86% of the patients in the Ministry trial were resistant to 3 or more drugs[34]), the Ministry's one-size-fits-all drug treatment plan would not be effective against MDRTB, and would be likely to exacerbate the spread of drug-resistant disease.

By mid-1999, it was clear that the PIH/SES treatments were curing drug-resistant TB. At that time, PIH/SES reported that 85% of the 80 drug-resistant patients who had completed individualized 18- to 24-month treatment protocols remained smear and culture-negative. A few months later as Peruvian health authorities analyzed the ministry's trial data, it appeared that the fears the NGO physicians expressed about the government trial were valid. Less than a third of the first cohort completing the Ministry's trial were cured.[35] After that, the Ministry joined forces with the PIH/SES team to treat MDRTB, an effort that was greatly aided by new funding from the Gates Foundation. In 2003, PIH reported a "probable cure" rate of 83% for ambulatory patients who completed at least 4 months of therapy. The first 75 patients treated in their ambulatory program had a wide range of drug-resistance profiles, and required 58 different drug combinations to achieve cures (Mitnick et al. 2003).

The findings that a standardized "one-size-fits-all" regimen results in such low cure rates for MDRTB patients presented a special challenge to WHO's communicable disease program. Another major challenge to international pro-tocols was illustrated by the differences in outpatient care in the 2 trials on Peruvian patients. To treat MDRTB, patients must take highly potent drugs for up to 18 to 24 months, which cause a myriad of side effects from upset stom-achs to dizziness, loss of appetite, and generalized aches and pains. Although both the PIH/SES and the initial Ministry trials for treating MDRTB were outpatient programs, the levels of community-based services differed greatly. To deal with the serious side effects of the drugs, the PIH/SES program put great emphasis on training full-time, salaried health promoters who spent most of each day doing visits to patients' homes, where they observed them take their drugs, talking with them about symptoms and advising them on how to deal with problems. Promoters also worked with family members to establish a support system for the sick person.

In contrast, in the Ministry trial, MDRTB patients had to travel to the clos-est clinic each morning to get their drugs, and support services were provided at the clinic. Some Ministry clinics had volunteer health promoters who went to look for patients who missed treatments, but, as the PSNB study showed, the effectiveness and coverage of the Ministry's health promoter network was spotty. Dr. Bayona, of SES, worried that the lack of community-based outreach and support in the Ministry program would lead to a high dropout rate that could amplify existing resistance, writing a death sentence for such patients and putting their families and friends at risk. He noted that some patients simply would not be able to visit the clinic daily. "If you have MDRTB are you going to sit in your house or are you going to go to work? You have to support yourself. People with MDRTB are working as waiters, mechanics, bus drivers, etc. and they are spreading (drug-resistant) disease."

Dr. Robert Gilman, a U.S. physician who did research on TB with PRISMA, a Lima-based health NGO, concurred with Bayona about the long-term risks of MDRTB patients going untreated. He cited the WHO estimate that a drug-resistant patient who remains infectious continues to infect about 10 other people each year, one of whom, on average, will come down with active MDRTB. Gilman, who teaches at Johns Hopkins School of Hygiene and Public Health, in Baltimore, MD, then made a chilling observation about this frequently quoted statistic: "You have to remember that *the other nine who are infected with MDRTB, but who don't get the disease right away may get it later if their immune systems become weakened by malnutrition or other illnesses*" (emphasis added). In a country with the malnutrition and poverty rate of Peru, that prospect did indeed seem daunting.

The dilemma that MDRTB poses to international health experts is a Faustian one. If the international spread of MDRTB is to be checked, TB specialists need to turn to more community-based and education-intensive approaches that are more costly and complicated to implement, but the future costs of not acting may be far higher. More recent surveys of DOTS programs for TB around the world have supported the findings of the PIH team that effective DOTS programs must be "patient-centered" approaches that include other social and economic supports such as food supplements and aid with costs of transportation.

Yet, as Dr. Snider of the CDC pointed out in an interview, from an economic standpoint, governments and international agencies have not yet made a full commitment to curing drug-susceptible TB. Regrettably, the United States, one of the countries best able to fund new international health efforts, has a poor record of leadership on the global TB problem. In 1993, just as the CDC and the WHO were gearing up to confront resurgent TB, the USAID cut its entire overseas budget for TB control (Garrett 1995). New policies adopted by the Clinton White House in 1996 to deal with emerging disease threats focused heavily on surveillance for TB at the country's borders and education of travelers, but failed to address the core problem of financing responses to the global epidemic (Lederberg 1996).

A big step was taken in 2001 when the Global Fund to Fight AIDS, Tuberculosis, and Malaria was set up with the goal of raising $15 billion for the international infectious disease crisis. But the Fund has not been fully funded by governments, Such neglect of TB in international health has a long history. The rub, according to Snider is that, "where there's a large pool of MDRTB, and drug-resistant patients enter existing TB treatment programs without being cured, even good TB programs lose effectiveness. It hurts their reputation with the public."

For this reason, the physicians at PIH elected to undertake a rare advocacy effort with governments, agencies, drug companies, and private foundations, seeking increased funding to treat MDRTB and cheaper prices for capreomycin and other second-line TB drugs. While Farmer and Kim emphasized the humanitarian argument for curing MDRTB, they found that they made more headway with international health authorities once they began emphasizing that in "hot spots" for drug resistance, DOTS programs for drug-susceptible TB may perversely amplify resistance if patients drop out and then reenter the program. In part, as a result of these efforts, the WHO set up structures to authorize second-line drugs for health agencies that undertook to cure drug-resistant patients in MDRTB "hot spots," and by 2000, prices of some second-line drugs had fallen significantly.

Toward an "Integrated" Public Health:
The Need for Advocacy, Public Education,
and Community-Based Models

In both case studies, the building of effective DOT programs followed economic crises and political controversies that led to changes in health administrations (accompanied in Peru by a change in national government). Unlike epidemiology, a medical anthropology approach to analysis helps bring the critical role of political and economic factors, as well as the medical and public health cultures that shape programs, into view.

In New York City, where the average standard of living is far higher than in Peru, the populations most affected by the poorly run TB program were ghettoized and "invisible" from a public policy perspective, and public health authorities found it convenient during the retrenchment years of the 1980s to ignore epidemiological indicators of rising TB incidence among the marginalized poor. It took a belated intervention by the CDC, several deaths, adverse media coverage and the fears of middle class citizens at risk for drug-resistant disease (articulated through the media) before local or federal authorities backed changes in policy and renewed funding.

In Peru, the population affected by TB and other diseases of poverty is far larger, but advocacy for public health reforms was undermined, initially by militarism in the 1970s, then by neoliberal economic interventions promoted by international lenders (and national business elites) during the 1980s.

A strong program for TB in Peru grew out of the efforts of a group of reformist physicians, but funding and political support for the program was tied to Fujimori's efforts to restore Peru's image in the eyes of tourists and foreign investors after the war and the embarrassing cholera epidemic.

Whether in Lima or New York, one thing public health programs have in common is financial instability over time. The tendency of U.S. policy makers to discontinue disease-specific programs after the problem is contained has been dubbed the "U-shaped curve of concern" (Reichman 1997). Likewise, Cueto (1997) has noted a long-standing pattern in Latin America of health services being funded in spurts, in response to an immediate epidemic threat, and then declining.

Publicity about the epidemic was a key factor prompting political reforms in the New York case, underscoring how the CDC, which lacks regulatory authority, must rely on its reputation for competence and its ability to nurture relationships and fund collaborative projects at the state and local levels when confronted with an emerging or resurgent disease outbreak. As Foreman (1994:27) has noted, in the United States, "the response to emergent public health hazards may be federalized, but it is not centralized."

On the international scene, the WHO, lacking a large budget or any regulatory authority, relies heavily on the reputation of its professional medical staff and a limited capacity to fund specific programs (e.g., diarrhea control, AIDS prevention, TB control, essential drugs), for its influence and leverage in member countries. The WHO's capacity to monitor a country's DOTS programs for TB is limited, as the organization has played a relatively minor role in assisting Ministries of Health with strategic planning or management of health services (De Cock 1999; Walt 1994).

Central to sustainability in any health program must be strong advocacy on the part of public health authorities to maintain support for prevention and screening infrastructure, and for rapid responses to rising rates of disease. Notably, in both New York City and Lima in the early 1990s, constructive criticism and leadership for reforms in TB programs often came from unconventional players, and depended on strong political advocacy both within the health community and in the larger political arena. Recent advocacy from PIH is likewise promising to be one of the most important factors in persuading the WHO and Peruvian government authorities to confront the problem of drug resistance. In these situations, advocacy was not a substitute for epidemiological data, but served as an impetus to doing the necessary studies and acting on the findings.

Nevertheless, in situations with low advocacy (e.g., New York City's TB Bureau in the 1980s) or with little pressure for accountability (e.g., Peru's National TB Program after receiving WHO recognition in 1996), conservative interpretations of epidemiological risks often become substitutes for evidence-based decision making. PSNB's critical study of Peru's clinic-based DOTS program such a short time after the WHO accolades also raises questions about the criteria used by the WHO to evaluate DOTS initiatives in developing countries. In how many other settings are the shortcomings of clinic-based DOTS being glossed over by development experts in the name of maintaining goodwill with national leaders?

The complacency that Peruvian health workers complained about in administration of the National TB Program seemed to reflect fear that, given the recent neoliberal zeal to cut social programs, critical debate about TB services would upset the applecart of a "good program"—even though, given Peru's poverty and MDRTB problem, the program was clearly not good enough.

Interestingly, in Congressional hearings held on the New York TB crisis in December 1991, Congressman Ted Weiss (D-N.Y.) charged that federal, state, and municipal agencies had all been complacent about TB funding, even after signs of rising TB incidence. He chided the public health authorities in the room for failing to advocate strongly enough when funds for programs like TB control were cut back. Alan Hinman, who at the time headed the CDC's National Center for Prevention Services, noted that funding for prevention often depended on public attention being drawn to a disease threat. But Weiss countered that it was the job of public health authorities, not Congress or the public, to assess threats to public health and advocate for new programs when they are needed.

While Weiss was certainly grandstanding in this opportunity to impugn Republican budget-cutters, it is true that studies of the history of U.S. public health point to a legacy of weak advocacy and lax enforcement of regulations, in part because of the beleaguered position of public health vis-a-vis private medicine and other interest groups (Weiss 1997). Some TB experts interviewed at the CDC for this study expressed discomfort about advocacy in the public arena. Snider, who pushed for the CDC's TB eradication program in the 1980s, pointed out that advocacy often involves overstating one's case, using hyperbole, and confronting authority—positions that seem at odds with the scientific stance of objectivity. In recent years, in response to the many "emerging" or "resurgent" infectious disease outbreaks, the CDC began to develop educational materials on how to better advocate about health concerns, with politicians, the press, and the public. But in a world in which TB causes a quarter of all preventable deaths[36] (with prospects for tens of millions more as MDRTB spreads and works its deadly synergy with AIDS[37]), these efforts are only the beginning of what is needed.

Advocacy goes hand-in-hand with public education. In an ideal world, said Snider, "public health ought to be pro-active—in regular contact with radio stations, with the Hispanic community, with gay men ...." As neglected as it is, especially when funds are short, public education about health risks may also be central to developing a strong constituency for sustaining health programs. Public education efforts on TB developed in New York City in the mid-1990s serve as a model for urban programs. The TB Bureau's Web site is a font of clearly written information presented in a question-and-answer format. Outreach workers took witty comic books on TB into communities. Unfortunately, in the United States, despite the advent of the so-called "information age" and clear evidence that the public is concerned about health issues, public education about preventive health has remained a low priority.

This was also true in Peru, where National TB Program workers lamented the lack of resources for promotion of public information on TB. Other than banners over a couple of highways, there was little to indicate government concern. Dr. Pablo Campos, who studied infectious disease at Cayetano Heredia University in Lima, noted that this is especially risky in a country where so many people are illiterate. "There is no popular concept of TB or AIDS in Peru," he said, but noted that he was hopeful about a new program to incorporate health education into the schools. At Daniel Carrion Hospital, Bonilla worried about what effect the lack of public awareness has on TB case finding. "The extreme poor don't go to clinics, and the middle class has a very low awareness of TB. Yet as the program progresses, we see more and more atypical patients. It's not just 'pobrecitos' who come into our clinics with TB nowadays."

One of the best approaches to public education may be to follow the PSNB recommendations (and the SES example) and put resources into community-based health outreach work. Dr. Campos agreed: "We need to redefine the roles of health promoters. They should be more involved in promoting the rights of the patient, instead of working as medical assistants."

Conclusion

Interestingly, many of the ingredients of academic proposals for a more "integrated" public health dovetail with the goals of community-based DOT, in that there is a heavy emphasis on education (of health workers and the public), and on improving communication and participation, both within the health system and with patients. Such programs require investment in people, and an embrace of longer-term futures and a more complex social and epidemiological big picture than is usually acknowledged in individualized, curative care models or in neoliberal political ideologies.

TB is spread by poverty, but by striking men and women in their prime, it also *creates* poverty. It is convenient for the developed world that most of the global TB epidemic is elsewhere. But, in the words of Farmer and Kim (1998) "local epidemics don't stay local." MDRTB recently turned up in 34 out of 35 countries surveyed (Pablos-Mendez et al. 1998) and there are now several documented cases of TB transmission on airliners.[38] Bifani, Plikaytis, and Kapur (1996) and Farmer (1999b) cite multiple cases of MDRTB strains making their way across borders and between U.S. cities. Clearly, in the era of globalization and "free trade," we are all in this together, and closing the borders simply isn't a practical (or humanitarian) solution.

We have had the means to cure TB for 50 years. But just as magic-bullet approaches fail to see the social and epidemiological forest for the individual trees, now, with MDRTB, we are seeing that international public health models also have to change—and bring the trees (and quality of care!) back into their concept of the forest. But structural barriers to care, and to funding of TB control, are usually at the root of bad programs, however they are designed. If TB is to be cured, the welfare of *people*, in all their aggregate and individual complexities, will have to be at the forefront of health planning, funding, and advocacy. The success of New York City's DOT program and the encouraging outcomes to date from the Socios en Salud program of community-based treatment for MDRTB demonstrate that this can be achieved in the Third World as well as in the First.

Acknowledgments

This chapter is a revised version of a paper that was first published in the book *Emerging Diseases and Society: Negotiating the Public Health Agenda*, edited by Randall M. Packard, Peter J. Brown, Ruth L. Berkelman, and Howard Frumkin, Baltimore and London: Johns Hopkins University Press, 2004, pp. 253–290. An earlier article on the Peru case study was published in *Medical Anthropology* Vol. 24 (3) July–September 2005. This research was made possible by a Mellon-Sawyer Post-Doctoral Fellowship at the Center for the Study of Health, Culture and Society, Rollins School of Public Health, Emory University during the Spring Semester, 1999; and by a Ford Foundation Peru Academic Exchange Fellowship, administered through the Duke University–University of North Carolina Program in Latin American Studies in June–July 1999. I would like to express special thanks to the staffs of PIH and Socios en Salud; and to the many other public health workers, scholars, and TB patients who shared their knowledge and experience with me during interviews in Atlanta, Boston, New York City, and Lima, Peru.

Notes

1. MDRTB is defined as resistance to at least 2 drugs, rifampicin and isoniazid, the 2 antibiotics in first-line TB treatment protocols.

2. Friedland, Sandra 1992 New Jersey Q & A: Dr. Lee B. Reichman, in "Waging a War on Drug-Resistant TB" *New York Times* Section, May 10, Section 13NJ, p.3.

3. See ALA 1996, Sbarbaro 1996, and Reichman 1997.

4. See Ryan 1992, p. 390 and Reichman 1997.

5. Interview with Dr. Karen Brudney, February 1999.

6. After Snider's plan became accepted at the CDC, the division was renamed Division of Tuberculosis Elimination.

7. Interview with Dr. Dixie Snider, Atlanta, Ga., April 1999; see also CDC 1989 and CDC 1996. In 1987, CDC officials estimated that it would cost $36 million a year to eradicate TB by 2010, but after the severity of the disease in inner cities was recognized in 1992, the agency revised its estimate radically upward, asking for $540 million a year. In contrast, the amount the Bush Administration requested for TB was only $12.3 million in 1992 and $35 million in 1993. See Specter, Michael, "Tuberculosis: A Killer Returns" *The New York Times*, October 11, 1992, p. 1.

8. Hilts, Philip J. 1990 "Victory Over TB Seen as Thwarted by Budget Unit" *New York Times*, February 28, Section A, p. 24.

9. Rosenthal, Elisabeth 1990 "The Return of TB: A Special Report—Tuberculosis Germs Resurging as Risk to Public Health" *New York Times*, July 15, Section 1, p.1.

10. Navarrro, Mireya 1992 "New York Asks U.S. for Help in Tracking New TB Cases" *New York Times*, January 24, Section B, p. 6.

11. Ministry of Health 1982 Situacion Actual de la Enfermedades Transmisibles en el Pais—1982, Unpublished internal document.

12. Interview with Dr. Marcos Cueto, Lima, Peru, June 1999.

13. Interview with Dr. Pedro Suarez, Director, National Program of Tuberculosis Control, Ministry of Health, Lima, June 1999.

14. Interviews by author in Lima, 1999.

15. Interview with Dr. Jack Adler, New York City, February 1999.

16. Phone interview with Dr. Barron Lerner, 1999.

17. Rosenthal 1990; ibid.

18. Brudney 1999; ibid.

19. Interview with Margaret Hamburg, 1999.

20. Weiss 1991; Interview with Dr. Margaret Hamburg, 1999.

21. Interview with Dr. Jim Curran, Dean of the Rollins School of Public Health, Emory University, and former director of AIDS research at the CDC, 2000.

22. In 1991, the CDC was using about $10 million in HIV funds for TB activities (testimony by Alan Hinman before the House of Representatives Human Resources and Intergovernmental Relations Subcommittee of the Committee on Government Relations, December 18, 1991.)

23. Two-thirds of New York City's TB cases were managed through community-based DOT under Health Department supervision, while one-third of the cases were managed in clinics and private practices, in collaboration with municipal health authorities. Most of these received their drugs in a clinic-based DOT program, using multidisciplinary health teams overseen by the Health Department (Fujiwara et al. 1997).

24. Interview with Dr. Paula Fujiwara, New York City, February 1999.

25. For example, in the 1993 fiscal year, at the height of the city's response to the epidemic, New York City's health department spent more than $100 million on TB control.

26. Interview with Dr. Rubin de Celis, Lima, Peru, June 1999.

27. Interview with Dr. Julio Castro, Lima, Peru, June 1999.

28. Interview with Beth Yeager, researcher on the Proyeto Salud y Nutricion Basica, Lima, Peru, June 1999.

29. The extent of the drug-resistant TB problem in Lima remains unclear because so much of the data is based on the patients who come to clinics or hospitals. As of

mid-1999, Dr. Robert Gilman, a U.S.-trained TB specialist at PRISMA (a Lima-based NGO), reported that pediatric TB rates had not risen, which was a good sign. Also, unlike U.S. urban centers and Africa, relatively few TB patients in Peru were co-infected with HIV. On the other hand, in the Social Security Hospital where he worked, Gilman reported that about 50% of AIDS patients were contracting active TB, and about 50% of those came down with MDRTB.

30. Interviews with PIH researchers and Ministry of Health staff.

31. Interviews and and background materials provided by Drs. Paul Farmer and Jim Yong Kim, Boston, February 1999.

32. I conducted interviews with patients, health professionals, and community health workers during a 2-day visit to Socios en Salud, Carabayllo, Peru, June 1999, where I accompanied a health promoter on his daily rounds to patients' homes. I also visited an SES primary care clinic in a poor barrio.

33. Interview with Dr. Robert Canales of the Ministry's Technical Unit for TB, June 1999.

34. Interviews with SES administrators in Lima and Dr. Paul Farmer in 2000.

35. Interviews with Canales in Lima, June 1999; and Farmer 2000.

36. Alan Hinman, cited in Hilts, Philip J. "Victory over TB seen as Thwarted by Budget Unit" *The New York Times* February 27, 1990, p. 24.

37. An HIV-positive person who is exposed to (drug-susceptible or drug-resistant) TB has a far higher chance of becoming infected, and of coming down with active disease, compared to HIV-negative persons. Once an HIV-positive person tests positive for TB on a skin test, that individual runs a 10% chance of coming down with active TB within a year. (Interview with Curran 2000; ibid.)

38. See MMWR 1995 for a CDC review of 6 such cases.

References

ALA (1996) Maintaining momentum: America's TB challenge. A public policy brief of the American Lung Association.

Bayer R, Stayton C, Desvarieux M, Healton C, Landesman S, Tsai WY (1998) Directly observed therapy and treatment completion in the United States: Is universal supervised therapy necessary? *American Journal of Public Health* 88(7):1052–1058.

Bayer R, Wilkinson D (1995) Directly observed therapy for tuberculosis: History of an idea. *Lancet* 345:1545–1548.

Becerra MC, Bayona J, Freeman J, Farmer PE, Kim JY (2000) Redefining MDR-TB transmission "hot spots." *International Journal of Tuberculosis and Lung Disease* 4(5):387–394.

Berkelman R, Bryan RT, Osterholm MT, LeDuc JW, Hughes JM (1994) Infectious disease surveillance: A crumbling foundation. *Science* 264:368–370.

Bifani PJ, Plikaytis BB, Kapur V (1996) Origin and interstate spread of a New York City multidrug resistant: *Mycobacterium tuberculosis* clone family. *Journal of the American Medical Association* 275:452–457.

Brudney K, Dobkin J (1991) A tale of two cities: Tuberculosis control in Nicaragua and New York City. *Seminars in Infectious Disease* 6(4):261–272.

CDC (1989) A strategic plan for the elimination of tuberculosis in the United States. *Morbidity and Mortality Weekly Report Supplement* 38(S-3), Centers for Disease Control and Prevention.

CDC (1996) Tuberculosis morbidity—United States, 1995. *Morbidity and Mortality Weekly Report* 45(18), Centers for Disease Control and Prevention, pp. 365–388.

Chossudovsky M (1997) "IMF Shock Treatment in Peru." In: *The Globablisation of Poverty: Impacts of IMF and World Bank Reforms*, M Chossudovsky, ed. London: Zed Books.

Cohn D, Bustreo F, Raviglione M (1997) Drug resistant tuberculosis: Review of the worldwide situation and the WHO/IUATLD Global Surveillance Project. *Clinical Infectious Diseases* 24(Suppl 1):S121–S130.

Cortez R, Calvo C (1996–1997) La Nutricion Infantil en el Peru. *Punto de Equilibrio* No. 46, Ano 6. Dic/Enero.

Cueto M (1997) *El Regreso de las Epidemias: Salud y Sociedad en el Peru del Siglo XX*. Lima: Instituto de Estudios Peruanos.

Davidson H, Smirnoff M, Klein S, Burdick E (1999) Patient satisfaction with care at directly observed therapy programs for tuberculosis in New York City. *American Journal of Public Health* 89(10):1567–1570.

De Cock K (1999) International Responses to HIV/AIDS. Presentation in Sawyer Seminar on Emerging Illnesses and Institutional Responses, Rollins School of Public Health, Emory University, April 2.

DeSalle R (1999) *Epidemic!: The World of Infectious Disease*. New York: The New Press.

Dubos R, Dubos J (1952) *The White Plague: Tuberculosis, Man and Society*. Boston: Little, Brown and Company.

Fairchild AL, Oppenheimer GM (1998) Public health nihilism vs. pragmatism: History, politics and the control of tuberculosis. *American Journal of Public Health* 88:1105–1117.

Farmer P (1999a) *Infections and Inequalities: The Modern Plagues*. Berkeley: University of California Press.

Farmer P (1999b) Hidden Epidemics of Tuberculosis. Working Paper No. 239, Latin American Program, Woodrow Wilson International Center for Scholars.

Farmer P, Kim JY (1998) Community-based approaches to the control of multi-drug resistant tuberculosis: Introducing DOTS-plus. *British Medical Journal* 317:671–674.

Farmer P, Nardell E (1998) Editorial: Nihilism and pragmatism in tuberculosis control. *American Journal of Public Health* 88(7):1014–1015.

Foreman CH, Jr. (1994) *Plagues, Products and Politics: Emergent Public Health Hazards and National Policymaking*. Washington, DC: The Brookings Institution.

Frieden T, Fujiwara P, Hamburg M, Ruggiero, D, Henning, K (1994) Tuberculosis clinics. *American Journal of Respiratory and Critical Care Medicine* 150:893–894.

Frieden T, Fujiwara P, Washko R, Hamburg MA (1995) Tuberculosis in New York City—turning the tide. *The New England Journal of Medicine* 333(4):229–233.

Frieden T, Sterling, T, Pablos-Mendez, A, Kilburn, J, Cauthen, G, Dooley, S (1993) The emergence of drug-resistant tuberculosis in New York City. *The New England Journal of Medicine* 328(8):521–526.

Fujiwara P, Larkin C, Frieden T (1997) Directly observed therapy in New York City: History, implementation, results, and challenges. *Clinics in Chest Medicine* 18(1):135–148.

Gandy M, Zumla A (2003) *The Return of the White Plague: Global Poverty and the "New" Tuberculosis*. New York City: Verso.

Garrett L (1995) *The Coming Plague: Newly Emerging Diseases in a World Out of Balance*. New York: Penguin Books.

Harantani J, Hernandez D (1991) *Cholera in Peru: A Rapid Assessment of the Country's Water and Sanitation Infrastructure.* Washington, DC: USAID Mission to Peru.

Hopewell P, Ganter B, Baron R, Sanchez-Hernandez, M (1985) Operational evaluation of treatment for tuberculosis: Results of 8- and 12-month regimens in Peru. *American Review of Respiratory Disease* 132(4):737–741.

Hopewell P, Sanchez-Hernandez M, Baron R, Ganter, B (1984) Operational evaluation of treatment for tuberculosis: Results of a "standard" 12-month regimen in Peru. *American Review of Respiratory Disease* 129:439–443.

IUATLD (1997) Anti-Tuberculosis Resistance in the World. Report published by the International Union Against Tuberculosis and Lung Diseases and the World Health Organization.

Kim JY, Shakow A, Bayona J, Rhatigan J, Rubin de Celis EL (2000) "Sickness Amidst Recovery: Public Debt and Private Suffering in Peru." In: *Dying for Growth: Global Inequality and the Health of the Poor.* JY Kim, JV Millen, A Irwin, J Gershman, eds. Monroe, Maine: Common Courage Press, pp. 127–153.

Kopanoff D, Snider D, Jr., Johnson M (1988) Recurrent tuberculosis: Why do patients develop disease again? A United States public health service cooperative survey. *American Journal of Public Health* 78(1):30–33.

Laszlo A, Kantor IN (1994) A random sample survey of initial drug resistance among tuberculosis cases in Latin America. *Bulletin of the World Health Organization* 72(4):603–610.

Lederberg J (1996) Infectious disease—a threat to global health and security. *Journal of the American Medical Association* 276(5):417–419.

Lerner BH (1993) New York City's tuberculosis control efforts: The historical limitations of the "War on Consumption." *American Journal of Public Health* 83(5):758–766.

Liu Z, Shilkret KL, Finelli L (1998) Initial drug regimens for the treatment of tuberculosis: Evaluation of physician prescribing practices in New Jersey, 1994–1995. *Chest* 113(6):1446–1451.

McClintock C (1989) "Peru's Sendero Luminoso Rebellion: Origins and Trajectory." In: *Power and Popular Protest: Latin American Social Movements.* S Eckstein, ed. Berkeley: University of California Press, pp. 61–101.

McKenna, M, McCray, E, Onorato, I (1995) The epidemiology of tuberculosis among foreign-born persons in the United states, 1986–1994. *New England Journal of Medicine* 332:1071–1076.

Ministry of Health (1983) Cuadro No. 5 Mortalidad y Morbilidad por tuberculosis, *Informe Estadistico Anual de Enfermedades Transmisibles*, 1963–1983, OGIE.

Mitnick C, Bayona J, Palacios E, Shin S, Furin J, Alcántara F, et al. (2003) Community-based therapy for multi-drug resistant tuberculosis in Lima, Peru. *New England Journal of Medicine* 348:119–128.

Nader L (1974) "Up the Anthropologist—Perspectives Gained from Studying Up." In: *Reinventing Anthropology.* D Hymes, ed. New York: Vintage Books, pp. 284–311.

Nolan C (1997) Topics for our times: The increasing demand for tuberculosis services—a new encumbrance on tuberculosis control programs. *American Journal of Public Health* 87(4):551–553.

Ott K (1996) *Fevered Lives: Tuberculosis in American Culture Since 1870.* Cambridge, MA: Harvard University Press.

Pablos-Mendez A, Raviglione M, Laszlo A, Binkin N, Rieder HL, Bustreo F, et al. (1998) Global surveillance for antituberculosis-drug resistance, 1994–1997. *New England Journal of Medicine* 338(23):1641–1649.

PSNB (1998) Estudio Sociomedico sobre la Tuberculosis: Lima. Informes de Investigacion 12, Proyecto Salud y Nutricion Basica, Lima, Peru.

Reichman L (1997) Defending the public's health against tuberculosis. *Journal of the American Medical Association* 278(10):865–867.

Reichman L (2002) *Timebomb: The Global Epidemic of Multi-Drug-Resistant Tuberculosis.* New York: McGraw Hill and Co.

Ryan F (1992) *The Forgotten Plague.* Boston: Little, Brown and Co.

Sanghavi DM, Gilman RH, Lescano-Guevara AG, Checkley W, Cabrera L, Cardenas V (1998) Hyperendemic pulmonary tuberculosis in a Peruvian shantytown. *American Journal of Epidemiology* 148(4):384–389.

Sbarbaro JA (1996) Commentary on tuberculosis surveillance. *Public Health Reports* 111(January–February):32–33.

Starr P (1982) *The Social Transformation of American Medicine.* New York: Basic Books.

Turshen M (1989) *The Politics of Public Health.* New Brunswick, NJ: Rutgers University Press.

Wallace R, Wallace D (1998) *A Plague on Your Houses: How New York was Burned Down and Public Health Crumbled.* New York: Verso.

Walt G (1994) *Health Policy: An Introduction to Process and Power.* London: Zed Books.

Weiss L (1997) *Private Medicine and Public Health: Profit, Politics, and Prejudice in the American Health Care Enterprise.* Boulder, CO: Westview Press.

Weiss T (1991) Testimony in "Tuberculosis in New York City: An Epidemic Returns": Proceedings of a hearing before the Human Resources and Intergovernmental Relations Subcommittee of the Committee on Governmental Operations, U.S. House of Representatives, December 18.

WHO (1997) *Treatment of Tuberculosis: Guidelines for National Programmes.* 2nd ed. Geneva: World Health Organization.

22

Biological Citizenship After Chernobyl

ADRIANA PETRYNA

Introduction: The Event

On April 26, 1986, Unit Four of the Chernobyl nuclear reactor exploded in Ukraine, damaging human immunities, the genetic structure of cells, and contaminating soils and waterways. The main reason for the accident is well documented by now. Soviet engineers wanted to test how long generators of Unit Four could operate without steam supply in the case of a power failure (IAEA 1986). During the test, operators sharply reduced power, and blocked steam to the reactor's generators and disabled many of its safety systems. A huge power surge followed, and at 1:23 AM, the unit exploded once and then again. Large-scale pressure gradients carried the radioactive plume to as high as 8 km by some estimates. The graphite core burned for days. Helicopter pilots dropped over 5,000 tons of boron carbide, dolomite, sand, clay, and lead in an attempt to suffocate the flames of the reactor's burning core. These interventions are now known to have compounded risk and uncertainty. With suffocation, the temperature of the nuclear core increased. This in turn caused radioactive substances to ascend more rapidly, forming a radioactive cloud that spread over Belarus, Ukraine, Russia, Europe, and other areas of the Northern Hemisphere.[1]

Eighteen days elapsed before Mikhail Gorbachev, then general secretary, appeared on Soviet television and acknowledged the nuclear release to the general population. Within that period, tens of thousands of people were either knowingly or unknowingly exposed to radioactive iodine-131, absorbed rapidly in the thyroid and resulting, among other things, in a sudden and massive onset of thyroid cancers in children and adults as early as 4 years after the exposure.[2] Such onsets could have been curtailed had the government distributed nonradioactive iodine pills within the first week of the disaster.[3] Contradicting assessments generated by English and American meteorological groups, Soviet administrators downplayed the extent of the plume and characterized Chernobyl as a controlled biomedical crisis. Soviet medical efforts focused on a group of 237 victims selected at the disaster site by Dr. Angelina Guskova; they were airlifted to the acute radiation sickness ward of the Institute of Biophysics in Moscow. Of those, 134 were diagnosed with acute radiation syndrome. Official reports set the death toll at 31 workers (IAEA 1991a,b; WHO 1996).[4] Behind such seemingly definite numbers lies a web of scientific, moral, and political uncertainties.

Over the next decade, 600,000 or more soldiers, firemen, and other workers, men and women, continued to be exposed to radiation.[5] Many were dispatched to the disaster site to carry out cleanup work ranging from bulldozing and disposing of contaminated topsoil to working in 1-minute intervals on the roof of an adjacent unit and shoveling radioactive debris into the mouth of the ruined one. Some of these so-called volunteers referred to themselves as "bio-robots," a term that suggests that the 1-minute rule was not well enforced. Others were relatively well paid to construct the so-called Sarcophagus (*Sarkofag*, now called the Shelter), a structure enclosing the ruined fourth unit of the reactor and containing 216 tons of uranium and plutonium. Currently, 15,000 people work at the now decommissioned power plant or are paid to provide technical assistance in the Zone of Exclusion. The Zone is an area 30 km in diameter circumscribing the disaster site. Access to the Zone is restricted to the plant's maintenance workers, engineers, health professionals, and researchers.

In 1992, during my first visit to Ukraine, I met one of the maintenance workers who was on a 2-week break from work in the Zone. He lived in a housing complex in Kyiv, Ukraine's capital, located about 110 km south of the disaster site. Filled with anger, he said: "Now I'm a 'sufferer.'" He used the word "sufferer" in reference to a legal category introduced the previous year by a newly independent Ukrainian state for persons affected by the Chernobyl disaster. "I get five dollars a month compensation. What can I buy for that?" He said he had no other option but to continue working in the Zone. Because of his work history, no firm would hire him. "This is from radiation," he said. He lifted his pant-leg and stuck his cigarette through a ring made of skin that had puckered up above his ankle. It was the result, he said, of direct contact with a radiation source, and what clinicians would call a "local skin burn." "This happened in the Zone ... We're people no one understands, in hospitals, in clinics." He characterized himself as one of the "living dead." "Our memory is gone. You forget everything—we walk like corpses."

In spite of the country's publicized efforts to improve safety standards in the Zone, the Director of the Shelter complex told me in an interview in 2000, "There are no norms of radiation safety here." The country's Ministry of Health sets annual allowable norms of dose exposures, but, according to the director, these norms are not strictly adhered to. That is because in Ukraine's period of sharp economic instability, employment in the Zone is considered premium. Referring to the plant workers, he told me, "Taking this risk is their individual problem. No one else is responsible for it." When I asked him to compare his country's enforcement of worker safety norms with those of Western Europe, he told me quite somberly, "No one has ever defined the price of a dose exposure here. No one has ever defined the value of a person here."[6] In a situation where economic forces drive people to become preoccupied with physical survival, the effects of leaving the value of a person undefined are far reaching. In such a world, physical risks, abuses, and uncertainties escalate. The labor of the biorobot appears ever more acceptable, desirable, and even normal.

In the effort to map environmental contamination, to measure individual and populationwide exposures, and to arbitrate claims of illness, government and scientific interventions have recast the Chernobyl aftermath as a complex political and health experience with its own bureaucratic and legal contours. The initial—and contested—scientific and medical assessments of the disaster's scope and human impact, the choice to delay public announcement, and the economic incentives to work in the Zone have uniquely shaped Chernobyl as a *tekhnohenna katastrofa* (a technogenic catastrophe), in the words of many of my informants, including people fighting for disability status, local physicians, and scientists. This term suggests that not only excessive exposures to radiation but policy interventions also have caused new uncertainties. These interventions have exacerbated the biological and social problems they were intended to resolve, and have even generated new ones. The processes in which the state responded to the crisis by assessing exposure and calculating compensation, in turn, contributes to further uncertainty concerning a resolution to the crisis, an increase in illness claims, and social suffering among affected individuals and groups.[7]

The Aftermath

My particular focus is on Ukraine, a country that inherited the destroyed nuclear power plant—along with an unresolved Chernobyl crisis—when it declared independence from the Soviet Union in 1991. Most of the Exclusion Zone is located in Ukraine. Approximately 8.9% of Ukraine's territory is considered contaminated. During the period of my field research (1992–1997, 2000), the country witnessed a rapid growth of a population claiming radiation exposure that made them eligible for some form of social protection. Social protection includes cash subsidies, family allowances, free medical care and education, and pension benefits for sufferers and the disabled. This new population, legally designated as *poterpili* (sufferers), numbers 3.5 million and constitutes a full 5% of the Ukrainian population.

On average, Ukraine expends about 5% of its budget on costs related to the Chernobyl aftermath, including the cleanup and technical maintenance of the ruined reactor. In 1995, over 65% of those costs were spent on social compensation for sufferers and on maintaining a massive legal–medical, scientific, and welfare apparatus. Neighboring Belarus, by contrast, spends considerably less per capita on the social welfare of its sufferers than Ukraine does and has limited the number of Chernobyl claimants. Twenty-three percent of this country's territory is considered contaminated, roughly three times the percentage of contaminated Ukrainian land. The Belarussian government has tended to suppress or ignore scientific research; it downplays the extent of the disaster and fails to provide enough funds for the medical surveillance of nearly 2 million people who live in contaminated areas.

Unlike Belarus, Ukraine has used the legacy of Chernobyl as a means of signaling its domestic and international legitimacy and staking territorial claims. It developed a politics of national autonomy through the Chernobyl crisis, characterizing Soviet responses to the disaster as negligent. The state established new social welfare and scientific institutions dedicated to a Chernobyl population and began to provide sufferers and disabled populations relatively generous cash entitlements drawn from a statewide Chernobyl tax. Moreover, the new government defined new and ambitious safety measures for workers in the so-called Zone. This meant stabilizing the deteriorating Shelter, following norms of workers' safety, mitigating future contamination, and closing the last remaining working units of the Chernobyl plant. The implementation of this new program had also become a key asset in Ukraine's foreign policy. Based on these efforts, Western European countries and the United States continue to promise Ukraine further technical assistance, loans, and potential trading partnerships. Such exchanges have legitimated a new political-economic arena in which profit, political influence, and corruption loom in the already powerful and tax-evading energy sector.

Ukraine's rational–technical response to the Chernobyl legacy is unique in that it blends humanism with strategies of governance and state building, and market strategies with forms of economic and political corruption. Such interrelated processes have generated new kinds of formal and informal social networks and economies that have allowed some segments of the population to survive and benefit from politically guaranteed subsidies. I worked in clinical and laboratory settings and in the now sizable social welfare apparatus dedicated to a Chernobyl-affected population—in its state agencies, and in the offices of nongovernmental interest groups in Kyiv. Together, these sites make up a subsystem of the state's public health and welfare infrastructure where increasingly poor citizens—former and current workers of the Chernobyl plant and populations resettled from contaminated zones—mobilize around their claims to radiation-induced injuries.

I term this complex bureaucratic process by which a population attempts to establish a status as harmfully exposed and deserving of compensation a "biological citizenship." In Ukraine, where an emergent democracy is yoked to a harsh market transition, the damaged biology of a population has become grounds for social membership and the basis for staking citizenship claims. By examining how state-operated research and clinical institutions and non-governmental organizations of "the disabled" (*invalidy*) respond to individual and collective claims to biological damage, I show how rights and entitlement claims are established and contested. I also delineate the ways prior Soviet interventions into the lives of affected populations have shaped these dynamics. One can describe biological citizenship as a massive demand for, but selective access to, a form of social welfare based on medical, scientific, and legal criteria that acknowledge and compensate biological injury. Such demands are formulated in the context of fundamental losses—losses of primary securities such as employment and state-sponsored health care. Struggles over scarce medical goods and over the criteria that constitute a legitimate claim to citizenship are part of postsocialism's uncharted terrain. Informal orders of exclusion and inclusion now coexist with more formal discourses on human rights.

The Known and the Unknown

The scale of the Chernobyl aftermath and its long-term health effects have been subjects of intense dispute and controversy. International scientific organizations insist that contamination from the Chernobyl reactor has been successfully contained but argue the need for ongoing technical surveillance and informational exchange (IAEA 1991a; "Chernobyl's Legacy" 1996). The UN Scientific Committee on the Effects of Atomic Radiation, which relies on data from the IAEA, has acknowledged the sudden increase in thyroid cancers among children living in affected areas. International biomedical and social scientific literatures have characterized most other disorders as products of "informational stress" (Sergeev 1988; WHO 1996), "somatization of fear" (Guskova 1995; Rumiantseva 1996), or lack of proper "risk perception" (Bromet and Havenaar 2007; Drottz-Sjoberg 1995). Ukrainian scientists and clinicians acknowledge rampant stress among affected populations but have criticized international health assessments for ignoring the contribution radiation makes—even in low doses—to adverse physiological change (Noshchenko et al. 2002; Pilinskaya 1999).

Much of the disagreement between UN and local scientists centers on the significance of *proven* versus *expected* health outcomes. Based on studies conducted after Hiroshima and Nagasaki, an "excess" of 6,600 cancer deaths, including 470 leukemia cases were expected. Other Japan-based studies on incidence and mortality of cancer indicate that the risk of cancer varies according to cancer type. The highest risk is observed for leukemia, breast cancer, thyroid cancer, lung cancer, and some cancers of the gastrointestinal tract. There is considerable disagreement between UN-affiliated scientists and their counterparts in Ukraine and Belarus regarding Chernobyl-related cancer rates. Leukemia estimates in particular vary widely. While UN agencies find no epidemiological evidence of a linkage between exposure and cancer risk, including leukemia, Prysyazhnyuk and colleagues (1999, 2007) indicate that for all cancers combined, statistically significant higher incidence rates were found among the most heavily exposed cleanup workers in Ukraine.[8] A team of Belarussian physicians concluded that leukemia rates among the most heavily exposed cleanup workers are 4 times the Belarusian national average (Pearce 2000:12; also Stone 2001). Gennady Lazjuk of the Institute for Hereditary Diseases in Minsk, along with collaborators in Japan and Europe, found that radiation exposure accounted for a 12% increase in birth defects in heavily contaminated areas in Belarus (Lazjuk Nikolaev, and Khmel 2000). Notwithstanding the recognized increase in thyroid cancers in children, the IAEA and the UN Scientific Committee on the Effects of Atomic Radiation found inconclusive evidence about radiation-related congenital malformations, both of which have been anticipated on the basis of research on survivors of the Hiroshima and Nagasaki bombing survivors (Pierce, Shimizu, Preston, Vaeth, and Mabuchi 1996).

UN scientists and local experts also disagree over where research emphasis should be placed or at what level biological changes should be detected. Human radiation effects vary according to whether they are deterministic or stochastic. Deterministic effects occur when levels of absorbed radiation doses are significant enough to kill cells that, if not adequately replaced, produce clinically observable pathologies. The severity of the effect is dependent on the radiation dose, with steep linear dose–effect relationships. This is opposed to stochastic effects, which, based on gene damage, confer a probability or chance that a harmful outcome will develop. In contrast with deterministic effects, stochastic effects are nonlinear in terms of the kinds of harm they can produce, but are most commonly associated with cancer and leukemia induction. Unlike deterministic effects, they increase the probability rather than the severity of a given pathology (Gofman 1981). Recent collaborations among post-Soviet and Western scientists, some of whom are unaffiliated with international radiological committees and agencies, have yielded new data related to stochastic effects. Using techniques far more sophisticated than those available at the time of the Hiroshima and Nagasaki studies, researchers have shown increases in human germ line alterations under conditions of low-dose irradiation among children born in 1994 in Mogilev, Belarus, in comparison with a control population in Britain (Dubrova et al. 1996). Others have noted significant increases in the frequency of chromosomal aberrations and other genetic markers of radiation effects in children living in contaminated areas (Pilinskaya and Dibskiy 2000). Clearly, the science of the human health effects of Chernobyl is an evolving one. As new technologies and research funds become available, new fields of knowledge are established. But at the present moment, what we know of the precise figures of damage is far from complete (Cardis et al. 2006; Kesminiene and Cardis 2007).

What we can conclude with some certainty, however, is that the process of making scientific knowledge is inextricable from the forms of power those processes legitimate, and even provide solutions for (Shapin and Schaffer 1985:15). How scientific knowledge is valued and the level at which it is said to hold significance can affect the planning of state interventions and medical surveillance, the size of populations considered to be at risk, and the courses of suffering and illnesses those populations experience. Moreover, interventions are predicated, in part, on policymakers' understandings of the relationship between radiation dose and bodily harm. The so-called linear hypothesis states that harm is proportional to dose and that radiation is harmful at any dose. Here it is not a question of whether harmful effects such as additional cancers exist but whether there are technologies available that are sufficiently powerful enough to make those effects demonstrable and whether governments desire to invest in or make use of such technologies. Hence, the issues raised by the linear hypothesis are of an ethical, political, and economic nature.

Policymakers have several intervention options at their disposal. At one end, those options can be described as "low-tech" and minimally interventionist. The rationale here is that because it is impossible to detect the small increases in cancer deaths predicted by the linear hypothesis, cancers—or, for that matter, many other diseases—should not be singled out as radiogenic. In the Chernobyl case, this rationale influenced the size of affected cohorts receiving intervention. Soviet officials claimed that except for the initial group of cleanup workers sent into the Zone, the radiation exposures that populations received were insignificant to their health. Indeed, there are many experts who remain committed to the idea that the primary health effects of Chernobyl are of a mental or psychosocial nature. In line with this reasoning, Soviet interventions focused on information dissemination (as in, for example, the state's battle against "radiophobia") and on the introduction of therapeutic and surveillance regimes to address psychosomatic ailments, characterized as products of individual psychological weakness and self-induction. Psychosocial medical categories were applied to exclude the majority of medical claims.

An alternative course of action would involve a state's immediate full disclosure about what is known and is not known about the complexity of health outcomes (including an acknowledgement of those health outcomes as being some combination of clinically observable, stochastic, and psychological effects). This kind of approach informed Ukraine's management of the aftermath and led, for example, to an improvement of the state's public health surveillance system. Lifting constraints on international collaboration and foreign aid, the state made a variety of research technologies, ranging from the epidemiological to the clinical and molecular biological, available to researchers assessing the disaster's health impact. A number of local scientists, in collaboration with a number of molecular biologists and geneticists from Western Europe, the United States, and Japan, are still sorting out the genetic causes of radiation-induced cancers.

Both the Soviet and post-Soviet/Ukrainian approaches entail social and political trade-offs and risks. If in the first case, Soviet policymakers can be accused of undermedicalizing or denying the health effects of the disaster altogether, Ukrainian policymakers can be accused for overmedicalizing their constituencies, and of creating a health system that fosters abuse. My purpose, however, is not to allocate blame but to paint a clearer picture of the dynamic interplay between scientific and social orders, and how those orders come to define actual conditions of health: those aspects that protect or undermine it and the moral and ethical discourses surrounding its rights and responsibilities. Following Veena Das' (1995:138) characterization of the aftermath of the Bhopal chemical disaster, it is imperative to understand how "pain and suffering are experiences that are actively created and distributed" within scientific/social orders themselves.

The number, novelty, physical variability, and duration of the kinds of particles that were released in the Chernobyl explosion make the open-endedness of the disaster's health effects hard to deny. This open-endedness necessitates further reflection on the ways the scientific research process itself contributes to the spread of pain and suffering by searching for easy answers and simple closures. In discerning the "true" causes of their subjects' suffering, researchers themselves have constructed categories of authentic and inauthentic suffering, thus marginalizing those who happen to fall into the latter category. So as not to contribute to this marginalizing, I avoided pigeonholing people affected by the disaster as either suffering from "hard" biologically induced symptoms or "soft" psychological ones—though their reasons for claiming the primacy of one etiology over another often entail moral and epistemological claims.

My decision to abstain from judgment is also supported on empirical grounds. Scientific understanding along with policy decisions, popular pressures, and availability of technological resources, can shift the frames of what is considered evidence of the physical impact of the disaster. What becomes central to this analysis is the different social contexts in which scientific knowledge is placed and the ethical values it is used to support. Worlds of science, statistics, bureaucracy, suffering, power, and biological processes co-evolve here in particular and unstable ways. How to discern their patterns as locally observable realities that affect specific health experiences and the negotiation of health categories and health care is a major creative challenge of this work.

The Anthropology of Human Disaster

Between 1992 and 1997, I conducted archival and field research in Ukraine, Russia, and the United States. In Ukraine, I worked with resettled families, mothers of exposed children, and radiation-exposed workers. I followed them to public events in the Kyiv area and sat in on their meetings with state administrators at the Parliamentary Commission on Human Rights where they negotiated the broadening of Chernobyl-related social and health care mandates. My data collection was oriented around these key questions: (1) How does the Ukrainian government administer individuals and populations claiming to be affected by radiation exposure? (2) What scientific knowledge and administrative policies are applied in the categorization of risk groups and in the formulation of compensation laws? (3) What scientific knowledge and political strategies are deployed by groups pressing for compensation and social justice on the basis of their Chernobyl condition? I carried out interviews with members of the country's Chernobyl Ministry (now defunct), responsible among other things for attracting relief organizations and humanitarian aid; coordinating international efforts for financing and maintaining the Shelter unit; funding environmental monitoring and new building construction such as homes for persons and families resettled from contaminated areas; coordinating the work of central and local state bodies and scientific and medical institutions; recommending policies for affected citizens; allocating finances for treatment and health care costs of affected populations; and distributing benefits and compensation. I was afforded access to memos and internal reports outlining the dynamics of social response to the disaster; rules of hygiene for living in contaminated areas; reports on patterns of media coverage; policy recommendations and medical criteria that Ministry of Health officials used in compensation decision making; and reports on emerging social psychological problems and methodological recommendations for rapid assessments of psychological status. Investigating how Chernobyl-related social mandates legitimated Ukrainian state-building processes, I collected data on Chernobyl welfare budgets and related them to national priorities for health and social protection spending in Ukraine, and gathered information on how and on what scientific bases laws of compensation for Chernobyl sufferers had been established and expanded since Ukraine's independence.

Along with my research at the level of state and civil society, I developed a brief social history of the scientific knowledge and technical experience that Soviet, American, and Ukrainian experts gained in the immediate and long-term management of Chernobyl. It became apparent that to do a fair analysis of the lived experience of Chernobyl I had to do multisited work. That meant becoming scientifically literate—inquiring into the circulation and assimilation of scientific knowledge at national, international, and local levels as well as exploring their tensions. I conducted interviews with key scientific and political players in both Kyiv and Moscow, comparing scientific norms of biological risk and safety in Soviet and post-Soviet administrations of the aftermath. I also looked into expert claims at the IAEA and at government laboratories in the United States. At Lawrence Berkeley Laboratory (whose work is unrelated to Chernobyl issues), I learned some of the basic radiobiological techniques for assessing the biological impact of radiation at the cellular and DNA levels. But, as one radiation scientist told me, the difference between the manipulable animal environment on which these assessments are made and populationwide exposures to low-dose radiation remains a "black box." Though causal links between high doses of radiation and human biological effects have been well established, the same cannot be said for continuous human exposure to low doses. It is no surprise that health predictions made by international health experts have often contradicted people's lived experience. The calculus of cost and criteria of assessment of injury are, given the state of knowledge, open-ended and contestable.

In the absence of agreed-upon standards of scientific assessment, a new social and political space had been opened in Ukraine. I learned in my long-term work with civil servants of the Chernobyl welfare apparatus that disputes over the scope of injury in this disaster, and over how to model it, continue to affect policy, social mobilizations, and not least the very nature of the course of illnesses in the affected populations I worked with. From the field, I could also observe that different scientific approaches (psychometric versus biological; laboratory versus field-based research), different funding priorities, and different senses of urgency concerning the unknown health effects of the disaster were not simply at odds with each other; nor were they simply waiting to be assessed for their suitability or unsuitability. Their confrontation and juxtaposition engendered a new environment—or, more precisely, a political economy of claims around radiation illness. Developing alongside the new scientific, biomedical, and legal institutions promoting "safe living" in Ukraine was another social phenomenon that caught my attention. It was the boom of civic organizations called *fondy* (funds) that administered international charity and the compensation claims of the Zone workers. Also, since these more than 500 Funds are tax exempt, they have sparked a large informal economy based on imports of a variety of goods, including pharmaceuticals, cars, foodstuffs, and so on.

In this political economy of Chernobyl-related illnesses, it was common knowledge that a person categorized as "disabled" was far better compensated than a mere "sufferer." Persons completely outside the system of Chernobyl sufferers knew they had little chance of getting decent social protections from the state. In this economy, scientific knowledge became a crucial medium of everyday life. The effectiveness of relating one's dose exposures to radiation-related symptoms, experiences, and work histories in the Zone determined the position one could occupy in the hierarchy of sufferers, and the extent to which one could wield capital that could further guarantee state protections. Post-socialist Ukraine presented a unique constellation in which state-building, social movements, and market developments were intertwined, generating new institutions and social arrangements through which citizenship and ethics were being transformed.

When I returned to Kyiv for year-long field research in 1996, my key field site became the Radiation Research Center. The Center was founded in June 1986 as the clinical research branch of the All-Union Center of Radiation Medicine. The center's staff grew from 90 to more than 1,300 by 1991. These numbers reflect its growth in status as an important social institution; they also illustrate how in the context of economic crisis, government bureaucracies expand rather than contract to provide their own forms of social protection. The center monitors patients with acute radiation sickness and conducts research on the clinical outcomes of human exposures to ionizing radiation. What is most important, it houses the central medical–labor committee [*Ekspertiza*], a group of scientists, clinicians, and administrators who are responsible for evaluating the health of Chernobyl Zone workers, resettled families, and inhabitants of contaminated areas. Their job is to evaluate a patient's level of disability (or loss of labor capacity) and to either verify or disavow the etiology of that disability in radiation exposure due to Chernobyl. Members authorize the Chernobyl connection or "tie" (*sviaz*)—a legal document attesting to the link between certain illnesses and radiation exposure and entitling the bearer to state compensation in the form of pensions, health care, and even education benefits for children. This package of benefits is, comparatively speaking, much better than average pensions and is therefore very desirable. As of 2000, the state paid an average $12 per month for usual, non-Chernobyl-related social insurance. The poverty line was approximately $27 a month. For persons disabled by the Chernobyl accident, for the same period, pension benefits averaged between $54 and $90 per month, depending on the degree of disability. A sufferer, a person who does not have disability status but has the status of having suffered from the Chernobyl accident, received $20 per month, on average.

Through contacts with politically active groups of disabled Chernobyl Zone workers who frequented clinics, I obtained permission to conduct research in the clinical wing of the center (known as the Clinic). By 1996, the Clinic had become an epicenter of medical, scientific and legal wrangling. Physical examinations, scientific resources, and specialized medical treatment became precious assets in qualifying for lifetime compensations for patients who were fortunate enough to be there. I was allowed to observe interactions between physicians, nurses, and patients; to attend decision-making meetings related to compensation claims; and to examine current research, particularly in the Clinic's Division of Nervous Pathologies.

The choice of this division as a research setting was intentional on my part. Medical–Labor committee members told me that the majority of disability claims were channeled through neurological wards on account of a variety of nervous system disorders. Yet, it was unclear whether these disorders stemmed from social stress owing to the country's dire economic situation or to radiation exposure, or from some combination of both. In addition to talking to scientists, health workers, and administrators, I conducted extended interviews with 60 male and female patients (aged 35–55) and had access to their medical records. I documented the course of their illnesses, diagnosis, and progress in obtaining disability status (*oformyty hrupu* which means to "make the group"). I also worked with 3 of the Chernobyl Funds, tracing the history of their membership and looking into their strategic relationships with the Clinic and the medical–labor committee. A final part of my work involved following the everyday activities of 5 of the Clinic's male patients and their wives and children. I was interested in how these men's introduction into this novel political economy of illness was changing their identities as breadwinners and father figures, as well as affecting their mental health. I was particularly interested in these men's changing sense of *lichnost'*, a Soviet concept of personhood that was expressed in individual commitment to work and to the labor collective, and in how married couples were using radiation illness as a means of subsistence in the new economy.

Navigating the Chernobyl Unknown

In what follows, I outline how international scientists and Soviet and post-Soviet public policymakers cast the scope of the Chernobyl disaster over time and how related compensation strategies were defined. My purpose is to highlight how indeterminacy of scientific knowledge about the illnesses people face and about the nature of atomic catastrophe materializes here as both a curse and a source of leverage. Elements such as atmospheric dispersion maps, international scientific cooperation, and local scientific responses, as well as people's involvement in bureaucratic and testing procedures, led up to what can be called a "technical and political course of illness." Examples of people's engagement with and influence on such courses themselves will then be discussed.

Most scientists today would agree that given the state of technology at the time of the disaster, specialists were unable to make an objective appraisal of what had happened (Medvedev 1990). Tom Sullivan, who until recently directed the Atmospheric Release Advisory Capability (ARAC) group at Lawrence Livermore Laboratory in Livermore, California, agrees with this general appraisal. Before the Chernobyl disaster, Sullivan's ARAC team had generated atmospheric dispersion models of the size and movement of nuclear plumes resulting from American and Chinese above-ground nuclear weapons tests and the Three Mile Island accident. "A 200 by 200 kilometer area had been sufficient to model prior radiation releases," he told me. "We did the imaging near the Chernobyl plant using this 200 kilometer square grid, but the grid was so saturated, I mean, you couldn't even make sense of it because every place had these enormously high radiation values ... *Our codes were not prepared for an event of this magnitude.*"

Soviet scientists, too, were unprepared, but they did not admit this in an August 1986 meeting with the IAEA. There they presented a crude analysis of the distribution of radiation in the Exclusion Zone and in the Soviet Union: "assessments were made of the actual and future radiation doses received by the populations of towns, villages, and other inhabited places. As a result of these and other measures, *it proved possible to keep exposures within the established limits*" (USSR State Committee on the Utilization of Atomic Energy 1986:38).

The issue at stake is the state's capacity to disinform or, rather, to create a state of ignorance to maintain political order. Historian Loren Graham (1998), for example, has written on how "false" sciences such as Lysenkoism, which denied the existence of the gene and advocated labor-intensive methods of accelerating crop yields, have been instrumental in shaping work psychology and social life in the socialist project. The fact is that limited Soviet maps of the Chernobyl fall-out justified limited forms of radiological surveillance and resettlement actions. Non-knowledge became essential to the deployment of authoritative knowledge. High doses absorbed by at least 200,000 Chernobyl workers between 1986 and 1987 were insufficiently documented. This was due, in part, to a lack of available functioning dosimeters. One biochemist whom I met in 1996 told me that many of the clean-up workers "received 6–8 times the lethal dose of radiation" (at 400 rem, bone marrow failure sets in).[9] "They are alive," he told me. "[The workers] know that they didn't die. *But they don't know how they survived.*" His statement speaks to the extent to which not only knowledge but also ignorance was constructed and used as a state method of upholding public order. As historian of science Robert Proctor tells us in his informative book on how politics shapes cancer science, ignorance "is not just a natural consequence of the ever shifting boundary between the known and the unknown." It is a "political consequence" of decisions concerning how to approach what could and should be done to mitigate danger or disease (1995:7). Policymakers distorted knowledge to avoid their responsibility to care for the population.

Chernobyl also became a venue for unprecedented international scientific cooperation and human research. President Mikhail Gorbachev personally invited a team of American oncologists led by leukemia specialist Robert Gale to conduct experimental bone marrow transplantations upon individuals whose exposures were beyond the lethal limit and for whom these transplantations were deemed appropriate. Additionally, 400 workers selected by Dr. Guskova and others received a genetically engineered hematopoietic growth factor molecule (rhGM-CSF), thought to regenerate stem cell growth. Though both the transplantations and the trial proved unsuccessful, the medical work on this cohort (and the objective indices created around them) helped consolidate an image of a biomedical crisis that was being contained by cutting-edge scientific applications. In an effort to alleviate the public's fear, Dr. Gale appeared live on television, walking barefoot in the zone with one of his children.

As this internationalization of science surrounding Chernobyl ensued, however, the physical management of contamination at the accident site was retained in the sphere of Soviet state control. One policy statement released by the Soviet Health Ministry at the height of this cooperation, for example, directed medical examiners in the Exclusion Zone to classify workers who have received a maximum dose as having "vegetovascular dystonia," that is, a kind of panic disorder, and a novel psychosocial disorder called "radiophobia" (or the fear of the biological influence of radiation). These categories were used to filter out the majority of disability claims.[10] Substantial challenges to this Soviet management came from certain labor sectors in subsequent years. At the end of 1989 only 130 additional persons were granted disability; by 1990, 2,753 more cases had been considered, of which 50% were authorized for neurological disorders. The levels of political influence of certain labor sectors are reflected in the order in which they received Chernobyl-related disability: coal miners, then workers of the Ministry of Internal Affairs (the police), then Transport Ministry workers. These various labor groups would soon realize that in the Ukrainian management of Chernobyl, forms of political leveraging had to be coupled with medical–scientific know-how.

Arguably the new Ukrainian accounting of the Chernobyl unknown was part and parcel of new strategies of "knowledge-based" governance and social mobilization. In 1991 and in its first set of laws, the new parliament denounced the preceding Soviet management of Chernobyl as "an act of genocide." The new nation–state viewed the disaster as (among other things) a key means for instituting domestic and international authority. Legislators assailed the Soviet standard for determining biological risk to populations. The Soviets had established a high 35 rem (a unit of absorbed dose), spread over an individual's lifetime (understood as a 70-year span) as the threshold of allowable radiation dose intakes. This high threshold dose minimized the scale of resettlement actions. Ukrainian law lowered the Soviet threshold dose to 7 rem over a lifetime, comparable to what an average American would be exposed to in his/her lifetime. In effect, these lowered measures for safe living increased the size of the labor forces going to the zone (since workers had to work shorter amounts of time if they were to avoid exceeding the stricter dose standards). The measures also expanded territories considered contaminated. A significant new sector of the population would want to claim itself as part of a state-protected post-Soviet polity. One biophysicist responsible for conducting retrospective dose assays on resettlers told me: "Long lines of resettlers extended from our laboratory doors. It wasn't enough that they were evacuated to 'clean' areas. People got entangled in the category of victim, by law. They had unpredictable futures and *each of them wanted to know their dose.*"

Stories of Suffering

Ivan Nimenko learned how to navigate the new times. He was moving up the social welfare ranks from sufferer to disabled person. While working in the state militia in the first weeks following the accident, he was ordered to evacuate the residents of Pripyat, a city of 50,000, housing nuclear plant workers and their families, within 36 hours after the disaster. I met him in the Radiation Research Center. Once closed to foreigners, it is a highly charged bureaucratic and clinical institution in which workers' occupational injury claims are made and stamped as authentic. Nimenko, like any prospective disabled person, sought the Chernobyl "tie"—a document that, as he put it, asserts that his illnesses are not "general," but are rather attributable to a Chernobyl-based cause. As he put it, "this is the document I need for my health."

Nimenko was admitted to the center's Division of Nervous Pathologies with a diagnosis that read "cerebral arteriosclerosis with arterial hypertension, osteochondrosis, gastritis, and hypochondriacal syndrome." This complex of diagnoses was not uncommon, and suggested that he was possibly a mere "psycho-social" case, therefore expendable from the compensation system. He needed to remove that possibility and replace it with an unconditional radiation-based etiology. Fundamental to this task was a radiation dose assessment that he had fought hard to get. Nimenko knew that according to international nuclear industry standards, a worker can incur up to 25 rem over his entire lifetime. He had incurred at least 25 rem in just 10 years. Nimenko had managed through a brother-in-law, a laboratory director, to enter the system, to get a coveted hospital bed, and to receive an examination with the medical examiner. He could count on affinal connections and old Soviet (primarily urban-based) informal exchange networks and relations known as "*blat*" to establish his legal status in the new state.[11] He was successful.

Like many others, Nimenko maintained that he was historically unaccounted for in the Soviet administration of the disaster. Referring to the lax radiation monitoring of Chernobyl workers, he said, "Regarding our individual cases," he said, "they wrote nothing. If there was any distinctive mark written about us in the registers, it read 0.0 (*nul'-nul'*), whatever the unit of measurement was." In characterizing his dose exposure as *nul'-nul'*, Nimenko recognized himself as having no legal force, or no consequence or value, during his Chernobyl work. For Nimenko, this Soviet 0.0 symbolized false accountability. Until today, scientists involved in executing the Soviet state's disaster response maintain that only 237 people with known doses are legitimate acute accident victims, and that only 30 of those died. These kinds of squared-off facts defined the scope of the disaster's consequences and foreclosed compensations to many like Nimenko who had potentially sustained future injuries. Nimenko knew these numbers by heart.

New gender dynamics were also at stake in this new legal and moral environment. In 1996, another representative of a fund told me the first words he said to his wife and son when he returned home from work, "Get away from me, I am contaminated!" Kulyk was a mere 38-year-old when I met him, but he looked to be at least 60 years old. Kulyk lay on a living room couch, a kind of centerpiece, surrounded by members of his fund. As he spoke, his wife mocked her husband's "stupid sense of duty." She was left to take care of a deteriorating person, "He was a party secretary, and now he is a skeleton. His stupid sense of duty is now killing everyone!" Tania explained Kulyk had experienced all signs of acute radiation sickness, "He lost consciousness constantly, coughed, and vomited blood .... He is alive, and that's all I know. I don't want to know what is inside his body." Every village, every housing block, every work collective knew a bio-robot, or someone who had died.

Many who had done less dangerous labor, like Nimenko, saw these bio-robots as political kin. Unlike Kulyk, Nimenko remained physically and socially mobile. He had mastered a language of symptoms and science, and was also part of a disabled persons' fund mediating the claims of other clean-up workers. He was scientifically literate and had a strong sense of the value of science. He knew how to read cytogenetic tests indicating chromosomal aberrations in his cells. He used the ambiguities of radiation science—and there are many—to facilitate his chances of having his case reassessed in a way that would favor his claim for compensation. These were not mundane clinical affairs; they were political actions. Patient/workers like Nimenko are the carriers of an unaccounted-for past, but they are also vectors of new social organization and practices of personhood. Nimenko was reestablishing his legal and moral value in the new state.

In this daily bureaucratic instantiation of Chernobyl, relations between workers of the Zone, resettled persons and families, scientists, physicians, legislators, and civil servants intensified. Together, these groups became invested in a new social and moral contract between state and civil society, a contract guaranteeing them the right to know their risk levels and use legal means to obtain medical care and monitoring. The sufferers and their administrators were also supported by nonsuffering citizens, who paid a 12% tax on their salaries to support compensations and assistance to the ruined reactor site. The hybrid quality of this post-socialist state and social contract comes into view. On the one hand, the Ukrainian government rejected Western neoliberal prescriptions to *downsize* its social welfare domain; on the other hand, it presented itself as informed by the principles of a modern risk society. Moreover, these Chernobyl laws allowed for unprecedented civic organizing; they also became distinct venues of corruption through which informal practices of providing or selling access to state privileges and protections expanded.

Here is another instance of how these dynamics operated in the everyday life: the country's eminent expert on matters related to the disaster, Symon Lavrov, was well regarded internationally for having developed computerized fallout models and calculating populationwide doses in the post-Soviet period. He told me, however, that "when a crying mother comes to my laboratory and asks me, Professor Lavrov, 'tell me what's wrong with my child?' I assign her a dose and say nothing more. I double it, as much as I can." The offer of a higher dose increased the likelihood that the mother would be able to secure social protection on account of her potentially sick child. The point is the following: the mother could offer her child a dose, a protective tie with the state, a biological tie, which is founded on a probability of sickness. What she could offer, perhaps the most precious thing she could offer her child in that context, is a specific knowledge, history, and category. The child's "exposure" and the knowledge that would make that exposure an empirical fact were not things to be repressed or denied (as had been tried in the Soviet model) but rather something to be made into a resource and then distributed through informal means.

Counter-politics

Specific cases illustrate how these economic and state processes, combined with the technical dynamics already described, have laid the groundwork for a "counter-politics" (Gordon 1991:5). Citizens have come to depend on obtainable technologies and legal procedures to gain political recognition and admission to some form of welfare inclusion. Aware that they had fewer chances for finding employment and health in the new market economy, these citizens accounted for elements in their lives (measures, numbers, symptoms) that could be linked to a state, scientific, and bureaucratic history of mismanagement and risk. The tighter the connection that could be drawn, the greater the chance of securing economic and social entitlement. This dimension of illness as counter-politics suggests that sufferers are aware of the way politics shapes what they know and don't know about their illnesses and that they are put in a role of having to use these politics to curb further deteriorations of their health, which they see as resulting, in part, from a collapsing state health system and loss of adequate legal protections.

Probability in relation to radiation-related disease became a central resource for local scientific research. This play with probability was being projected back into nature, so to speak, through an intricate local science. Young neuropsychiatrists made the best of the inescapability of their political circumstance (they could not get visas to leave the country) as they integrated international medical taxonomies into Soviet ones and developed classifications of mental and nervous disorders for dose ranges that in some expert literatures were considered far too low to make any significant biological contribution. For example, neuropsychiatrists were involved in a project designed to find and assess cases of mental retardation in children exposed in utero in the first year after the disaster. In the case of one such child, a limping 9-year-old boy, researchers and parents pooled their knowledge to reconstruct the child's disorder as having a radiation origin. His mother was an emergency doctor who elected to work in the zone until late in her pregnancy. Even though the boy's radiation dose was low, he was given the status of sufferer because of his mother's occupation-related exposure and also because a positron emission tomography (PET) scan did reveal a cerebral lesion that was never hypothesized as being related to anything other than radiation. (It could have been birth trauma). As researchers constructed a human research cohort, they were also constructing a destiny for the newly designated human research subjects. It was precisely the destiny that the parents were intent on offering to this child—a biological citizenship.

Illness as Work

Radiation-related claims and practices constituted a form of work in this market transition. A clinical administrator concurred that claims to radiation illness among the Ukrainian population amounted to a form of "market compensation." He told me, "If people could improve their family budgets, there would be a lot less illness. People are now oriented towards one thing. They believe that only through the constitution of illnesses, and particularly difficult illnesses, incurable ones, can they improve their family budgets." Administrators of the Radiation Research Center told me they are not to be "blamed too much" for fueling an informal economy of diagnoses and entitlements. Complicities could be found at every level, and the moral conflicts they entailed were publicly discussed. One administrator who authenticated compensation claims, Dr. Ihor Demeshko, told me illnesses had become a form of currency. "There are a lot of people out of work," he said. "People don't have enough money to eat. The state doesn't give medicines for free anymore. Drugs stores are commercialized." He likened his work to that of a bank. "The diagnosis we write is money."

The importance of these diagnoses to everyday people cannot be stressed enough. "There's pressure from the invalids to write a Chernobyl-related diagnosis. The demands on the state are increasing with every instant. People working in the Zones who have high-risk jobs sign up for work knowing about that risk. They reason, 'I get sick, I get this much money. I die, my family will get this much money.'" While illness after Chernobyl has become the great social leveler, providing access to biological citizenship for some, the gates to these democratic pastures open and close at random. The apparent randomness of the law (in the form of denials of access, exclusions, postponements) combined with the economic instability is precisely what insures the system's mobility and a collective drive toward illness.

Dr. Demeshko allowed me to take notes and to ask questions of claimants entering his office over 5 days. By 1996, the laws on procuring the Chernobyl tie were getting more restrictive. The following office interactions are intended to capture a flow of appeals and the repertoire of patient strategies. Many female clients, for example, staked their claim to privileges on the basis of deceased husbands, or children or grandchildren alleged to have been *in utero* at the time of the disaster. Many male clients invoked the number of days they worked in the Zone to indicate exposure, or the number of days they have not worked at all, to indicate their degree of illness. Many of the claimants lived on less than $40 a month. Their names and their family members' names were registered in a state-operated registry of Chernobyl sufferers. Some wanted to discontinue work in the Zone and receive a disability status (these workers tended to have disproportionately high salaries). Others who had already worked in the Zone wanted to ascend to a higher disability grade to increase their pension. And others wanted to register their children or grandchildren as disabled.

We can also observe how the sick role and privileges were allocated and/ or denied, and the effects these allocations or denials generated. Allocation in one case was based on the wealth the client can pass onto the research center. In another case, Demeshko perceived the claimant to be "on the border with death." Denials were often based on poorly documented evidence of exposure, or on the principal that the claimants' illnesses developed beyond the limits of acceptable timetables. But in essence, few formal rules guided the allocation of these privileges. Some clients had to beg for them; others were given advice about informal clinical procedures to expedite their claims.

The mother of a child *in utero* at the time of the disaster enters Demeshko's office. Her husband is a level three disabled person; she is a level two. She claims her daughter is "not developing properly." The child "used to be quick, now her legs hurt." The daughter has thyroid cancer. Someone's head peers through the door. Demeshko says, "A decision hasn't been made for you yet."

A middle-aged rural woman walks in. She was evacuated from her village in Zone Two. When she says that her daughter was pregnant at the time of the disaster, she starts to cry. "The little girl," she says, "now 10 years old, has a dry mouth, weakness; she's weak, her thinking is slow, her thyroid is swollen, her legs hurt, her blood is poor." The woman said the girl would be interned in the gastroenterological ward of the Clinic for monitoring. She works hard to elicit sympathy from Demeshko, who will eventually decide whether the girl will become a state-protected invalid on the basis of her diagnostic paperwork. Demeshko interrupts the grandmother and tells her that she is in the wrong place and should go to the Chernobyl children's hospital for the evaluation of the child's status.

A man in his mid-50s enters. He says that he has worked at the reactor site since 1978, and that he regularly interns himself at the center and at the local clinic of the Chernobyl plant for monitoring and treatment. The man keeps careful records of his illnesses. He shows documentary evidence of his dose, a high 73 rem. When I asked him why he was seeing Demeshko now he says, "I'm sick." Demeshko then asks him, "And before?" The man answered that he was sick, but that he "hid it." When I asked him why he hid it, he answers, "So I could work in the Zone, I'm used to working." "How much do you make?" Demeshko asks him. "$270 a month." He then turns to the seated woman: "How much do you make?" he asks, and her answer is "$27 a month." When I ask the worker whether he could say more about what brought him to the clinic, he answered in a cynical way, "Head spins."

A tired-looking elderly man comes in and throws his documents toward Demeshko, who then asked him where he works. The man replies that he does not work, and that he lives on a pension. He says that he evacuated people from the zones when he worked for the city taxi service. Demeshko, without reason or explanation, does not accept the documents and tells him to go to another hospital.

A man in his mid-50s walks in. After Demeshko inquires, he says he worked in the Zone "for one day, on May 18, 1986." He doesn't know his dose. The man worked as a driver and claims to have fallen ill in 1995, 9 years after the disaster, with rheumatism, stenocardia, cardiosclerosis, and arrhythmia. "They gave me the Chernobyl tie because of my heart arrhythmia," he tells me. He also says that he no longer works and has been living on a disability pension that provides him with $27 a month. The man wants to accede to a higher Chernobyl disability rank. When he leaves the office, Demeshko guesses that the man "bought" a disability tie because, he says, the claimant's illnesses appeared "after the acceptable timetable for arrhythmia … . His disability status will expire and he won't be able to renew it." The man's physical condition, regardless of whether it is Chernobyl-induced, allegedly prevents him from working. His having based his claim on 1 day of work at Chernobyl means either that the man is driven by desperation or that his expectations of compensation are unrealistic, or both.

A well-dressed man entered and without introductions reports that he was previously a patient in the cardiological ward. He says that he worked in the Zone for 6 days in 1986, "building the *Sarkofag*." In 1993, he allegedly fell ill with stenocardia. Demeshko asks him where he works. He says he is a director of the Kyiv Energy Company. He gives an account of his lost work capacity, "I haven't worked 26 days in 5 weeks," and says he thinks he can't work any more. Demeshko told him "to go see the center's financial manager."

After the man leaves, Demeshko says that his stenocardia appeared after the accepted timetable for stenocardia. The limit is 5 years. "He got his illness 7 years after the disaster. He got sick too late. By law, we can't give him disability status. But because he is a director, we might be able to get some *humanitarka* (a donation or payment) out of him."

A woman enters, a widow, representing her deceased husband. "I submitted his medical documents last year," she says. "A decision hasn't been made yet on your husband's matter," Demeshko answers. She leaves, saying little else about her case. Demeshko apparently knows her situation and is delaying decision making.

A middle-aged rural woman enters the office. She says that her "husband-invalid" (*cholovik-invalid*) died 3 days ago and that she is seeking additional social protections. Her husband, a driver by profession, worked in the Zone in 2-week shifts, transporting contaminated building materials from the reactor to "burial pits" scattered throughout the Exclusion Zone. She lives on a pension of $26. He collected a pension of $75 before his cancer-related death. Demeshko then asks her, "Was there a Chernobyl pension already calculated in his regular pension?"

"Yes, an added $16 a month for work in the Zone," she answers.
"Did you get compensation for his death?" Demeshko asks.

"Just for his funeral," she says.

"What do you want here?" Demeshko asked.

The woman answers, "My husband said to me, 'When I die, get the Chernobyl privileges.'"

In this case, the deceased calculated in advance the benefits to his family of his Chernobyl-related death. His wife "inherited" his medical documents with which she is advocating for more social protections from the state. She claims his disability is linked to his death (*zviaz po smerti*, or "in connection with death").

A man enters the room. He says that in June 1986, he worked for 2 weeks in the Zone, cutting down the surrounding contaminated forests: "Our whole factory went," he says. He says he doesn't know his dose. He receives a pension of $26 a month as a sufferer. He says he needs disability status so that he could pay for his thyroid operation and treatments of thyroid replacement hormone. He seems desperate, depressed, and resigned to the vagaries of bureaucracy. Demeshko accepts his documents for review.

A woman enters and says without any introduction, "My husband was a disabled person (level one), a professional. He died of kidney cancer. His dose was 25 rem. He received $325 in pension payments." She wants the death tie. When she leaves, Demeshko says, "This woman isn't going to get any more money. The Ministry of Social Welfare has already given her money for his funeral."

A man enters. He is receiving a pension of $32 and wants disability status. He says that his wife, a Zone worker, died recently and he says he needed to "protect himself." He doesn't know his dose.

A woman enters. She is wearing a black dress and a black scarf. Her husband died just 3 days ago. She wanted the privileges associated with his Chernobyl-related death. Her husband worked as an engineer. His dose was an extremely high 180 rem, and he died of lung cancer.

A woman enters. She was evacuated from Pripyat in the Zone on April 27, 1986. She was laid off from work at a bread factory, where her salary was $37 a month. She lists her illnesses for Demeshko. In 1987, she was diagnosed with vegetovascular dystonia and discirculatory encephalopathy—both nervous disorders. She has 3 children to support. "Can you protect your family?" Demeshko asks her.

"No," she says.

"What will you do next?" I ask her.

"Trade, sell whatever I can. The state doesn't pay anything."

Demeshko sends her to the local polyclinic. "Go there and they will write a referral to the neurological ward here. That will get you the Chernobyl tie."

A man enters. He shows Demeshko documents from a specialized examination that the medical-labor committee required him to undergo. The man worked at the Chernobyl plant for 8 months starting in May 1986. He wants his disability. He alleges that he has eczema, and invokes the authority of Dr. Angelina Guskova when he claims his eczema "has turned into acute radiation dermatitis—diagnosed in Moscow." Demeshko tells him that there are no privileges associated with acute radiation dermatitis. The diagnosis he will need to be considered for disability is skin cancer. After the man leaves, Demeshko explains that Guskova repealed any acute radiation sickness-related diagnoses in 1988. "In general, disability is no longer given for acute radiation sickness. However, if a person shows complications from the effects of acute radiation sickness, he would be entitled to consideration. Skin cancer would count."

A man enters; he looks sallow and exhausted. He puts a document on the table that shows evidence of his dose. "Here's an estimation of my dose." The estimation was made on the basis of the roads that he traveled to get to the Zone and their levels of contamination. "I worked in the *mohyl'nyky* [irradiated materials garbage pits]." He says that he suffers from hypotonia and has had 2 heart attacks. Demeshko asks him to show documentation of his hospital stays starting in 1990. The man answers that he failed to have his diagnoses registered from year to year. "You will get no tie," Demeshko tells him. "But people are busy harvesting their potatoes now," he added, "so maybe there's a bed available for you in the neurology ward. You can get a diagnosis there." The man leaves; Demeshko tells me, "He's on the border with death, we have many like that."

Depression, exhaustion, and defeat fill this newly renovated office. So many women in black dresses make the same claims—their relatives or spouses have died. The legacy of Chernobyl is being remade as an intractable marriage between life and death. Yet, the Chernobyl death has no distinct biological markers. What distinguishes it is the life that preceded it. That life has a specific medical profile and a specific relation with the state. It is subject to a particular type of experience of citizenship and social inclusion. By the time of his or her death, the Chernobyl sufferer will have been the subject of a massive amount of writing. He or she will leave behind a stack of mostly illegible medical records, hospital referrals, signatures, institutional rubber stamps, dose assessments, diagnoses, corrections to diagnoses, more diagnoses, and other papers conferring his/her Chernobyl identity.

Everyday Violence

In the ever-widening gulf between exact and inexact sciences, probable and improbable causes and, exact and inexact criteria of blame, an entire social transformation took place and occasioned new forms of desperation and bureaucratic dependence. The story of Anton and Halia (both aged 42 in 1997) gives evidence of the ways such desperation and dependence were at work in the most personal arenas. The new institutions, procedures, and actors at work at the state level, at the research clinic, and at the level of civic organizations were making their way into the couple's home. Anton's identity as a worker, his sense of masculinity, and his role as a father and breadwinner were being violently dislocated and altered in the process. In 1986, the state recruited Anton to work for 6 months in the Zone, transporting bags of lead oxide, sand, and gravel to the reactor sight. The bags were airlifted and deposited using helicopters. He had no idea how much radiation he absorbed in those 6 months. From 1991 on, Anton routinely passed through the clinical system and, like any "prospective" invalid, was monitored. His symptoms mounted over time. He had chronic headaches, lost his short-term memory, exhibited antisocial behavior, developed a speech disorder, and experienced seizures and impotence, as well as many other problems. Despite the growing number and intensity of his symptoms, his diagnosis did not "progress" from an initial listing as a "psychosocial" case.

When I met Anton and his wife, Halia, they were trying to manage on a small pension he received as a sufferer. Anton saw himself as bankrupt, morally as well as economically: "The state took my life away. Ripped me off, gone. What to be happy about? An honorable man cannot survive now. For what? For what? We had a life. We had butter. We had milk. I can't buy a clothes iron. Before I could buy fifty irons. The money was there. My wife's salary is less than the cost of one iron." He told me that he didn't know "how to trade goods" or to sell petty goods on the market. Persuaded by his wife, Anton found himself confronting the shameful option of breadwinning with his illness in the Chernobyl compensation system or of facing poverty. Over time, and in a concerted effort to remove his psychosocial label, the couple befriended a leader of a disabled workers' activist group in a clinic. Through him they met a neurologist who knew the director of the local medical-labor committee. The couple hoped this individual would provide support for Anton's (ultimately successful) bid for Chernobyl-related disability.

The economic motives for his actions were clear enough. Yet, it was difficult for me to see this person giving up everything he knew and thought about himself to prove that his diffuse symptoms had an organic basis. Neurology was a key gateway to disability; neurological disorders were most ambiguous but most possible to prove using diagnostic technologies, self-induced symptoms, and bodily display. At each step, Anton was mentally breaking down; he fell into a pattern of domestic violence. His legal–medical gamble—this gaining of life in the new market economy through illness—reflected the practices of an entire citizenry lacking money or the means of generating it. This approach has become a commonsensical survival tactic. Common sense, in Clifford Geertz's formulation, is that which is "left over when all [the] more articulated sorts of symbol systems have exhausted their tasks" (1983:92).

Yet this mode of survival is by no means normal, but part and parcel of a reality of structural violence (Farmer 1999). Lack of health care, limited treatment interventions, and persistent social inequalities that are intensified by social and economic policies have contributed to worldwide epidemics of preventable infectious diseases such as multidrug resistant tuberculosis. In the Ukrainian context, efforts to assess and remediate the Chernobyl aftermath contributed to social indeterminacy and novel formations of power. Suffering—its experiences and interpretations—has been patterned and realized through the interventions that were meant to remediate Chernobyl over time. Citizens, acutely aware of themselves as having lesser prospects for work and health in a market economy, inventoried those elements in their lives (measures, numbers, symptoms) that could connect to a broader history of error, mismanagement, and risk. The tighter the connections that could be drawn, the greater the probability of economic and social entitlement—at least in the short term. Sufferers were aware of the way "politics shapes what they know and don't know" (Proctor 1995:7) about their illnesses, and that they are willing to exploit these politics to limit further assaults on their well-being, which they see as resulting from a collapsing state health system and loss of adequate legal protections.

Informal economies of knowledge, codified symptoms, differential medical access, a continuum of diagnoses, and "Chernobyl ties" were mobilized and began to function as institutions in parallel with the state's official legal social protection system. These new resources functioned more like advances of credit, ensuring social protections in the uncertain future for people whose temporal horizons were short. The deep intrusion of illness into personal lives fostered a type of violence that went beyond the line of what could be policed. There was no place that provided natural immunity from these unnatural and technical forces. This state of unprotectedness constituted a baseline from which people were refashioning themselves as persons to be protected in the new sociopolitical environment in which they now lived.

Conclusion

The lives of Chernobyl-affected populations are interwoven with the Soviet Union's collapse and the harsh political–economic restructuring that followed. Their collective experiences do not lend themselves to easy psychological labeling. Nor can they be reduced to assessments of isolated individuals' perceptions or related to some optimal mode of social adaptation. Yet, scientific agencies continue to promulgate the idea that the health effects of Chernobyl are primarily psychological in nature. A recent report states that the public health effects "were not nearly as substantial as had at first been feared." It notes "persistent myths," "misperceptions" and a "'paralyzing fatalism' among residents of affected areas."[12] These psychological interpretations can easily obscure the political contexts in which such apparent fatalism took shape. As Dr. Ilya Likhtarev, a leading Ukrainian radiation specialist, told me in 1997, "We have learned that tragedy is not defined by the numbers who have died." He suggested that the "truth" of Chernobyl was much more somber than what numbers can say.

As I have shown here and in my book, *Life Exposed* (2002), public health policies in both the Soviet and post-Soviet period turned the Chernobyl aftermath into a complex political and social experience with its own bureaucratic and legal contours. The cumulative impact of these policies is that the claims and social suffering continue among affected individuals and groups. Some might be tempted to link this trend to a paralyzing fatalism. I call it biological citizenship. Mediated by scientific research centers, public health bureaucracies, and activist organizations, it is a massive demand for, but selective access to, a form of social welfare based on scientific and legal criteria that acknowledges injury and compensates for it. To engage this form of citizenship, sufferers manipulated those elements in their lives that could link their diseases to a history of error, mismanagement, and risk, and that could afford them a probability of short term economic and social entitlement. These dynamics of survival produced their own spiraling effects, disrupting family lives, creating senses of injustice and insecurity, and shaping individual life chances and interpersonal and political negotiations.

The Chernobyl aftermath is by no means a phenomenon that is confined to the past or interpretable as mere psychological trauma. Indeed, public health experts have defined and quantified the aftermath via specialized scientific fields; but their isolated facts have obscured its more general dimensions. Anthropologists need to study the public health aspects linked to disasters from a holistic standpoint. That is, they need to analyze how people incorporate scientific facts, even in their partiality, into an everyday struggle for life—conveyed here as a complex and often painful interplay between technical visions for handling the accident's effects and lived individual and social disturbances. Such an approach would better account for the experiences of afflicted populations on their own terms. It would also call to account how policymakers, through their actions and decisions, have molded these experiences over time, for better and for worse. Health in this context cannot simply be a matter of "adapting healthier lifestyles" in contaminated zones.[13] It is a product of history as well as a contested way of being in the world.

Acknowledgments

I am grateful to Marcia Inhorn, Robert Hahn, and João Biehl for their insights and commentaries on this essay, which was adapted from my book, *Life Exposed: Biological Citizens after Chernobyl* (2002).

Notes

1. See Sich 1996. With these and all other compounding factors, "estimates of the long-term health consequences of the Chernobyl accident are uncertain even as to the order of magnitude" (von Hippel 1991:235; also see von Hippel 2000).

2. Thirteen thousand children in affected regions absorbed a radiation dose to the thyroid of more than twice the maximum allowable dose for nuclear workers for an entire year. See Shcherbak 1996.

3. Iodine pills raise the amount of iodide in the bloodstream so that the thyroid cannot absorb more. The radioactive iodine to which a person is exposed is excreted in the urine.

4. This figure was recently revised to 56 fatalities attributable to the disaster.

5. Estimates vary from 600,000 to 800,000. These workers were recruited from all over the Soviet Union. But the labor pool drew most heavily from Ukrainian and Russian populations.

6. Such values are calculated on the basis of "rem-expenditures" workers absorb; their amounts are limited by international standards. Despite the existence of such standards, norms of worker exposures are being decided locally and within the constraints of local economies that "undervalue" workers' lives by overexposing them to more risk for less pay.

7. Social suffering "results from what political, economic, and institutional power does to people, and, reciprocally, from how these forms of power themselves influence responses to social problems" (Kleinman, Das, and Lock 1996:xi).

8. In 2005, a UN report wrote, "Apart from the dramatic increase in thyroid cancer incidence among those exposed at a young age, there is no clearly demonstrated increase in the incidence of solid cancers or leukemia due to radiation in the most affected populations" (Chernobyl Forum 2005:7).

9. Symptoms of acute radiation sickness begin at 200 rem. At 400 rem, bone marrow failure sets in. Lethal dose (LD_{100}) is a dose exposure that causes 100% of the death of cells or death of the human. $LD_{50/30}$ is a dose exposure that causes 50% of the death of cells or the human being within 30 days.

10. In my interviews I heard about instances of workers mimicking symptoms of ARS (vomiting, for example). This indicates the level of desperation on the part of some of them to receive permission to leave the zone.

11. On *blat*, see Ledeneva 1998.

12. See Chernobyl: the true scale of the accident. 20 Years Later a UN Report Provides Definitive Answers and Ways to Repair Lives. http://www.who.int/mediacentre/news/releases/2005/pr38/en/index.html downloaded November 1, 2007. Information draws from findings of the report "Chernobyl's Legacy: Health, Environmental and Socio-Economic Impacts," released by the UN Chernobyl Forum's Health Effects of the Chernobyl Accident and Special Health Care Programmes. Geneva: WHO 2006.

13. Ibid.

References

Bromet, Evelyn J, Havenaar, Johan M (2007) Psychological and perceived health effects of the Chernobyl disaster: A 20-year review. *Health Physics* 93(5):516–521.

Cardis Elisabeth, Geoffrey Howe, Elaine Ron, Vladimir Bebeshko, Tetyana Bogdanova, Andre Bouville, et al. (2006) Cancer consequences of the Chernobyl accident: 20 years on. *Journal of Radiological Protection* 26:127–140.

Chernobyl Forum (2005) Chernobyl's legacy health, environmental and socio-economic impacts. www.iaea.org/Publications/Booklets/Chernobyl/chernobyl.pdf

Chernobyl's legacy to science (1996) *Nature* 380:653.

Das V (1995) *Critical Events: An Anthropological Perspective on Contemporary India.* New York: Oxford University Press.

Drottz-Sjoberg BM (1995) "Risk Perception Research and Disaster." In: *Mental Health Consequences of the Chernobyl Disaster: Current State and Future Prospects.* K Loganovsky, K Yuriev, eds. Kyiv: Physicians of Chernobyl.

Dubrova YE, Nesterov VN, Krouchinsky NG, Ostapenko VA, Neumann R, Neil DL et al. (1996) Human minisatellite rate after the Chernobyl accident. *Nature* 380:683–686.

Farmer P (1999) *Infections and Inequalities: The Modern Plagues.* Berkeley, CA: University of California Press.

Geertz C (1983) *Local Knowledge: Further Essays in Interpretive Anthropology.* New York: Basic Books.

Gofman J (1981) *Radiation and Human Health.* San Francisco: Sierra Club Books.

Gordon C (1991) "Government Rationality: An Introduction." In: *The Foucault Effect: Studies in Governmentality.* G Burchell, C Gordon, and P Miller, eds. Chicago, IL: University of Chicago Press, pp. 1–52.

Graham L (1998) *What Have We Learned about Science and Technology from the Russian Experience?* Stanford, CA: Stanford University Press.

Guskova A (1995) "Radiation and the Brain." In: *Mental Health Consequences of the Chernobyl Disaster: Current State and Future Prospects.* K Loganovsky, K Yuriev, eds. Kyiv: Physicians of Chernobyl.

International Atomic Energy Agency (IAEA) (1986) Soviet State Committee on the Utilization of Atomic Energy, Report to the IAEA. Vienna: IAEA.

International Atomic Energy Agency (1991a) The International Chernobyl Project: Assessment of Radiological Consequences and Evaluation of Protective Measures. Report by an International Advisory Committee, Vienna.

International Atomic Energy Agency (1991b) The International Chernobyl Project: Proceedings of an International Conference, Vienna.

International Atomic Energy Agency (1996) *One Decade After Chernobyl: Summing Up the Consequences of the Accident.* Lanham, MD: Bernan Associates.

Kesminiene A, Cardis E (2007) Cancer epidemiology after the Chernobyl accident. *Bulletin du Cancer* 94(5):423–430.

Kleinman A, Das, V, Lock, M (1996) Introduction. *Daedalus* 125(1):xi–xx.

Lazjuk GI, Nikolaev DI, Khmel RD (2000) Epidemiology of Congenital Malformations in Belarus and the Chernobyl Accident. *American Journal of Human Genetics* 67(4):214.

Ledeneva A (1998) *Russia's Economy of Favours: Blat, Networking, and Informal Exchange.* Cambridge, UK: Cambridge University Press.

Medvedev Z (1990) *The Legacy of Chernobyl.* New York: WW Norton.

Noshchenko AG, Zamostyan PV, Bondar OY, Drozdova VD (2002) Radiation-induced leukemia risk among those aged 0–20 at the time of the Chernobyl accident: A case-control study in the Ukraine. *International Journal of Cancer* 99: 609–18.

Pearce F (2000) Chernobyl: The political fall-out continues. *UNESCO Courier,* October 10.

Petryna A (2002) *Life Exposed: Biological Citizens After Chernobyl.* Princeton, NJ: Princeton University Press.

Pierce DA, Shimizu Y, Preston DL, Vaeth M, Mabuchi K (1996) Studies of the mortality of atomic bomb survivors. *Radiation Research* 146:1–27.

Pilinskaya MA (1999) Cytogenetic effects in somatic cells of Chernobyl accident survivors as bio-marker of low radiation doses exposure. *International Journal of Radiation Medicine* 2(2):83–95.

Pilinskaya MA, Dibskiy CC (2000) The frequency of chromosome exchanges in critical groups of Chernobyl accident victims. *International Journal of Radiation Medicine* 1(5):83–95.

Proctor R (1995) *Cancer Wars: How Politics Shapes What We Know and Don't Know about Cancer.* New York: Basic Books.

Prysyazhnyuk AY Gristchenko V, Gulak L, Fedorenko Z, Fuzik M (1999) Epidemiological study of cancer in population affected after the Chernobyl accident: Results, problems, perspectives. *International Journal of Radiation Medicine* 2(2):42–50.

Prysyazhnyuk AY, Gristchenko V, Fedorenko Z, Gulak L, Fuzik M, Slipenyuk K et al. (2007) Twenty years after the Chernobyl accident: Solid cancer incidence in various groups of the Ukrainian population. *Radiation and Environmental Biophysics* 46(1):43–51.

Rumiantseva GM (1996) "Dynamics of Social-Psychological Consequences Ten Years after Chernobyl." In: *The Radiological Consequences of the Chernobyl Accident.* Brussels: European Commission, pp. 529–535.

Sergeev GV (1988) Mediko-Sanitarnye Meropriiatiia po Likvidatsii Posledstvii Avarii na Chernobyl'skoi Atomnoi Elektrostantsii. In: *Meditsinskii Aspekti Avarii na Chernobyl'skoi AES.* Kyiv: Zdorov'ia, pp. 15–26.

Shapin S, Schaffer S (1985) *Leviathan and the Air-Pump: Hobbes, Boyle, and the Experimental Life.* Princeton, NJ: Princeton University Press.

Shcherbak Y (1996) Ten years of the Chernobyl era. *Scientific American* April:45–49.

Sich A (1996) The denial syndrome. *Bulletin of Atomic Scientists* 52(3):38–40.

Stone R (2001) Living in the shadow of Chernobyl. *Science* 292(5376):420–424.

UN Chernobyl Forum (2006) *Health Effects of the Chernobyl Accident and Special Health Care Programmes.* Geneva: WHO.

USSR State Committee on the Utilization of Atomic Energy (1986) The Accident at the Chernobyl Nuclear Power Plant and its Consequences. Information compiled for the IAEA Expert's Meeting, August 25–29, 1986, Vienna. Working Document for the Post-Accident Review Meeting.

Von Hippel F (1991) *Citizen Scientist.* New York: American Institute of Physics.

Von Hippel F (2000) "Radiation risk and ethics": Health hazards, prevention costs, and radiophobia. *Physics Today* April:11.

World Health Organization (1996) *Health Consequences of the Chernobyl Accident. Results of the IPHECA Pilot Projects and Related National Programmes.* Geneva: WHO.

23

An Ethnographic Evaluation of Post-Alma Ata Health System Reforms in Mongolia: Lessons for Addressing Health Inequities in Poor Communities

CRAIG R. JANES

Introduction

Observers of global health-care reform identify 3 waves of activity: post-World War II (WWII) vertical disease control and eradication, coupled with investment in urban, tertiary care hospitals; the "health for all" revolution launched at Alma Ata in 1978, which brought comprehensive, community-oriented primary care to the fore; and the 1980s and 1990s push to bring models of economic rationality and evidence-based medicine to bear on health reform, resulting in the transformation of comprehensive primary care in the control of communities to selective care in control of experts. Throughout these 3 waves, attention to fundamental ethical and moral issues have waxed and waned. Immediate postwar disease control activities were undoubtedly motivated by beneficence and a sense of obligation to address the serious burden of disease in the newly emerging states of the global South. Health care outside of the major urban, tertiary care centers was often provided by missionary relief organizations (Litsios 2002, 2004). The Health for All movement proceeded from an emerging commitment to social justice, health as a human right, and a challenge to biomedical authority (Cueto 2004). These principles were largely eclipsed by the ascendancy of economic rationality as the driving conceptual framework of health reform (Janes 2004).

A new millennium has brought global health scholars and advocates to the brink of a fourth wave of health reform, where a growing movement to define global health ethics has reintroduced principles of equity and fairness into the organization of health care services (Gwatkin 2000, 2001; Kickbush 2004; Kickbush and Buse 2001; Roberts, Hsiao, Berman, and Reich 2004). The challenge facing reformers today is the lack of a strong evidence base concerning what kinds of intervention options work for reaching the poor. While epidemiologic and macrolevel health system researchers can contribute to building this evidence base, it seems clear that the most relevant and useful evaluation of such interventions must occur at the level where users interact with the health care system. Anthropologists, who typically work at this critical interface, are particularly well positioned to contribute to the fourth wave of health reform.

In this chapter, I discuss the conceptual and organizational foundations of late twentieth and early twenty-first century health reforms, identifying what I consider the key questions for further research and analysis. I then apply these questions to the consideration of a particularly apt case study of health reform: the introduction of World Bank scripted third-wave reforms to post-socialist Mongolia in the 1990s (Janes, Chuluundorj, Hilliard, Rak, and Janchiv 2005). This case study shows how the organizational features of efficiency-driven reform come into conflict with principles of equity and fairness. The study also suggests intervention options that would substantially improve the system's ability to effectively reach the most vulnerable and poor. I conclude by drawing lessons for countries in the global South that are currently struggling with the social consequences of third-wave reform.

Health System Reforms: A Brief History

The Origins of Primary Health Care

In the immediate post-WWII era, health care was mainly provided in the context of large urban hospitals, with sizeable sectors of the rural population deprived of access entirely (World Health Organization 2000). This system, characterized by Halfdan Mahler, Director General of the World Health Organization (WHO) from 1973 to 1988, as one based on expensive and largely inaccessible "disease palaces," gave way to one of the more revolutionary movements in global health: the introduction of universal, comprehensive primary care as a pillar of global attempts to bring "health for all" by the end of the twentieth century.

Origins of the universal approach to comprehensive primary care had many antecedents, and the road to Alma Ata, where the agreement on the primary care was finally concluded in 1978, was not easily traversed (Litsios 2002). Cueto (2004) links the Alma Ata declaration to a coalescence of 4 disparate influences: the failure of vertical programs and the misallocation of health funds to expensive and cost-inefficient tertiary care hospitals; mounting critiques of biomedicine and the rise of the "new" public health paradigm, which advanced a perspective that emphasized the multilevel determinants of health; the leadership of Halfdan Mahler, who many consider to be a dynamic and charismatic leader who espoused communitarian and social justice approaches to the provision of health services; and the existence of successful models of rural primary care in several resource-poor settings. Chief among these was the success of China's rural reform movement, based on community health workers ("barefoot doctors") and local financing (Sidel 1972). Politically, the emergence of newly independent nations, especially in Africa, fostered an environment conducive to more community-based and less technically oriented solutions.

The cornerstone of primary health care as it was conceived at Alma Ata was its explicit orientation to accessible, affordable, and technologically appropriate care, including curative as well as preventive services (World Health Organization 2000). Its orientation to community also represented opposition to biomedical elitism (Cueto 2004). Well in advance of the World Bank's later movement into the health sector (World Bank 1993) and report of the Macroeconomic Commission on Health (Commission on Macroeconomics and Health 2001), the Alma Ata declaration also advanced the argument that population health was an important determinant of economic development (Cueto 2004).

A central theme in the Alma Ata declaration was the focus on health care in the context of community participation and development (Rifkin and Walt 1986). Although the technical and allocative inefficiencies[1] of comprehensive primary health care emerged as significant problems shortly after it was introduced, community participation and the challenge to biomedical authority inherent to the model have remained underappreciated and to some degree forgotten strengths of the approach. Certainly it was a theme that attracted the interest of anthropologists, who, among the social and health scientists working in international health, were most likely to engage with grassroots development. Several key volumes and essays written by anthropologists over the past 2 decades engage critically the concept of community development and participation, especially in the context of local, national, and global political–economic processes (Coreil and Mull 1990; Janes 2004; Morgan 1990, 2001; Nichter and Nichter 1996). Current writers suggest that the grassroots orientation of primary health care remains one of its chief, unheralded, and often overlooked contributions to health development, and is essential to delivering accessible and effective health care, especially in rural areas (Atkinson et al. 1999; Fritzen 2007; Petersen and Swartz 2002). Writing about the importance of community-based approaches to HIV/AIDS prevention and treatment, Petersen and Swartz (2002:1011) observe that "measurable technical interventions should not be at the expense of an empowering, developmental approach to care at the primary level ...."

Challenges to Comprehensive Primary Health Care

Almost immediately after it was launched the primary care initiative became the focus of critical review by several scholars, foundations, and institutions. A highly influential review of primary health care published in the *New England Journal of Medicine* in 1979 by Kenneth Warren and Julia Walsh laid out an alternative, interim strategy to primary care which, instead of focusing broadly on basic health services at the community level, argued for a focus instead on those conditions leading to the greatest levels of preventable mortality and morbidity (Walsh and Warren 1979). Glossed as "selective primary care," the approach involved the provision of a low-cost package of health services, intended primarily for mothers and children, and including most notably the well-known "GOBI" interventions: growth monitoring, oral rehydration therapy, breast-feeding, and immunization (later this was expanded to "GOBI-FF" with the addition of family planning and food supplementation) (Mull 1990).

Selective care was immediately touted as an alternative or interim strategy to achieving fully comprehensive primary health care in low-income settings. As comprehensive primary health care was developed in several countries it became apparent, especially to international donors desiring a decent health return for their investments, that the selective approach had much to recommend it. Comprehensive primary health-care programs were often inadequately funded, staffed, organized, and managed, leading to the observation by many critics that it should be termed "primitive" rather than "primary" health care (World Health Organization 2000). Inadequate funding of these programs was in part due to the continuing preference on the part of international donors to fund specific, vertical interventions, or interventions that would produce measurable health outcomes over short-term project cycles (Petersen and Swartz 2002). Program design aside, a more significant cause of the demise of community-based primary health care was the global debt crisis of the 1980s, structural adjustment, and the push by international institutions, especially the World Bank, for market-oriented reforms to health and social service systems more generally (Castro and Singer 2004; Janes 2004; Kickbush and Buse 2001; Walt, Pavignani, Gilson, and Buse 1999; Whiteford and Nixon 2000; Zwi and Yach 2002).

Third-Generation Reforms: The "New" Universalism

The selective approach to primary health care is the foundation for what the WHO in its 2000 report on health systems refers to as the "new universalism." The new universalism involves provision of an essential, but restricted, package of health services to all. The guiding blueprint for this vision of health care is the World Bank's 1993 *World Development Report*, subtitled *Investing in Health*. Through a careful cost–utility analysis of interventions, the Bank built a case for investing resources in the most cost-effective and thus "essential" packages of primary health care and public health interventions. The Bank further argued that direct government provision of services is inefficient, and advocated a role for the government that is principally regulatory: applying policy instruments to provide and regulate insurance, social or private, stimulate competition, and permit privatization.

It is not possible to overemphasize the importance of this document. It represents a watershed in global health policy and marks the ascent of the World Bank as one of the major, if not primary, actors in global health, clearly eclipsing the WHO by the end of the millennium (Abbasi 1999). The advocacy for a public guarantee of a package of essential clinical and public health services, delivered outside direct government control, and the stimulation of the private sector for provision of nonessential services represented the final death knell for comprehensive primary care as envisioned by the framers at Alma Ata. It also marked the ascendancy of the "third generation" of health reform (World Health Organization 2000). Nearly all reports on health reform or health system performance published since 1993 employ some version of the cost–efficiency analysis developed in the World Development Report, or accept the logic that the role of the public sector in health provision is through the guarantee of a selective package of "essential" services.

Bringing Ethics to Health-Care Reform

From the late 1990s there has been growing concern that third-wave reforms, by virtue of their foundation in cost–efficiency analysis, market fundamentalism, and reduced role of the state in providing services, would lead to serious inequities in access to health care. Recent studies suggest that the new universalism tends to increase choices and access for those who can pay, while reducing access to the most poor and vulnerable, suggesting a need for a new wave of equity-oriented health reforms (Gwatkin 2001). The principle of equity as it is used in these studies is defined as the fair allocation of health-care resources according to need, according to ability to pay, and in recognition of the potentially devastating effects of catastrophic illness in the most poor and vulnerable (Janes et al. 2005).

Growing concern over fairness, equity, and social justice in global health has resulted in a more forthright and explicit application of normative ethical theory to health system reform (Roberts and Reich 2002; Roberts et al. 2004). This exercise highlights the degree to which health reform has been operationalized with little if any reference to ethics, leaving moral concerns implicit and/or unaddressed. Roberts and colleagues (2004), in their important how-to book on health system reform, argue that reformers typically apply utilitarian, liberal, or communitarian ethics. According to them (Roberts et al. 2004), modern "objective" utilitarianism rests on an assumption that individual choices are unreliable, and argues instead for judgments to be made by experts. The development and application of the Disability Adjusted Life Years (DALY) framework in cost–utility analyses conducted by the World Bank and others is a good example of this approach. The main problem with the utilitarian approach is that it sacrifices the needs of individuals for outcomes measured at the population level—inevitably some groups become means for others' ends. Rational in economic terms (though not necessarily in the eyes of specific groups or communities), utilitarianism may be ruthless in its goal of producing the largest gain for the available resources. Writes Roberts and colleagues (2004:48), "Utilitarian policymakers can disregard patients who are too expensive to save, and can sacrifice the few for the sake of the many. Following utilitarian logic, passengers who are starving on a lifeboat could kill and eat a few of their fellows, provided the gains exceed the losses." Given this inherent logic of utilitarianism, it is not surprising that efficiency-driven reform has been found to produce inequitable outcomes.

The main alternative to utilitarianism is liberalism. Rooted historically in the philosophy of Kant, modern "egalitarian" liberals argue that individuals have the right to make their own decisions as to how to live. Key to the liberal argument is the idea of rights or "claims that individuals can make on each other by virtue of their humanity" (Roberts et al. 2004:49). To many liberals who argue from a social justice perspective, everyone is considered to have a right to the minimum level of resources needed to exercise meaningful life choices. This argument implies redistribution of resources so as to ensure that each individual has an opportunity for making the choices that would lead to a meaningful life, including choices to use health care. Liberalism is thus inherently oriented to judgments about fairness in the distribution of resources, and is the underlying principle of health services in many of the modern welfare states.

Whereas liberalism and utilitarianism describe universal frameworks—that there should be a single moral standard framework that applies to all societies—those who ascribe to a communitarian framework, particularly as informed by cultural relativism, recognize the contingent nature of ethics and morality. Consistent with the anthropological perspective, communitarians privilege local theories about what constitutes a good society, an acceptable level and kind of service, and the core functions of public health within a community (i.e., is tobacco use ethically objectionable in a health conscious society, or is it an individual choice?). Ideas about fairness and equity would, according to this perspective, require contextualization in terms of local cultural traditions, beliefs, and values.

In reality, researchers and policymakers, even when making their ethical assumptions explicit, tend to blend the different ethical frameworks, depending on their goals and research orientation. Many, if not most, in public health subscribe to a rights-based liberal approach to health care (e.g., fairness dictates that everyone in a society with the same need should have access to the same level of services), but might also apply a utilitarian framework to issues of population health policy (e.g., legal measures to constrain accessibility of tobacco and alcohol). Most liberals would also ascribe to the idea that there may be some variability, depending on cultural context, in what constitutes fundamental rights. Anthropologists, who may find relativist perspectives on morality to be more consistent with their focus on local, lived experience, also recognize the limits of relativism. Most will apply relativism as a theoretical perspective and research orientation rather than as a strict moral principle in terms of advocating policy. Despite such mixing of perspectives, and a tendency for ethics to remain implicit in policy, recognition of the normative foundations of health reform has an important consequence for research and practice: it helps identify points at which inequities or injustices might emerge—for example, in the de facto rationing of health care, or in the decisions made to resolve the conflict between public health and individual choice. In other words, it helps guide research into the consequences of health care reform.

Gwatkin (2001:722), in acknowledging the poor equity performance of modern health sector reform, suggests a need for "deeper" reforms. However, a significant barrier to implementing such reforms is a relative lack of evidence concerning the equity consequences of particular interventions. He writes:

> The work to date has produced significant increases in knowledge about the magnitude and nature of health inequalities, and has resulted in valuable conceptual frameworks for approaching these issues. But it has not yet reached the heart of the matter; the identification of measures that can effectively deal with the inequalities that have been uncovered.

Gwatkin concludes that new research which has as its main goal the identification and evaluation of specific policy measures is needed before "deeper" reform can proceed. By extension, such research should focus closely on how existing initiatives reach the poor, particularly through examining how the system looks from the perspective of the poor themselves. This was the objective of our study of health reform in Mongolia.

Health Sector Reform and Equity in Post-Socialist Mongolia

Unlike many countries of the global South, before the disintegration of socialism in the early 1990s Mongolia had little experience with Western-led development. From 1921 to 1990 Mongolia was a socialist state linked politically and economically to the former Soviet Union and Eastern European commonwealth. It had applied Soviet and Cuban models to the development of its health care system (the "Semashko" model). This system, though heavily hospital based and inefficient in modern terms, had made substantial improvements to public health by 1990. There were approximately 750 hospital beds and 240 physicians per 100,000 population. Though there were some urban–rural differences in quality and access to care, overall the system was considered to have been highly equitable. Between 1960 and 1990, life expectancy increased from 47 to 63 years (United Nations Development Programme 2000). By 1990, 96% of the population was literate. Women shared equally in these gains; by the end of the socialist era 40% of university graduates were women, and even today, enrollment rates of women at all levels of the educational system exceed rates for men (United Nations Development Programme 2003).

A democratic reform movement developed in the 1980s, resulting in agreement by the ruling party to hold multiparty elections and open up the centrally planned economy to market economic reforms. In the 1990s, Mongolia became something of a "poster country" for capitalist development, subject to the "shock therapy" that was then advocated by the USAID and the Harvard Institute for Economic Development (Griffin 2001; Rossabi 2005). Although touted as a "star pupil of liberal development economics" (Griffin 2001:1), Mongolia was thrown into social chaos and brought to the verge of economic collapse (Janes and Chuluundorj 2004). Sizeable economic subsidies from the former Soviet Union and other Eastern block countries were terminated, contributing to a sharp drop in GDP. Industrial production was curtailed, resulting in high rates of unemployment in urban areas, and for a short time, an unprecedented wave of urban-to-rural migration as poor and desperate urbanites attempted to take up the then more economically secure occupation of livestock herding (Humphrey and Sneath 1999; Griffin 2001). Per capita income declined precipitously over the decade from 1989 to 1999, from US$1,643 to US$374 (in constant 1993 dollars; Government of Mongolia 2000). Although it appears that unemployment rates have now stabilized with the partial recovery of the industrial sector and the growth of a service sector in the capital, economic growth has been disappointing (United Nations Development Programme 2003). Over one-third of the population remains under the government-established poverty line, and the depth and severity of poverty has increased (United Nations Development Programme 2003).

Economic reforms were coupled with reforms to government: over objections of the democratic reformers who led the transition in the 1990s, Mongolia was forced by external institutions to accept a "weak state" solution, decentralizing and privatizing many of its essential services (Rossabi 2005). Coupled with the loss of Soviet subsidies, which accounted for nearly 30% of GDP, the result of these political and economic reforms was a serious deterioration of rural health and education infrastructures. Doctors and teachers went unpaid, there were shortages of medicines and supplies and even basic food and energy commodities. Many physicians took up herding or left the health service entirely. The former herding and state farm collectives, or *negdel*, which had governed social and economic activities and protected locals from environmental risks and economic shocks, disappeared overnight, generating a large class of rural, vulnerable poor. Sharp increases in maternal mortality, especially in the rural countryside, were one result (Janes and Chuluundorj 2004).

Recovery of the health services from the shocks of the early 1990s has only been partial and enabled primarily by the investment of considerable external financing from the Asian Development Bank (ADB). The ADB has now completed two waves of health sector reform focusing on the following five goals: development of an essential services package of primary health services; downsizing secondary and tertiary care hospitals; increasing private sector participation in health-care provision; "rationalizing" of health personnel by controlling the kind and number of providers trained; and introduction of a new payment scheme, based on a mix of fee-for-service and risk-adjusted capitation, to support growth of the private sector in health care (ADB 2002). To pave the way for ADB reforms, the government of Mongolia formally adopted a primary health care strategy as the core of its health system, legislating universal access by all citizens to primary care services. A single-payer national health insurance system, based on the European social insurance model, was established in 1994. Various policy changes have been made to the social insurance fund over the years to protect so-called vulnerable subgroups (e.g., pregnant women and minor children). To date, health reform has not entirely erased the Soviet-style Semashko system,[2] which is still very much in evidence in rural areas, at the hospital level, and in the ways in which payments are made to primary health care providers (World Bank 2007). But there have been several key changes to the system.

First, despite a continued reliance on hospital-based care, Mongolia has built an impressive system of primary health-care centers in its cities and provincial capitals, now covering about two-thirds of the population. The system, similar to the general practice system in the United Kingdom, provides care through a network of family physicians. These physicians are organized into small practices comprised of 2-to-4 physicians and 1-to-2 nurses. Each practice is responsible for providing care to a specified catchment area or community ranging in population from 1,200 to 1,500 people. At present there are a total of 238 group practices with 835 doctors and 762 nurses (World Bank 2007). Each practice is considered a private entity, funded by capitation-based contracts with local government. Capitation payments are adjusted to provide an incentive for serving the poor: for each poor person a family practice receives 3,200 Mongolian togrogs (about US$3) per year, and for each nonpoor person, the practice receives 2,300 Mongolian togrogs (about US$2 per year). Ideally, the family doctor provides essential clinical services to its community, concentrating on care for women and children, some minor acute care services, and long-term care for the chronically ill. The family doctor also serves as a source of referrals to and gatekeeper for secondary levels of care which are provided by district or provincial hospitals. Family physicians have access to only simple diagnostic tools and though they can prescribe drugs which are partly subsidized by the social insurance fund they cannot provide any other than emergency drugs directly to their patients.

Second, stimulation of the private sector through changes to legislation and financing has resulted in an explosion of private hospitals and clinics. There are now over 500 registered private health care organizations, and the number is growing rapidly. Many are small clinics, often with a few beds, offering specialty services. Private obstetrics-gynecology and traditional medicine clinics are greatest in number (Janes and Hilliard 2008). Registered private organizations are able to bill the social insurance for services rendered, though they also charge sometimes substantial copayments or user fees. In addition, public hospitals are moving increasingly toward a private model (contracting out services, management functions, etc.). There is substantial concern that without some regulation, the private system will soon be out of control, siphoning off scarce funds and personnel from the public and primary care systems. Even the World Bank warns of impending chaos, suggesting that privatization will result in a 2-tiered system: high-quality private care for the middle income and above and low-quality care for the poor (World Bank 2007).

Third, the introduction of social insurance and the expansion of the primary care system has changed the way that health care is provided and paid for. Depending on one's status, the social insurance fund covers only a portion of expenses at private clinics, and tertiary and secondary care settings.[3] While primary care is universally accessible and free to the user, referral out of the primary care sector may impose significant financial burdens and opportunity costs on the poor. Lack of integration of primary care with other levels of care further sharpens this divide.

Outside of cities and provincial capitals health reform has not made any significant inroads into the poorly staffed and supplied rural sector. Many doctors and nurses have left service, either retiring or moving to towns or cities where salaries are higher and working conditions are perceived to be better. At present, county-level health care is provided in the context of a *soum* or county clinic, typically an 8-to-10 bed facility staffed by one or more physicians and support staff. Each clinic serves a population of between 2,000 and 3,000 individuals. The clinic is funded from the county budget and by the social insurance fund, and authority for overseeing the clinic has been largely decentralized to county administrators. Each county also manages a revolving drug fund.[4] County clinics include on staff several community health workers, or *feldshers*, who provide very basic care primarily to herding families in the more remote areas. The third phase of health reform in Mongolia is intended to enhance the quality of rural health care, particularly in strengthening the role of the *feldshers*.

Research Setting and Methodology

In the research my colleagues and I have undertaken in Mongolia, we have been most concerned with understanding how the economic and political transition described above has affected rural communities and the poor (Janes 2004; Janes and Chuluundorj 2004; Janes and Hilliard 2008; Janes et al. 2005). Our interest in understanding the impact of health reform began with our analysis of health system collapse and its impact on maternal mortality (Janes and Chuluundorj 2004). We have also examined the development of traditional Mongolian medicine (Janes and Hilliard 2008), and are currently conducting a study of factors affecting vulnerability among rural herders (Janes in Press). Most relevant to this chapter is a project we conducted between 2002 and 2004 at the height of the implementation of the family group practice experiment. Our main research questions focused on identifying those processes that affected access to health care from the perspective of communities, emphasizing the experiences of the urban poor (Janes et al. 2005). Our focus was on assessing whether third-generation reforms, ostensibly designed according to the guidelines of the "new universalism," produced equity in funding and access. As we operationalized it, equity in the distribution of health care was defined on the basis of 3 socioeconomic processes: (1) fair mobilization of resources to pay for everyone's health care (often termed "vertical" equity); (2) fair needs-based distribution of health services—in terms of access, quality, and type of care (those with equal needs, and of equal status receive equal services; that is, "horizontal" equity); and (3) fair protection afforded to individuals and families from the consequences of catastrophic illness (Hsiao and Liu 2001).

During the summer and early fall months of 2002, and during June and July in 2004, we engaged in a mixed method and multilevel study of health reform as it was experienced by individuals and their primary care physicians at the community level. The core methodology of the study was a survey of households. The sample was a multistage, cluster-type, random sample of households in low-income suburbs of Ulaanbaatar, and in 2 rural provinces in northwestern Mongolia (see Figures 23.1 and Figure 23.2). Our goal was not to select a representative sample of all Mongolians but to identify those whose incomes were at the lower end of the income range, and for whom health care costs and access would be expected to be of some concern. We selected a sample of

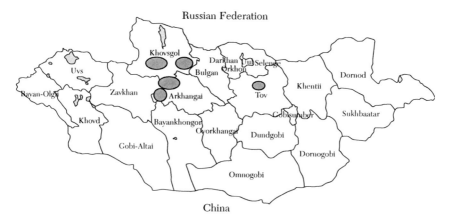

Figure 23.1. Map of Mongolia showing provinces. Shaded ovals indicate research sites.

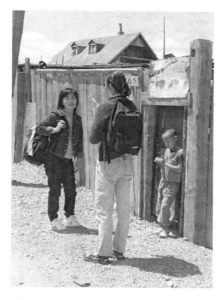

Figure 23.2. Research assistants canvassing urban Mongolian households. (Photo by Kitty K. Corbett)

73 households from 3 districts in periurban Ulaanbaatar. These districts were identified by Mongolian health officials as being comprised of large numbers of poor and vulnerable families. To compare the experience of urban and rural communities we drew a sample of 33 households from 5 counties (counties and

households both selected randomly) in 2 rural provinces, and from the provincial capital of a rural province (Khovsgol) where health reform efforts had been ongoing for several years. The total number of households interviewed numbered 106, representing the health and health-seeking experiences of 542 individuals.

In each household we interviewed the male and/or female head, depending on who was present. We asked questions concerning the size and composition of the household, household economics, food security, maternal and child health, reproductive health, and health care utilization, costs, and barriers to access experienced over the past year. Because it is often difficult to reduce the complexities of particular illness episodes to quantifiable categories, particularly if an illness requires multiple visits to different practitioners, we supplemented the quantitative information gathered in the structured household survey with qualitative narratives of illness and resulting attempts at treatment. In these narratives, individuals told us the "story" of an illness episode up to the time of the interview. We prompted for specific experiences concerning access, cost, as well as reflections on the quality of care received.

To understand health reform from the perspective of those in the healthcare system itself we interviewed and observed practitioners and policymakers from all levels of the health system in Mongolia. Data collection activities included the following: (1) 2 focus groups ($N = 8$ in each group) with family doctors from the study districts of Ulaanbaatar; (2) interviews of the heads of 3 family group practices in Ulaanbaatar, 2 family group practices in the provincial capital of Khovsgol, and physicians and/or nursing staff from each of the 5 rural county (*soum*) level clinics we visited in Khovsgol and Arkhangai provinces; (3) interviews of 58 practitioners in secondary/tertiary inpatient hospitals in Ulaanbaatar and the provincial capital of Khovsgol; and (4) observations of clinical treatment in 5 family group practices: 3 in Ulaanbaatar, and 2 in Khovsgol. Data on access to health care were also collected from secondary sources, mainly agencies of the Mongolia Ministry of Health.

Quantitative Findings

Figure 23.2, based on official Ministry of Health data, indicates variability in inpatient hospitalization by socioeconomic status. Figures 23.3, 23.4, and 23.5 drawn from analysis of the quantitative portion of our interview study, show that perceived barriers to care and amount of household income paid for care also varies by socioeconomic status. Most affected are the poorest of the poor, which in our study are defined as those below the poverty line who report food insecurity.[5] Between 30% and 43% of those below the poverty line reported that they failed to follow health care advice or delayed seeking care because

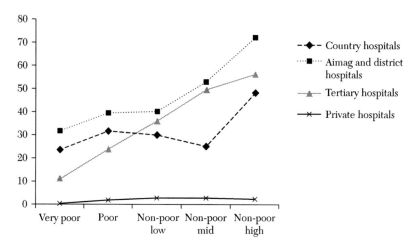

Figure 23.3. Hospital admissions by socioeconomic status, Mongolia, 2004.
Source: Mongolia Ministry of Health.

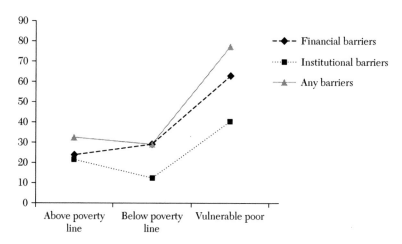

Figure 23.4. Percent in income category reporting barriers to health care versus households reporting illness in the last year.

of financial concerns. Between 19% and 25% of those in the poor categories reported that health care costs had threatened the economic security of their households (Janes et al. 2005:17).

Multiple logistic regression was used to evaluate the relative contribution of poverty, rural or urban residence, and other social and economic indicators to barriers and their consequences (Janes et al. 2005). After adjusting for household size, residence, education, age, and gender of the household head, those in the vulnerable poor category were about 4 to 11 times more likely to

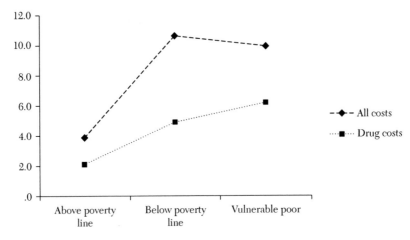

Figure 23.5. Percent of household per capita income spent on health care versus households reporting illness in the last year.

report financial and institutional barriers to access, delaying health care, and a real or anticipated threat to household economic security as a consequence of health care costs.

We concluded from our analyses of the quantitative data that there were substantial organizational and economic barriers that prevented the poor from accessing desired health care services. Indeed, health care reform in Mongolia failed to meet any of our equity criteria: health care costs were not fairly shared, health resources were unfairly distributed in the community, and poor families were especially vulnerable to impoverishment caused by serious illness.

Qualitative and Ethnographic Findings

While the quantitative data clearly indicate that the Mongolian health system fails on several equity criteria, they do not indicate why this is so. Our ethnographic and qualitative evaluation of health care reform, from the perspectives of both community members and health care providers, provides insight into the principal barriers to access. Analysis of this qualitative information points to 4 predominant themes: (1) high costs and overall difficulties associated with what were perceived to be unnecessary referral practices; (2) failure of the primary care system to provide appropriate care for the chronically ill and disabled; (3) problems associated with an increasingly complex and chaotic health system, especially rampant privatization of formerly public services; and (4) difficulties faced by the practitioners themselves, including especially those associated with changing nature of their practice as the more affluent individuals increasingly opt for private care, and the excessive bureaucratization of the hybrid public/private funding model. I address each of these in turn.

First, individuals expressed a great deal of concern regarding the sometimes hidden or unanticipated costs of health care. These costs are of 2 types: opportunity costs associated with loss of time, days off work, and time needed to accompany a sick family member, and indirect costs associated with transportation and related expenses for individuals having to travel to obtain secondary or tertiary care. Indirect costs are of particular concern in rural areas and in cases of catastrophic illness. Both opportunity and indirect costs may be associated with the common practice at the primary care level of excessive referral.

Observation of primary care settings suggested that in the absence of drugs, diagnostic tools, and in many cases appropriate expertise, the family doctor is primarily a referral rather than a treatment resource. In the vast majority of cases we observed in family practice clinics patients were given a slip of paper to take to a provider somewhere else. Because access to secondary and tertiary care services requires health insurance, and usually formal copayments or informal "gifts" to providers, those without health insurance or with little cash are often not able to act on a family doctor's referral.

The social insurance law does contain provisions for waiving copays for "vulnerable" populations, provided that members of these groups have insurance in the first place. However, vulnerability in Mongolia is defined by age (children and the retired) and gender/reproductive status (pregnant women) rather than by poverty status. Although coverage by social insurance has expanded significantly over the past several years, at present the Government of Mongolia reports that about 20% of the population, among which the poor and unemployed are disproportionately represented, are uninsured. These data were consistent with our interview study: 20% of individuals overall were uninsured and about 25% of those in the poorest families were uninsured. Those most likely to be uninsured were males of working age who were unemployed.

In addition to costly referral practices from family doctors to specialists, individuals are often given multiple prescriptions for drugs, which then have to be purchased from private pharmacies. Although drugs on the insurance formulary are subsidized from insurance funds, out-of-pocket payments are always required. In the most resource-poor settings patients are put into the position of deciding how much of what kind of drug to buy resulting in the potentially dangerous misuse of drugs.

This theme of costs associated with referral practices was discussed at length by most of our interviewees, for example:

> Family doctors are too expensive because they always send you somewhere where you have to buy drugs or pay for tests. If their diagnosis is wrong, you've spent money for nothing. (Household head)

Insurance doesn't work, you still have to spend a lot of money. So why buy it at all? (Household head)

Our patients are just too poor to buy the medicines they need. (Family doctor)

Patients without insurance are unable to have diagnostic tests done or to buy medications. They just keep coming back to us, and we keep referring them for things they can't afford. (Family doctor)

Emergency transportation and other indirect health costs are not covered by social insurance. We identified several cases where indirect expenses incurred as a result of catastrophic illness had impoverished whole extended families. As is the case worldwide, health care costs have been identified to be among the top causes of poverty in Mongolia (Mearns 2004; Narayan, Chambers, and Kaul 2000). The case study presented below illustrates this problem.

In addition to the costs associated with referral, patients find the referral practices themselves to be time-consuming, ineffective, and often confusing. Primary care is often insufficiently comprehensive in scope and of suspect quality, requiring expensive referrals to secondary and tertiary-care providers. Except for basic preventive care, individuals with sufficient financial resources will often bypass family doctors and go straight to those who can provide what are perceived to be better or more appropriate services. The following statements are representative:

Family doctors are just a referral service; they can't do anything but send you somewhere else. All they do is refer and prescribe, so it's best to bypass them whenever you can. You might as will go somewhere else directly and save the time. (Household head)

Family doctor services are poor; there isn't much they can do for you except send you somewhere else where you have to pay. I just go directly to a private doctor. (Household head)

The wealthy can easily bypass the family doctor, so why shouldn't the rest of us do this as well? Why shouldn't we go directly to those we know can help us? (Household head)

As a result of deficiencies in the attenuated, essential care model implemented in Mongolia it is clear from the preceding comments that hospitals and private clinics continue as the main providers of primary health care services. The primary care model introduced into Mongolia is, as our respondents observed, a form of attenuated care that provides little service. Because it is the primary, if not only, resource for the poor, there are serious equity consequences.

Second, although family doctors are intended to provide long-term care for those who suffer from chronic illness or disability, their inability to provide drugs or anything other than the most simple of diagnostic tests considerably complicates this task. Long-term use of essential medications was difficult for the poorest patients, where regular expenditures for drugs compete with other household needs. Among the chronically ill in poor households there was a tendency to suspend treatment, or to undertake treatment only when symptoms affected performance of regular activities. Given that in Mongolia infectious diseases are no longer the primary cause of death, with cardiovascular disease, stroke, cancer, hypertension, and diabetes comprising the main health threats, the lack of effective strategies at the primary care level to address such chronic conditions is of serious concern (World Health Organization 2005).

> I only take my blood pressure medication when I have the symptoms (headache, dizziness, blurry vision); I can't afford to buy the medications all the time. (Household head)

> Care of our chronically ill mother has taken nearly all of the income of our entire extended family. This isn't right. (Household head)

Third, many individuals and providers complained about the increasingly confusing health sector in Ulaanbaatar. Rampant privatization and hospital reorganization has made the health system increasingly complex, and it is sometimes unclear to patients until they are presented a bill for payment whether they are in a public or private sector facility. Within many large public hospitals and clinics doctors have opened their own private clinics operating parallel to the public clinics they staff during regular working hours. In some public hospitals even patients with health insurance are asked to pay considerable sums of money out-of-pocket for what should be covered services. As has happened in many similar contexts worldwide, uncontrolled privatization not only makes for an increasingly chaotic and fragmented system, it tends to divert essential resources away from where they are needed most (World Bank 2007):

> Even with insurance the costs of surgery and laboratory tests are too high; there's no way I can afford to pay for it. They told me that it would cost over 100,000 *togrogs* (US$ 100—an "informal payment" to the provider is often required for any surgery) to repair my child's perforated eardrum. (Household head)

> The family doctor kept referring us for x-rays to a private clinic; it turned out this was the clinic of a "friend" she was trying to help. (Household head)

> We were sent from one hospital to the next, spending all of our money in the process. (Household head)

> It's sometimes hard to get good care unless you give "gifts" to the doctor. (Household head)

Fourth, primary health care providers expressed a great deal of frustration over their inability to provide what they considered to be appropriate care. They were frustrated by their lack of access to drugs and diagnostic resources. In this regard, providers also recognized that access to medical care had increasingly become differentiated by social privilege. Thus, the patients who needed drugs or diagnostic services the most—the poor and uninsured—were precisely those for whom they could do the least. They knew that their referrals would mostly go unheeded, and their prescriptions unfilled or only partially filled. Cynicism, declining morale, and frustration were compounded by inefficiencies in the quasi-private payment system. Bureaucratic issues, partial payments, and heavy-handed financial "discipline" of family doctors by district bureaucrats resulted in partial and delayed salary payments. Salaries to family doctors have turned out to be rather low, much less than they can make in the private sector, and there is now serious concern with the long-term sustainability of the system (World Bank 2007):

> We believe we must provide care to all of the poor people in our district, but they are usually not insured and don't have the money to buy medicines. (Family doctor)
>
> Our middle class patients just ignore us; they go to private doctors. We provide care only for the poor. (Family doctor)
>
> We are not reimbursed for providing care to unregistered people (usually new immigrants from the rural countryside), but for moral and ethical reasons we must provide them services. (Family doctor)
>
> The district administration cuts our funds for inappropriate reasons, and without warning or notice. (Family doctor)
>
> We go weeks, often months, without salary. (Family doctor)

Case Studies

The process through which these interrelated factors produce health inequities are most clearly revealed in the consideration of case studies of families facing serious illness. What follows are 3 vignettes, each illustrating one or more of the themes explicated here.

Case One: Informal Payments and Inequitable Access to Surgical Services

Narantsetseg is a 45-year-old woman who lives with her husband, their 4 children, 1 grandchild, a niece and nephew, and her adult brother. In the month before the interview Narantsetseg had gone to her family doctor complaining of chest pains and uncontrollable anger. The illness prevented her from performing her household duties for about 2 weeks, though her unemployed daughter was able to help out. After listening to her symptoms, the family doctor referred her to the district hospital to see a specialist. He performed an ultrasound, for which she was charged US$5, and told her that she had an enlarged thyroid. She was then referred to an endocrinologist for surgery. Narantseseg did not have insurance at the time, and knowing that surgery would be expensive purchased insurance before seeing the endocrinologist. The insurance cost her a bit more than US$9, which she had to borrow from her sister-in-law. Unfortunately, and despite having her insurance papers, she was asked to pay US$62 in advance. There was no way she could afford this so she has been unable to have the surgery. She is now "just hoping to find money somewhere," maybe from her sister-in-law, but she just does not know. As with many of the people we talked to during the study, Narantseseg likes her family doctor, and appreciates having her close by. However, she also knows that the family doctor can do little for her when her symptoms worsen, and cannot advocate on her behalf when she has to go to specialists, whom she distrusts deeply.

Case Two: The Costs of Privatization

Lutbat is a 48-year-old male who lives alone in a small wooden house in one of the suburbs of Ulaanbaatar. He suffers from a number of chronic illnesses and unhealed injuries. Although Lutbat receives a disability pension and carries health insurance, he has been unable to obtain regular treatment for his conditions. His main complaint is that he cannot afford the treatments that his physicians tell him that he needs.

In 1983, while working Lutbat suffered a back injury that led to partial paralysis below the waist. He was bedridden for 3 years. During this time (the socialist period) he received regular massage and acupuncture treatments at a rehabilitation facility built by the Russians in a rural area near the capital. Lutbat claims that the treatments were very effective and after 3 years of rehabilitation he regained feeling in his legs and was able to walk again, although he still has no feeling below the knees and his gait is awkward. He went back to work this time as an "advisor," avoiding any physical labor. Unfortunately, as was the case with many industries during the post-transition period, in 1996 the company went bankrupt and he was laid off from his job. Given his physical limitations he has been unable to find employment. He was declared disabled by the state in 1997, and receives a regular monthly pension of about US$30. He also receives subsidized health insurance. He regularly sees his family doctor and his insurance fully covers annual visits to several specialists and lab tests. His insurance, however, does not cover all of the costs of prescribed treatment, which in this case consists primarily of massage therapy and acupuncture. These treatments are provided primarily within traditional Mongolian medicine hospitals and clinics, one of the most thoroughly privatized sectors of the health system (Janes and Hilliard 2008). These services are expensive, even with insurance, and Lutbat cannot afford them on his small pension. He has tried for years to no avail to find a doctor or hospital that will take his insurance and waive copayment. He complains that "everything has been privatized." While he likes and respects his family doctor he also acknowledges that she can do very little for him.

Given the limitations to his mobility, Lutbat also has difficulty getting to and from specialty clinics. With help from neighbors he can make it to the bus stop, but getting on and off the often crowded buses is a challenge. In January of 2002 Lutbat dislocated his kneecap falling from a bus. Although he was able to manually relocate it there at the bus stop, he still suffers chronic pain from the injury. He went to his family doctor who referred him to the local trauma hospital, but for some reason not clear to Lutbat they refused to take his insurance and demanded cash payment. This injury has gone untreated. On the advice of a neighbor, he now treats his knee through regular applications of cold, salty tea.

Case Three: The Tragedy of Catastrophic Illness

We interviewed members of a 2-household nomadic herding family in remote rural Khovsgol province. The family consists of a couple in their late 40s, their 2 daughters and 2 sons, the husband of the oldest daughter, and 1 grandchild.

This particular family lost nearly all of their 200 animals in the winter disaster of 2001. Called "*dzud*," these disasters result from heavy snow and/or severe cold which causes animals to starve or freeze to death; it is the major climate risk faced by rural herders in Mongolia. Subsequent to the disaster they were contacted by an international NGO and offered the opportunity to participate in a special restocking program where they would be given "starter herds" over a 3-year period (big animals the first year, smaller animals the next 2 years). These adult animals have to be "repaid"—not in cash but in equivalent animal units—over a 5-year period. They are entitled to keep the "natural increase" of these animals. This is a common strategy for restocking herds in disaster-prone areas and is considered to be sustainable over long periods, although participating households may not be able to manage subsequent risks, like illness, which may affect their ability to repay the initial loan of animals.

About a year after the disaster, the 23-year-old wife of one of the sons of the family developed symptoms of fatigue that became so debilitating that the family rented a car to take her to the local county clinic. The county doctors could not find anything wrong, and so referred her to the provincial hospital. There a blood test showed that she was very anemic: "her blood was clear like water." Diagnosing leukemia, the doctor at the provincial doctor recommended that the young woman be taken immediately to the appropriate tertiary care hospital in Ulaanbaatar. She was so weak that she was unable to take the bus. The family had to sell several of their large animals to pay for plane tickets for her and an accompanying family member, and to pay the living expenses for that family member while she was being treated in Ulaanbaatar. In Ulaanbaatar she was hospitalized for 45 days during which she was given blood transfusions and other treatments. Although the hospitalization itself was free, the family had to pay US$400 for the blood treatments. Finally, having exhausted treatment opportunities, the woman was sent home. She died at home 20 days later. The costs of treatment and transportation together totaled nearly US$1,000, or about 2 year's income for this family. They were forced to sell off a good portion of their loan animals to pay for this treatment. Although the family has no regrets about having spent this money, and they have no complaints about the quality of care they received, they also recognize that they are highly vulnerable to complete impoverishment. They worry that any economic shock will force them to liquidate their remaining livestock and migrate to the province center where they would face an uncertain future. As has been documented in Mongolia and elsewhere, such instances of catastrophic illness are one of the main determinants of poverty (Narayan et al. 2000).

Summary: The Conceptual and Structural Deficiencies of Third-Generation Reform

The findings presented here point to 2 serious conceptual flaws that characterize most third-generation reforms worldwide. First, although the focus of primary care is to provide fully accessible and essential services to all citizens regardless of their ability to pay, this ostensibly egalitarian liberal position is compromised by the fact that the overall approach to health reform is strongly utilitarian: primary health care is designed as a means to reduce the "inefficient" use of hospital services. Primary care providers are set up as gatekeepers and the leveling of copayment requirements at secondary and tertiary levels is designed to reduce utilization of these more expensive alternatives. However, if a full array of health services is not available at the community level then those with the social capital and economic resources will bypass the primary care level and go straight to the hospital. It is only the poor, then, who find themselves restricted by necessity to use the facilities of a poorly functioning primary care sector. One conclusion that can be drawn from our study is that it is only through adequate development of high-quality comprehensive primary care—that looks something more like what was intended at Alma Ata and is rooted in the principle of social solidarity—that the ruthlessness of utilitarian health reform is mitigated and some measure of fairness is assured.

Second, an important consequence of utilitarian reforms involves segmenting of the health care system into primary, secondary, and tertiary care levels with relatively little attention given to the paths that individuals must take to navigate between them. As is the case with many third-generation reforms, the application of varying rules of access and payment schemes to different levels of care imposes significant informational and opportunity costs, erects bureaucratic barriers, and produces additional financial risks for patients. As described above, patients often complained not only of the superficial and often unnecessary referrals given by family doctors but also of the difficulty they have navigating district hospitals, where insurance documentation and copayments were required, and where the highly bureaucratic organization of diagnostic and treatment services was often bewildering. Individuals reported being given the wrong tests, going to the wrong clinic, only to be referred along elsewhere, and occasionally finding themselves in a private clinic where substantially greater out-of-pocket fees were requested. These factors tended to exacerbate inequities in the system, erecting a number of nearly insurmountable barriers for the poor. In circumstances of catastrophic illness where individuals have little choice but to pay high fees and accept huge indirect costs, the consequences may be dire.

These problems are not isolated to Mongolia. In one evaluation of primary care by the World Health Organization it was found that the practice of separating publicly available but "selective" primary health care from other levels of care resulted in tiered, fragmented systems that were found to unfairly discriminate against the most poor and vulnerable. Importantly, and consistent with the Mongolian case, in countries where chronic, noninfectious diseases have increased in importance, fragmentation impairs effective management of diseases such as diabetes and hypertension (World Health Organization 2003).

The logic of this critique suggests that there are several points at which intervention might improve equity and fairness. Most importantly, the breadth and quality of primary health care must be addressed. The selective or attenuated model of primary health care that is featured prominently in many third-generation reforms must give way to comprehensive care providing a wider array of desired services including access to essential drugs and routine diagnostic testing. Services should ideally include maternal and child health care services; long-term treatment of chronic diseases, especially hypertension and diabetes; palliative and supportive care for the terminally ill; management of mental health conditions; and a range of health promotion, disease prevention, and disease surveillance activities. In Mongolia, these might be expanded to include interventions related to the prevention of sexually transmitted infections, diet, smoking, alcohol use, and intimate partner violence.

To introduce a more substantive model of primary care providers must engage, or reengage, the communities they serve. The utilitarian model of health reform typically locates decision making in the hands of experts, and attention to community-defined needs often falls by the wayside. While the role of experts is critical to the delivery of appropriate services, the opinions of experts must be balanced with the needs of communities. The wisdom of Alma Ata, increasingly appreciated, clearly lay in its attention to local community context (Fritzen 2007; Mosely and Chen 1984; Petersen and Swartz 2002). In a more communitarian model of primary care, providers would engage in active outreach to the families they serve so that they may come to understand health needs in the context of their day-to-day lives. It is through such active outreach that appropriate public health education can be provided. Conversely, residents of the local area served by a clinic must have the means for evaluating it, and the political power to demand that a clinic respond to their needs.

Finally, organizational flaws produced in large part by the utilitarian model of reform should be corrected. The segmentation of care must be addressed in order to insure, from the perspective of the patient, a more seamless transition from one level of care to the next. Elimination of copayments, user fees, and information and bureaucratic barriers that discriminate against the very poor, coupled with a more comprehensive and higher quality primary care system, would go a long way in repairing the divisions between primary care and specialty levels of care (Janes 2004).

In my years of working in Mongolia I have tried to articulate to policymakers and donors how the processes documented here tend to produce and exacerbate inequity. Results have been conveyed in written white papers, talks, and meetings with key stakeholders, though not without some resistance (Janes 2003). Throughout I have tried to orient policymakers to community concerns and needs, and to help them see things from the perspective of poor individuals struggling with multiple challenges to their own and their families' well-being. I do not know whether I have been successful, though I find it gratifying to note that WHO and the World Bank in Mongolia are now advocating for improvements to primary care, including building shared diagnostic facilities for family group practices, increasing salaries of family doctors to attract more and better doctors to service, and giving family doctors access to and control of essential drug formularies (e.g., World Bank 2007). The Bank now seems ready to acknowledge that greater public investment and a stronger regulatory presence by the state in the health sector is required.

Conclusion: Toward Fourth-Generation Reforms

It may seem naïve to readers knowledgeable of the failure of Alma Ata to advocate, in part, a return to some of its basic principles. And while I am fully cognizant of the many problems that compromised its effective implementation, my research suggests that a return to its basic tenets, in particular its core communitarian and liberal ethics, would remedy many of the flaws inherent in third-generation reforms. Utilitarian approaches will always be to some extent required in an area of social service where resources are scarce and economizing obligatory. Yet, such approaches must be balanced with rights-based frameworks that bring to the forefront issues of justice and fairness. This can be accomplished by placing technically sufficient services squarely within the overview of communities, responsive to community needs, and consistent with the principles of social solidarity.

Realist critics of this approach will wonder whether fairness or equity as goals can or should supersede efficiency and economic rationality. My research suggests that the distinction often drawn between equity and efficiency is an artificial one. If high-quality services are provided effectively and fairly at the primary care level, which involves some involvement with and oversight by a local community, then the demand for expensive hospital-based services will be reduced. If services are organized according to a principle of social solidarity, where everyone regardless of class is entitled to the same array of services, there is less need for an inefficient, parallel system of care (i.e., a private sector) and an adequate pooling of risk is ensured (Roberts et al. 2004; Waitzkin 2003). Health care inequities may also contribute to the persistence in populations of reservoirs of untreated or ineffectively treated infections, thus posing a serious challenge to population health (i.e., the global problem with antibiotic resistance) (Farmer 1999; Farmer 2003; Radyowijati and Haak 2003). It is also increasingly recognized that serious illness often leads to impoverishment and, if ineffectively managed by extant social and health systems, may impede economic development (Commission on Macroeconomics and Health 2001; Evans, Whitehead, Diderichson, Bhuiya, and Wirth 2001; Narayan et al. 2000). Equity would thus seem to be fundamental to efficiency rather than at odds with it.

The research presented here suggests that a fourth generation of health reform is in order. It is rooted in the moral argument that fairness and justice should be the central organizing tenets of health systems. It takes up some of the core principles of Alma Ata, in particular its emphasis on the empowerment of communities and its locally focused participatory approach, without losing sight of the need to ensure that primary health care is given the technical resources it needs to address local health needs fully and effectively. It does not set aside efficiency as a goal, but locates it within a moral and ethical framework. An anthropological approach to health reform, with its focus on community participation and empowerment, is an effective tool for realizing this vision.

Notes

1. Technical efficiency, also called production efficiency, refers to the provision of a good or service at a minimum cost. It refers primarily to *how* something is produced. In the context of health care it describes the cost-effective provision of a particular

health service. Allocative efficiency refers to whether the right collection of outputs is produced to achieve overall health goals or status gains. Together these 2 concepts integrate the concepts of cost utility, quality, and accessibility.

2. "In this model, the state is responsible for both the financing and delivery of health care. The system emphasized the provision of health services mainly through hospitals, and as a result, Mongolia has inherited a large, inefficient hospital network that provides a low quality of care. Mongolia has more hospital beds than almost any country in the world" (World Bank 2007:i).

3. Vulnerable groups, which include pregnant women, young children, the retired, and disabled, are not subject to copayment requirements or user fees at the point of service in the tertiary or secondary care setting.

4. Revolving drug funds were established by WHO/UNICEF in the late 1980s to improve access to essential drugs in poor, primarily rural settings. Termed the "Bamako Initiative," the program provides a stock of basic medications to a hospital or clinic, which are in turn sold at the local level to raise sufficient funds to replenish supplies.

5. Food security was assessed by asking household heads whether and how frequently the household had experienced food shortages, or worried about experiencing such shortages, in the year before the interview.

References

Abbasi K (1999) Changing sides: The World Bank and world health. *British Medical Journal* 318:865–869.

ADB (2002) *Social Impact Assessment Report: Second Health Sector Development Project*. Ulaanbaatar, Mongolia: Asian Development Bank & the Mongolian Ministry of Health.

Atkinson S, Ngwengwe A, Macwan'gi M, Ngulube TJ, Harpham T, O'Connell A (1999) The referral process and urban health care in sub-Saharan Africa: The case of Lusaka, Zambia. *Social Science and Medicine* 49:27–38.

Castro A, Singer M, eds. (2004) *Unhealthy Health Policy: A Critical Anthropological Examination*. Walnut Creek, CA: Altamira Press.

Commission on Macroeconomics and Health (2001) *Macroeconomics and Health: Investing in Health for Economic Development*. Geneva: World Health Organization.

Coreil M, Mull DJ, eds. (1990) *Anthropology and Primary Health Care*. Boulder, CO: Westview Press.

Cueto M (2004) The origins of primary health care and selective primary health care. *American Journal of Public Health* 94:1864–1874.

Evans T, Whitehead M, Diderichson F, Bhuiya A, Wirth M, eds. (2001) "Introduction." In: *Challenging Inequities in Health: From Ethics to Action*. New York: Oxford University Press.

Farmer P (1999) *Infections and Inequalities*. Berkeley, CA: University of California Press.

Farmer P (2003) *Pathologies of Power*. Berkeley, CA: University of California Press.

Fritzen SA (2007) Legacies of primary health care in an age of health sector reform: Vietnam's commune clinics in transition. *Social Science and Medicine* 64:1611–1623.

Government of Mongolia (2000) National Statistical Report 2000. Ulaanbaatar, Mongolia: National Statistics Office, Government of Mongolia.

Griffin K (2001) *A Strategy for Poverty Reduction in Mongolia.* Ulaanbaatar, Mongolia: United Nations Development Programme.

Gwatkin DR (2000) Health inequalities and the health of the poor: What do we know? What can we do? *Bulletin of the World Health Organization* 78:3–18.

Gwatkin DR (2001) The need for equity-oriented health sector reforms. *International Journal of Epidemiology* 30:720–723.

Hsiao W, Liu Y (2001) "Health Care Financing: Assessing Its Relationship to Health Equity." In: *Challenging Inequities in Health: From Ethics to Action.* T Evans, M Whitehead, F Diderichsen, A Bhuiva, M Wirth, eds. New York: Oxford University Press.

Humphrey C, Sneath D (1999) *The End of Nomadism? Society, State and the Environment in Inner Asia.* Durham, NC: Duke University Press.

Janes CR (2003) Criticizing with impunity? Bridging the widening gulf between academic discourse and action anthropology in global health. *Social Analysis* 47:90–95.

Janes CR (2004) Going global in century XXI: Medical anthropology and the new primary health care. *Human Organization* 63:457–471.

Janes CR (In Press) "Spatial Mobility and Health in Post-socialist Mongolia." In: *Space Movement and Health.* KR Hampshire, SM Coleman, eds. Oxford, UK: Berghahn Books.

Janes CR, Chuluundorj O (2004) Free markets and dead mothers: The social ecology of maternal mortality in post-socialist Mongolia. *Medical Anthropology Quarterly* 18:102–129.

Janes CR, Chuluundorj O, Hilliard C, Rak K, Janchiv K (2005) Poor medicine for poor people? Assessing the impact of neoliberal reform on health care equity in a post-socialist context. *Global Public Health* 1:5–30.

Janes CR, Hilliard C (2008) "Inventing Tradition: Tibetan Medicine in the Post-socialist Contexts of China and Mongolia." In: *Exploring Tibetan Medicine in Contemporary Context.* L Pordie, ed. London: Routledge.

Kickbush I (2004) From charity to rights: Proposal for five action areas of global health. *Journal of Epidemiology and Community Health* 58:630–631.

Kickbush I, Buse K (2001) "Global Influences and Global Responses: International Health at the Turn of the 21st Century." In: *International Public Health.* MH Merson, RE Black, AJ Mills, eds. Gaithersberg, MD: Aspen Pubs.

Litsios S (2002) The long and difficult road to Alma-Ata: A personal reflection. *International Journal of Health Services* 32:709–732.

Litsios S (2004) The Christian Medical Commission and the development of the World Health Organization's primary health care approach. *American Journal of Public Health* 94:1884–1893.

Mearns R (2004) Sustainable livelihoods on Mongolia's pastoral commons: Insights from a participatory poverty assessment. *Development and Change* 35:107–139.

Morgan LM (1990) International politics and primary health care in Costa Rica. *Social Science and Medicine* 30:211–219.

Morgan LM (2001) Community participation in health: Perpetual allure, persistent challenge. *Health Policy and Planning* 16:221–230.

Mosely WH, Chen LC (1984) "An Analytical Framework for the Study of Child Survival in Developing Countries." In: *Child Survival: Strategies for Research.*

WH Mosley, LC Chen, eds. Supplement to Population and Development Review 10, pp. 25–45.

Mull DJ (1990) "The Primary Health Care Dialectic: History, Rhetoric, and Reality." In: *Anthropology and Primary Health Care*. J Coreil, DJ Mull, eds. Boulder, CO: Westview.

Narayan D, Chambers R, Kaul M (2000) *Voices of the Poor: Crying Out for Change*. New York: Oxford University Press (for the World Bank).

Nichter M, Nichter M, eds. (1996) *Anthropology and International Health: Asian Case Studies*. 2nd edition. Amsterdam: Gordon and Breach.

Petersen I, Swartz L (2002) Primary health care in the era of HIV/AIDS: Some implications for health systems reform. *Social Science and Medicine* 55:1005–1013.

Radyowijati A, Haak H (2003) Improving antibiotic use in low-income countries: An overview of evidence on determinants. *Social Science and Medicine* 57:733–744.

Rifkin SB, Walt G (1986) Why health improves: Defining the issues concerning "comprehensive primary health care" and "selective primary health care." *Social Science and Medicine* 23:559–566.

Roberts MJ, Hsiao W, Berman P, Reich MR (2004) *Getting Health Reform Right: A Guide to Improving Performance and Equity*. New York: Oxford University Press.

Roberts MJ, Reich MR (2002) Ethical analysis in public health. *Lancet* 359:1055–1059.

Rossabi M (2005) *Modern Mongolia: From Khans to Commissars to Capitalists*. Berkeley, CA: UC Press.

Sidel V (1972) The barefoot doctors of the People's Republic of China. *New England Journal of Medicine* 286:1292–1300.

United Nations Development Programme (2000) *Human Development Report, Mongolia 2000*. Ulaanbaatar, Mongolia: United Nations Development Programme.

United Nations Development Programme (2003) *Human Development Report Mongolia 2003*. Ulaanbaatar, Mongolia: United Nations Development Programme.

Waitzkin H (2003) Report of the WHO commission on macroeconomics and health: A summary and critique. *Lancet* 361:523–526.

Walsh JA, Warren KS (1979) Selective primary health care: An interim strategy for disease control in developing countries. *New England Journal of Medicine* 301:967–974.

Walt G, Pavignani E, Gilson L, Buse K (1999) Health sector development: From aid coordination to resource management. *Health Policy Plan* 14:207–218.

Whiteford LM, Nixon LL (2000) "Comparative Health Systems: Emerging Convergences and Globalization." In: *The Handbook of Social Studies in Health and Medicine*. GL Albrecht, R Fitzpatrick, SC Scrimshaw, eds. London: Sage Publications.

World Bank (1993) *Investing in Health: World Development Report 1993*. New York: Oxford University Press (for the World Bank).

World Bank (2007) The Mongolian Health System at a Crossroad: An Incomplete Transition to a Post-Semashko Model. Working Paper Series No. 2007–1, Human Development Sector Unit, East Asian and the Pacific Region. Washington, DC: World Bank.

World Health Organization (2000) *The World Health Report 2000: Health Systems*. Geneva: World Health Organization.

World Health Organization (2003) A global review of primary health care: Emerging messages. Geneva: Noncommunicable Diseases and Mental Health, Evidence and Information for Policy, World Health Organization.

World Health Organization (2005) Preparing a health care workforce for the 21st century: The challenge of chronic conditions. Geneva: WHO, Noncommunicable Diseases and Mental Health Cluster. Chronic Diseases and Health Promotion Department.

Zwi AB, Yach D (2002) International health in the 21st century: Trends and challenges. *Social Science and Medicine* 54:1615–1620.

24

Bureaucratic Aspects of International Health Programs

GEORGE M. FOSTER

Introduction

Since the end of World War II, great strides have been made in meeting health needs, particularly in Third World countries, which have historically lagged behind industrialized regions. Death rates have fallen significantly, longevity has markedly increased, environmental sanitation has improved, maternal and child health facilities have multiplied, immunization programs increasingly protect children against common childhood diseases, and the incidence of many other diseases, such as malaria, has been notably lowered.

At the same time, enormous health problems still confront most of the world, and it is widely recognized that "Health for All by the Year 2000" was never achieved (WHO 1979). Why? In public health, we have long since acquired the skills needed to provide pure water and environmental sanitation, to immunize against common childhood diseases, to design nutritionally balanced diets, and to teach personal hygiene and food safety. These skills, as Ramalingaswami (1986:1097) notes, "were largely responsible for the great transformation in health that took place in the industrialized world at the time of the First Industrial Revolution." They are also the skills that can affect a comparable revolution in Third World health conditions. But we are failing to utilize these skills fully, according to Ramalingaswami, because of political, cultural, ethical, and bureaucratic factors.

681

These factors are marked by a common characteristic: they are all sociocultural. Not one is primarily medical. In other words, medical knowledge and medical research alone cannot bring health for all. Our problems lie in the fields of politics and commitment, of planning for health needs, and of administration of programs and projects.

This is not the first time in history that administrative and planning talents have been called on to help meet perceived health needs. Perhaps the earliest "international" health agencies were the Public Health Boards established by north Italian city–states to meet the threat of the Black Death (1347–1351). Not only did the boards monitor the incidence and progress of illness within their boundaries but they also exchanged information with their counterparts in other cities with a view to establishing quarantine measures. Considering the low level of medical knowledge at that time, it is perhaps not surprising that

> the rise and development of the Health Boards and of related health legislation were not so much the brainchild of the medical profession as they were the products of the administrative talents of Italian Renaissance society. ... From their beginnings the Boards were in the hands not of the medical men but of administrators who, of course, made use of the knowledge and skills of physicians and surgeons whenever the situation demanded (Cipolla 1976:20–21).

History repeats itself today, for knowledge and skills beyond those of medicine are needed to make progress in meeting health needs. Specifically, administrative, political, economic, sociocultural, and ethical factors must be taken into account in the planning and conduct of health programs. Within the field of international health, this fact is appreciated in varying degrees. Thus, it is generally agreed that knowledge of the sociocultural characteristics of recipient groups is essential to the best planning and execution of health programs. Less widely accepted is the fact that the structural and dynamic characteristics of health agencies profoundly influence the planning and mode of operations of international health programs. Health bureaucracies are therefore just as logical objects of scientific investigation as traditional communities.

To study bureaucracies, of course, is hardly a novel idea. Since the time of the German sociologist Max Weber (1864–1920), social scientists have studied administrative organizations to understand how their structure and dynamics influence the societies of which they are a part. Empirical research has confirmed the obvious: informal relations and unofficial practices are widespread in all bureaucracies, and are essential to their activities. Far from detracting from the efficiency of the organization (as Weber's model postulated), these relationships and practices often contribute to more efficient operations (e.g., see discussion of Simmons, below).

Although the health field has provided the arena for a number of studies of bureaucracies and the health professions within national boundaries, relatively little research on health agencies—in contrast to the communities they serve—has been carried out in the international setting. Among exceptions is Simmons's early analysis of the clinical team in a Chilean health center, which revealed the highly useful but unofficial function health center nurses performed in mediating between doctors and patients (Simmons 1955). When in a routine administrative shift of duties the nurses were assigned full-time to home visiting, communication between doctors and patients virtually broke down. Equally revealing is Philips's review of the Rockefeller Foundation's hookworm campaign in Ceylon from 1916 to 1922 (Philips 1955). The study is important because it demonstrates how the physicians' misconceptions about appropriate innovative roles and their lack of knowledge of what their activities meant to the tea coolies were responsible for the failure of the program. Practically all of the problems in planning and operating international health programs encountered 50 years later in the post-World War II period emerged during those 6 years.

Methodology

This study is based on information acquired through participant observation. In common anthropological usage, the term implies that researchers speak the language of and participate as fully as possible in the life of the members of a group—a peasant community, urban ghetto residents, staff of a hospital, or a government agency—with specific goals in mind, such as writing a scientific monograph, a popular book, or a committee report. Information gathered in this fashion tends to be "interpreted" rather than "analyzed." Anthropologists ask of their data, "What does this all add up to? What do the data tell us about human behavior, about social organization and culture?" Competing interpretations are the rule; there are no ways to repeat a study under controlled conditions duplicating the first anthropologist's work, no simple way to prove or disprove a hypothesis. The interpretation that seems most plausible to most anthropologists is generally accepted until and unless a more plausible hypothesis appears.

Reflection on 40 years of personal observations and experiences in the field of technical aid, especially international health programs, augmented by examination of the published record and discussions with colleagues in many fields, has led to the conclusions in this study. During my professional life, I have observed and participated in the development of a number of international multi- and bilateral technical aid programs, beginning in 1943 when, as a "social science analyst," I joined the U.S. Institute of Inter-American Affairs (IIAA), which had been established a year earlier to help Latin American countries develop their agricultural, health, and educational systems. The IIAA was the forerunner and prototype of today's United States Agency for International Development (USAID). In 1946, after 2 years as a Smithsonian Institution (SI) visiting professor in Mexico City, I returned to Washington. There, in 1951, my contact with the IIAA was renewed when SI colleagues in several Latin American countries and I carried out an initial study of aspects of the institute's work in public health. Our report (Foster 1951), which stressed the cultural and social "barriers" that inhibited acceptance of much of the American program, was enthusiastically received by IIAA health personnel. It appeared to answer many questions that had puzzled them, especially why new public health centers failed to attract the clients for whom they were designed. As a result, the SI anthropologists were invited to join an IIAA evaluation team formed to appraise the results of the first 10 years of its health programs (Foster 1953, 1982a).

In 1953 I accepted a professorship in the Department of Anthropology at the University of California, Berkeley, where, during the following 30 years, I served as consultant in a number of overseas technical aid projects and programs: for USAID in community development (CD) and health education in India, Pakistan, the Philippines, Indonesia, Afghanistan, Nepal, and Northern Rhodesia (today Zambia), for periods of several weeks to 6 months; for the United Nations Children's Fund (UNICEF) and, especially, the World Health Organization (WHO), for periods of 2 weeks to 3 months in Geneva, Indonesia,

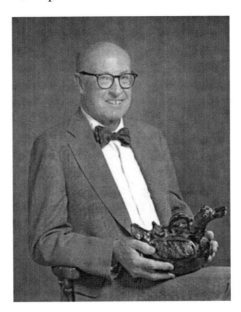

Figure 24.1 George M. Foster, Professor of Anthropology at University of California, Berkeley, 1953–1979. Professor Foster is widely regarded as an important founder of the field of medical anthropology. He died in 2006. (Photo by G. Paul Bishop, uc Berkeley News Service.)

India, Sri Lanka, Malaysia, Thailand, and the Philippines, with shorter stays in Nepal, Nigeria, Cameroon, and Kenya.

A considerable number of stateside and international workshops, committee memberships, and meetings also gave me opportunity to interact with international health specialists, and to observe them in action. All these experiences added to my understanding of the bureaucratic aspects of international health agencies and programs.

Types of International Health Agencies

Organizations working in the international field may be classified as follows:

1. Multilateral organizations, exemplified by the specialized United Nations agencies such as the WHO and UNICEF. The critical characteristic of these agencies is that membership is open to all countries, whose representatives collectively set policy.
2. Bilateral governmental agencies such as USAID, based on working agreements between the donor organization and the ministries of health of recipient countries. Although improved health is also the goal of such agencies, basic policy is set largely by the donor organization, and its activities constitute an arm of the foreign policy of the supporting government.
3. Private secular organizations such as the Rockefeller, Ford, and other large, multipurpose foundations, and myriad smaller and more specialized groups that depend on charitable contributions for support. Historically, these organizations have stressed preventive medicine and public health measures rather than clinical activities.
4. Private religious organizations such as the medical missions that have been supported by Western European and North American Christian denominations for a century and a half. Historically, medical missions have been more concerned with curative activities than with preventive measures. They differ from the other organizations in that meeting health needs often is not a primary aim in itself, but rather a strategy to help achieve the ultimate goal of making converts. Medical missions and private secular organizations are usually grouped under the rubric private voluntary organizations (PVOs) or nongovernmental organizations (NGOs).

This chapter focuses on the multi- and bilateral organizations. Although distinctive in important ways, as huge bureaucracies conforming essentially to the procedures of governments, they are sufficiently similar to one another to permit joint analysis and comparison. Almost without exception, they conform to a "donor–recipient" pattern in which specialists from technologically advanced countries work with "counterparts" in less developed countries in improving health services in the latter regions. This pattern is largely a product of the past 50 years.

By the end of World War II it was clear that war-ravaged Europe required major financial help to rebuild. This came largely in the form of Marshall Plan aid from the United States. It was also clear that during the war the rest of the world had changed significantly, and that even greater changes were an immediate prospect. European colonies were soon to become independent. They, and other countries little, if at all, industrialized, would need major financial and technological help in their developmental efforts, essential to achieve higher standards of living and, it was hoped, political stability. Thus was born the concept of huge technical aid programs in such fields as health, agriculture, and education, as a major arm of foreign policy of the industrialized countries, and as a field of cooperation within the United Nations and its specialized agencies (Basch 1978).

Evolving Models of Technical Aid

From their beginning, technical assistance programs have been based on underlying assumptions judged to be self-evident by the program personnel. Tendler (1975:10) states the basic assumption:

> Development assistance was established on the premise that the developed world possessed both the talent and the capital for helping backward countries to develop. Development know-how was spoken about as if it were like capital—a stock of goods capable of being transferred from its owners to the less privileged.

It logically follows that if some people have "know-how" and others do not, then those with the know-how are the proper ones to plan and execute the transfer. Technical aid and developmental planning in general are, as Korten and Alfonso (1981:2) point out,

> based on an organizational model which assumes that the major planning decisions will be made centrally based on economic analyses prepared by highly trained technicians. ... The decisions are made by experts far removed from the people and their needs, and implemented through structures intended to be more responsive to central direction than local reality.

Premises change over time. This is as true of premises underlying international health organizations as of other large bureaucracies. Over the past 50 years, 3 sequential models of the perception of problems encountered in delivering technical aid can be identified: the "silver platter" model, the sociocultural model, and the bureaucratic model.

The Silver Platter Model

In the early years of technical aid, planners and technical specialists—health personnel included—felt that their task was to attack problems with the techniques and institutional forms that worked well in industrialized countries. Although speaking only of higher education in (then) British Africa, Ashby (1966:244) aptly described the picture for all technical aid:

> Underlying British enterprise in providing higher education for her people overseas was one massive assumption: that the pattern of university appropriate for Manchester, Exeter and Hull was ipso facto appropriate for Ibadan, Kampala, and Singapore .... As with cars, so with universities: we willingly made minor modifications to suit the climate, but we proposed no radical change in design, and we did not regard it as our business to enquire whether French or American models might be more suitable.

The result was universities often poorly suited to the needs of developing countries. In the history of international health programs, the same underlying assumption repeats itself continually: the health strategies that have served the West are universals, equally suited to Boston or Bombay. Health programs have been seen as exercises in the transfer of techniques, in the implantation of educational, preventive, and curative services based on the biomedical model, in which the major challenge is to persuade people to abandon their traditional beliefs and practices in favor of the new. As with British higher education, this assumption often has produced inappropriate and ineffective health services in Third World countries.

It was further assumed that people in less developed countries, the recipients of help, would immediately appreciate the advantages of the new ways, once exposed to them, and that given the opportunity they would quickly adopt them. The errors underlying this "transfer of techniques" approach are beautifully illustrated by the early health program of the US Institute of Inter-American Affairs, established in 1942. The centerpiece of the program was American-type public health centers, emphasizing preventive activities in such fields as maternal and child health care and environmental sanitation. Initially these centers failed to attract anticipated patronage. Behavioral research revealed that in countries where people have limited access to modern health care, they are uninterested in prevention until their first priority (treatment of illness) has been satisfied. Only after curative services—initially lacking—were added did health centers begin to play an important health role (Foster 1952).

The Sociocultural Model

By the mid-1950s this early ethnocentric view of technical aid began to give way to a new approach that postulated that the major problems in the transfer of advanced technologies, including those of the health sciences, are rooted in the society and culture of the recipient peoples, and that programs and projects aimed at redressing poverty, poor health, inefficient agriculture, and illiteracy must be designed to fit the needs and expectations of these people. The populations toward whom these programs are pointed, it is argued, want to raise their standards of living and are willing to modify their behavior when they perceive advantage in the new ways. But psychological, social, and cultural "barriers" inhibit these changes. Consequently, if these barriers can be identified through sociocultural research, and if the motivations to change can be identified, then developmental assistance can be presented in such a way that client populations will eagerly accept it. This model represents an enormous advance over the silver platter model. As far as it goes, it is correct. Without an understanding of the local community, its worldview and its comprehension of the innovative alternatives presented to it, planners and technical specialists are working blindly.

The Bureaucratic Model

Even the most sophisticated applications of the sociocultural model, however, often failed to produce the desired results. Little by little, we have come to realize that not only is it important to understand the recipient's culture but it is also equally important to understand the sociocultural forms of innovating organizations. Just as barriers to change are found in peasant communities, so are they found in the structure, values, and operating procedures of development bureaucracies, and in the individual personal qualities of planners and change agents. In other words, the bureaucratic model says that to develop the most effective aid programs it is essential to understand the culture of the agency developing and guiding a program, as well as the national and international assumptions (both conscious and unconscious) that shape bureaucratic cultures.

For many reasons, the bureaucratic model has been less completely accepted than the sociocultural model; many health personnel still reject it, insisting that the community, and the community alone, is the problem. It is easy to see why the sociocultural model has been so readily accepted: it is nonthreatening to agency personnel, for the problem is defined as "out there," away from the centers of policy, planning, and program operations. No one in the innovating organization need feel responsible, or on the spot, in accepting this model.

Even for those who realize the validity of the bureaucratic model, it is often difficult to admit that "we are a part of the problem." Not all reluctance to attempt the innovative action that the bureaucratic model calls for, of course, is psychological. Staff members of bureaucracies fully understand the limits of their organizations, of their inherent rigidity, and of the many constraints they place on reflective thinking and action. Since efforts to bring about major organizational changes so often seem futile, staff members find it easier to accept organizational norms as a given, and to place their hopes on changes in community forms that will make clients more receptive to their programs. Perhaps they are realistic in taking this position. Certainly the changes in traditional communities since the end of World War II suggest that they can indeed change more rapidly than entrenched bureaucracies.

Bureaucracies as Sociocultural Systems

In their structural and dynamic aspects, bureaucracies are much like communities. Normally they are composed of people of both sexes and different ages, organized in a hierarchy of authority, responsibility, obligations, and functional tasks. They also have social structures that define the relationships, roles, and statuses of their members. Through formal and informal educational methods, new members of bureaucratic societies learn appropriate role behavior and the values, routines, and premises that guide the organization.

Bureaucracies further resemble communities in that they are integrated, functional units in which the parts fit closely together; consequently, no change occurs in isolation, without rearrangement in the role relationships of the members, without increasing the responsibilities and authority of some and diminishing those of others. Like community members, the personnel of large organizations jealously guard their traditional perquisites and privileges; they do not easily surrender their vested interests, except in exchange for something as good or better. They rationalize their positions by assuring themselves that what is good for them is best for the organization.

Bureaucracies also resemble communities in that, within norms of behavior and values, individual members exhibit great variation in ability, character, personality, views, and judgment. The personnel of bureaucracies are not simply carriers of their organizational cultures; they are also psychological beings who need ego gratification and satisfaction from their performances. They are characterized by emotional securities and insecurities, likes and dislikes, and hopes and doubts. Sometimes they feel successful in their accomplishments, and at other times they feel threatened or rejected. To understand the working of bureaucracies, it is essential to pay attention to the ever-present psychological dimension of personnel.

Evaluating International Health Agencies

The identification and evaluation of the strengths and weaknesses of international health organizations is a highly subjective exercise. A pessimist will look at the world's unmet health needs and conclude that, a half century after their founding, these agencies fall far short of what was expected of them. An optimist, comparing contemporary world health levels with those prevailing at the end of World War II, can only conclude that the agencies have accomplished much more than what might have been anticipated. For the fact is, as pointed out earlier, enormous strides have been made in meeting the world's health needs, particularly in developing countries. That much remains to be done is more an indication of the magnitude of the task than of the shortcomings of health organizations.

International health agencies have helped significantly in raising world health levels by a variety of means: they have attracted able and dedicated administrators and technical specialists and have drawn on the latest biomedical knowledge of the world's medical research institutions. By means of travel grants, traineeships, and fellowships for Third World health personnel, they have helped strengthen indigenous ministries of health and health care facilities in the countries concerned.

It is widely assumed that multilateral agencies have major advantages over bilateral ones. In the case of WHO, for example, all member nations can feel that this is our organization, no longer dominated (as in the early years) by the West. In the WHO annual General Assembly there is opportunity for broader input and discussion of a wider variety of concerns and ideas than in any bilateral program. Moreover, the continuing interaction of personnel from many countries in the same office permits dialogue on a wide spectrum of ideas that cannot be achieved in an organization largely representing a single cultural tradition.

Worldwide campaigns such as smallpox eradication, immunization against childhood illnesses, and oral rehydration therapy to treat infant diarrheal diseases can be pursued with a vigor and degree of support impossible for any bilateral agency. And, with respect to educational and legal efforts to persuade mothers to nurse rather than bottle-feed their infants, the multilateral organizations do not suffer the political constraints imposed on some of the bilateral agencies. There are problems, of course, as when member nations insist that specific diseases are not found within their borders. For example, when the first cases of AIDS were recognized in 1983, many African governments refused to acknowledge cases within their borders. Yet, it has proven easier for WHO to persuade these countries that they must be involved in AIDS control than it would have been for any bilateral agency.

For reasons like these, increased channeling of health aid through multilateral institutions has emerged as an attractive solution to many of the problems encountered in bilateral programs. Yet the evidence is not all one-sided. Basch states the problem: "This step, it is asserted, would reduce many of the tensions and obligations implicit in bilateral arrangements, distribute aid on the basis of need rather than political loyalty, and make assistance contingent on policy reforms backed by world opinion." Yet, he continues, "while this may be so, multilateralization introduces into the ODA [official development assistance] picture at least a third bureaucracy with its inherent red-tapism, delay, and administrative expense, and it blurs the special relationships and specific mutual interests of the parties concerned" (Basch 1978:339). Moreover, at times, bilateral organizations can innovate in ways that the multinational organizations, for all their strengths, cannot attempt for policy reasons.

Problems Encountered in International Health Agencies

In considering the problems encountered in international health agencies, and in looking for ways in which their effectiveness may be increased, we are dealing with "the art of the possible" (Ramalingaswami 1986:1097). Some of the factors that prevent health agencies from realizing their full potential are inherent in all bureaucracies, and little can be done about them. Other problems, however, seem self-imposed; with innovative action from within the organization they can be significantly reduced, to the benefit of the agency and its clients. Examples of both follow.

Rationalizing Budgets

Agencies never have all the financial resources they believe they can spend profitably. Hence, officials of all bureaucracies do the natural thing: in requesting funds for future activities they cast their past achievements in the best possible light and describe future plans in the most glowing terms. International health agencies are not immune to this exercise. To justify their budget requests they need quick results, especially results that can be counted: numbers of latrines installed, children vaccinated, and family planning methods demonstrated. Long-range strategies that take time to produce results suffer in comparison to programs such as these. Again, the need to show that the organization is forward looking creates pressure to generate new projects simply for their own sake, often without adequate research and evaluation of all of the implications of the proposal. Moreover, the launching of new projects may necessitate the dropping of promising ongoing projects before they have had time to fully demonstrate their potential.

Limited Corporate Memories

Health agencies, like other corporate groups, often seem marked by what can be called a "limited corporate memory"; only with difficulty do they learn from their own past, and they fail to draw on the relevant prior experience of others. For example, by the end of World War II the history of medical missions and data from the early Rockefeller international health programs and other crosscultural health activities contained invaluable information about strategies most likely to produce results in designing and carrying out health projects in developing countries. Yet, when the major multilateral and bilateral agencies began their work 50 years ago, they paid little attention to this wealth of experience. Consequently, they repeated mistakes made many times in the past, mistakes that might have been avoided.

More recently, the concept of primary health care (PHC) offers a similar picture: the reinvention of the CD wheel of 20 years earlier. In this process international health agencies have made many of the same mistakes and suffered the same disappointments as the earlier enthusiastic CD advocates (Foster 1982b; Muhondwa 1986). As Bichmann (1983:7) writes,

> There are surprising analogies between the PHC and the CD approach ... but in the documents promoting the PHC-strategy, no clear reference to this fact is given. ... AS PHC with its comprehensive approach encompasses sector-external health-related subjects like agricultural development, road infrastructure, education, etc. so did the CD programmes of the fifties and sixties aim at integrated rural development including health-related activities. ... Generally speaking, CD did not yield the expected results on a nation-wide scale. ... Why then should PHC produce a better outcome than CD?

It is difficult to tell whether failure to consider prior relevant experience is inherent in bureaucratic structures, or whether it reflects a reluctance of personnel to diminish the appearance of their creativity by giving credit to others. Whatever the explanation, in contrast to budgeting problems, which appear insoluble, appropriate research resources can improve the corporate memory problem. After all, learning from experience is commonplace.

Constraints Imposed by Agency Doctrines

Bureaucracies must usually develop policy in the absence of much of the information that should ideally be available. The dangers inherent in this situation can be guarded against partially by periodic reviews of progress and by keeping policy as flexible as possible so that course corrections can be made as needed. Policies, like engineering designs, should not be frozen until all the problems have been solved. In international health agencies, however, it sometimes looks as if ideologically attractive but untested policies are raised to the level of doctrine more because of the enthusiasms and special professional interests of those in a position to make such decisions than because of objective consideration of what is known. And, once policy becomes doctrine, it is the rare staff member who can afford to question it. The life expectancy of whistle-blowers in bureaucracies is not long.

The concept of community participation (CP) as a major component in PHC strategies illustrates this point. First broached as a promising PHC approach in 1975 in WHO's widely quoted Health by the People (Newell 1975) and in the study Alternative Approaches to Meeting Basic Health Needs in Developing Countries (Djukanovic and Mach 1975), CP was elevated to the level of doctrine on the basis of the 1977 UNICEF-WHO Joint Committee on Health Policy report, "Community Involvement in Primary Health Care: A Study of the Process of Community Motivation and Continued Participation" (WHO 1977).

This study illustrates a common bureaucratic practice: the use of "research" to legitimize previously decided-upon policies rather than to provide data for judging the desirability of the policies. There are good things about the study. It analyzes, and draws conclusions from, case studies of projects in each of 9 countries in which it can be argued that the community had indeed been "involved." However, a tenth case study was excluded from the final draft because its findings were contrary to the desired conclusions. In fact, in no sense was the sample random and no serious effort was made to consider negative evidence. The study disingenuously notes that "time did not permit an exhaustive study," and the methodological weaknesses of the report are made clear. In spite of these obvious limitations, the report was accepted as the solid evidence on which the role of CP was spelled out in the 1978 Alma-Ata Conference on Primary Health Care (WHO 1978).

CP has been the subject of a number of subsequent WHO meetings and studies, none of which has seriously questioned the validity of the idea. It continues to receive ritual obeisance within the organization, in spite of the fact that this approach—as with CD—usually has produced meager results in the Third World.

Constraints Imposed by Western Ideologies

In international health agencies, basic policies, program priorities, and doctrines are presumed to reflect the considered judgment of objective and dispassionate health professionals. Often they do. Yet, there are always supraorganizational influences underlying the policy-determining process, the impact of which is not always appreciated. Stone (1989) suggests that the "cultural imprint of the West" is manifest and expressed in "the rhetoric and the fads," and in the style and approach of development. "It is as though the world of international development, although ostensibly geared toward maximizing its relevance to the poor of the Third World, has become like a mirror in which the values, interests and philosophies of the West are found reflected" (Stone 1989:206). CP, which "now stands as an established development strategy," is an example: the concept entails the Western values of self-reliance, equality, and individualism, values to which most of us subscribe. Yet, she points out that it is a mistake to assume that these values equally characterize Third World communities.

Contemporary international concerns with nutrition and interest in "women in development" (WID) also reflect a contemporary Western ideology, Stone believes. According to Stone (1989:206),

> Nutrition is now a major and growing focus in development programs. And regardless of the scientific soundness of this focus, the fact remains that nutrition loomed as a major thrust in international development circles at the same time as "nutrition" became a subject of great popular fascination in the United States. Nutrition programs multiplied in the Third World around the time that the Americans began to criticize their junk food, measure their cholesterol, and to perceive sound nutrition as a solution to their problems.
>
> Another, perhaps more pointed, case is "Women in Development" (WID), now a major concern within virtually every development agency in the world. Again, regardless of the value or soundness of WID programs, they did not arise from the expressed interests and felt needs of the masses of the Third World poor. Rather, a development focus on women grew from the fact that the status of women and attendant questions of sexual equality became burning issues in the West.

Of course, the cultural ideology of the West as reflected in the international health agencies goes far beyond CP, nutrition, and WID. It constitutes a basic statement about a sociopolitical and economic system, the correctness of which is self-evident to its leaders and most of its people. The bilateral health agencies must operate within the constraints of this ideology. They must be cautious in advocating policies such as major land reform and wealth redistribution, even though sociopolitical and economic changes in much of the world are seen by program planners as necessary to achieve higher health levels. The multilateral organizations are somewhat more flexible on these points; they can advocate socialist as well as capitalist responses to health needs. Yet, they, too, can go only so far, since withdrawal of the financial support of the West would render them impotent; they must walk a fine line indeed.

Constraints Imposed by Professional and Personal Characteristics of Agency Personnel

Bureaucrats do not, and cannot be expected to, function with formalistic impersonality. They have likes and dislikes, prejudices, friendships, and enmities. These, and many other personal characteristics, influence their role performances, and hence the functioning of their organizations. Personality traits like these are individual. Other personality traits may be thought of as group based, characterizing the members of professions and professionals as a class. They also affect the performance of individuals and, consequently, organizational activities. Competent professionals have a positive self-image; they have confidence in their ability and take pride in their work. Some professionals can work quietly, satisfied with the knowledge that they are doing a good job. But many more exhibit—or conceal with varying degrees of success—a need for ego gratification, which comes from recognition by their peers. Hence, they like to promote activities in which they can demonstrate their professional skills. Sometimes this leads to confusion between personal and organizational needs.

Pride in performance and a positive self-image obviously are important elements in stimulating the best possible work. But when present in excess, in projects where cooperative efforts and intersectoral policies are desirable, these personal–professional factors can jeopardize planning and program operations. For, carried away with enthusiasm, some professionals readily believe that their contributions are the key to program success and that they should have first call on resources. In PHC, for example, lip service is paid to the importance of integrated programs that include agriculture, education, access roads, and the like. Yet few, whose primary field is health, doubt that health activities and particularly their own specialties should receive first attention.

The policies, programs, and priorities of large organizations, including those concerned with international health, reflect a pair of processes: a public and explicit planning mechanism, and the often private, professional concerns and enthusiasms of powerful individuals and groups within the organization.

Competition for Clients

Bureaucracies, international health agencies included, need clients to justify their existence. The worst thing that can happen to such a bureaucracy is to solve the problems it was set up to solve, and thus to be left without clients. At least 2 groups of clients of international health agencies can be identified. The first is the individual community member, a human being in need of health protection and care. There are adequate numbers of these clients, enough for everyone searching for a client, and the supply will not dry up. But help to community members is filtered through intermediate clients, the health ministries and services of the countries receiving developmental aid. In contrast to community members, these clients are limited in number; there are not always enough of them to satisfy the needs of all organizations involved in international health work. This leads to competition among donor agencies, with results sometimes inimical to the host country's best interests.

Sterling (1976:14) gives a vivid picture of such competition in Kathmandu in the mid-1970s:

> At last count when I was there, about 700 missionaries of progress were racketing around town in their Land Rovers and Toyota jeeps, representing some fifty donor states and agencies, all urging assorted projects on a nation the size of Arkansas. Among the foreign benefactors are USAID, the Indian Cooperation Mission, the Chinese, Russians, British, Canadians, Australians, New Zealanders, Pakistanis, and Swiss, the Japanese Overseas Cooperation Volunteers, the German Volunteer service, the Ford Foundation, the Rockefeller Foundation, the Dooley Foundation (using volunteer airline hostesses who take six months off for good works), Anglia University, Cornell University, [and] the World Bank.

And these are only a few examples. Such an abundance of foreign aid stresses the capacity of many Third World governments to provide the counterpart services and personnel expected by most development agencies.

The Workshop Syndrome

Meetings are the lifeblood of bureaucracies. The simplest form is that well-known bureaucratic phenomenon, the staff meeting. At higher levels, meetings take the form of longer regional and international conferences and workshops. The numbers, varieties, and frequencies of such meetings in international health organizations are quite dazzling: USAID meetings in Washington, UNICEF meetings in New York, and WHO meetings at headquarters in Geneva and in the regional offices.

One is led to speculate as to their raison d'être. Some justifications are obvious: it is important that world leaders in various health fields meet and discuss common concerns, that they assess the gravity of health threats (such as AIDS), that they take stock of progress in controlling diarrheal diseases, and that they plan future activities. Major workshops can play another important role, that of validating organization policies and programs. For example, Justice writes of Nepal that "Kathmandu officials place great importance on high-level conferences because they are a visible activity that extends legitimacy to programs such as ICHP [Integrated Community Health Program]" (Justice 1986:78).

Beyond these obvious justifications there are latent reasons why the pattern is so popular, particularly in multilateral organizations. This has to do with the nature of professional employment in Third World countries, and with the attraction of a career in the United Nations agencies. In developed countries, employment in international health organizations can be challenging and interesting, and professionally desirable. But whether the agency is public or private, compensation is comparable to that in many other lines of work. To land a job with USAID is not, for an American, a particular financial plum and if, for any reason, a technical specialist leaves the organization, comparable employment elsewhere is a reasonable expectation.

But the picture is quite different in WHO, for example, where a majority of the professional jobs are now held by physicians and other health specialists from Third World countries. For them a WHO (or UNICEF, or World Bank) appointment is a financial plum. At international salary levels, they enjoy a standard of living far above what they might otherwise expect, in addition to early retirement, a generous pension, international travel, and association with colleagues on a regional and worldwide basis. Consequently, such appointments are eagerly sought after. In comparison to professional colleagues in their home countries, Third World UN staff members are a highly privileged group. They are, however, vulnerable: to dismissal because of poor performance, or performance deemed dangerous to the well-being of the organization, and to the envy of their less fortunate national colleagues.

Vulnerability, of course, leads to cautious behavior. Tendler illustrates this point in her analysis of USAID, where she found that "outpost-level" employees responding to the uncertainties of Washington political and interagency constraints opted for "a kind of safe-for-all-occasions, problem-avoiding" approach to their jobs (Tendler 1975:25). But what is safe behavior? Talk and discussion rather more than vigorous action. I believe that multilateral health organization meetings, many on the same topic, repeating similar general recommendations (always calling for further study of the problem), at least to some extent fulfill the role of providing visible evidence of concern with health problems, in an activity that carries minimal risk to participants.

I have noted, particularly in the regional offices of WHO, that in addition to providing safe-for-all-occasions activities for permanent staff members, conferences and workshops also fulfill an envy-reducing role vis-a-vis national colleagues who would like to, but do not, hold similar appointments. For the latter group, occasional participation in WHO regional meetings is attractive for financial and prestige reasons. Temporary appointees receive both a daily honorarium for services rendered and a per diem to cover away-from-home expenses. These payments are very attractive to health personnel in many Third World countries, where salary scales are low by international standards. Especially when participants stay with local friends (often the case), thus saving most of the per diem, payment for a 2-week meeting may equal regular salary of several months. National participants in regional meetings also have the satisfaction of feeling that they are a part of the international action and that, although they lack the status and salary of permanent WHO employees, at least they share peripherally in the good life provided by the organization.

Unfortunately, this pattern of sharing may reflect patronage behavior not consistent with the highest levels of professional practice. Since regional conference participants usually are nominated by national health authorities rather than the meeting organizers, administrators often appoint faithful staff members whose turn to travel has come, rather than individuals whose qualifications best fit the conference specifications. Consequently, workshop participants often have little notion as to the goals of the meeting; at best they are dead weight, and at worst they squander valuable time with extraneous talk.

Poor Quality of Behavioral Research

A good deal of the behavioral research carried out by international health organizations has been of poor quality. I have described (Foster 1987) how in WHO in the early 1980s bureaucratic constraints and the research assumptions of the medical profession significantly inhibited first-class investigations. I suggested that "even the most comprehensive statements on the importance of behavioral research stress communities, not health services. Health bureaucracies operate on the assumption that the purpose of behavioral research is to find out how to persuade target populations to change their behavior more nearly to conform to what health projects call for" (Foster 1987:711). It is taken for granted that health care delivery programs, in spite of minor shortcomings, are the appropriate vehicle for raising health levels.

Probably it is unrealistic to expect that behavioral analysis will ever play much of a role in policy and planning activities. One part of the problem is that behavioral research rarely is concerned with administrative organizations. To illustrate, the concept of "community participation," an often-enunciated international health doctrine, sounds attractive as a basic policy. What could be more democratic than inviting villagers to join government administrators and planners in deciding how best to meet local health needs? Yet, experience shows that those in positions of power in centralized governmental systems are rarely willing to surrender authority in the interest of democratic participation. More often than not the concept of CP is diametrically opposed to administrative policies, which do not change easily.

A second part of the problem is how to incorporate behavioral information into the planning process. Time constraints inherent in the bureaucratic process place a premium on rapid decisions. Although good behavioral research can be done more rapidly than is sometimes thought, it takes time for this information to work its way up the ladder. In any event, high-level officials often doubt the utility of behavioral information. To illustrate, in Nepal, Justice (1986:111) found that officials in donor agencies and in government "generally agreed that cultural information is rarely used in planning." Among the reasons given was the belief that such information was not available, and "when it was available, it was not very useful." In the case of USAID's project paper outlining its Nepal health and family planning programs, Justice found that the "social soundness analysis" was condensed to 3 pages (plus 8 in the appendix). "Agency representatives whom I interviewed implied that it was included primarily as a formality to fulfill the requirements specified by Congress" (Justice 1986:116).

For reasons such as these, behavioral research in international health organizations probably will continue to play a minor role, largely limited to the identification of social and cultural factors that are relevant to community acceptance or rejection of health programs decided on by distant planners, programs in which the community has had little input.

Rebuilding Agencies for International Health

This chapter raises a number of questions that must be addressed by international health agencies if they are to improve their performances significantly. They include, but by no means are limited to, the following:

1. Can the reflexive bureaucratic model be institutionalized so that more realistic premises will underlie the definition of problems in health program planning?
2. How can corporate memories be strengthened? How can the necessary resources be built into large organizations so that they are better able to profit from their own experience and from relevant experiences of other organizations?
3. How can the dangers of the early enunciation of policy doctrines restricting innovative thinking in international health organizations be avoided?
4. How can the threat of attempting to satisfy Western ideological concerns by incorporating them into international health planning be controlled?
5. To what extent do professional–personality factors impinge on planning processes? Does overall balance in projects suffer because of the influence of powerful personalities? Or is an occasionally adversarial process the appropriate way to determine organizational policies?
6. How serious is the "competition for clients" syndrome in development assistance programs? Can, or should, anything be done about this problem?
7. Does the "workshop syndrome" divert international health agencies' personnel from other activities to the extent that overall goals of the institutions are compromised? Should the number of meetings be limited?

8. How can the scope of behavioral research in international health agencies be broadened to include not only client groups but also the agencies that plan and carry out assistance programs? What can be done to ensure greater use of such research in setting policy and in program operations?

Acknowledgment

This chapter is a revision of an article first published in *Social Science and Medicine* 25 (1987):1039–1048. The chapter was also included in the first edition of this volume.

References

Ashby E (1966) *Universities: British, Indian, African. A Study in the Ecology of Higher Education.* Cambridge, MA: Harvard University Press.
Basch PH (1978) *International Health.* New York: Oxford University Press.
Bichmann W (1983) Primary health care: A new strategy? Lessons to learn from community participation. Paper presented at the workshop "Primary Health Care in the Developing World," 10th International Congress of Preventive and Social Medicine, Heidelberg/Mannheim, September 27–October 1.
Cipolla CM (1976) *Public Health and the Medical Profession in the Renaissance.* Cambridge, UK: Cambridge University Press.
Djukanovic V, Mach EP (1975) *Alternative Approaches to Meeting Basic Health Needs in Developing Countries.* Geneva: World Health Organization.
Foster GM, ed. (1951) A cross-cultural anthropological analysis of a technical aid program. Washington, DC: Smithsonian Institution, July 25. [Mimeo]
Foster GM (1952) Relationships between theoretical and applied anthropology: A public health program analysis. *Human Organization* 11:5–16.
Foster GM (1953) Use of anthropological methods and data in planning and operation (10-year evaluation of the bilateral health programs of the Institute of Inter-American Affairs). *Public Health Reports* 68:841–857.
Foster GM (1982a) Applied anthropology and international health: Retrospect and prospect. *Human Organization* 41:189–197.
Foster GM (1982b) Community development and primary health care: Their conceptual similarities. *Medical Anthropology* 183–195.
Foster GM (1987) World Health Organization behavioral science research: Problems and prospects. *Social Science and Medicine* 24:709–717.
Justice J (1986) *Policies, Plans and People: Culture and Health Development in Nepal.* Berkeley, CA: University of California Press.
Korten DC, Alfonso FB (1981) *Bureaucracy and the Poor: Closing the Gap.* Singapore: McGraw-Hill.
Muhondwa EPY (1986) Rural development and primary health care in less developed countries. *Social Science and Medicine* 22:1237–1256.

Newell KW (1975) *Health by the People*. Geneva: World Health Organization.

Philips J (1955) "The Hookworm Campaign in Ceylon." In: *Hands across Frontiers*. HM Teaf Jr., PG Franck, eds. Ithaca, NY: Cornell University Press, pp. 265–305.

Ramalingaswami V (1986) The art of the possible. *Social Science and Medicine* 22:1097–1103.

Simmons O (1955) "The Clinical Team in a Chilean Health Center." In: *Health, Culture and Community*. B Paul, ed. New York: Russell Sage Foundation, pp. 325–348.

Sterling C (1976) Nepal. *Atlantic Monthly* October:14–25.

Stone L (1989) Cultural crossroads of community participation in development: A case from Nepal. *Human Organization* 48:206–213.

Tendler J (1975) *Inside Foreign Aid*. Baltimore, MD: Johns Hopkins Press.

WHO (1977) Community Involvement in Primary Health Care. A Study of the Process of Community Motivation and Continued Participation. Report for the 1977 UNICEF-WHO Joint Committee on Health Policy. Geneva: World Health Organization. JC21/UNICEF–WHO/77.2.

WHO (1978) Primary Health Care. Report of International Conference on Primary Health Care, Alma-Ata, USSR, September 6–12. Geneva: World Health Organization.

WHO (1979) *Formulating Strategies for Health for All by the Year 2000*. Geneva: World Health Organization.

Index

Note: Page numbers in *italics* denote tables or figures.

CPSIA information can be obtained at www.ICGtesting.com
Printed in the USA
BVOW03s0640070814

361925BV00003B/4/P